FOURTH EDITION

Hodson and Geddes'
Cystic Fibrosis

FOURTH EDITION

Hodson and Geddes'
Cystic Fibrosis

EDITED BY

Andrew Bush MB BS (HONS) MA MD FRCP FRCPCH FERS
PROFESSOR OF PAEDIATRICS AND HEAD OF SECTION (PAEDIATRICS), IMPERIAL COLLEGE
PROFESSOR OF PAEDIATRIC RESPIROLOGY, NATIONAL HEART AND LUNG INSTITUTE
CONSULTANT PAEDIATRIC CHEST PHYSICIAN, ROYAL BROMPTON & HAREFIELD NHS FOUNDATION TRUST
LONDON, UK

Diana Bilton MD FRCP
CONSULTANT PHYSICIAN AND ADJUNCT PROFESSOR, IMPERIAL COLLEGE, DEPARTMENT OF RESPIRATORY MEDICINE,
ROYAL BROMPTON & HAREFIELD NHS FOUNDATION TRUST
LONDON, UK

Margaret Hodson OBE MD MSC MA FRCP DMED.ED
EMERITUS PROFESSOR OF RESPIRATORY MEDICINE, IMPERIAL COLLEGE LONDON
HONORARY CONSULTANT PHYSICIAN, ROYAL BROMPTON AND HAREFIELD NHS TRUST
LONDON, UK

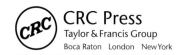

CRC Press
Taylor & Francis Group
Boca Raton   London   New York

CRC Press is an imprint of the
Taylor & Francis Group, an **informa** business

CRC Press
Taylor & Francis Group
6000 Broken Sound Parkway NW, Suite 300
Boca Raton, FL 33487-2742

© 2016 by Taylor & Francis Group, LLC
CRC Press is an imprint of Taylor & Francis Group, an Informa business

Printed and bound in India by Replika Press Pvt. Ltd.

No claim to original U.S. Government works

Printed on acid-free paper
Version Date: 20150511

International Standard Book Number-13: 978-1-4441-8000-8 (Pack - Book and Ebook)

Visit the Taylor & Francis Web site at
http://www.taylorandfrancis.com

and the CRC Press Web site at
http://www.crcpress.com

Contents

Preface

"Go and look it up in *Hodson and Geddes*" must be among the most common phrases heard in the CF clinic or ward round over the last many years. Duncan Geddes has stepped down as editor of this edition, and it will also be Margaret Hodson's last volume. So in honor of these two giants in the field, this edition has been renamed *Hodson and Geddes' Cystic Fibrosis*. This change was greeted with universal approval by all who were consulted, other than the two professors themselves, who were adamantly opposed to the change. For perhaps the only time in the life of the CF community, their views were ignored—and rightly so!

So why a new edition? This is an era of change in CF; new diagnostic methods—the advance of newborn screening, the recognition of milder and atypical phenotypes; new diagnostic techniques such as molecular microbiology; new approaches to conventional problems, and, more excitingly, the age of targeting the upstream defect, with gene therapy and designer molecular treatments, with their incredible benefit and even more incredible expense; and novel animal models—what will the ferret and pig teach us? So a big focus of this volume is clinical trials work; what we have got right, what went wrong, and what we can learn so we can do better in the future.

There are many innovations in this edition. Most obviously, for the first time we have a companion eBook. This eBook is automatically available to individuals who purchase the print book at no additional charge. To avoid any confusion, both versions are identical.

We have also included classic chapters from the previous edition—James M. Littlewood on the history of CF and Philip Robinson on the Melbourne approach to the newborn screened baby—both of which are well worth rereading and are found in the appendices. And two exciting new chapters that take a fresh look at these topics have been added; Kris De Boeck on the journey starting with the discovery of the CF gene and an account of a UK protocol for the education visit for newborn screening. We have also shuffled the pack of our authors, making some of them stretch to write new chapters, as well as bidding a grateful and fond farewell to others; this has allowed us to bring in new contributors to challenge our thinking. A totally new innovation is a chapter written by patients and families—without doubt the most informative and challenging in the book. A special mention to Jessica Harrison—teenage girls get a bad press, but hers was the first contribution to be submitted, length perfect, and word perfect. Let no one badmouth teenagers ever again; would that some senior professorial persons (no names, but you know who you are, and so do we!) had followed her example! We sincerely hope that this combination of the best of the conventional, with the new horizons, makes this book a worthwhile read.

We must thank the publishers, and in particular Rachael Russell, for unfailing patience (even when taxed beyond the limit), enthusiasm, and support. The credit for the quality of the work is theirs; the blame for any errors which have slipped through belongs solely to us.

Finally, we want to mark with sadness the passing of a giant in the field, Gerd Döring. He has contributed to this and previous editions; his contributions to the field have been well-rehearsed elsewhere; suffice to say he will be sadly missed. As with another great German hero, Oscar Schindler, he is mourned in every continent.

Diana Bilton
Royal Brompton Hospital
London, United Kingdom

Andy Bush
Royal Brompton Hospital
London, United Kingdom

Contributors

Penny Agent, BSc (Hons), DMS, MCSP
Director of Rehabilitation and Therapies
Royal Brompton and Harefield NHS Foundation Trust
London, United Kingdom

Eric W.F.W. Alton, MA, MD, FRCP, FMedSci
Professor of Gene Therapy and Respiratory Medicine
Imperial College London
and
Royal Brompton Hospital
London, United Kingdom

Robert M. Aris, MD
Professor of Medicine
Division of Pulmonary and Critical Care Medicine
University of North Carolina at Chapel Hill
Chapel Hill, North Carolina

Paul Aurora, BSc, MB, BS, MSc, PhD, MRCP, MRCPCH
Consultant in Paediatric Respiratory Medicine and Lung
Transplantation
Cardiothoracic Transplant and Respiratory Units
Great Ormond Street Hospital for Children NHS
Foundation Trust
and
Honorary Senior Lecturer
Portex Respiratory Unit
UCL Institute of Child Health
London, United Kingdom

Ian M. Balfour-Lynn, MD
Consultant in Paediatric Respiratory Medicine
Royal Brompton and Harefield NHS Foundation Trust
London, United Kingdom

Helen Benn
London, United Kingdom

Matt Benn
London, United Kingdom

Siân Bentley, BPharm (Hons), MRPharmS, DipPP
Specialist Pharmacist, Paediatrics
Pharmacy Department
Royal Brompton and Harefield NHS Foundation Trust
London, United Kingdom

Diana Bilton, MD, FRCP
Consultant Physician/Honorary Senior Lecturer
Department of Respiratory Medicine Royal Brompton
Hospital
London, United Kingdom

Kris De Boeck, MD, PhD
Department of Paediatrics
University of Leuven
Leuven, Belgium

Richard C. Boucher, MD
Cystic Fibrosis Research and Treatment Center
University of North Carolina at Chapel Hill
Chapel Hill, North Carolina

Nicola Bridges, DM, FRCPCH
Consultant Pediatric Endocrinologist
Department of Paediatrics
Chelsea and Westminster Hospital
and
Royal Brompton and Harefield NHS Trust
London, United Kingdom

Andrew Bush, MD, FRCP, FRCPCH, FERS
Professor of Paediatrics and Head of Section (Paediatrics)
Imperial College London
National Heart and Lung Institute
Royal Brompton and Harefield NHS
Foundation Trust
London, United Kingdom

Martin Carby, MD, MBBS, BSc, FRCP
Consultant Respiratory and Transplant Physician
Clinical Tutor
Cardiothoracic Transplant Unit
Harefield Hospital
Harefield, Middlesex, United Kingdom

Sanjay H. Chotirmall, MD, PhD
Assistant Professor of Molecular Medicine
Lee Kong Chian School of Medicine
Nanyang Technological University
Republic of Singapore

Nicola Collins, BSc (Hons), MCSP
Clinical Lead Physiotherapist Paediatrics
Paediatric Physiotherapy
Royal Brompton and Harefield NHS Foundation Trust
London, United Kingdom

Sarah Collins, MSc
CF Specialist Dietitian
Royal Brompton and Harefield NHS Foundation Trust
London, United Kingdom

Finella Craig, MD
Consultant in Paediatric Palliative Medicine
The Louis Dundas Centre
Great Ormond Street Hospital for Children NHS
Foundation Trust
London, United Kingdom

Kamilla Dack, RBN, MSc
CF Clinical Nurse Specialist
Royal Brompton and Harefield NHS
Foundation Trust
London, United Kingdom

R.J. Darrah, MS, PhD
Assistant Professor
Assistant Director of the Genetic Counseling Training
Program
Frances Payne Bolton School of Nursing
Case Western Reserve University
Cleveland, Ohio

Jane C. Davies, MD
Professor of Paediatric Respirology and Experimental
Medicine
Department of Gene Therapy
National Heart and Lung Institute
Imperial College London
and
Department of Respiratory Medicine
Royal Brompton and Harefield NHS Foundation Trust
London, United Kingdom

Gerd Döring (deceased)
Institute of Medical Microbiology and Hygiene
Universitätsklinikum Tübingen
Tübingen, Germany

M.L. Drumm, PhD
Professor and Vice Chair of Research, Department of
Pediatrics
and
Department of Genetics and Genome Sciences
Case Western Reserve University
Cleveland, Ohio

Alistair J.A. Duff, MA, MSc, DClinPsy, FRCP Edin
Consultant Clinical Psychologist
Leeds Teaching Hospitals NHS Trust
University of Leeds
Leeds, United Kingdom

J. Stuart Elborn, MD
Professor of Respiratory Medicine and Dean,
School of Medicine, Dentistry, and Biomedical
Sciences
Queens University Belfast
Belfast, United Kingdom

Pascale Fanen, MD, PhD
Professor of Biochemistry and Molecular Biology
Department of Genetics
Henri Mondor University Hospital
Paris, France

Brigitte Fauroux, MD, PhD
Professor in Pediatrics, Head of the Pediatric
Noninvasive Ventilation and Sleep Unit
Necker University Hospital
Paris, France

Patrick A. Flume, MD
Professor of Medicine and Pediatrics
Director, MUSC Cystic Fibrosis Center
Departments of Medicine and Pediatrics
Medical University of South Carolina
Charleston, South Carolina

Jackie Francis EN(G), RN, RSCN, BSc (Hon)
Royal Brompton and Harefield NHS
Foundation Trust
London, United Kingdom

Joshua N. Freedman, MD
Assistant Professor of Pediatrics
Emory University
Atlanta, Georgia

Christina Gagliardo, MD
Director of Pediatric Infectious Diseases
Maimonides Medical Center
Infants & Children's Hospital
Brooklyn, New York

Duncan Geddes, MD, FRCP
Professor of Respiratory Medicine
Royal Brompton and Harefield NHS
Foundation Trust
London, United Kingdom

Jennifer L. Goralski, MD
Clinical Instructor of Medicine and Pediatrics
Division of Pulmonary and Critical Care Medicine
University of North Carolina at Chapel Hill
Chapel Hill, North Carolina

Christopher H. Goss, MD, MS
Professor of Medicine
Division of Pulmonary and Critical Care Medicine
Department of Medicine
University of Washington Medical Center
Seattle, Washington

Frances Pearce Gould
Cambridge Corporate Consultants Limited
Cambridge, United Kingdom

Rupert Pearce Gould
Cambridge Corporate Consultants Limited
Cambridge, United Kingdom

William E. Grant, MCh, FRCSI, FRCSEd, FRCS(ORL)
Consultant Otorhinolaryngologist
Charing Cross and Chelsea and Westminster
Hospitals
London, United Kingdom

Uta Griesenbach, PhD, Dipl-Biol
Reader/Associate Professor in Molecular Medicine
Imperial College London
London, United Kingdom

Khin Ma Gyi, MBBS, FRCP, DTM&H
Consultant Respiratory Physician/ Honorary
Senior Lecturer
Royal Brompton and Harefield NHS
Foundation Trust
London, United Kingdom

Jess Harrison
London, United Kingdom

Margaret Hodson, MD, MSc, FRCP
Professor of Respiratory Medicine
Imperial School of Medicine
National Heart and Lung Institute
and
Royal Brompton Hospital
London, United Kingdom

Emily Hoyle
Cystic Fibrosis Patient at the Royal Bromtpon
Hospital, London
London, UK

Andrew M. Jones, MD
Consultant Physician and Honorary Reader
Manchester Adult Cystic Fibrosis Centre
University Hospitals South Manchester NHS
Foundation Trust
Manchester, United Kingdom

Mary Jurd, BSc (Hons), RD
Paediatric Respiratory Dietitian
Royal Brompton Hospital
London, United Kingdom

Shahid A. Khan, BSc, MB, BS, PhD, FRCP
Clinical Senior Lecturer and Consultant Physician
Department of Hepatology and
Gastroenterology
Imperial College London
London, United Kingdom

Sonia Khirani, PhD
Armand Trousseau Hospital
Gennevilliers, France
and
Noninvasive Ventilation and Sleep Unit
Necker University Hospital
Paris, France

Romana Kuchai, MRCS, DLO, MD, FRCS (ORL-HNS)
Consultant Otorhinolaryngologist
Charing Cross and St. Mary's Hospitals
London, United Kingdom

James M. Littlewood, OBE, MB, ChB, MD, FRCP, FRCPE, FRCPCH, DCH
Honorary President
UK Cystic Fibrosis Trust
Leeds, United Kingdom

Stephanie J. MacNeill, PhD
Research Fellow in Medical Statistics
Department of Respiratory Epidemiology, Occupational
Medicine and Public Health
Imperial College London National Heart and Lung
Institute
London, United Kingdom

Susan Madge, SRN, RSCN, MSc, PhD
Consultant Nurse
Royal Brompton and Harefield NHS
Foundation Trust
London, United Kingdom

Noel G. McElvaney, MB, FRCPI
Professor of Medicine RCSI
Respiratory Research Division
Department of Medicine
Royal College of Surgeons in Ireland
and
Education and Research Center
Beaumont Hospital
Dublin, Ireland

Kevin Molloy, MB, Bch, BAO, MRCPI
Clinical Research Fellow
Respiratory Research Division
Department of Medicine
Royal College of Surgeons in Ireland
and
Education and Research Center
Beaumont Hospital
Dublin, Ireland

Michelle A. Murray, MD, MRCPI, MSc (Clin Ed)
Respiratory Specialist Registrar
Respiratory Research Division
Department of Medicine
Royal College of Surgeons in Ireland
and
Education and Research Center
Beaumont Hospital
Dublin, Ireland

Arlette Odink, MD, PhD
Thoracic Radiologist
Department of Radiology
Erasmus MC
Rotterdam, the Netherlands

David Orenstein, MD, MA
Antonio J. and Janet Palumbo Professor of Cystic Fibrosis
Pediatric Pulmonology
Children's Hospital of Pittsburgh of UPMC
Pittsburgh, Pennsylvania

Catherine M. Owens, BSc, MBBS, MRCP, FRCR
Consultant Paediatric Radiologist and Honorary
Reader UCL
Institute of Child Health and Great Ormond Street
Hospital for Children NHS Foundation Trust
London, United Kingdom

Helen Oxley, BSc, MSc, CPsychol
Consultant Clinical Psychologist
Manchester Adult Cystic Fibrosis Centre,
Wythenshawe Hospital
Manchester, United Kingdom

Helen Parrott, BSc
Clinical Specialty Lead—Adult CF Therapies
Royal Brompton and Harefield NHS Foundation
Trust
London, United Kingdom

Kevin Passey
Patient Advocate
Royal Brompton Hospital
London, United Kingdom

Michele Puckey, BSc, MSc (Hons)
Consultant Paediatric Clinical Psychologist
Royal Brompton and Harefield NHS
Foundation Trust
London, United Kingdom

Bradley S. Quon MD, MS, MBA
Assistant Professor of Medicine
UBC James Hogg Centre for Cardiovascular and
Pulmonary Research
Institute for Heart and Lung Health
St. Paul's Hospital
Vancouver, British Columbia, Canada

Sarath Ranganathan, MB, ChB, MRCP, FRCPCH, FRACP, PhD
Assistant Professor
Department of Respiratory Medicine
Royal Children's Hospital
and
Department of Pediatrics
University of Melbourne, Australia

Felix Ratjen, MD, PhD, FRCP(C), FERS
Head, Division of Respiratory Medicine
Sellers Chair of Cystic Fibrosis
Hospital for Sick Children, Toronto
University of Toronto
Toronto, Ontario, Canada

Philip Robinson BMedSc, PhD, MD, MBBS, FRACP
Director, Cystic Fibrosis Unit
Department of Respiratory Medicine
Royal Children's Hospital
Melbourne, Australia

Geraint B. Rogers, MD
Associate Professor
SAHMRI Infection and Immunity Theme
School of Medicine
Flinders University
Adelaide, Australia

Mark Rosenthal, MD, FRCP, FRCPCH
Consultant in Paediatric Respiratory Medicine
Royal Brompton Hospital
London, United Kingdom

Rachel Rowe
Manchester Adult Cystic Fibrosis Unit
Wythenshawe Hospital
Manchester, United Kingdom

Bruce K. Rubin, MEngr, MD, MBA, FRCPC
Jesse Ball DuPont Distinguished Professor
and Chair, Department of Pediatrics
Professor of Engineering
Virginia Commonwealth University School
of Medicine
and
Children's Hospital of Richmond at Virginia
Commonwealth University
Richmond, Virginia

Lisa Saiman, MD, MPH
Professor of Pediatrics
Department of Pediatrics
Columbia University Medical Center
and
Department of Infection Prevention and Control
NewYork-Presbyterian Hospital
New York City, New York

Michael S. Schechter, MD, MPH
Professor of Pediatrics
Virginia Commonwealth University
Richmond, Virginia

Hiran Selvadurai, MBBS, PhD, FRACP
Associate Professor and Director of Respiratory Medicine
Department of Respiratory Medicine
Discipline of Pediatrics and Child Health
The Children's Hospital, Westmead
Sydney, Australia

Isabelle Sermet-Gaudelus, MD, PhD
Professor
Department of Pediatrics
Université Paris Sorbonne
Paris, France

Christopher Sheldon, DM, FRCP
Consultant Physician, Respiratory Medicine
Royal Devon and Exeter Hospital (Wonford)
Exeter, United Kingdom

Nicholas J. Simmonds, MD
Consultant Adult Cystic Fibrosis Physician
Royal Brompton Hospital and Imperial
College London
London, United Kingdom

André Simon
Cardiothoracic Transplant Unit
Harefield Hospital
Harefield, Middlesex, United Kingdom

Samatha Sonnappa, MBBS, MD, DCH, MRCP, FRCPCH, PhD
Clinician Scientist and Honorary Consultant
Portex Unit: Respiratory Medicine and Physiology
UCL Institute of Child Health
and
Great Ormond Street Hospital for Children NHS
Foundation Trust
London, United Kingdom

Kevin Southern, PhD, FRCPCH, MBChB
Reader in Paediatric Respiratory Medicine
Department of Women's and Children's Health
University of Liverpool
Liverpool, United Kingdom

Alan Steel, MD
Consultant Gastroenterologist
Chelsea and Westminster Hospital NHS Foundation Trust
London, United Kingdom

Anna-Marie Stevens, RN, MSc
Macmillan Nurse Consultant Palliative Care
The Royal Marsden and Royal Brompton Palliative Care
Service
The Royal Marsden NHS Foundation Trust
London, United Kingdom

Stephen M. Stick, MD, PhD
Pediatric Pulmonologist
Department of Respiratory Medicine
Princess Margaret Hospital for Children
Perth, Australia

Pat Stringer, RGN, RSCN, BsC (Hons)
Specialist Practitioner in Community Children's Nursing
Clinical Nurse Specialist in Children's Cystic Fibrosis Home
Care
Royal Brompton Hospital
London, United Kingdom

Padmaja Subbarao, MD, MSc (Epid), FRCP(C)
Director, Pulmonary Function Laboratory
Clinician-Scientist, Respirologist
Division of Respiratory Medicine
Hospital for Sick Children
University of Toronto
Toronto, Ontario, Canada

J. Guy Thorpe-Beeston MA, MD, FRCOG
Consultant Obstetrician and Gynecologist
Department of Obstetrics and Gynecology
Chelsea and Westminster Healthcare NHS Foundation Trust
London, United Kingdom

Harm A.W.M. Tiddens, MD, PhD
Pediatric Pulmonologist
Department of Pediatric Pulmonology and Allergology
Erasmus MC-Sophia Children's Hospital
and
Department of Radiology
Erasmus MC
Rotterdam, the Netherlands

Donald R. VanDevanter, PhD
Adjunct Associate Professor of Pediatrics
Department of Pediatrics
Case Western Reserve University School of Medicine
Cleveland, Ohio

Marcel van Straten, PhD
Clinical Physicist
Department of Radiology
Erasmus MC
Rotterdam, the Netherlands

Claire Wainwright, MBBS, MRCP, FRACP, MD
Respiratory Physician and Lead for Cystic Fibrosis Services
Queensland Children's Medical Research Institute
and
School of Medicine
University of Queensland
Brisbane, Australia
and
Department of Respiratory and Sleep Medicine
Lady Cilento Children's Hospital
South Brisbane, Australia

Michael Waller, MD
Senior Clinical Research Fellow in Cystic Fibrosis
Department of Gene Therapy
Imperial College London and Royal Brompton Hospital
London, United Kingdom

Colin Wallis, MD, MRCP, FRCPCH, FCP, DCH
Consultant in Respiratory Pediatrics and Honorary Reader
Great Ormond Street Hospital for Children NHS
Foundation Trust
and
UCL Institute of Child Health
London, United Kingdom

David Westaby, MD
Consultant Gastroenterologist
Hammersmith Hospital
Imperial College Healthcare NHS Trust
London, United Kingdom

Ronald W. Williams, MD
Assistant Professor
Division of Pediatric Pulmonary
Department of Pediatrics
Virginia Commonwealth University School of Medicine
Children's Hospital of Richmond at VCU
Richmond, Virginia

Sue Wolfe, RD, BSc(hons), Dipdiet
Consultant Dietitian (Paediatric Cystic Fibrosis)
Regional Paediatric Cystic Fibrosis Unit
Clarendon Wing
The Leeds Children's Hospital
Leeds, United Kingdom

PART 1

Introduction: What is cystic fibrosis?

Introduction: From the discovery of the *CFTR* gene in 1989 through to 2014

KRIS DE BOECK

The previous edition of this book commenced with a history of cystic fibrosis (CF) by Dr. Littlewood, up until the discovery of cystic fibrosis transmembrane conductance regulator (*CFTR*). This is available in the e-book form and has been further extended and is also available online via http://cfmedicine.com/history. This chapter will rather describe how, slowly, the entire field of CF was transformed by a continuous stream of knowledge, a new look at the diagnosis of CF, reorganization of clinical research, clinical care, and partnering.

A selection of the plenary lectures at the European cystic fibrosis conferences can serve as a guide for the shift in focus over the years (Table 1.1). The plenary lectures at the North American cystic fibrosis conferences, listed in Table 1.2, describe the parallel story on the other side of the Atlantic.

I describe how the European CF clinician experienced this period. It is difficult to understand that there indeed was a time when we treated patients with CF without knowing anything about the *CFTR* gene nor much about the basic defect in CF. Very many people contributed to the successes, but I will mention only a few people specifically. It is obvious that I have to oversimplify the story. For both facts, I apologize in advance.

KNOWLEDGE: CF CLINICIANS LEARN ABOUT THE *CFTR* GENE, THE CFTR PROTEIN, AND CELL BIOLOGY

CFTR GENE CODE WAS FINALLY BROKEN

The knowledge of the entire base sequence of the *CFTR* gene and the description of the common mutation *F508del* brought a lot of excitement in the early 1990s, including the belief that a cure via gene therapy would soon be available. However, many hurdles to gene therapy lined up. In patients with CF, efficient gene transfer proved difficult and was not

without risk: the large size of the *CFTR* gene is problematic, adenoviral vectors can cause severe inflammation, antibodies to viral vectors impair efficacy with repeated administration, and adenoviral receptors are located mainly at the less exposed basolateral epithelial cell surface. The hype leading to the belief that gene therapy would soon (within the 1990s) bring the solution for patients with CF ebbed down.

NUMEROUS *CFTR* MUTATIONS WERE REPORTED

CFTR mutation after *CFTR* mutation was being described. The enormous genetic heterogeneity of the disease was recognized. Although this led to explaining part of the heterogeneity in disease severity, a landmark paper from Eitan Kerem et al.[1] shattered the notion of a simple correlation between genotype and phenotype. Pancreatic phenotype seemed largely driven by genotype, but individual homozygous *F508del* patients appeared to have a vast difference in lung disease severity, pointing from the start to the importance of genetic modifiers and the environment.

Given this genetic heterogeneity, gene therapy remained an attractive option, especially to improve CF lung disease, an organ accessible via aerosol inhalation. So, a few groups, the UK gene therapy consortium most prominently, continued in this field of gene therapy and explored the use of nonviral vectors. Their effort led to the phase 2b trial with monthly applications of gene therapy in 200 patients, a landmark trial from which the first results are eagerly awaited.

FIRST CARTOONS OF THE CFTR PROTEIN EMERGE

The rather unexpected great complexity of applying gene therapy in CF had shifted much of the focus to the CFTR protein. The resemblance of the 'anticipated' structure of the CFTR protein to the ABC transporters made the chloride

Table 1.1 ECFS plenary lectures

Year	City	Plenary title	Speaker
1991	Copenhagen	Gene therapy in CF	Crystal RG
1993	Madrid	Spectrum of mutations in cystic fibrosis	Estivill X
1994	Paris	Gene therapy: Results of first clinical trials	Crystal R
		Pharmacotherapy for abnormal ion transport in CF: Aerosolized amiloride and uridine triphosphate	Knowles M
1995	Brussels	CF in the mouse and gene therapy in man	Porteus DJ
		Changes in genetic counseling strategies for CF	Brock DJH
1997	Davos		
1998	Berlin	Gene therapy	Geddes D
		Gene targeting: Prospects for CF gene therapy	Gruenert DC
1999	The Hague	How do we link CF ion transport defects to CF lung disease?	Boucher RC
2000	Stockholm	The CFTR protein: Function and dysfunction, processing and misprocessing	Riordan JR
2001	Vienna	The *CFTR* gene	Cutting G
		Genetic modifiers of CF—the emerging picture	Zielenski J
		Gene therapy—where we are, where are we going?	Hyde S
2002	Genoa	Patients' segregation pros	Koch C
		Patients' segregation cons	Geddes D
2003	Belfast	How should we screen for CF?	Farrel P
		New treatments for CF	Geddes D
2004	Birmingham	Atypical CF	Knowles M
		Phenotype: Genes or environment	Cutting G
		Genetic counseling	Super M
2005	Crete	The latest CFTR research	Amaral M
		How to correct the basic CF defect in mice	Gulbins E
		How pathogens cause lung infection and inflammation	Döring G
		How to treat airway infection in the future	Høiby N
2006	Copenhagen	Therapy for CF based on a rational understanding of CFTR	Sheppard D
2007	Belek	Anti-inflammatory treatment: How far can we go?	Elborn S
		How do we assess therapeutic benefits?	De Boeck K
		Is newborn screening for CF a basic human right?	Farrell P
2008	Prague	What do we still need to know to stop CF lung damage:	
		CFTR dysfunction	Amaral M
		Infection	Döring G
		Inflammation	Accurso F
		Options to treat	Davies J
2009	Brest	Clinical trials: Priorities and challenges	Tiddens H
		Patient organizations' contributions to clinical research	Dufour F
2010	Valencia	Restoring CFTR function in CF airways	Boucher R
		Current treatments for CF to prevent disease progression	Stick S
2011	Hamburg	Models of inflammation: From bench to bedside	Mall M
		Genotype-phenotype in CF: Implications in CF care	Durie P
2012	Dublin	Inflammation and infection, lessons from the CF pig model	McCray P
		Potentiating and correcting CFTR	De Boeck K
2013	Lisbon	CFTR2 The importance of understanding genotype	Cutting G
		Delivering quality care in CF. New challenges and solutions?	Bilton D
2014	Gothenburg	Mucus – The central problem in CF	Hansson GC
		Preventing and treating pulmonary exacerbations	Flume P

Source: Courtesy of H. Riley and C. Dubois, ECFS office.

Table 1.2 Plenary lectures at the North American cystic fibrosis conferences

Year	Plenary title	Speaker
1989	The CF gene	Collins FS, Riordan J, Tsui L-C
	Advances in medical treatment of cystic fibrosis	Rosenstein BJ
	A look toward the future	Boucher RC, Wilson JM
1990	The CF gene one year later	Collins FS, Riordan J, Tsui L-C
	Gene therapy and model systems	Caskey CT, Crystal RG
	Immunopathology and new approaches to therapy	Berger M, Hoiby N, Moss R, Suter S
1991	The CF gene two years later: Progress and projections	Collins FS
	New frontiers in therapy	Crystal RG
1992	The CF gene: Perceptions, puzzles and promises	Collins FS
	The new pharmacology: Tools to arrest CF lung disease	Boucher RC
	Gene therapy in CF: Progress and prognosis:	
	In vivo gene transfer strategies for the respiratory manifestations of cystic fibrosis	Crystal RG
	Strategies for gene therapy of CF	Wilson JM
1993	The CF gene: Old questions, new insights	Collins FS
	CF: Electrolyte transport revisited	Welsh MJ
	Gene therapy for CF: A glimpse into the future	Boucher RC, Crystal RC, Whitsett JA, Wilson JM
1994	Understanding cystic fibrosis: Accomplishments and challenges on the road to a cure	Welsh MJ
	Advances in clinical science and management	Davis PB
	Prospects for human gene therapy of cystic fibrosis	Wilson JM
1995	1995: The year in review	Collins FS
	Clinical advances in CF: Recognizing the cure	Davis PB
	Human gene therapy for CF: Lessons learned & hurdles to success	Crystal RG
1996	CF research: Highlights of 1996	Collins FS
	The immune system: The devil within of the good guy?	Wilson CB
	On track with CF gene delivery vehicles	Wilson JM
1997	CF research: The best of 1997	Collins FS
	New clinical developments in CF: From the test tube to the bedside	Ramsey BW
	Gene therapy for CF: Where have we been and where are we going?	Crystal RG
1998	The best of 1998	Taussig LM, Tsui LC
	CFTR structure & function: pathophysiologic insights & novel targets for pharmacotherapies	Guggino WB, Hanrahan JW
	The CF cure: How close are we?	Cantin AM, Davis PB
1999	The best of 1999	Boucher RC
	The process of drug discovery—an enlightened journey	Beall RJ, Campbell PW
	New clinical interventions	Ramsey BW
2000	The best of 2000	Wine JJ
	CFF mission and vision	Beall RJ, Campbell PW
	Solving the puzzle: CF clinical research 2000	Accurso FJ
2001	The best of 2001	Welsh MJ
	Why won't they do what we tell them to do? Understanding families and understanding adherence	Bluebond-Langner Myra, Lask B
	CF clinical research: A journey with a destination	Cantin AM
2002	CF airways pathophysiology: CFTR & beyond	Boucher RC
	Changes in the natural history of CF from a GI perspective	Durie PR
	Developing better therapies for patients with CF: 2002 Progress report	Ramsey BW
2003	From genes to drugs: The CF master plan	Collins, Beall RJ, Ashlock MA
	Providing exemplary care: A partnership for change	O'Connor, Marshall BC
	Disease progression in CF: Can we gain the upper hand?	Moss RD

(Continued)

Table 1.2 (*Continued*) Plenary lectures at the North American cystic fibrosis conferences

Year	Plenary title	Speaker
2004	Developing CF therapies: From the laboratory to the patient	Davis PB, Konstan MW
	How do we recognize a clinically effective new treatment?	Alton E
	Care providers and people with CF: Together we can make great things happen!	Batalden P, Acton JD, Page HO
2005	50 years of CF: Milestones to a cure	Campbell PW, Beall RJ
	50 Years of CF clinical trials research: Accelerating the progress	Goss CH
	CF nutrition: Opportunities for the scientist & the care team	Borowitz D
2006	Promises to keep: Turning discoveries into drugs	Davis PB
	Clinical research: Our compass to a cure	Clancy JP
	CF pulmonary care: Measuring & improving our effectiveness	Yankaskas JR
2007	From basic science to the clinic: Where are we and what is still missing?	Amaral MD
	CF drug development: What's new?	Ratjen F
	Improving patient outcomes using the tools we have now	Boyle MP
2008	Preventing CF lung disease	Wine JJ
	The CFF pipeline: The amazing story of progress, hope, and challenge	Campbell PW
	Taking the CF battle to the extremes: Healthy starts with newborn screening; healthy aging with improved adult care	Farrell PM, Simon RH
2009	Two decades of CFTR research: From gene discovery to therapeutic target	Collins FS, Rowe SM
	Inflammation & infection: Update on the pipeline	Konstan MW
	Early airway infection in young children with CF—what is the optimal therapy?	Ramsey BW, Retsch-Bogart G, Wainwright CE
2010	Pipeline: Airway surface liquid modulation	Sorscher E
	Animal models	Stolz DA
	Transforming CF healthcare: Partnership for life	Berwick D, Marshall BC
2011	CFTR modulation—25 years of NACFC progress	Mall MA
	CFTR 2—a research & clinical practice tool	Cutting GR, Sosnay P
	Pulmonary exacerbations	Flume PA
2012	Reversing the basic defect: A vision for the future	Rowe SM, Skach W
	Advances in GI aspects of CF	Borowitz D
	Adherence ... Where's the app for that?	Riekert KA
2013	Restoring CFTR Function: Roadmap to a Cure (Part 1)	Donaldson SH
	Roadmap to a Cure (Part 2) Clinical Research Pathway to Ensure That All Patients With CF Benefit From Novel Therapies	Ramsey BW
		Engelhardt JF
	CFRD: From Bench to Bedside & Back Again (Care)	Kelly A
2014	Scaling the Mountain: The Journey to Delivering Transformational CF Therapeutics	Boyle M
	CF Microbiology Past, Present, Future	LiPuma J
	CF Advisory Board Track: From Codman to Collaboratories: A Care Model for CF That's Fit for the Future	Nelson E

Source: Courtesy of P. Campbell and CFF office

transport function logical and confirmed the previously documented chloride impermeable epithelium as (one of) the basic defects in CF. The presence of an R domain, unique in the ABC transporters, led to speculation about its function in opening and closing the channel pore. We saw the first cartoons depicting the CFTR protein (Figure 1.1): two membrane-spanning domains (MSDs), two nucleotide-binding domains (NBDs), and the enigmatic R domain. We heard the cell biologists discuss whether the protein is expressed at the cell surface as a monomer, a dimer, or even a tetramer.

NEW KNOWLEDGE LED TO THE PARADIGM OF CYSTIC FIBROSIS PATHOPHYSIOLOGY

The pathophysiologic cascade of CF was described: from faulty *CFTR* gene, via abnormal CFTR protein, over disturbed ion flux, dehydrated airway surface liquid, and impaired mucociliary clearance to cycles of airway obstruction, chronic lung infection, and excessive inflammation, ultimately leading to organ dysfunction. This useful

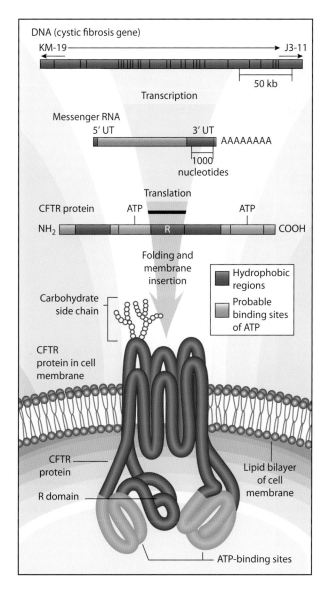

DNA (cystic fibrosis gene)

KM-19 ⟶ J3-11

50 kb

Transcription

Messenger RNA

5′ UT   3′ UT

AAAAAAAA

1000 nucleotides

Translation

CFTR protein   ATP   ATP

NH₂   R   COOH

Folding and membrane insertion

Carbohydrate side chain

CFTR protein in cell membrane

CFTR protein

R domain

Lipid bilayer of cell membrane

ATP-binding sites

Hydrophobic regions

Probable binding sites of ATP

Figure 1.1 Early cartoon depicting the different domains of the cystic fibrosis transmembrane conductance regulator protein.

paradigm has remained a constant feature in CF presentations (Figure 1.2). The beauty was that a putative or existing therapy could be put at every level. Each individual scientist or clinician could position his project in this "cascade" without forgetting the overall picture. Increasingly as time went by, therapeutic targets have been focused upstream toward the basic defect as you will read here.

Viscous secretions and disturbed mucociliary clearance gave credence to the disease's old name of "mucoviscidosis." The clinicians left it to the basic scientists to unravel whether the "low volume" or the "high salt" hypothesis could explain the dehydrated airway surface liquid.[2,3] In the high salt hypothesis, a hypertonic airway surface liquid destroys the salt-sensitive natural antimicrobial molecules or defensins, thereby linking the dehydrated epithelium to CF's impaired lung defense. Attempts to measure the exact salt concentration in the epithelial lining fluid left room

were fraught with difficulty, and the results were controversial. Currently, the low volume hypothesis is favored.

But the CFTR was discovered to be more than just a chloride channel: bicarbonate, hypothiocyanate, and other anions were also transported.[4-6]

IMPORTANCE OF ION CHANNELS OTHER THAN CFTR WAS RECOGNIZED

Because the CFTR protein is embedded in the cell membrane next to other ion channels, the hierarchy in this potpourri of receptors was studied. Manipulating CFTR's partners became a new therapeutic goal. The first attempts were to manipulate the epithelial sodium channel ENaC, overactive in the absence of CFTR and amenable to down-regulation by blockers such as amiloride. But the first clinical trial failed, the failure being attributed to amiloride's short-lived action.[7] Although, in recent years, the CF pig model questions the theory of ENaC hyperactivity,[8] the search for safe and effective long-acting ENaC blockers continues. The pioneering work on ENaC by the German group with Greger, Kunzelmann, and Mall culminating in the development of a β-ENaC overexpressing mouse model deserves specific mention.[9] In an interventional study with amiloride in this mouse model, they pointed out that efficacy was only seen with preventive therapy and not with rescue therapy.

In addition, a mistaken hypothesis in a previous paper came to light. In the presence of amiloride, nucleosides applied to the cell surface were found to activate the defective chloride transport path in CF, possibly via the CFTR protein itself.[10] Because it was later found that in "classic CF" the CFTR protein is not present at the cell membrane, this stimulation could only occur via "alternative" chloride channels. A new drug target was born. Denufosol, a purinergic (P_2Y_2) agonist stimulating chloride secretion via these alternative chloride channels, seemed promising in phase 2, but robust clinical efficacy was absent in phase 3 studies.[11,12] In the mean time, these alternative chloride channels have been nailed down as the TMEM16A proteins.[13]

CFTR MUTATION CLASSES: THE LINK BETWEEN MUTATIONS AND PROTEIN

CFTR mutations were grouped in six classes according to their effect on the synthesis and function of the CFTR protein.[14] Another classic CF slide was introduced (Figure 1.3). Because the most common mutation *F508del* belongs to class 2, whereby protein misfolding leads to degradation in the proteasome, an intense study of CFTR folding started, including the formation of a CFTR folding consortium. This had the enormous advantage of bringing in existing knowledge such as "high throughput screening," as well as building CFTR-specific knowledge.

Clinicians embarked on genotype–phenotype studies to link mutation class to disease pattern.[15] We learned

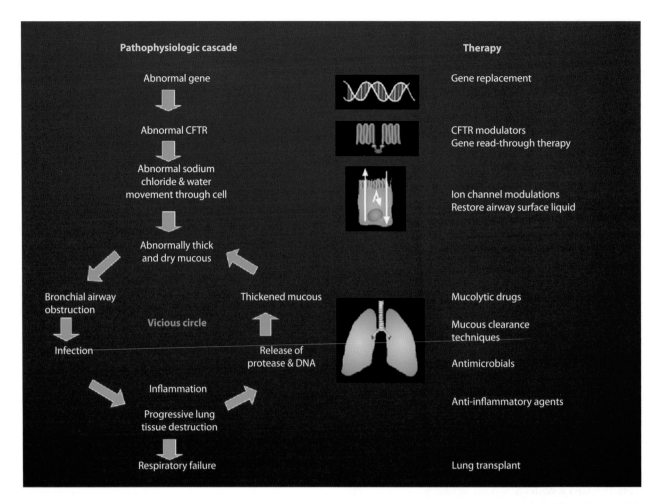

Figure 1.2 Paradigm of cystic fibrosis pathophysiology plus listing of putative and existing therapies to improve or prevent lung disease.

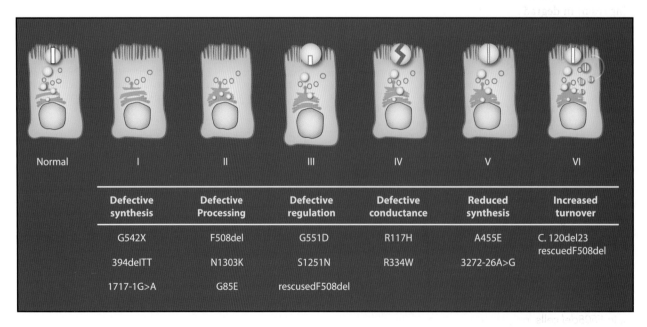

Figure 1.3 Cystic fibrosis transmembrane conductance regulator (*CFTR*) mutations are grouped in classes according to how the *CFTR* mutation interferes with CFTR protein synthesis or function. (Adapted from Amaral, M, and CM Farinha, *Curr Pharm Des*, 19(19), 3497–508, 2013.)

that having at least one class IV or V mutation can attenuate the clinical picture. Plausible, because in classes IV and V, CFTR protein is present at the cell membrane, be it either with decreased conductance (class IV) or in reduced amount (class V). Unfortunately, patients with two so-called "severe" mutations, namely, classes I (no synthesis), II (degradation), and III (no channel opening), greatly outnumber patients with at least one "mild" mutation of class IV or V.

Although useful for group predictions, the heterogeneity between individuals in the same mutation class proved to be vast, again pointing toward the importance of gene modifiers and the environment. Cleverly designed twin and sibling studies quantified the relative impact of these.[16,17] Different groups uncovered several modifier genes, but in later years genome-wide association studies were performed.[18] So far, these revealed few modifier genes with a major impact on disease outcome. The real challenge is of course to transpose the knowledge on modifier genes (and environment) to new therapeutic strategies.

WE LANDED IN THE EXCITING ERA OF CORRECTORS AND POTENTIATORS

The complex folding and trafficking process of CFTR protein soon became an intense object of study by many, including a group in Lisbon headed by Margarida Amaral. En route through the endoplasmic reticulum, the immature CFTR protein is first partially (band B) and then fully glycosylated and recognized as "band C" in western blot (Figure 1.4). CFTR undergoes folding during synthesis. The protein encounters multiple checkpoints and makes contact with multiple binding partners or chaperones as well as nonchaperones. The description of the entire CFTR interactome was a major step forward.[19] Errors in CFTR processing result in degradation via the proteasome. The huge complexity of CFTR folding during transcription and post transcription has meant that correcting this proves to be a much more major task than was first thought.

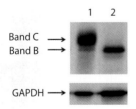

Figure 1.4 Western blot of cystic fibrosis transmembrane conductance regulator (CFTR) protein. Western blot of wild type (left) and *F508del* (right) CFTR protein expressed in BHK cells. In wild-type CFTR expressing cells, a prominent upper band, also called band C (corresponding to the fully glycosylated or mature form of CFTR), and a lower band, also called band B (corresponding to the immature, only partially glycosylated CFTR protein), are seen. In *F508del* cells, only band B is present (band C is absent), indicating that the mutant protein has not undergone maturation. (From Amaral M and CM Farinha, *Curr Pharm* Des, 2013; 19(19): 3497–508.)

In *F508del CFTR* cell lines, the protein is not present at the cell's brush border but remains distributed diffusely in the cytoplasm. Increased appearance of CFTR protein at the cell surface after exposure in vitro to cold (23°C) was a first step in the search for "correctors," compounds that increase the amount of CFTR at the cell surface.[20] The technique of high throughput screening based on advances in robotics and high-speed computer technology greatly helped the search for effective correctors: in these automated systems and by coupling CFTR to a yellow fluorescent protein-based halide sensor, thousands of chemical compounds could be tested overnight for their ability to activate CFTR chloride transport in, e.g., *F508del* cell lines. In Europe, Luis Gallieta was very active in this search for CFTR modulators. Several chemical correctors were evaluated such as phenylbutyrate, sildenafil, vardenafil, and genistein; the latter was later on considered as a potentiator. These compounds made it to the first stages of clinical development, but their efficacy was only modest. Eventually, the more potent corrector VX-809 was developed. After proof of concept in phase 2, this compound was being tested in phase 3 clinical trials, in conjunction with the potentiator VX-770. Indeed, when the F508del CFTR protein was "rescued" to the cell surface by corrector VX-809, the rescued protein channel's open probability is decreased and this can be enhanced in vitro by potentiator VX-770. In patients with CF and *F508del* mutations combined therapy with corrector plus potentiator has modest efficacy.[21]

According to recent information, very efficient correction of misfolding may require at least a two-step correction approach: improving the folding and thermal stability of the protein as well as improving the linking of MSDs with NBDs via the intracytoplasmic loops (ICLs).[22,23] Apparently, the absence of phenylalanine at position 508 in NBD1 leaves a pocket that needs to be filled to restore the interface between NBD1 and ICL4. For optimal efficacy, other interactions, e.g., between NBD2 and MSD1 and between NBD1 and NBD2, may also need to be corrected. The mechanism of action of correctors identified via high throughput screening is mostly unknown. It is reassuring that an "intelligent" search for correctors with additive mechanisms of action, complementing the high throughput screens, has already started.

The highly dynamic process of opening and closing the CFTR protein was also being studied in great detail. The group in Bristol headed by David Sheppard made major contributions in this field. For a recent discussion of adenosine triphosphate (ATP)-dependent as well as ATP-independent mechanisms of CFTR channel opening and new insights into the configuration of the CFTR pore, see the study by Hwang and Kirk.[6] Clinicians learned about the classical "nutcracker" theory of opening the CFTR pore. Phosphorylation brings more structure to the bulky R domain, which thereby "moves out of the way." Phosphorylation and ATP binding and hydrolysis at the NBDs lead to their dimerization. This in turn transmits—via the intracytoplasmic loops—a configurational change driving the MSDs apart: chloride or other anions can then pass. But this passage is short-lived: the reverse process takes place by dimerization of MSDs and opening of NBDs until a new cycle starts. But channel opening is apparently much more complex and can also occur independently of ATP binding.

The discovery of VX-770 (later named ivacaftor), a CFTR potentiator that increases the CFTR channel's open probability, was a major breakthrough. The compound's in vitro efficacy was confirmed in vivo (Kalydeco®) in patients carrying at least one *G551D* mutation, the most common class III mutation.[24] Ivacaftor became the first drug on the market that improves patient outcome by improving the basic defect of CF, a true milestone in CF drug development and the first piece in the difficult puzzle of "curing CF". Although it should be noted that pancreatic insufficiency remains in these patients and whether ivacaftor will prevent the development of later complications, such as CF-related diabetes and bone disease, remains to be seen.

Efficacy of ivacaftor has been proven in other class III mutations, which are responsive in vitro.[25-27] But there may be more indications for treatment with potentiators than patients with class III mutations only. In vitro ivacaftor potentiates wild-type *CFTR* and several mutant forms of *CFTR* of classes IV and V. The mutation class theory thereby needs revision. Many mutations have indeed characteristics of more than one conventional mutation class. In a new paradigm (Figure 1.5), we think of CFTR function as the product of the number of CFTR channels (typically disturbed in classes I, II, and V) and the function of the CFTR channel, the latter being dependent on the open channel probability (disturbed in class III and in rescued mutant *CFTR*) and the channel conductance (typically disturbed in class IV). Correctors and stop codon read-through drugs increase the number of CFTR proteins, and potentiators increase CFTR function opening. Strategies that target the *F508del* mutation at the mRNA level are also under development. Thus, multiple novel therapies may need to be tailored to individual mutations.

Also for patients with premature stop codon mutations, correction by ataluren, a compound aimed at overreading these premature stop codons, is being pursued.[26,28] In the phase 3 clinical trial the primary outcome of improvement in FEV1 was not reached.[29]

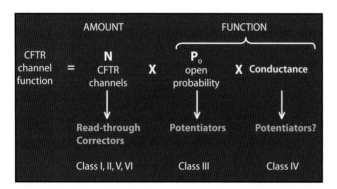

Figure 1.5 Current paradigm linking defects in cystic fibrosis transmembrane conductance regulator (CFTR) protein function or synthesis and *CFTR* mutation classes with potential therapies by CFTR modulators.

MODEL SYSTEMS: THE CF MOUSE, THE CF PIG, THE CF FERRET, AND ORGANOIDS

After the discovery of the *CFTR* gene, a CF mouse model was developed. Although it brought knowledge on inflammation and infection in CF lung disease, the fact that the CF mouse does not spontaneously develop lung disease was a major drawback. The CF pig, CF ferret, and CF rat took a much longer time to develop but proved to be excellent animal models for early CF lung disease, as they reflect lung disease in humans much better compared to the CF mouse model.[30] The CF pig becomes infected with a myriad of bacteria,[31] has abnormal airway cartilage,[32] and has a disturbed growth hormone axis.[33] These same abnormalities were documented in infants with CF. The CF pig model points toward the importance of bicarbonate not only in the gut but also in the lung surface liquid.[34] This knowledge will likely lead to new therapeutic options.

In the past year, an exciting new tool surfaced in the Netherlands: organoids, grown from rectal biopsies in patients.[35] This might open the possibility of individualized assessment of the efficacy of CFTR modulators in patients with rare *CFTR* mutations.

DIAGNOSIS OF CYSTIC FIBROSIS NEEDED TO BE REVISED

DIAGNOSTIC CONSENSUS, DIAGNOSTIC ALGORITHM, AND CFTR-RELATED DISORDERS

The diversity of *CFTR* mutations raised a new question: "what is cystic fibrosis?" The old definition of CF as a severe autosomal recessive disease characterized by changes in the lung, gastrointestinal tract, sweat gland, and male reproductive tract proved insufficient. *CFTR* mutations had been described even in adults with minimal disease expression or single organ disease. How much disease expression should be there before it is warranted to state that a person is suffering from CF? Indeed, labeling a person with the diagnosis of CF impacts not only health and treatment but also social functioning and well-being. A new definition of CF was proposed and revised later on with small differences between the United States and Europe.[36-38] But all agreed that the diagnosis must be supported by the presence of classical CF symptoms (or a sibling with CF or a positive newborn screening [NBS] test) plus two positive pilocarpine sweat tests (or the presence of two CF disease–causing mutations or an abnormal nasal potential difference or intestinal current measurement).

Because several diagnostic tests became available, a European algorithm was drafted to guide the clinician in the CF diagnostic pathway.[37] Some were unhappy with these algorithms, because in difficult cases results of diagnostic tests may be discordant and because "CF is a continuum rather than a yes/no condition."

The CFTR2 project (www.CFTR2.org) led by Garry Cutting was set up to answer some of the uncertainties about "CF-causing mutations," by exploring existing patient registries and describing the phenotype of patients with *CFTR* mutations with a frequency above 0.01%.

More confusing was the notion of "CFTR-related disorders," the term used for subjects with symptoms suggestive of CF but who do not meet diagnostic criteria.[39]

NEWBORN SCREENING FOR CYSTIC FIBROSIS BECOMES THE STANDARD

NBS for CF was carried out prior to knowledge of *CFTR* mutations. Long-standing programs based on immunoreactive trypsin (IRT) measurements had proved the feasibility of NBS, as well as its long-term benefit on nutritional outcome.[40] Algorithms combining IRT with DNA analysis for the most common *CFTR* mutations in the target region greatly improved the efficacy of the program, by avoiding recall of many patients with falsely elevated IRT. In parallel, the advantages and lack of disadvantages of NBS became clearer. Algorithms for NBS were adopted in an increasing number of countries. European guidelines were drafted for how to organize NBS as well as how to manage infants with CF.[41,42] Opinions and governments differ in their approach to CF carrier detection. Some see it as an advantage if used for cascade screening and others as a disadvantage if revealing the carrier status of a baby is considered unethical.[43] A three-tier algorithm with IRT, DNA, and pancreas-associated protein greatly reduces detection of carriers and can also be considered.[44]

But there is no progress without new questions resulting. An unexpectedly high number of babies detected via NBS had the genotype *R117H-7T/F508del* and did not develop symptoms during childhood.[45] And what to do with babies who are screen positive but have an equivocal diagnosis of CF?[46] Do they truly deserve the strange name of "CFTR-related metabolic syndrome" chosen on the other side of the Atlantic?[47] And, although CF screening uses excellent and increasingly sophisticated methods, they are screening and not diagnostic tests.[48] Clinicians must remember that some patients will be missed by NBS.

CYSTIC FIBROSIS CLINICAL RESEARCH HAS METAMORPHOSED

A MASTER PLAN APPROACH CHANGES CLINICAL RESEARCH

Over the past 25 years, CF clinical research has changed from artisan patchwork to an entrepreneurial exercise with full attention to decisiveness. For too long, clinical research had mainly been thought provoking. Bright research ideas were put forward, but the unequivocal proof of evidence was often lacking.[49] A good example of a large-scale CF trial of the modern era was the study of the efficacy of rhDNase.[50]

Efficient translation of the improving knowledge about CF to better treatments demanded a different approach. The birth of the therapeutic development network (TDN) in the United States in 1998 was a giant step in a new direction.[51] Large-scale, well-designed clinical trials with decisive answers became the new standard: among others, inhaled tobramycin, DNase used as early intervention, oral azithromycin, and EPIC.[52-55] A European example of research organization, the UK gene therapy consortium, was founded in 2001 (http://www.cfgenetherapy.org.uk). Inspired by the successful TDN, the European Cystic Fibrosis Society Clinical Trials Network (ECFS-CTN) (www.ecfs.eu/ctn) was formed in 2008. This initiative of the European Cystic Fibrosis Society received great support from the Cystic Fibrosis Foundation (CFF) and from the CFF-TDN. It was also supported by the European CF patient associations. Similarly, in Australia a CF-specific research network was formed with focus on disease in the preschool child (http://arestcf.org).

A master plan approach to clinical research became the obvious need. First, CF patient data registries were explored and the major challenges in CF, such as the age at fastest lung deterioration, impact of pulmonary exacerbations on lung disease progression, and identification of the most important CF complications, were defined. Second, CFF built a therapeutic pipeline (www.CFF.org) and prioritized the research of CFTR modulators.

NEED FOR NEW OUTCOME MEASURES IS RECOGNIZED

The rational approach to clinical research was accompanied by a much closer attention to outcome parameters: standard operating procedures, adequate assessment of study feasibility, and power calculation.[56]

With improved CF treatments, we became the victims of our own success. Because the rate of lung function decline had become small, forced expiratory volume in 1 second (FEV_1) was no longer an easy to use surrogate outcome parameter.[57,58] More sensitive outcome measures were studied in great detail. Proving the usefulness of computerized chest tomography with quantification of bronchiectasis, air trapping, and bronchial wall thickening became the mission of the Dutch group headed by Harm Tiddens.[59] Lung clearance index, a parameter of gas mixing efficiency, more sensitive than routine spirometry, was introduced in the field of CF by Per Gustafsson.[60] With drugs that attack the basic CF defect, there was a resurgence of interest in biomarkers of CFTR function such as the sweat chloride, nasal potential difference measurement, and intestinal current measurements.[61] To better study the first steps in CF lung disease, the in vivo study of mucociliary clearance was also reenergized.[62]

CENTRALIZED CARE BY MULTIDISCIPLINARY TEAMS FOR PATIENTS WITH CYSTIC FIBROSIS

GUIDELINES AND CONSENSUS STRIVE FOR EVIDENCE-BASED CYSTIC FIBROSIS CARE

In many places, in 1989 the care for patients with CF was solely in the hands of a motivated clinician trying to do his best. But the insight to the basic defect boosted improvements in patient care. The importance of care in a CF center with appropriately staffed multidisciplinary teams was increasingly recognized and aspired to.[63,64] At present, optimal centralized CF care implies that all CF team members bring in their specific expertise (nurse, physiotherapist, social worker, psychologist, dietician, administrative support, and if possible pharmacist) for the full benefit of the patient.[65] All work under the coordination and with the support of the CF center director.

The results of several seminal trials led to a better evidence base for the treatment of CF lung disease. Treatment with rhDNase, inhaled tobramycin, and azithromycin became standard care. To align thoughts on optimal treatment strategies, several consensuses were drafted by the CFF. Under the momentum of Gerd Doering (ECFS president from 1998 to 2006), a series of European consensus documents were prepared, discussed in beautiful Artimino, and published.[65–70] Equally successful consensus conferences were held at Lake Garda, organized by Carlo Castellani, with a focus on *CFTR* mutation analysis,[71] CF NBS,[36] and carrier screening.[72]

POPULATION OF CYSTIC FIBROSIS PATIENTS CHANGES

The improved care was first noticeable in the pediatric population. Maintaining good nutrition and treating airway obstruction and infection intensively transformed not only how children with CF looked but also the atmosphere on the pediatric wards. The CF wards were a place where many children and adolescents repeatedly spent several weeks on end. They inevitably got to know each other and befriended and adored hanging out together. On many occasions, they even got themselves into mischievous behavior. The need for segregation according to type of bacterial infection hit this population like a bomb. But, over time, nearly every pediatric clinic saw a decrease in the number and duration of hospital admissions for children with CF. Sadly, many of the usual residents on the wards died. Some reached adult age with or without lung transplant. The newer generations of children with CF never needed this high number of hospital admissions. Increasingly, home intravenous antibiotic therapy became an alternative for in-hospital treatment. The importance of patient segregation was much better understood and accepted by newer generations of patients.

Good nutritional status and a normal median FEV_1 until adolescence was achieved, were reasonably satisfied with the early CF disease course. In addition, in an increasing number of countries NBS allowed optimal CF care from birth onward. But despite this optimal start, Australian researchers demonstrated that up to half of the patients already had bronchiectasis during preschool years.[73] Airway inflammation and infection start very early in life.[74] There is thus an obvious need for even better management of young children with CF.

More and more, CF was no longer a disease of mainly children and adolescents. The number of adults with CF increased steadily, with more patients surviving until adult age with or without lung transplant, as well as with new diagnoses of CF in adults. In many CF clinics, adults now equal or outnumber the children. Still, the mean age of expected survival (around 50 years) for current birth cohorts and the, at present, median age at death (around 30 years) are much below any nation's average. The increasing number of adults is so far not paralleled by the necessary number of physicians and facilities for adult CF care. In many clinics, a transition program to adult care is not available and pediatricians continue to treat adults with CF. Because this increase in adult patients is anticipated to continue,[75] training adult specialists in CF is a key action point that will be taken up by a joint ECFS and European Respiratory Society task force.

LUNG TRANSPLANT BECOMES AN OPTION FOR END-STAGE LUNG DISEASE

Lung transplant, first performed in Stanford in 1981 and first applied in CF around the time the *CFTR* gene was discovered, became a valid option for patients with end-stage lung disease.[76] Techniques evolved from heart–lung transplant, double lung transplant, and sequential single lung transplant with clam shell incision to sequential single lung with isolated submammary incision, mostly without the need for cardiopulmonary bypass. The outcome after transplant is better for CF than for other indications. In the best centers, 10-year survival post lung transplant for patients with CF is up to 80%. Still, the availability of transplant services differs greatly between countries and despite an improved quality of life patients face new complications post transplant such as rejection, obliterative bronchiolitis, medication side effects, and malignancy, as well as needing to continue many CF medications from before transplantation.

WE GAIN MAJOR NEW INSIGHTS INTO AIRWAY MICROBIOLOGY

Over time and with more patients attaining adult age, we gained major new insights into airway microbiology. In Europe, *Pseudomonas* lung infection had always been in the center of attention. Niels Hoiby and the Copenhagen

CF center were in the vanguard of this research. For years, there was a transatlantic disagreement about the importance of *Pseudomonas*: pro and con debates were regular features at CF meetings. But with increasing proof of patient–patient transmission and lung deterioration after *Pseudomonas* acquisition, the transatlantic dispute about the importance of *Pseudomonas* lung infection was finally settled. All eventually agreed that it is necessary to eradicate early *Pseudomonas* infection and to segregate patients with *Pseudomonas* lung infection from patients without *Pseudomonas* infection: this was the end of summer holiday camps, beginning of patient segregation, and start of excessive fear of water, with the hope of avoiding *Pseudomonas* infection.[70] As a result of eradication of early *Pseudomonas* infection, chronic *Pseudomonas* infection in children with CF has decreased from more than 50% to around 10%.[77,78]

The metabolism of *Pseudomonas* in patients with CF was better understood, especially the switch to the mucoid "biofilm mode" in the reduced oxygen concentrations in airway mucus.[79] New pathogens other than the well-known *Staphylococcus aureus* and *Pseudomonas aeruginosa* were described: *Burkholderia cenocepacia*, capable of suddenly decimating patients; members of an ever-growing group of closely related bacteria, *Stenotrophomonas maltophilia*; and more recently *Achromobacter xylosoxidans*. But clinicians also appreciated the importance of nontuberculous mycobacteria, with *Mycobacterium abscessus* being the most feared, and a growing list of fungi from the well-known *Aspergillus fumigatus* to the lesser known *Scedosporium apiospermum* and black yeast, *Exophiala dermatitidis*.[80,81]

Systematic study of the lung microbiota taught that even the normal lung is not sterile.[82] The lung microbiota in CF is infinitely complex with a very vast spectrum of potential pathogens including countless anaerobic bacteria.[83] With increasing patient illness, the diversity of lung microbiota decreases.[84] So, appropriately, CF treatment diversified in attention from mainly *S. aureus* and *P. aeruginosa* to any potential pathogen in the CF lung and the interactions between microorganisms, which may be adverse, beneficial, or neutral.

Because pulmonary exacerbations lead to lung function decline, definition, frequency, risk factors, and treatment were studied intensely.[85–87]

CYSTIC FIBROSIS REGISTRIES BECOME EVEN MORE IMPORTANT TOOLS

As patients with CF become older, many CF-specific complications emerge or their prevalence is better appreciated. A few are named here: CF-related diabetes, kidney stones, osteoporosis, and intestinal malignancies.[88–91] Not only as outcome parameters in clinical trials, but, also in the clinic more attention went to patient well-being, especially in adults. The new research fields of pain and anxiety were opened.[92,93]

Although CF registries predate the discovery of the *CFTR* gene, there was a boost in exploring cross-sectional and longitudinal patient data for obvious health economic reasons,

to have robust data on the natural history of the disease and define priorities in research, to learn about CF-specific complications, to study outcome parameters, to understand the diversity and geographic distribution of *CFTR* mutations, and also for benchmarking and identification of best practice models by comparing outcome between centers to lead to quality improvement.[94]

PARTNERING MOVED THE CYSTIC FIBROSIS FIELD FORWARD

More than before, academic groups joined forces. This was facilitated by the new means of communication available: e-mail, teleconferencing, websites, Skype, drop boxes, and "clouds." Further, contacts between scientific as well as patient/parent CF organizations around the world have become closer.

In Europe, the increasing importance of CF research and care translated into a growth in the membership of the ECFS. The yearly ECFS meetings transformed from the gathering of CF "addicts" fitting in a small auditorium to a full-size conference with parallel sessions and well over 2000 attendees. The ECFS gained visibility via a website and via the foundation of the *Journal of Cystic Fibrosis* in 2001. During the leadership of Stuart Elborn, the activities of the ECFS expanded further. The ECFS-CTN was founded in 2008. The registry working group was transformed to the European Cystic Fibrosis Society Patient Registry in December 2010. Existing European working groups such as the Cystic Fibrosis Newborn Screening Group and the Diagnostic Network obtained better support, and several new working groups were formed (ECFS Exercise Working Group, ECFS Gene Modifier Working Group, ECFS Lung Microbiome Working Group, and ECFS Non-Tuberculous Mycobacteria Working Group).

Early on, the CFF had already taken the initiative of partnering with companies. Their initiative of supplying major research funding to companies boosted innovative drug development for CF. And this initiative was broadened: CF clinicians brought input into the clinical phase of drug development. Their background knowledge of CF and the clinical trial networks facilitated a more efficient clinical phase of drug development.

CF physicians came into closer contact with health authorities. Bringing new drugs with a favorable risk–benefit balance to the market requires careful evaluation. Here again, the background knowledge of CF physicians was increasingly appreciated to assist in the correct assessment. CF physicians familiarize themselves with the complex clinical trial directives and regulations. Discussions between CF clinicians, pharmaceutical company representatives, patients, and the European Medicines Agency all aim for more efficient and safe clinical research.

Patients and patient representatives became more assertive and became involved in several aspects of CF care and research. Their vision on life changed from "hoping to survive" to "hoping to see the cure of CF."

ALL PARTIES ARE AWARE OF MAJOR CHALLENGES AHEAD

Although better treatments are available, they are continuously added to the existing ones so that the treatment burden becomes extremely high and is a risk factor for low treatment adherence.[95] Comparative effectiveness research initiated by academia becomes more and more important. This type of clinical trials should be facilitated by separate rules for "low intervention clinical trials" (e.g., a marketed drug with a good safety profile being tested off-label), a new category recently put forward in the new European Clinical Trial Regulation (http://ec.europa.eu/health/files/clinicaltrials/2012_07_/proposal_en.pdf). Let us hope that the European funding organizations will empower this regulation with the necessary finances. The ever increasing number of adults with CF needs to be paralleled with the necessary number of adult-trained physicians.

In Europe, the gap in outcome between patients with CF in high- and low-income countries is large.[96] Lobbying for more financial support and better access to care in every country should be a priority.

Even in high-income countries, affordability of care should be preserved. The very high cost of new molecules is a concern, especially in the current economically challenging times. We cannot develop medicines that cannot be afforded by those who need them.[97]

A SPECIAL HOMAGE TO CFF AND CFF-TDN

I discussed the change in the field of CF from 1989 until present from the perspective of the European CF clinician. But to put this entire period into the correct perspective, a specific mention of the importance of the work in North America is needed. From the discovery of the *CFTR* gene until the present time, many major new insights in CF were gained in the United States. Without the CFF, the field of CF would not be what it is today. The CFF was a major financer of not only research in the United States but also selected projects outside the United States. The visionary role of Bob Beall cannot be emphasized sufficiently. He was most likely the first to believe in the possibility of a cure for CF. He worked tirelessly toward that goal by facilitating CF research and promoting excellence in CF care. Bob Beall surrounded himself with equally brilliant people like Preston Campbell and Bruce Marshall. Together with excellent clinical researchers headed by Bonnie Ramsey, Bob Beall saw the importance of a specific clinical trial network dedicated to CF research. His and their example has inspired us all to give the best for patients with CF, be it in research or in clinical care.

REFERENCES

1. Kerem E, Corey M, Kerem BS et al. The relation between genotype and phenotype in cystic fibrosis—analysis of the most common mutation (delta F508). *New Engl J Med* 1990; **323**: 1517–22.
2. Goldman MJ, Anderson GM, Stolzenberg ED et al. Human beta-defensin-1 is a salt-sensitive antibiotic in lung that is inactivated in cystic fibrosis. *Cell* 1997; **85**: 229–36.
3. Matsui H, Grubb BR, Tarran R et al. Evidence for periciliaryliquid layer depletion, not abnormal ion composition, in the pathogenesis of cystic fibrosis airway disease. *Cell* 1998; **95**: 1005–15.
4. Tate S, MacGregor G, Davis M et al. Airways in cystic fibrosis are acidified: Detection by exhaled breath condensate. *Thorax* 2002; **57**: 926–9.
5. Moskwa P, Lorentzen D, Excoffon KJ et al. A novel host defense system of airways is defective in cystic fibrosis. *Am J Resp Crit Care* 2007; **175**: 174–83.
6. Hwang TC, Kirk KL. The CFTR ion channel: Gating, regulation, and anion permeation. *Cold Spring Harb Perspect Med* 2013 Jan 1; **3**(1). doi: pii: a009498. 10.1101/cshperspect.a009498.
7. Pons G, Marchand MC, d'Athis P et al. French multicentre randomized double-blind placebo-controlled trial on nebulized amiloride in cystic fibrosis patients. The Amiloride-AFLM Collaborative Study Group. *Pediatr Pulm* 2000; **30**: 25–31.
8. Chen JH, Stoltz DA, Karp PH et al. Loss of anion transport without increased sodium absorption characterizes newborn porcine cystic fibrosis airway epithelia. *Cell* 2010; **143**: 911–23.
9. Zhou Z, Treis D, Schubert SC et al. Preventive but not late amiloride therapy reduces morbidity and mortality of lung disease in betaENaC-overexpressing mice. *Am J Respir Crit Care Med* 2008; **178**: 1245–56.
10. Knowles MR, Clarke LL, Boucher RC. Activation by extracellular nucleotides of chloride secretion in the airway epithelia of patients with cystic fibrosis. *New Engl J Med* 1991; **325**: 533–8.
11. Accurso FJ, Moss RB, Wilmott RW et al. Denufosol tetrasodium in patients with cystic fibrosis and normal to mildly impaired lung function. *Am J Respir Crit Care Med* 2011; **183**: 627–34.
12. Ratjen F, Durham T, Navratil T et al. Long term effects of denufosol tetrasodium in patients with cystic fibrosis. *J Cyst Fibros* 2012; **11**: 539–49.
13. Huang F, Rock JR, Harfe BD et al. Studies on expression and function of the TMEM16A calcium-activated chloride channel. *P Natl Acad Sci USA* 2009; **15**: 21413–8.
14. Amaral M, Farinha CM. Rescuing mutant CFTR: A multi-task approach to a better outcome in treating cystic fibrosis. *Curr Pharm Des* 2013; 19(19): 3497–508.

15. Koch C, Cuppens H, Rainisio et al. European Epidemiologic Registry of Cystic Fibrosis (ERCF): Comparison of major disease manifestations between patients with different classes of mutations. *Pediatr Pulm* 2001; **31**: 1–12.

16. Mekus F, Ballmann M, Bronsveld I et al. Categories of deltaF508 homozygous cystic fibrosis twin and sibling pairs with distinct phenotypic characteristics. *Twin Research* 2000; **3**: 277–93.

17. Vascoy LL, Blackman SM, Collaco JM et al. Heritability of lung disease severity in cystic fibrosis. *Am J Respir Crit Care Med* 2007; **175**: 1036–43.

18. Wright FA, Strug LJ, Doshi VK. *et al*. Genome-wide association and linkage identify modifier loci of lung disease severity in cystic fibrosis at 11p13 and 20q13.2. *Nat Genet* 2011; **43**: 539–46.

19. Wang X, Venable J, LaPointe P et al. Hsp90 cochaperone Aha1 downregulation rescues misfolding of CFTR in cystic fibrosis. *Cell* 2006; **127**: 803–15.

20. Denning GM, Anderson MP, Amara JF et al. Processing of mutant cystic fibrosis transmembrane conductance regulator is temperature-sensitive. *Nature* 1992; **358**: 761–4.

21. Wainwright CE, Elborn JS, Ramsey BW et al. Efficacy and safety of a CFTR corrector (lumacaftor) in combination with a CFTR potentiator (ivacaftor) in patients with cystic fibrosis who are homozygous for F508del-CFTR: Phase 3 TRAFFIC and TRANSPORT studies. *New Engl J Med* in press.

22. Rabeh WM, Bossard F, Xu H et al. Correction of both NBD1 energetics and domain interface is required to restore F508CFTR folding and function. *Cell* 2012; **148**: 150–63.

23. Mendoza JL, Schmidt A, Li Q et al. Requirements for efficient correction of F508 CFTR revealed by analyses of evolved sequences. *Cell* 2012; **148**: 164–74.

24. Ramsey BW, Davies J, McElvaney NG et al. A CFTR potentiator in patients with cystic fibrosis and the G551D mutation. *New Engl J Med* 2011; **365**: 1663–72.

25. Yu H, Burton B, Huang CJ et al. Ivacaftor potentiation of multiple CFTR channels with gating mutations. *J Cyst Fibros* 2012; **11**: 237–45.

26. Kerem E, Hirawat S, Armoni S et al. Effectiveness of PTC124 treatment of cystic fibrosis caused by nonsense mutations: A prospective phase II trial. *Lancet* 2008; **372**: 719–27.

27. De Boeck K, Munck A, Walker S, Faro A, Hiatt P, Gilmartin G, Higgins M. Efficacy and safety of ivacaftor in patients with cystic fibrosis and a non-G551D gating mutation. *J Cyst Fibros* 2014 Dec;13(6):674–80. doi: 10.1016/j.jcf.2014.09.005. Epub 2014 Sep 26.

28. Sermet-Gaudelus I, De Boeck K, Casimir GJ et al. Ataluren (PTC124) induces cystic fibrosis transmembrane conductance regulator protein expression and activity in children with nonsense mutation cystic fibrosis. *Am J Respir Crit Care Med* 2012; **15**: 1262–72.

29. Stoltz DA, Meyerholz DK, Pezzulo et al. Cystic fibrosis pigs develop lung disease and exhibit defective bacterial eradication at birth. *Sci Transl Med* 2010; **2**: 29ra31.

30. Kerem E, Konstan MW, De Boeck K, Accurso FJ et al. Ataluren for the treatment of nonsense-mutation cystic fibrosis: A randomised, double-blind, placebo-controlled phase 3 trial. *Lancet Respir Med* 2014 Jul;2(7):539–47. doi: 10.1016/S2213-2600(14)70100-6. Epub 2014 May 15.

31. Stoltz DA, Meyerholz DK, Welsh MJ. Origins of cystic fibrosis lung disease. *N Engl J Med* 2015 Jan 22;372(4):351-62. doi: 10.1056/NEJMra1300109.

32. Meyerholz DK, Stoltz DA, Namati E et al. Loss of cystic fibrosis transmembrane conductance regulator function produces abnormalities in tracheal development in neonatal pigs and young children. *American Journal of Respiratory Critical Care Medicine* 2010; **182**: 1251–61.

33. Rogan MP, Reznikov LR, Pezzulo AA et al. Pigs and humans with cystic fibrosis have reduced insulin-like growth factor 1 (IGF1) levels at birth. *Proc Natl Acad Sci USA* 2010; **107**: 20571–5.

34. Pezzulo AA, Tang XX, Hoegger MJ et al. Reduced airway surface pH impairs bacterial killing in the porcine cystic fibrosis lung. *Nature* 2012; **487**: 109–13.

35. Dekkers JF, Wiegerinck CL, de Jonge HR et al. A functional CFTR assay using primary cystic fibrosis intestinal organoids. *Nat Med* 2013 Jul;19(7):939–45. doi: 10.1038/nm.3201. Epub 2013 Jun 2.

36. Rosenstein BJ, Cutting GR. The diagnosis of cystic fibrosis: A consensus statement. Cystic Fibrosis Foundation Consensus Panel. *J Pediatr* 1998; **132**: 589–95.

37. De Boeck K, Wilschanski M, Castellani C et al. Cystic fibrosis: Terminology and diagnostic algorithms. *Thorax* 2006; **61**: 627–35.

38. Farrell PM, Rosenstein BJ, White TB et al. Guidelines for diagnosis of cystic fibrosis in newborns through older adults: Cystic Fibrosis Foundation consensus report. *J Pediatr* 2008; **153**: S4–14.

39. Bombieri C, Claustres M, De Boeck et al. Recommendations for the classification of disease as CFTR-related disorders. *J Cyst Fibros* 2011; **10**: S86–102.

40. Calvin J, Hogg SL, McShane D et al. Thirty years of screening for cystic fibrosis in East Anglia. *Arch Dis Child* 2012; **97**: 1043–7.

41. Castellani C, Southern KW, Brownlee K et al. European best practice guidelines for cystic fibrosis neonatal screening. *J Cyst Fibros* 2009; **8**: 153–73.

42. Sermet-Gaudelus I, Mayell SJ, Southern KW et al. Guidelines on the early management of infants diagnosed with cystic fibrosis following newborn screening. *J Cyst Fibros* 2010; **9**: 323–9.

43. Duguépéroux I, Audrézet MP, Parent P et al. Cascade testing in families of carriers identified through newborn screening in Western Brittany (France). *J Cyst Fibros* 2013 Jul;12(4):338–44. doi: 10.1016/j.jcf.2012.11.009. Epub 2012 Dec 28.

44. Vernooy-van Langen AM, Loeber JG, Elvers B et al. Novel strategies in newborn screening for cystic fibrosis: A prospective controlled study. *Thorax* 2012; **67**: 289–95.

45. Scotet V, Audrézet MP, Roussey M et al. Immunoreactive trypsin/DNA newborn screening for cystic fibrosis: Should the R117H variant be included in CFTR mutation panels? *Pediatrics* 2006; **118**: 523–9.

46. Mayell SJ, Munck A, Craig JV et al. A European consensus for the evaluation and management of infants with an equivocal diagnosis following newborn screening for cystic fibrosis. *J Cyst Fibros* 2009; **8**: 71–8.

47. Cystic Fibrosis Foundation, Borowitz D, Parad, RB et al. Cystic Fibrosis Foundation practice guidelines for the management of infants with cystic fibrosis transmembrane conductance regulator-related metabolic syndrome during the first two years of life and beyond. *J Pediatr* 2009; **155**: S106–16.

48. Rock MJ, Levy H, Zaleski C, Farrell PM. Factors accounting for a missed diagnosis of cystic fibrosis after newborn screening. *Pediatr Pulm* 2011; **46**: 1166–74.

49. Cheng K, Smyth RL, Motley J et al. Randomized controlled trials in cystic fibrosis (1966–1997) categorized by time, design, and intervention. *Pediatr Pulm* 2000; **29**: 1–7.

50. Fuchs HJ, Borowitz DS, Christiansen DH et al. Effect of aerosolized recombinant human DNase on exacerbations of respiratory symptoms and on pulmonary function in patients with cystic fibrosis. The Pulmozyme Study Group. *New Engl J Med* 1994; **331**: 637–42.

51. Goss CH, Mayer-Hamblett N, Kronmal RA, Ramsey BW. The cystic fibrosis therapeutics development network (CF TDN): A paradigm of a clinical trials network for genetic and orphan diseases. *Adv Drug Deliver Rev* 2002; **5**: 1505–25.

52. Ramsey BW, Pepe MS, Quan JM et al. Intermittent administration of inhaled tobramycin in patients with cystic fibrosis. Cystic Fibrosis Inhaled Tobramycin Study Group. *New Engl J Med* 1999; **7**: 23–30.

53. Quan JM, Tiddens HA, Sy JP, McKenzie SG et al. A two-year randomized, placebo-controlled trial of dornase alfa in young patients with cystic fibrosis with mild lung function abnormalities. *J Pediatr* 2001; **139**: 813–20.

54. Saiman L, Marshall BC, Mayer-Hamblett N, Burns JL et al. Azithromycin in patients with cystic fibrosis chronically infected with *Pseudomonas aeruginosa*: A randomized controlled trial. *J Am Med Assoc* 2003; **290**: 1749–56.

55. Treggiari MM, Retsch-Bogart G, Mayer-Hamblett N et al. Comparative efficacy and safety of 4 randomized regimens to treat early *Pseudomonas aeruginosa* infection in children with cystic fibrosis. *Arch Pediatr Adolesc Med* 2011; **165**: 847–56.

56. Rosenfeld M. An overview of endpoints for cystic fibrosis clinical trials: One size does not fit all. *Proc Am Thorac Soc* 2007; **4**: 299–301.

57. Que C, Cullinan P, Geddes D. Improving rate of decline of FEV$_1$ in young adults with cystic fibrosis. *Thorax* 2006; **61**: 155–7.

58. Liou TG, Elkin EP, Pasta DJ, Jacobs JR et al. Year-to-year changes in lung function in individuals with cystic fibrosis. *J Cyst Fibros* 2010; **9**: 250–6.

59. Tiddens HA, de Jong PA. Imaging and clinical trials in cystic fibrosis. *Proc Am Thorac Soc* 2007; **4**: 343–6.

60. Robinson PD, Goldman MD, Gustafsson PM. Inert gas washout: Theoretical background and clinical utility in respiratory disease. *Respiration* 2009; **78**: 339–55.

61. De Boeck K, Kent L, Davies J et al. CFTR biomarkers: Time for promotion to surrogate end-point. *Eur Respir J* 2013; **41**: 203–16.

62. Donaldson SH, Corcoran TE, Laube BL, Bennett WD. Mucociliary clearance as an outcome measure for cystic fibrosis clinical research. *Proc Am Thorac Soc* 2007; **1**: 399–405.

63. van Koolwijk LM, Uiterwaal CS, van der Laag J et al. Treatment of children with cystic fibrosis: Central, local or both? *Acta Paediatr* 2002; **9**: 972–7.

64. Lebecque P, Leonard A, De Boeck K et al. Early referral to cystic fibrosis specialist centre impacts on respiratory outcome. *J Cyst Fibros* 2009; **8**: 26–30.

65. Kerem E, Conway S, Elborn S, Heijerman H for the Consensus Committee. Standards of care for patients with cystic fibrosis: A European consensus. *J Cyst Fibros* 2005; **4**: 7–26.

66. Sinaasappel M, Stern M, Littlewood J et al. Nutrition in patients with cystic fibrosis: A European consensus. *J Cyst Fibros* 2002; **1**: 67–91.

67. Döring G, Høiby N for the Consensus Study Group. Early intervention and prevention of lung disease in cystic fibrosis: A European consensus. *J Cyst Fibros* 2004; **3**: 67–91.

68. Döring G, Elborn JS, Johannesson M et al. Clinical trials in cystic fibrosis. *J Cyst Fibros* 2007; **6**: 85–90.

69. Heijermann H, Westerman E, Conway S et al. Inhaled medication and inhalation devices for lung disease in patients with cystic fibrosis: A European consensus. *J Cyst Fibros* 2009; **8**: 295–315.

70. Döring G, Flume P, Heijerman H et al. Treatment of lung infection in patients with cystic fibrosis: Current and future strategies. *J Cyst Fibros* 2012; **11**: 461–79.

71. Castellani C, Cuppens H, Macek M Jr et al. Consensus on the use and interpretation of cystic fibrosis mutation analysis in clinical practice. *J Cyst Fibros* 2008; **7**: 179–96.

72. Castellani C, Macek M Jr, Cassiman JJ et al. Benchmarks for cystic fibrosis carrier screening: A European consensus document. *J Cyst Fibros* 2010; **9**: 165–78.

73. Wainwright CE, Vidmar S, Armstrong DS et al. Effect of bronchoalveolar lavage-directed therapy on *Pseudomonas aeruginosa* infection and structural lung injury in children with cystic fibrosis: A randomized trial. *J Am Med Assoc* 2011; **306**: 163–71.

74. Belessis Y, Dixon B, Hawkins G et al. Early cystic fibrosis lung disease detected by bronchoalveolar lavage and lung clearance index. *Am J Respir Crit Care Med* 2012; **185**: 862–73.

75. Tuchman LK, Schwartz LA, Sawicki GS et al. Cystic fibrosis and transition to adult medical care. *Pediatrics* 2010; **125**: 2009–791.

76. Braun AT, Merlo CA. Cystic fibrosis lung transplantation. *Curr Opin Pulm Med* 2011; **17**: 467–72.

77. Proesmans M, Balinska-Miskiewicz W, Dupont L et al. Evaluating the "Leeds criteria" for *Pseudomonas aeruginosa* infection in a cystic fibrosis centre. *Eur Respir J* 2006; **27**: 937–43.

78. Lebecque P, Leal T, Zylberberg K et al. Towards zero prevalence of chronic *Pseudomonas aeruginosa* infection in children with cystic fibrosis. *J Cyst Fibros* 2006; **5**: 237–44.

79. Worlitzsch D, Tarran R, Ulrich M et al. Effects of reduced mucus oxygen concentration in airway *Pseudomonas* infections of cystic fibrosis patients. *J Clin Invest* 2002; **109**: 317–25.

80. Pihet M, Carrere J, Cimon B et al. Occurrence and relevance of filamentous fungi in respiratory secretions of patients with cystic fibrosis—a review. *Med Mycol* 2009; **47**: 387–97.

81. Lebecque P, Leonard A, Huang D et al. Exophiala (Wangiella) dermatitidis and cystic fibrosis—prevalence and risk factors. *Med Mycol* 2010; **48**: S4–9.

82. Beck JM, Young VB, Huffnagle GB. The microbiome of the lung. *Transl Res* 2012; **160**: 258–66.

83. Delhaes L, Monchy S, Fréalle E et al. The airway microbiota in cystic fibrosis: A complex fungal and bacterial community—implications for therapeutic management. *PLoS One* 2012; **7**: e36313.

84. Filkins LM, Hampton TH, Gifford AH et al. Prevalence of streptococci and increased polymicrobial diversity associated with cystic fibrosis patient stability. *J Bacteriol* 2012; **194**: 4709–17.

85. Goss CH, Burns JL. Exacerbations in cystic fibrosis. 1: Epidemiology and pathogenesis. *Thorax* 2007; **62**: 360–7.

86. Bell SC, Robinson PJ. Exacerbations in cystic fibrosis. 2: Prevention. *Thorax* 2007; **62**: 723–32.

87. Smyth A, Elborn JS. Exacerbations in cystic fibrosis: 3—Management. *Thorax* 2008; **63**: 180–4.

88. Moran A, Brunzell C, Cohen RC et al. Clinical care guidelines for cystic fibrosis-related diabetes: A position statement of the American Diabetes Association and a clinical practice guideline of the Cystic Fibrosis Foundation, endorsed by the Pediatric Endocrine Society. *Diabetes Care* 2010; **33**: 2697–708.

89. Gibney EM, Goldfarb DS. The association of nephrolithiasis with cystic fibrosis. *Am J Kidney Dis* 2003; **42**: 1–11.

90. Javier RM, Jacquot J. Bone disease in cystic fibrosis: What's new? *Joint Bone Spine* 2011; **78**: 445–50.

91. Maisonneuve P, Marshall BC, Knapp EA, Lowenfels AB et al. Cancer risk in cystic fibrosis: A 20-year nationwide study from the United States. *J Natl Cancer I* 2013; **105**: 122–9.

92. Festini F, Ballarin S, Codamo T et al. Prevalence of pain in adults with cystic fibrosis. *J Cyst Fibros.* 2004; **3**: 51–7.

93. Cruz I, Marciel KK, Quittner AL, Schechter MS. Anxiety and depression in cystic fibrosis. *Sem Resp Crit Care M* 2009; **30**: 569–78.

94. Stern M. The use of a cystic fibrosis patient registry to assess outcomes and improve cystic fibrosis care in Germany. *Curr Opin Pulm Med* 2011; **17**: 473–7.

95. Sawicki GS, Ren CL, Konstan MW et al. Treatment complexity in cystic fibrosis: Trends over time and associations with site-specific outcomes. *J Cyst Fibros* 2013 Sep;12(5):461–7. doi: 10.1016/j.jcf.2012.12.009. Epub 2013 Jan 24.

96. McCormick J, Mehta G, Olesen HV et al. Comparative demographics of the European cystic fibrosis population: A cross-sectional database analysis. *Lancet* 2010; **20**: 1007–13.

97. Bush A, Simmonds NJ. Hot off the breath: 'I've a cost for'—the 64 million dollar question. *Thorax* 2012; **67**: 382–4.

2

Epidemiology of cystic fibrosis

STEPHANIE J. MACNEILL

INTRODUCTION

This chapter explores the epidemiology of cystic fibrosis (CF), including the influence of the different genotypes and mutation classes associated with the disease, its incidence and prevalence, patient survival, demographic and clinical characteristics, and factors influencing prognosis.

Describing the health of large patient populations is made possible in part through the use of national disease registries. As such, we have made use of the 2011 annual reports from the Cystic Fibrosis Foundation (CFF) in the United States,[1] Cystic Fibrosis Trust in the United Kingdom,[2] Cystic Fibrosis Canada,[3] and 2008–2009 data from the European CF Society.[4] We also included 2009 data from Australia published by Bell et al.[5] Comparisons between countries, however, should be made cautiously as countries will have different health-care systems and treatment practices and registries will differ in the way data are collected (annual reviews or encounter based, for example), levels of completeness, and reference values used for nutritional and pulmonary outcomes. Additionally, it is worth noting that registry studies—like all observational studies—are prone to ascertainment bias where all patients are not represented equally in the cohort. In relation to registry studies, this may stem from national screening practices (or lack thereof) where patients with certain genotypes are less likely to be identified. Registries based on being treated at specialist centers are also at risk of bias if there are groups of patients who are unable to access such services. This may be for reasons of geography or ability to pay, for example. Given this potential for bias, it is important when interpreting results to be mindful of how patients are identified for such registries and their estimated coverage. For example, the 2011 annual report produced by the Cystic Fibrosis Trust in the United Kingdom—where there exists a universal access health-care system and all CF patients are seen at specialist centers—included data on 89% of the patients registered at these centers. Data from Italy, however, which are included in the European Cystic Fibrosis Society's report, cover only an estimated 14% of patients.

BIRTH AND POPULATION PREVALENCE

BIRTH PREVALENCE

The birth prevalence of CF in different populations is described in Table 2.1 and illustrates how CF varies greatly by region and population. It is most common in northern European and Caucasian North Americans and Ashkenazi Jews, although it has also been identified in Asia, South and Central America, and Africa. Within a country, differences are frequently observed reflecting the ethnic diversity of the population. In California, for example, researchers observed a birth prevalence of 1:5025 across all births, yet when split by ethnic group it varied from 1:2577 in Caucasians to only 1:5848 among African-Americans.[6] It should thus be emphasized that the old cliché of CF being purely a disease of white races can firmly be laid to rest.

Caution must be exerted, however, when making comparisons between countries and between studies. Identification of patients with CF will vary between studies, from the use of national patient registries with established neonatal screening to surveys at single centers. Also, the methods used for diagnosing patients with CF will vary over time and, in some cases, between countries.

Underdiagnosis in some countries can lead to underestimates in incidence. This may stem from limited availability of newborn screening or deaths prior to diagnosis. For example, when using data from national registries across Europe, McCormick et al.[43] observed that the size of the CF populations in non–EU countries was lower than in EU countries within Europe. While striking, the authors highlighted that this disparity may be due in part to underdiagnosis and higher rates of early infant mortality in these countries and therefore urged caution in the interpretation of these results.

Table 2.1 Birth prevalence of CF by country and population[a]

Population	Incidence	Details
Africa		
South Africa—black population [7]	784 to 13,924	Predicted based on carrier frequency
South Africa—Cape Town [8]		Based on the number of new patients and live births during a 4-year period at a children's hospital
White population	2,000	
Black population	12,000	
Asia		
Japan [9]	350,000	Based on reported cases and live births after 1980
Australia		
Australia [5]	2,986	Registry study using data averaged over 5 years to 2008
Australia—Victoria [10]	3,139	Based on live births in Victoria between 1989 and 2008
New Zealand (non-Maori) [11]	3,179	Based on data collected between 1960 and 1983
Europe		
Austria [12]	3,500	Review of studies using survey or registry data
Austria [13]	3,436	Review of newborn screening program in 2004
Belgium [12]	2,850	Review of studies using survey or registry data
Belgium—Wallonia [13]	7,509	Review of newborn screening program in 2004
Bulgaria [12]	2,500	Review of studies using survey or registry data
Cyprus [12]	7,914	Review of studies using survey or registry data
Czech Republic [12]	2,833	Review of studies using survey or registry data
Czech Republic—Western region [14]	9,100	Study of newborn screening programs between 2004 and 2005
Denmark [12]	4,700	Review of studies using survey or registry data
Denmark [15]	4,760	Based on data between 1945 and 1985
Denmark—Faroe Islands [16]	1,775	Based on data between 1954 and 1993
Estonia [12]	4,500	Review of studies using survey or registry data
Finland [12]	25,000	Review of studies using survey or registry data
France [12]	4,700	Review of studies using survey or registry data
France [13]	1:4,384	Review of newborn screening program in 2004
France—Brittany [17][b]	3,268	Analysis of births in Brittany 2009
Germany [12]	3,300	Review of studies using survey or registry data
Germany [13]	2,291	Review of newborn screening program in 2004
Greece [12]	3,500	Review of studies using survey or registry data
Ireland [12,18]	1,353	Review of studies using survey or registry data
Ireland [19]	1,838	Using national registry data and national health statistics
Italy [12,20]	4,238	Review of studies using survey or registry data
Italy [13]	4,618	Review of newborn screening program in 2004
Italy—regions [14]	2,650 to 5,200	Study of regional newborn screening programs between 2004 and 2005
Italy—Veneto/Trentino Alto-Adige [21]	3,540	Study of births between 1990 and 2005
Netherlands [12,22]	4,750	Review of studies using survey or registry data
Netherlands [23]	6,062	Study comparing two screening strategies between 2008 and 2009
Norway [24]	6,574	Study of screening program between 1982 and 1984
Poland [12]	5,000	Review of studies using survey or registry data
Portugal [12]	6,000	Review of studies using survey or registry data
Romania [12]	2,056	Review of studies using survey or registry data
Slovakia [12]	1,800	Review of studies using survey or registry data
Slovenia [12]	3,000	Review of studies using survey or registry data
Spain [12]	3,750	Review of studies using survey or registry data
Spain [13]	2,840	Review of newborn screening program in 2004

(Continued)

Table 2.1 (*Continued*) Birth prevalence of CF by country and population[a]

Population	Incidence	Details
Spain—regions [14]	4,000 to 10,500	Study of regional newborn screening programs between 2004 and 2005
Sweden [12,25]	5,600	Review of registry studies
Russia [13]	3,714	Review of newborn screening program in 2004
United Kingdom [26]	2,381	Analysis of national survey data and death certificates between 1968 and 1987
United Kingdom [27]	2,415	Average proportion of CF births between 1968 and 1987
United Kingdom—regions [14]	2,250 to 2,850	Study of regional newborn screening programs between 2004 and 2005
United Kingdom—East Anglia [28]	3,245	Data from neonatal screening in 1990
United Kingdom—Wales [13]	1,888	Assessment of newborn screening program in 2004
United Kingdom—Northern Ireland [29]	1,969	Based on identified cases and live births between 1961 and 1971
United Kingdom—Northern Ireland [30]	1,807	Assessment of newborn screening program between 1983 and 1987
United Kingdom—Scotland [13]	2,874	Assessment of newborn screening program in 2004
United Kingdom—Scotland [31]	1,984	Calculated from heterozygote frequencies in a cohort of women attending antenatal screening
Middle East		
Bahrain [32]	5,800	Based on diagnoses and population statistics
Israel: Ashkenazi Jews and Arabs [33]	1,800 to 4,000	Based on identified cases in Israel between 1946 and 1975
Jordan [34]	2,560	Based on newborn screening statistics
United Arab Emirates [35]	15,000	
North America		
Canada [36] 1971–1987 2000	2,714 3,608	Based on a study of temporal trends in CF birth prevalences
Canada—Saguenay-Lac-St.-Jean (Quebec) [37][c]	902	Based on data between 1975 and 1988
United States [38] Whites Non-whites	3,419 12,163	Using national registry data between 1989 and 1991 and statistical models to account for underdiagnosis due to death prior to diagnosis
United States—California [6]	5,025	Using data from state-wide newborn screening program
United States—Massachusetts [39]	2,908	Using data from newborn screening between 1999 and 2003
United States—Michigan [40]	3,198	Using data from newborn screening program between 2007 and 2008
United States—Wisconsin [30]	3,983	Using data from newborn screening program between 1994 and 2002
South America		
Brazil [41]	6,902	Based on known cases and population samples

Source: Daigneault J et al., *Hum Biol*, 64(1), 115–9, 1992.
[a] Expressed as the number of live births per incident case of CF.
[b] A number of studies have been conducted in Brittany studying its relatively high birth prevalence over time. Earlier studies have shown slightly higher birth rates [21,42] than that presented here for Brittany.
[c] The high prevalence in Saguenay-Lac St. Jean is thought to be due to founder effect and genetic drift.

TEMPORAL TRENDS IN INCIDENCE

Since the discovery of the CF gene, carrier testing has become possible and there has been some interest in assessing whether there have been subsequent changes in the birth prevalence of CF due, in part, to families choosing not to have children on learning of their carrier status. In northeastern Italy, a decrease in the birth prevalence of CF was observed between 1993 and 2007, which was greater in the eastern region where carrier testing is more widely available.[44] In Canada, the CF birth prevalence was stable between 1971 and 1987 and then from 1988—a year prior to the advent of carrier screening—there was a linear decline in birth prevalence until 2000.[36] In Victoria, Australia, researchers noted a decline in the live-birth prevalence of CF after the implementation of newborn screening,[45] and in Massachusetts researchers observed fewer children than expected identified with CF through newborn screening in 2003 through to 2006.[46] It was suggested that the provision of preconception and prenatal screening to the general population to identify carriers of CF might result in a decrease in the number of births of children with CF.[46]

In Brittany, France, where CF is relatively common (1:2948)[42] researchers noted a 30.5% difference in the 10-year birth prevalence (1992–2001) of CF depending on whether CF-affected pregnancies that were terminated during pregnancy were included.[47] The researchers concluded that prenatal diagnoses were responsible for this decrease. The region noted a 40% decline in incidence over a 35-year period until 2009.[17] Specifically, they noted a breakpoint in the late 1980s when prenatal diagnoses became more common after which the incident rate remained relatively stable.

POPULATION PREVALENCE

Population prevalence statistics are rarely presented in the literature, but they can be calculated with the use of specialist patient registries and official population statistics. These will still be influenced by the estimated coverage of the patient registries, however, which can vary greatly between countries. The 2008–2009 annual report for the European Cystic Fibrosis Society Patient Registry noted a wide variation in the estimated coverage of the data provided,[4] and many national registries noted coverage ranging from 14% to 100%. A summary is presented in Table 2.2 illustrating a wide variation in estimated prevalence across countries. CF was most common in Ireland and least common in Romania, Finland, and the Baltic countries of Latvia and Lithuania.

Farrell et al.[12] produced an extensive report of population prevalences for European countries using survey data and registry information. Combining data from all 27 EU countries, they estimated a population prevalence of 7.37 per 100,000 in 2004, which is only slightly lower than the 2011 prevalence in the United States, as described earlier.

Despite reductions in the birth prevalence of CF noted in some countries, there is evidence that the population prevalence is increasing. Since 2007, the number of new diagnoses in the United Kingdom exceeded the number of deaths by approximately 145 each year, suggesting an increase in prevalence of 0.2 per 100,000 population per year.[2] Similar trends emerge from US data from 2006.[2]

GENOTYPE DISTRIBUTION

An extensive international analysis by the Cystic Fibrosis Genetic Analysis Consortium published in 1995 described the distribution of *CFTR* genotypes and observed that the most commonly observed CF mutations were *F508del* (66.0%), followed by *G542X* (2.4%), *G551D* (1.6%), *N1303K* (1.3%), and *W1282X* (1.2%).[54]

Whereas *F508del* proved to be common, striking between- and within-country differences have been observed. Bobadilla et al.[55] conducted an international review of published genotype prevalences that illustrates this. Within Europe *F508del* was the most common, yet its prevalence varied from 87.5% in Denmark to only 31.0% in Lithuania. Within France, United Kingdom, and Italy, there are noted geographic differences. Ethnic differences were noted in the United Kingdom, where the prevalence of *F508del* mutation was only 19.2% in a Pakistani subpopulation compared to 75.3% across the country as a whole. In Africa and the Middle East, other mutations such as *W1282X* and *S549R* were most common among Ashkenazi Jews and in the United Arab Emirates, respectively. In other countries in this region, *F508del* remained the most common mutation but was less common than in Europe (17.6% in Tunisia, for example, compared with 75.3% in the United Kingdom). In South America, the prevalence of *F508del* varied from 25.0% in Ecuador to 58.6% in Argentina. In North America, there were clear within-country differences: in Lac St. Jean, Quebec, the prevalence of *F508del* was 59.0% compared to 71.4% in nearby Quebec City. In the United States the prevalence across the country was 68.6%, whereas it was only 48.0% among African-Americans.

It has been observed that some non-*F508del* mutations are more common in particular populations—*G542X* is seen more commonly in Mediterranean Europe and Africa; *G551D* in those of Celtic descent in Ireland, United Kingdom, and Brittany; *W1282X* in Ashkenazi Jews; *394delTT* in countries bordering the Baltic Sea; *3120+1G->T* in African-Americans; *621+1G->T* in Lac St. Jean; *R1162X* in US Native Americans; and *3849+10KbC->T* in US Hispanics.[55] The implication of this variation is that in heterogeneous populations screening for a wide array of genotypes is important. Furthermore, this has implications for health economics; a greater cost burden for expensive new molecules such as ivacaftor will fall on countries with a high prevalence of the *G551D* mutation.

With the discovery of the *CFTR* gene and subsequent delineation of the various mutations, there have been efforts to determine whether specific mutations—or functional classes—are associated with improved or worse outcomes. Although considerable variability within functional classes exists, some common trends have emerged. McKone et al.[56] observed lower mortality in patients with functional classes IV and V compared to those with homozygous *F508del*. When comparing classes I–III with IV and V, they observed a reduced mortality in the latter, which was not explained by forced expiratory volume in 1 second (FEV_1), body mass index (BMI), pseudomonas infection, or pancreatic sufficiency.[57] Similarly, de Garcia et al.[58] observed lower baseline spirometry and greater loss of lung function over follow-up in adults with *CFTR* mutation classes I or II on both chromosomes, and Koch[59] noted that a class IV *CFTR* mutation appeared to offer some protection against pancreatic insufficiency.

Table 2.2 Population prevalence of cystic fibrosis

Population	Population prevalence (per 100,000)	Year	Details
Australia			
Australia	14.07	2011	Based on the 2011 Australian CF registry annual report and official population statistics [48,49]
Europe			
Austria [12]	8.39	2004	Review of studies using survey or registry data
Belgium [12]	10.3	2004	Review of studies using survey or registry data
Belgium[a]	11.05	2009	Based on the 2008–2009 European Cystic Fibrosis Society Patient Registry Report and official population statistics [4,50]
Bulgaria [12]	2.26	2004	Review of studies using survey or registry data
Cyprus [12]	3.35	2004	Review of studies using survey or registry data
Czech Republic [12]	5.56	2004	Review of studies using survey or registry data
Czech Republic[a]	4.86	2009	Based on the 2008–2009 European Cystic Fibrosis Society Patient Registry Report and official population statistics [4,50]
Denmark [12]	7.61	2004	Review of studies using survey or registry data
Denmark[a]	8.18	2009	Based on the 2008–2009 European Cystic Fibrosis Society Patient Registry Report and official population statistics [4,50]
Estonia [12]	6.18	2004	Review of studies using survey or registry data
Finland [12]	1.23	2004	Review of studies using survey or registry data
France [12]	7.50	2004	Review of studies using survey or registry data
France[a]	9.74	2009	Based on the 2008–2009 European Cystic Fibrosis Society Patient Registry Report and official population statistics [4,50]
Germany [12]	8.29	2004	Review of studies using survey or registry data
Germany[a]	6.84	2008	Based on the 2008–2009 European Cystic Fibrosis Society Patient Registry Report and official population statistics [4,50]
Greece [12]	5.21	2004	Review of studies using survey or registry data
Hungary [12]	4.09	2004	Review of studies using survey or registry data
Hungary[a]	6.15	2009	Based on the 2008–2009 European Cystic Fibrosis Society Patient Registry Report and official population statistics [4,50]
Ireland [12]	29.8	2004	Review of studies using survey or registry data
Ireland[a]	25.78	2008	Based on the 2008–2009 European Cystic Fibrosis Society Patient Registry Report and official population statistics [4,50]
Italy [12]	8.72	2004	Review of studies using survey or registry data
Latvia [12]	1.04	2004	Review of studies using survey or registry data
Lithuania [12]	1.30	2004	Review of studies using survey or registry data
Luxembourg [12]	4.31	2004	Review of studies using survey or registry data
Malta [12]	5.79	2004	Review of studies using survey or registry data
Netherlands [12]	7.81	2004	Review of studies using survey or registry data
Netherlands	7.81	2009	Based on the 2008–2009 European Cystic Fibrosis Society Patient Registry Report and official population statistics [4,50]
Poland [12]	2.56	2004	Review of studies using survey or registry data
Portugal [12]	2.71	2004	Review of studies using survey or registry data
Romania [12]	1.06	2004	Review of studies using survey or registry data
Slovakia [12]	6.27	2004	Review of studies using survey or registry data
Slovenia [12]	3.28	2004	Review of studies using survey or registry data
Spain [12]	5.46	2004	Review of studies using survey or registry data
Sweden [12]	4.03	2004	Review of studies using survey or registry data
Sweden[a]	7.18	2009	Based on the 2008–2009 European Cystic Fibrosis Society Patient Registry Report and official population statistics [4,50]

Table 2.2 *(Continued)* Population prevalence of cystic fibrosis

Population	Population prevalence (per 100,000)	Year	Details
United Kingdom [12]	13.7	2004	Review of studies using survey or registry data
United Kingdom	15.47	2011	Based on the number of patients registered in the 2011 CF Trust Registry annual report and official population statistics [2,50]
Middle East			
Israel	7.91	2009	Based on the 2008–2009 European Cystic Fibrosis Society Patient Registry Report and official population statistics [4,51]
North America			
Canada	11.7	2011	Based on the 2011 Canadian Cystic Fibrosis Registry annual report and 2011 census data [3,52]
United States	8.7	2011	Based on the 2011 CF Foundation Registry annual report and estimated population size for 2011 [1,53]

[a] Where the population prevalence was estimated using data from the European Cystic Fibrosis Patient Registry report, the number of patients with CF was estimated from the number of patients seen that year and estimated registry coverage that year.

SURVIVAL

As in any life-threatening disease, much research has been conducted to understand patient survival—estimating current survival, temporal trends, and predictors. The way in which survival is measured, however, is varied as described later. The many factors influencing survival are discussed in the prognosis section of this chapter.

MORTALITY

Crude mortality rates for CF are often presented as the number of deaths per 1000 (or 100,000) population. In the general population, CF as a cause of death is rare—the crude CF mortality rate in the general population in 2012 was 0.16 per 100,000 in England and Wales.[50,60] Among young people aged 5–24 years, however, it represents 1.3% of all deaths.

When estimating the mortality rate in CF patients, it is important that reliable data on the size of the affected population are used and a complete ascertainment of deaths is available. National registries provide useful data in this respect. Using 2011 national registry data, the mortality rate among CF patients in the United States was measured at 16 per 1000 registered patients[1] and 12 per 1000 in the United Kingdom[2] and in Canada.[3]

Using a relatively new patient registry in France, researchers noted an improvement in the crude death rate from 21.6 per 1000 in 1994–1996 to 15.8 per 1000 in 2001–2003.[61] While not doubting these results, the researchers themselves highlighted that it was likely their registry was incomplete as they estimated that they only had 63% coverage of the total CF population assuming an incident rate of 1:4600.

Despite the flaws of the data used in the previous calculation, others have also noted a reduction in the CF mortality rate. In England and Wales, Panickar[62] noted that mortality rates in children declined between 1968 and 2000 and that the biggest change was in deaths among infants under the age of 1 year, probably at least in part a result of better surgical management of meconium ileus. Separately, Lewis[63] noted that once patients reached 20 years there was little difference in mortality rates when looking at 3-year cohorts of patients between 1947 and 1967.

MEDIAN AGE AT DEATH

Median age at death is a simple description of the ages of all patients who have died of CF. The calculation only uses data from those patients who have died and is not influenced by the current ages of those patients still living. As such, it is generally lower than the median survival (described in the section "Current Survival") as survivors are not included. It is dependent on the completeness of the data available, and in patient registries the issue of completeness relates to how well the registry captures the full patient population and therefore all deaths in that population. When using routinely collected death data, the completeness of the data relates to the coding of deaths and ensuring that non-CF deaths in CF patients are captured. It is also worth noting that median age at death in small populations can be unstable and therefore comparisons with other larger populations or over time must be performed with caution.

Mindful of these caveats, there have been significant increases in the median age at death in the last decades. In England and Wales, the median age at death increased from 0–4 years in 1959 to 25–29 years in 2008.[64] In Spain, the median age at death increased from 4.4 years in males and 3.8 years in females in 1981 to 20.1 years and 17.7 years in males and females, respectively, in 2004.[65] In Australia, the mean age at death increased from 13.3 years in 1979 to 26.6 years in 2005.[66]

Using the most up-to-date available national registry data, the median age at death was reported to be 27.1 years in the United States,[1] 26.0 years in the United Kingdom,[2] 34.0 years in Canada,[3] and 25.0 years across Europe.[4]

CURRENT SURVIVAL

Current survival is calculated based on age-specific mortality rates observed over a year and estimates life expectancy for a hypothetical population assuming that the current mortality rates reflect future rates and remain constant over time.[67] Current survival has been estimated to be 37.7 years in Italy[68] and 50.6 for males and 43.2 years in females in Canada.[3] In the United States and United Kingdom, who use similar methodology to estimate current survival, 2011 estimates of survival were 36.8 years in the former[1] and 41.5 years in the latter.[2]

COHORT SURVIVAL

Cohort survival is similar to current survival, but it is calculated for different birth cohorts of patients. The technical complexities of calculating current survival in smaller populations have been described by Jackson et al.,[69] who illustrated the effectiveness of a parametric model to estimate survival. Using this method to predict survival beyond the observed data, they estimated median survival in the United States and Ireland in two birth cohorts: patients born between 1980–1984 and 1985–1994. Their analyses showed an improvement between the two cohorts with improved survival in the latter. For patients born between 1980 and 1984, survival was estimated at 37.8 years in males and 31.5 years in females in the United States and 32.2 years and 24.7 years, respectively, in Ireland. In those born between 1985 and 1994, survival was estimated at 50.9 years in males and 42.4 years in females in the United States and 51.1 years and 39.0 years, respectively, in Ireland.[70] A separate study in the United Kingdom also noted improvements with successive birth cohorts when studying 3-year cohorts between 1968 and 1994.[26]

Being able to provide patients and their families with meaningful estimates of survival is important. Dodge[26] estimated that a male born in 2003 in the United Kingdom could expect to live to 42.6 years and a female to 36.9 years assuming that current age-specific mortality rates continue. Given that the researchers noted improvements, however, they suggest that it is not unrealistic to assume that median survival can surpass 50 years for patients born in 2000.

AGE DISTRIBUTION

The current CF patient population is split almost evenly between adults and children: 48.3% of CF patients in the United States[1] are 18 years of age and older compared to 49% in Australia,[5] 57.2% in Canada,[3] and 48% across Europe.[4] The median age of patients seen in 2011 in the United Kingdom was 18 years, and the full distribution is presented in Figure 2.1.

This distribution is in stark contrast to the population profile in the United States in 1990, where 31.7% were younger than 15 years and only 7.3% were older than 30 years.[71] The care of CF patients has evolved greatly with the development of specialized adult care, which takes into account their unique needs. Given that patients are surviving longer and that the number of new diagnoses of CF exceeds the number of deaths, the need for specialist adult CF care will only grow.

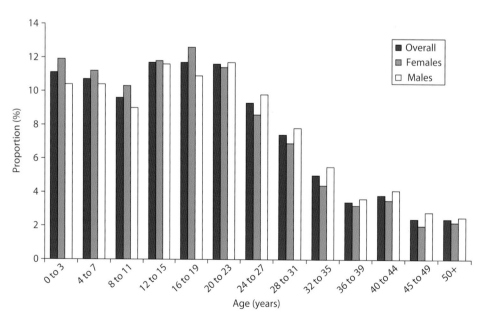

Figure 2.1 Age distribution of patients with cystic fibrosis seen at specialist centers in the United Kingdom in 2011. (From CF Trust, *Cystic Fibrosis Trust Annual Data Report 2011*, 2013.)

LONG-TERM SURVIVORS

As survival in CF has improved, an interest in studying those patients surviving to 40 years has developed—an arbitrary cutoff, yet one that has been adopted in a number of studies[72,73] (see Chapter 25). In 2011, 8.6% of patients seen in the United Kingdom were 40 years and older.[2] Studying a cohort of these long-term survivors at a specialist adult clinic in the United Kingdom,[74] researchers noted that although these patients were less likely to be pancreatic insufficient and less likely to be homozygous *F508dt* over three-quarters had at least one *F508del* allele. This suggests that these patients are not hugely dissimilar genetically from the rest of the CF population. On average, their lung function and BMI were well preserved and many were married and working, suggesting that the disease burden in these survivors is not as high as feared. Identifying predictors of long-term survival, however, has proved to be difficult and in a case-control study at the same UK clinic researchers only identified measures of good health at the time of transition to adult care as predictors.[72]

CHARACTERISTICS AT PRESENTATION

CF is often diagnosed by the presence of clinical signs and symptoms—including those of chronic sinopulmonary disease, gastrointestinal or nutritional anomalies, salt loss syndromes, or genital abnormalities—and then corroborated with laboratory results.[75] Newborn screening has become more widespread, and as such many patients are diagnosed prior to the development of these typical presentations.

AGE AT DIAGNOSIS

When examining recent cohorts of patients with CF, it was noted that most are diagnosed within the first year of life: the median ages at diagnosis of patients in 2011 were 5 months in the United States,[1] 7 months in Canada,[3] and 3 months in the United Kingdom.[2] In a survey of European countries in 2008–2009, the median age was 6 months, but this varied between contributing countries from 1.9 months in Italy to 1 year in Latvia and Portugal.[4] The presence or absence of newborn screening influences these figures. The distribution of age at diagnosis in the United Kingdom is presented in Figure 2.2.

NEONATAL SCREENING

Neonatal screening in CF typically begins with screening for high immunoreactive trypsinogen levels in the blood. High levels are then confirmed with a second test or DNA screening and then sweat chloride tests.[75] Protocols vary and are discussed in detail in Chapter 11. The proportion of current patients identified by newborn screening varies by country as newborn screening is not universally available. In 2009, 83% of new diagnoses in Australia were by newborn screening,[5] whereas in the United States this figure

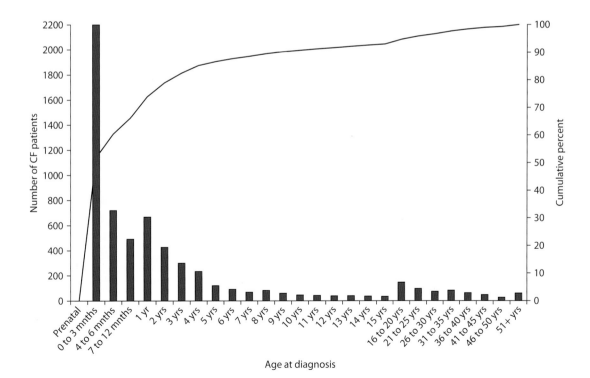

Figure 2.2 Distribution of age at diagnosis of patients seen in the United Kingdom in 2011 (including those diagnosed in 2011 and earlier). (From CF Trust, *Cystic Fibrosis Trust Annual Data Report 2011*, 2013.)

was 59%.[1] In a cross-sectional study of data from registries and specialist centers across Europe in 2008–2009, it was observed that 45% of children 5 years and younger were identified in newborn screening.[4] This figure, however, is skewed by the fact that newborn screening is not available in all contributing countries; thus, figures are likely to increase as access to newborn screening becomes more widespread.

ADULT PRESENTATIONS

Although most patients are diagnosed with CF in childhood, there is a growing proportion of patients who are first diagnosed as adults.[76,77] Although it is possible that, in some cases, the reasons for the delay in diagnosis may be a lack of access to specialist care, it has also been shown that patients diagnosed as adults have a different clinical presentation. They are less likely to present with typical gastrointestinal complications and are more likely to present with

respiratory disease,[76,77] being more likely to be pancreatic sufficient.[76–79] Sweat chloride levels in these patients also tended to be lower[76,77] and, while the presence of an *F508del* genotype was common, patients diagnosed as adults were less likely to be homozygote *F508del*.[76–79] A number of the non-*F508del* mutations more common in patients diagnosed as adults were classes IV to V.[76,78]

MODE OF PRESENTATION

The US Cystic Foundation (CFF) Registry routinely reports statistics on the clinical characteristics patients present at the time of diagnosis. In patients diagnosed in 2011, most were identified by newborn screening, DNA analysis, and respiratory abnormalities.[1] When taking into consideration the rest of the current patient population, a large proportion presented with malnutrition, malabsorption, or respiratory abnormalities, as illustrated in Figure 2.3.

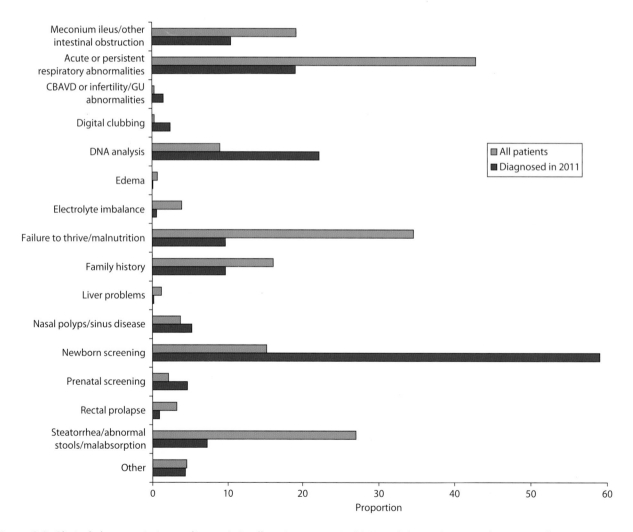

Figure 2.3 Clinical characteristics at diagnosis in all patients seen in 2011 and those diagnosed in 2011. Characteristics are not mutually exclusive and, as such, proportions do not add to 100. (From CF Foundation, Patient Registry 2011: Annual data report to the centre directors, 2012.)

CLINICAL FEATURES

LUNG FUNCTION

Lung function is routinely measured in CF patients from the age of 6 years, the earliest age at which such clinical measures are likely to be reliable. (Although in specialist research centers, lung function is measured at younger ages.) In 2011, the median FEV_1 (percentage predicted) was 74.7% for patients 6 years and older in the United Kingdom[2] and in the United States the mean was 77.1%.[1] In Canada and Australia, where these measures are summarized separately for adults and children, the median for children of 6–17 years was 91.7% in Canada[3] and 92.8% in Australia (2009).[5] For adults, these values were lower, 64.6% in Canada and 66.4% in Australia. This decline in FEV_1 with age was also seen in the United States[1] and is illustrated in Figure 2.4 using data from the UK registry. While this decline in FEV_1 with age is well documented, there is evidence to suggest that FEV_1 levels have improved over time. The US CFF presented a cross-sectional analysis of national data in 1991, 2001, and 2011 comparing median FEV_1 by age and found that while the decline with age was consistent in each period median FEV_1 values were higher in 2011 than in previous years. They also noted improvements in FEV_1 across successive birth cohorts.[1]

How lung function changes over time has been studied by a number of researchers, and recent work using large registry databases has provided useful information for clinicians. Taylor Robinson et al.[80] used longitudinal data from the Danish CF registry where monthly measures of FEV_1 on all patients (1969–2010) showed that a change in FEV_1 % predicted of more than 13% likely represents disease progression, whereas smaller changes are likely short-term fluctuations that patients may recover from. In this work, the authors also demonstrated that baseline FEV_1 % is a good predictor of future FEV_1 % up to 15 years later, although its predictive power decreases with time. *Pseudomonas aeruginosa* infection and pancreatic insufficiency were both associated with faster rates of decline in FEV_1, and there was a clear

difference in baseline and rate of decline by birth cohort with improved baseline lung function in later cohorts. Similar findings were observed in North America by Konstan et al.[81] using data from the Epidemiologic Study of Cystic Fibrosis (ESCF) (n = 24,863). They observed a number of factors that were associated with lung function decline in different age groups, but only three were significant across each age group: sex, the presence of crackles, and a higher baseline FEV_1. Interestingly, the observed effect of sex on lung function decline was not the same across all age groups. In 6- to 8-year-olds females had a higher rate of decline, whereas in 9- to 17-year-olds females had a lower rate of decline.

The age of transition from pediatric to adult care is variable, but it usually occurs between the ages of 16 and 18 years and there is concern in the clinical community that there is a deterioration in health after this critical stage. Using data from the ESCF, Vanden Branden et al.[82] observed that the rate of decline in FEV_1 in adolescence (14–17.4 years) is less than that in young adulthood (18.5–22 years).[82] Patients at a greater risk of decline include those who have had a slower rate of FEV_1 decline in adolescence, have greater FEV_1 variability, have greater BMI decline, are male, have chronic use of inhaled antibiotics, have *Haemophilus influenzae*, do not have multi-drug-resistant *P. aeruginosa*, and have lower than expected FEV_1 and BMI at 18. Cross-sectionally, there is some evidence that patients are reaching adulthood in better health. The CFF explored how the proportion of 18-year-olds with normal or mild, moderate, or severe obstruction varied over different birth cohorts[1] (Table 2.3). They noted that in 2011 most 18-year-olds reached adulthood with normal lung function or only mild obstruction, a large improvement compared to 1986 when the proportion was less than a third. Also of note was that in 2011 only 6.1% had severe obstruction compared to 29.2% in 1986.

GROWTH AND NUTRITION

The growth and nutrition of children with CF is usually measured in terms of height, weight, and BMI percentiles with appropriate reference populations. In the United States

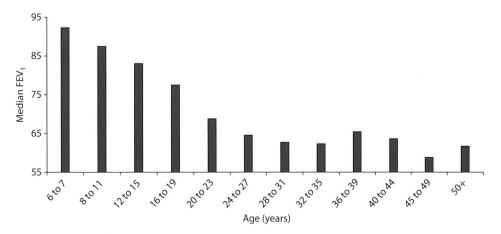

Figure 2.4 Median forced expiratory volume in 1 second percentage (FEV_1 %) predicted by age group. Note that the zero is suppressed. (From CF Trust, *Cystic Fibrosis Trust Annual Data Report 2011*, 2013.)

Table 2.3 Lung function distribution in 18-year-olds in 1986 and 2011

	18-Year-olds in 1986	18-Year-olds in 2011
Normal/mild obstruction (FEV$_1$ ≥ 70%)	31.9%	68.6%
Moderate obstruction (40% ≤ FEV$_1$ ≤ 69%)	38.9%	25.3%
Severe obstruction (FEV$_1$ < 40%)	29.2%	6.1%

Source: CF Foundation, Patient Registry 2011: Annual data report to the centre directors, 2012.

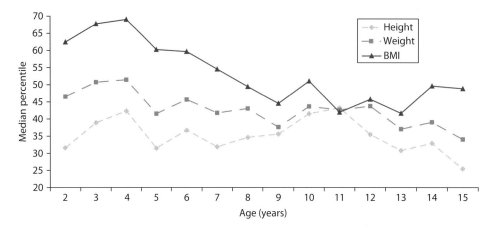

Figure 2.5 Median height, weight, and body mass index percentiles by age. (From CF Trust, *Cystic Fibrosis Trust Annual Data Report 2011*, 2013.)

and United Kingdom, national registry data showed that these measures tended to increase with age only up to 4 to 5 years and then decrease.[1,2] This is illustrated in the United Kingdom in Figure 2.5.

When summarized across ages, median height and weight percentiles in UK children (2–15 years) in 2011 were 34.8 and 42.9, respectively.[2] The median BMI percentile in this age band was 53.6 in the United Kingdom, 51.9 in the United States (2–19 years), and 44.4 in Canada (2–17 years).[3] The US CFF examined weight and height percentiles in successive cohorts by age and observed a trend toward small improvements in these measures across successive birth cohorts.[1]

Nutritional status in adults is generally measured by BMI, and median levels across national registries are broadly similar despite using slightly different age ranges: 22.0 in the United States,[1] 22.1 in Canada,[3] 22.5 in Australia,[5] and 21.6 in the United Kingdom.[2]

INFECTIONS

Patients with CF are prone to respiratory infections and are routinely tested for the presence of numerous respiratory microorganisms. In their annual reporting, each national registry describes infection rates for common microorganisms. Across the United Kingdom, United States, Australia, and Canada, the most commonly reported infections are to *Staphylococcus aureus* and *P. aeruginosa*. For the latter, the prevalence of infections increases with age such that by adulthood over half of patients currently report it.[1–3,5] Data from the United Kingdom are presented in Figure 2.6, which shows a steep increase in the proportion of patients infected up to early adulthood after which it stabilizes.

Interestingly, infection rates for different microorganisms vary considerably between and within countries. For example, in 2011, 25.9% of patients in the United States had MRSA[1] compared with 2.6% in the United Kingdom,[2] 4.2% in Australia,[5] and 5% in Canada.[3] Conversely, *Burkholderia cepacia* was least common in the United States, 2.6% compared with 3.8% in the United Kingdom, 4.6% in Australia, and 5% in Canada. Within countries, there are differences between specialist CF units. In the United States, unit-level infection rates in children range between 10% and 59.1%.[1]

Keeping patients infection free for as long as possible is important as it has been shown that lung disease worsens more quickly after *P. aeruginosa* infection.[83] It has been observed that in children *CFTR* genotype functionality is an important predictor of age of first acquisition of *P. aeruginosa*.[84] Additionally, in analyses adjusted for CFTR functional class, ethnicity, and newborn screening, patients using pancreatic enzymes had an earlier age of initial acquisition. Other studies noted that being female, homozygous *F508del*, and prior *S. aureus* infections are also important predictors of early acquisition of *P. aeurginosa*.[85] The effect of prophylactic antibiotics on *P. aeruginosa* acquisition is debated.

COMPLICATIONS

As well as the usual pulmonary and gastrointestinal complications traditionally associated with CF, patients with the disease can also experience other complications that are related to CF (such as cystic fibrosis–related diabetes [CFRD]). National CF registries collect data on a wide range of such complications. In the United Kingdom, the most common of

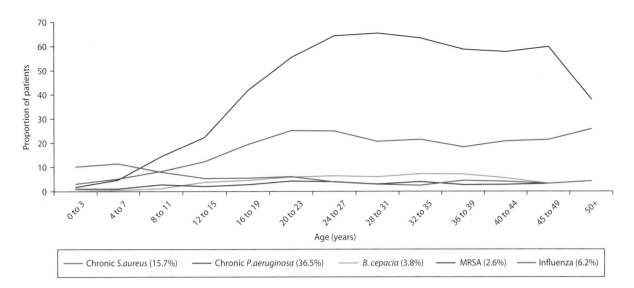

Figure 2.6 Age-specific prevalences of respiratory infections. (From CF Trust, *Cystic Fibrosis Trust Annual Data Report 2011*, 2013.)

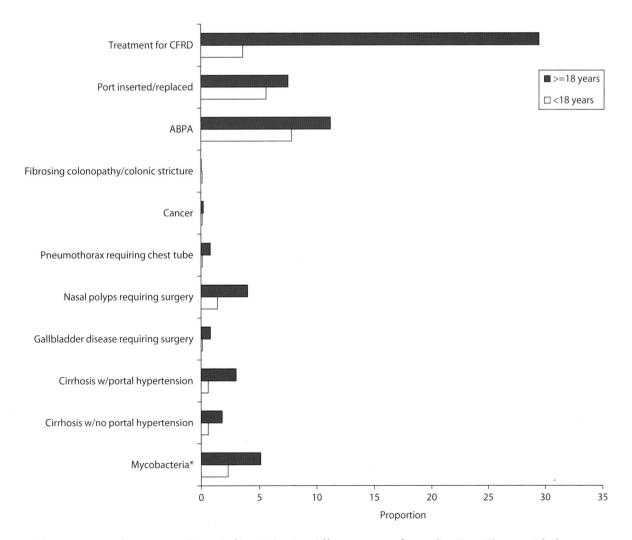

Figure 2.7 Proportion of patients with cystic fibrosis having different types of complications. The asterisk denotes nontuberculous or atypical. ABPA, allergic bronchopulmonary aspergillosis. (From CF Trust, *Cystic Fibrosis Trust Annual Data Report 2011*, 2013.)

these are CFRD and allergic bronchopulmonary aspergillosis[2] (Figure 2.7). In the United States, where a wider range of complications are reported by the CFF, the most common complications are sinus disease (29.2%), gastroesophageal reflux disease (28.9%), asthma (23.9%), and CFRD (18.9%).[1] When interpreting such data, it is worth considering the potential for ascertainment bias such that reported rates of complications may overestimate the true prevalence if patients with milder genotypes are not included, for example.

Many of the complications faced by CF patients become more common as patients grow older. As such, the improved survival of CF patients in recent years has meant that patients are facing health challenges uncommon in previous generations. Of the complications reported in the United Kingdom, only fibrosing colonopathy/colonic stricture was more common in children than adults. The US CFF reported that the proportion of patients reporting CFRD, bone disease, and depression increases with age[1] such that in patients 35 years and older at least a quarter of patients suffer from these conditions. A similar trend was documented in Canada for CFRD.[3]

EDUCATION AND EMPLOYMENT

As patients with CF move into adulthood, there have been efforts to monitor not only their physical health but also other social parameters including education and employment. Treatment regimes in CF can be extremely time consuming, and hospitalizations for exacerbations take patients away from their normal routine. As such, there has been a concern that CF can have a detrimental effect on patient's educational attainment, job opportunities, and functioning at work.

EDUCATION

The most extensive data available on educational attainment in CF patients can be obtained from national registry reports and a study conducted by Walters et al.,[86] who surveyed all UK adults with CF in 1990. In 2011, the US CFF reported that 92.4% of patients aged 18 years and older had at least obtained their high school diploma, with 33.8% obtaining a college diploma or completing a postgraduate degree.[1] In the United Kingdom in 1990, Walters et al.[86] showed that 85% of adults left school with some form of qualification, a result not dissimilar to the general population (in the 2001 Census survey, 81% of adults in England and Wales had some form of qualification; adapted from data from the Office for National Statistics licensed under the Open Government Licence v.1.0).

This positive experience was not universally observed, however. In a US study from the same era comparing adult patients with CF with healthy controls, CF patients were less likely to have a college degree than the healthy controls, although this difference did not reach statistical significance.[87] A number of smaller surveys at single centers have shown that some patients felt that they had to leave their studies due to CF.[88,89] This is supported by Walter et al.'s[86] study, which showed that the 15% of adults who left school without qualifications had higher symptom scores compared to those who stayed on.

EMPLOYMENT

Traditionally, with education—other factors remaining the same—come better employment opportunities. If CF patients are achieving academically, then it is worth exploring whether they are reaching their full potential in the workplace. In Walter et al.'s[86] large survey of adults with CF in the United Kingdom in 1990, 54% of adults were in paid employment. Twenty-one years later, 70.0% of patients aged 16 years and older in the United Kingdom reported being in work or study[2] and in the United States 58.4% of patients aged 18 years and older (the age by which most students will have completed high school) were in full- or part-time work or study.[1] In a recent large cross-sectional analysis of adult patients in Germany and Austria, researchers observed employment rates of 45.9% in 21- to 30-year-olds and 62.2% in 31- to 40-year-olds and 55.6% of patients over the age of 40 years had retired.[90] Other cross-sectional studies in the United States and elsewhere have noted varying levels of employment ranging from 48% to 72%.[88,91–93] Comparisons between countries and over long periods are obviously difficult, however, as local employment rates in the general population will differ. The results suggest, however, that most adults are in some form of employment or education.

Interestingly, patients in employment are not always in better health. In the United States, there was no evidence that FEV_1 differed by whether patients worked and both groups had low lung function.[92] It has been suggested that CF patients persist in working even with low lung function as it may serve as a distraction from their symptoms.[92] Other reasons for remaining in work despite low lung function include the opportunity to make a living and potentially benefit from health-care coverage through their employer. Conversely, in a small survey in Belgium, patients in work tended to have higher FEV_1 and were less likely to have P. aeruginosa.[94] Perhaps most convincing is a recent 15-year cohort study of adults using the United Kingdom's CF Registry database, which showed that those in employment tended to have higher BMI and FEV_1 and had spent less time in hospital.[95] As predictors of being in employment, however, the researchers showed that socioeconomic deprivation as measured at the postcode level modified the effect of FEV_1 such that FEV_1 had a smaller effect in the least deprived quintile and greatest effect in the most deprived.

When considering the type of work CF patients take on, it has been shown that they tend to take nonmanual jobs. Walters et al.[86] observed that adults with CF in work were more likely to be in nonmanual jobs compared to both the general population and their parents.[86] In a survey in the United States, 53.4% of adults in work were in professional,

approach has also been recently launched in Germany using patient registry data.[157]

These initiatives at local and national levels illustrate the desire within the CF community to learn and improve the care they deliver.

REFERENCES

1. CF Foundation. Patient Registry 2011: Annual data report to the centre directors. 2012.

2. CF Trust. *Cystic Fibrosis Trust Annual Data Report 2011*. 2013.

3. CF Canada. *Canadian Cystic Fibrosis Registry Annual Report 2011*. Toronto, Canada: Cystic Fibrosis Canada; 2011.

4. Viviani L, Zolin A, Olesen HV et al. *ECFSPR Annual Report 2008–2009*. 2012, Karup, Denmark: ECFS.

5. Bell SC, Bye PT, Cooper PJ, Martin AJ, McKay KO, Robinson PJ et al. Cystic fibrosis in Australia, 2009: Results from a data registry. *Med J Australia* 2011; **195**(7): 396–400. [Epub 2011/10/08].

6. Feuchtbaum L, Carter J, Dowray S, Currier RJ, Lorey F. Birth prevalence of disorders detectable through newborn screening by race/ethnicity. *Genet Med* 2012; **14**(11): 937–45.

7. Padoa C, Goldman A, Jenkins T, Ramsay M. Cystic fibrosis carrier frequencies in populations of African origin. *J Med Genet* 1999; **36**(1): 41–4.

8. Hill ID, MacDonald WB, Bowie MD, Ireland JD. Cystic fibrosis in Cape Town. *S Afr Med J* 1988; **73**(3): 147–9. [Epub 1988/02/06].

9. Yamashiro Y, Shimizu T, Oguchi S, Shioya T, Nagata S, Ohtsuka Y. The estimated incidence of cystic fibrosis in Japan. *J Pediatr Gastr Nutr* 1997; **24**(5): 544–7.

10. Massie RJ, Curnow L, Glazner J, Armstrong DS, Francis I. Lessons learned from 20 years of newborn screening for cystic fibrosis. *Med J Australia* 2012; **196**(1): 67–70. [Epub 2012/01/20].

11. Wesley AW, Stewart AW. Cystic fibrosis in New Zealand: Incidence and mortality. *New Zeal Med J* 1985; **98**(778): 321–3. [Epub 1985/05/08].

12. Farrell PM. The prevalence of cystic fibrosis in the European Union. *J Cyst Fibros* 2008; **7**(5): 450–3.

13. Loeber JG. Neonatal screening in Europe; the situation in 2004. *J Inherit Metab Dis* 2007; **30**(4): 430–8.

14. Southern KW, Munck A, Pollitt R, Travert G, Zanolla L, Dankert-Roelse J et al. A survey of newborn screening for cystic fibrosis in Europe. *J Cyst Fibros* 2007; **6**(1): 57–65.

15. Nielsen OH, Thomsen BL, Green A, Andersen PK, Hauge M, Schiotz PO. Cystic fibrosis in Denmark 1945 to 1985. An analysis of incidence, mortality and influence of centralized treatment on survival. *Acta Paediatr Scand* 1988; **77**(6): 836–41. [Epub 1988/11/01].

16. Schwartz M, Sorensen N, Brandt NJ, Hogdall E, Holm T. High incidence of cystic fibrosis on the Faroe Islands: A molecular and genealogical study. *Hum Genet* 1995; **95**(6): 703–6. [Epub 1995/06/01].

17. Scotet V, Dugueperoux I, Saliou P, Rault G, Roussey M, Audrezet M-P et al. Evidence for decline in the incidence of cystic fibrosis: A 35-year observational study in Brittany, France. *Orphanet J Rare Dis* 2012; **7**(1): 14.

18. Farrell P, Joffe S, Foley L, Canny GJ, Mayne P, Rosenberg M. Diagnosis of cystic fibrosis in the Republic of Ireland: Epidemiology and costs. *Irish Med J* 2007; **100**(8): 557–60. [Epub 2007/10/25].

19. Arce M, Mulherin D, McWilliam P, Lawler M, FitzGerald MX, Humphries P. Frequency of deletion 508 among Irish cystic fibrosis patients. *Hum Genet* 1990; **85**(4): 403–4.

20. Bossi A, Casazza G, Padoan R, Milani S. What is the incidence of cystic fibrosis in Italy? Data from the National Registry (1988–2001). *Hum Biol* 2004; **76**(3): 455–67. [Epub 2004/10/16].

21. Scotet V, Assael BM, Duguéperoux I, Tamanini A, Audrézet M-P, Férec C et al. Time trends in birth incidence of cystic fibrosis in two European areas: Data from newborn screening programs. *J Pediatr* 2008; **152**(1): 25–32.

22. Slieker MG, Uiterwaal CSPM, Sinaasappel M, Heijerman HGM, van der Laag J, van der Ent CK. Birth prevalence and survival in cystic fibrosis: A national cohort study in the Netherlands. *Chest J* 2005; **128**(4): 2309–15.

23. Vernooij-van Langen AMM, Loeber JG, Elvers B, Triepels RH, Gille JJP, Van der Ploeg CPB et al. Novel strategies in newborn screening for cystic fibrosis: A prospective controlled study. *Thorax* 2012; **67**(4): 289–95.

24. Edminson PD, Michalsen H, Aagenaes O, Lie SO. Screening for cystic fibrosis among newborns in Norway by measurement of serum/plasma trypsin-like immunoreactivity. Results of a 2 1/2-year pilot project. *Scand J Gastroentero Suppl* 1988; **143**: 13–8. [Epub 1988/01/01].

25. Lannefors L, Lindgren A. Demographic transition of the Swedish cystic fibrosis community—results of modern care. *Resp Med* 2002; **96**(9): 681–5. [Epub 2002/09/24].

26. Dodge JA, Lewis PA, Stanton M, Wilsher J. Cystic fibrosis mortality and survival in the UK: 1947–2003. *Eur Respir J* 2007; **29**(3): 522–6.

27. Dodge JA, Morison S, Lewis PA, Coles EC, Geddes D, Russell G et al. Incidence, population, and survival of cystic fibrosis in the UK, 1968–95. *Arch Disease Child* 1997; **77**(6): 493–6.

28. Green MR, Weaver LT, Heeley AF, Nicholson K, Kuzemko JA, Barton DE et al. Cystic fibrosis identified by neonatal screening: Incidence, genotype, and early natural history. *Arch Dis Child* 1993; **68**(4): 464–7. [Epub 1993/04/01].

29. Nevin GB, Nevin NC, Redmond AO. Prevalence and survival of patients with cystic fibrosis in Northern Ireland, 1961–1971. *Ulster Med J* 1983; **52**(2): 153–6. [Epub 1983/01/01].

30. Rock MJ, Hoffman G, Laessig RH, Kopish GJ, Litsheim TJ, Farrell PM. Newborn screening for cystic fibrosis in Wisconsin: Nine-year experience with routine trypsinogen/DNA testing. *J Pediatr* 2005; **147**(Suppl 3): S73–7.

31. Brock DJH, Gilfillan A, Holloway S. The incidence of cystic fibrosis in Scotland calculated from heterozygote frequencies. *Clin Genet* 1998; **53**(1): 47–9.

32. Al-Mahroos F. Cystic Fibrosis in Bahrain: Incidence, phenotype, and outcome. *J Trop Pediatr* 1998; **44**(1): 35–9.

33. Katznelson D, Ben-Yishay M. Cystic fibrosis in Israel: Clinical and genetic aspects. *Israel J Med Sci* 1978; **14**(2): 204–11. [Epub 1978/02/01].

34. Nazer HM. Early diagnosis of cystic fibrosis in Jordanian shildren. *J Trop Pediatr* 1992; **38**(3): 113–5.

35. Frossard PM, Girodon E, Dawson KP, Ghanem N, Plassa F, Lestringant GG et al. Identification of cystic fibrosis mutations in the United Arab Emirates. *Hum Mutat* 1998; **11**(5): 412–3.

36. Dupuis A, Hamilton D, Cole DEC, Corey M. Cystic fibrosis birth rates in Canada: A decreasing trend since the onset of genetic testing. *J Pediatr* 2005; **147**(3): 312–5.

37. Daigneault J, Aubin G, Simard F, De Braekeleer M. Incidence of cystic fibrosis in Saguenay-Lac-St.-Jean (Quebec, Canada). *Hum Biol* 1992; **64**(1): 115–9. [Epub 1992/02/01].

38. Kosorok MR, Wei WH, Farrell PM. The incidence of cystic fibrosis. *Stat Med* 1996; **15**(5): 449–62. [Epub 1996/03/15].

39. Comeau AM, Parad RB, Dorkin HL, Dovey M, Gerstle R, Haver K et al. Population-based newborn screening for genetic disorders when multiple mutation DNA testing is incorporated: A cystic fibrosis newborn screening model demonstrating increased sensitivity but more carrier detections. *Pediatrics* 2004; **113**(6): 1573–81.

40. Korzeniewski SJ, Young WI, Hawkins HC, Cavanagh K, Nasr SZ, Langbo C et al. Variation in immunoreactive trypsinogen concentrations among Michigan newborns and implications for cystic fibrosis newborn screening. *Pediatr Pulmonol* 2011; **46**(2): 125–30. [Epub 2010/09/18].

41. Cabello GM, Moreira AF, Horovitz D, Correia P, Santa Rosa A, Llerena J Jr et al. Cystic fibrosis: Low frequency of DF508 mutation in 2 population samples from Rio de Janeiro, Brazil. *Hum Biol* 1999; **71**(2): 189–96. [Epub 1999/05/01].

42. Scotet V, Gillet D, Duguépéroux I, Audrézet M-P, Bellis G, Garnier B et al. Spatial and temporal distribution of cystic fibrosis and of its mutations in Brittany, France: A retrospective study from 1960. *Hum Genet* 2002; **111**(3): 247–54.

43. McCormick J, Mehta G, Olesen HV, Viviani L, Macek Jr M, Mehta A. Comparative demographics of the European cystic fibrosis population: A cross-sectional database analysis. *Lancet* 2010; **375**(9719): 1007–13.

44. Castellani C, Picci L, Tamanini A, Girardi P, Rizzotti P, Assael BM. Association between carrier screening and incidence of cystic fibrosis. *JAMA* 2009; **302**(23): 2573–9.

45. Massie J, Curnow L, Gaffney L, Carlin J, Francis I. Declining prevalence of cystic fibrosis since the introduction of newborn screening. *Arch Dis Child* 2010; **95**(7): 531–3.

46. Hale JE, Parad RB, Comeau AM. Newborn screening showing decreasing incidence of cystic fibrosis. *New Engl J Med* 2008; **358**(9): 973–4.

47. Scotet V, Audrézet M-P, Roussey M, Rault G, Blayau M, Braekeleer M et al. Impact of public health strategies on the birth prevalence of cystic fibrosis in Brittany, France. *Hum Genet* 2003; **113**(3): 280–5.

48. ACFD Registry. *Cystic Fibrosis in Australia in 2011*. 14th Annual Report. Australia; 2012, Baulkham Hills, Australia: CF Australia.

49. Australian Bureau of Statistics. 3101.0—Australian Demographic Statistics, Mar 2013. 2013 [accessed October 27, 2013]; Available from: http://www.abs.gov.au/AUSSTATS/abs@.nsf/DetailsPage/3101.0Mar%202013?OpenDocument.

50. European Commission Eurostat. Population on 1 January. 2013 [accessed October 27, 2013]; Available from: http://epp.eurostat.ec.europa.eu/tgm/table.do?tab=table'language=en'pcode=tps00001'tableSelection=1'footnotes=yes'labeling=labels'plugin=1.

51. The World Bank. World Bank DataBank. 2013; Available from: http://databank.worldbank.org/data/views/reports/tableview.aspx.

52. Statistics Canada. Population and dwelling counts, for Canada, provinces and territories, 2011 and 2006 censuses. 2013 [accessed May 2, 2013]; Available from: http://www12.statcan.gc.ca/census-recensement/2011/dp-pd/hlt-fst/pd-pl/Table-Tableau.cfm?LANG=Eng'T=101'S=50'O=A.

53. United States Census Bureau. US and World Population Clock. 2010 [accessed May 2, 2013]; Available from: http://www.census.gov/popclock/.

54. Zielenski J, Tsui L. Cystic fibrosis: Genotypic and phenotypic variations. *Annu Rev Genet* 1995; **29**(1): 777–807.

55. Bobadilla JL, Macek M, Fine JP, Farrell PM. Cystic fibrosis: A worldwide analysis of CFTR mutations—correlation with incidence data and application to screening. *Hum Mutat* 2002; **19**(6): 575–606.

56. McKone EF, Emerson SS, Edwards KL, Aitken ML. Effect of genotype on phenotype and mortality in cystic fibrosis: A retrospective cohort study. *Lancet* 2003; **361**(9370): 1671–6.

57. McKone EF, Goss CH, Aitken ML. CFTR genotype as a predictor of prognosis in cystic fibrosis. *Chest J* 2006; **130**(5): 1441–7.

58. de Gracia J, Mata F, Álvarez A, Casals T, Gatner S, Vendrell M et al. Genotype-phenotype correlation for pulmonary function in cystic fibrosis. *Thorax* 2005; **60**(7): 558–63.

59. Koch C, Cuppens H, Rainisio M, Madessani U, Harms HK, Hodson ME et al. European Epidemiologic Registry of Cystic Fibrosis (ERCF): Comparison of major disease manifestations between patients with different classes of mutations. *Pediatr Pulmonol* 2001; **31**(1): 1–12.

60. ONS. Mortality Rates. 2013 [accessed October 27, 2013]; Available from: http://www.ons.gov.uk /ons/taxonomy/index.html?nscl=Mortality+ Rates#tab-data-tables.

61. Bellis G, Cazes M-H, Parant A, Gaimard M, Travers C, Le Roux E et al. Cystic fibrosis mortality trends in France. *J Cyst Fibros* 2007; **6**(3): 179–86.

62. Panickar JR, Dodd SR, Smyth RL, Couriel JM. Trends in deaths from respiratory illness in children in England and Wales from 1968 to 2000. *Thorax* 2005; **60**(12): 1035–8.

63. Lewis PA, Morison S, Dodge JA, Geddes D, Coles EC, Russell G et al. Survival estimates for adults with cystic fibrosis born in the United Kingdom between 1947 and 1967. *Thorax* 1999; **54**(5): 420–2.

64. Barr HL, Britton J, Smyth AR, Fogarty AW. Association between socioeconomic status, sex, and age at death from cystic fibrosis in England and Wales (1959 to 2008): Cross sectional study. *BMJ* 2011; **343**: d4662.

65. Ramalle-Gomara E, Perucha M, González M-Á, Quiñones C, Andrés J, Posada M. Cystic fibrosis mortality trends in Spain among infants and young children: 1981–2004. *Eur J Epidemiol* 2008; **23**(8): 523–9.

66. Reid DW, Blizzard CL, Shugg DM, Flowers C, Cash C, Greville HM. Changes in cystic fibrosis mortality in Australia, 1979–2005. *Med J Australia* 2011; **195**(7): 392–5. [Epub 2011/10/08].

67. Daly LE, Bourke GJ. *Interpretation and Uses of Medical Statistics.* Oxford, United Kingdom: Blackwell Science; 2000.

68. Assael BM, Castellani C, Ocampo MB, Iansa P, Callegaro A, Valsecchi MG. Epidemiology and survival analysis of cystic fibrosis in an area of intense neonatal screening over 30 years. *Am J Epidemiol* 2002; **156**(5): 397–401.

69. Jackson AD, Daly L, Jackson AL, Kelleher C, Marshall BC, Quinton HB et al. Validation and use of a parametric model for projecting cystic fibrosis survivorship beyond observed data: A birth cohort analysis. *Thorax* 2011; **66**(8): 674–9.

70. Jackson AD, Daly L, Kelleher C, Marshall BC, Quinton HB, Foley L et al. The application of current lifetable methods to compare cystic fibrosis median survival internationally is limited. *J Cyst Fibros* 2011; **10**(1): 62–5.

71. FitzSimmons SC. The changing epidemiology of cystic fibrosis. *J Pediatr* 1993; **122**(1): 1–9. [Epub 1993/01/01].

72. Simmonds NJ, MacNeill SJ, Cullinan P, Hodson ME. Cystic fibrosis and survival to 40 years: A case–control study. *Eur Respir J* 2010; **36**(6): 1277–83.

73. Hodson ME, Simmonds NJ, Warwick WJ, Tullis E, Castellani C, Assael B et al. An international/ multicentre report on patients with cystic fibrosis (CF) over the age of 40 years. *J Cyst Fibros* 2008; **7**(6): 537–42.

74. Simmonds NJ, Cullinan P, Hodson ME. Growing old with cystic fibrosis—the characteristics of long-term survivors of cystic fibrosis. *Resp Med* 2009; **103**(4): 629–35.

75. Farrell PM, Rosenstein BJ, White TB, Accurso FJ, Castellani C, Cutting GR et al. Guidelines for diagnosis of cystic fibrosis in newborns through older adults: Cystic Fibrosis Foundation consensus report. *J Pediatr* 2008; **153**(2): S4–14.

76. Keating CL, Liu X, DiMango EA. Classic respiratory disease but atypical diagnostic testing distinguishes adult presentation of cystic fibrosis. *Chest J* 2010; **137**(5): 1157–63.

77. Gilljam M, Ellis L, Corey M, Zielenski J, Durie P, Tullis DE. Clinical manifestations of cystic fibrosis among patients with diagnosis in adulthood. *Chest J* 2004; **126**(4): 1215–24.

78. Rodman DM, Polis JM, Heltshe SL, Sontag MK, Chacon C, Rodman RV et al. Late diagnosis defines a unique population of long-term survivors of cystic fibrosis. *Am J Resp Crit Care* 2005; **171**(6): 621–6.

79. Gan KH, Geus WP, Bakker W, Lamers CB, Heijerman HG. Genetic and clinical features of patients with cystic fibrosis diagnosed after the age of 16 years. *Thorax* 1995; **50**(12): 1301–4. [Epub 1995/12/01].

80. Taylor-Robinson D, Whitehead M, Diderichsen F, Olesen HV, Pressler T, Smyth RL et al. Understanding the natural progression in %FEV$_1$ decline in patients with cystic fibrosis: A longitudinal study. *Thorax* 2012; **67**(10): 860–6.

81. Konstan MW, Morgan WJ, Butler SM, Pasta DJ, Craib ML, Silva SJ et al. Risk factors for rate of decline in forced expiratory volume in one second in children and adolescents with cystic fibrosis. *J Pediatr* 2007; **151**(2): 134-9.e1.

82. VandenBranden SL, McMullen A, Schechter MS, Pasta DJ, Michaelis RL, Konstan MW et al. Lung function decline from adolescence to young adulthood in cystic fibrosis. *Pediatr Pulmonol* 2012; **47**(2): 135–43.

83. Kosorok MR, Zeng L, West SEH, Rock MJ, Splaingard ML, Laxova A et al. Acceleration of lung disease in children with cystic fibrosis after *Pseudomonas aeruginosa* acquisition. *Pediatr Pulmonol* 2001; **32**(4): 277–87.

84. Rosenfeld M, Emerson J, McNamara S, Thompson V, Ramsey BW, Morgan W et al. Risk factors for age at initial *Pseudomonas* acquisition in the cystic fibrosis epic observational cohort. *J Cyst Fibros* 2012; **11**(5): 446–53.

85. Maselli JH, Sontag MK, Norris JM, MacKenzie T, Wagener JS, Accurso FJ. Risk factors for initial acquisition of *Pseudomonas aeruginosa* in children with cystic fibrosis identified by newborn screening. *Pediatr Pulmonol* 2003; **35**(4): 257–62.

86. Walters S, Britton J, Hodson ME. Demographic and social characteristics of adults with cystic fibrosis in the United Kingdom. *BMJ* 1993; **306**(6877): 549–52. [Epub 1993/02/27].

87. Shepherd SL, Hovell MF, Harwood IR, Granger LE, Hofstetter CR, Molgaard C et al. A comparative study of the psychosocial assets of adults with cystic fibrosis and their healthy peers. *CHEST J* 1990; **97**(6): 1310–6.

88. Laborde-Castérot H, Donnay C, Chapron J, Burgel P-R, Kanaan R, Honoré I et al. Employment and work disability in adults with cystic fibrosis. *J Cyst Fibros* 2012; **11**(2): 137–43.

89. Penketh AR, Wise A, Mearns MB, Hodson ME, Batten JC. Cystic fibrosis in adolescents and adults. *Thorax* 1987; **42**(7): 526–32. [Epub 1987/07/01].

90. Besier T, Goldbeck L. Growing up with cystic fibrosis: Achievement, life satisfaction, and mental health. *Qual Life Res* 2012; **21**(10): 1829–35.

91. Hogg M, Braithwaite M, Bailey M, Kotsimbos T, Wilson JW. Work disability in adults with cystic fibrosis and its relationship to quality of life. *J Cyst Fibros* 2007; **6**(3): 223–7.

92. Burker EJ, Sedway J, Carone S. Psychological and educational factors: Better predictors of work status than FEV$_1$ in adults with cystic fibrosis. *Pediatr Pulmonol* 2004; **38**(5): 413–8.

93. Riekert KA, Bartlett SJ, Boyle MP, Krishnan JA, Rand CS. The association between depression, lung function, and health-related quality of life among adults with cystic fibrosis. *CHEST J* 2007; **132**(1): 231–7.

94. Havermans T, Colpaert K, Dupont LJ. Quality of life in patients with cystic fibrosis: Association with anxiety and depression. *J Cyst Fibros* 2008; **7**(6): 581–4.

95. Taylor-Robinson DC, Smyth R, Diggle PJ, Whitehead M. A longitudinal study of the impact of social deprivation and disease severity on employment status in the UK cystic fibrosis population. *PloS One* 2013; **8**(8): e73322.

96. Gillen M, Lallas D, Brown C, Yelin E, Blanc P. Work disability in adults with cystic fibrosis. *Am J Resp Crit Care* 1995; **152**(1): 153–6.

97. O'Connor GT, Quinton HB, Kahn R, Robichaud P, Maddock J, Lever T et al. Case-mix adjustment for evaluation of mortality in cystic fibrosis. *Pediatr Pulmonol* 2002; **33**(2): 99–105.

98. Courtney JM, Bradley J, McCaughan J, O'Connor TM, Shortt C, Bredin CP et al. Predictors of mortality in adults with cystic fibrosis. *Pediatr Pulmonol* 2007; **42**(6): 525–32. [Epub 2007/05/01].

99. Lai HJ, Cheng Y, Cho H, Kosorok MR, Farrell PM. Association between initial disease presentation, lung disease outcomes, and survival in patients with cystic fibrosis. *Am J Epidemiol* 2004; **159**(6): 537–46.

100. Rosenfeld M, Davis R, FitzSimmons S, Pepe M, Ramsey B. Gender gap in cystic fibrosis mortality. *Am J Epidemiol* 1997; **145**(9): 794–803.

101. Britton JR. Effects of social class, sex, and region of residence on age at death from cystic fibrosis. *BMJ* 1989; **298**(6672): 483–7. [Epub 1989/02/25].

102. Fogarty A, Hubbard R, Britton J. International comparison of median age at death from cystic fibrosis. *CHEST J* 2000; **117**(6): 1656–60.

103. Kerem E, Reisman J, Corey M, Canny GJ, Levison H. Prediction of mortality in patients with cystic fibrosis. *New Engl J Med* 1992; **326**(18): 1187–91.

104. Corey M, Farewell V. Determinants of mortality from cystic fibrosis in Canada, 1970–1989. *Am J Epidemiol* 1996; **143**(10): 1007–17.

105. Chamnan P, Shine BSF, Haworth CS, Bilton D, Adler AI. Diabetes as a determinant of mortality in cystic fibrosis. *Diabetes Care* 2010; **33**(2): 311–6.

106. Kulich M, Rosenfeld M, Goss CH, Wilmott R. Improved survival among young patients with cystic fibrosis. *J Pediatr* 2003; **142**(6): 631–6.

107. Liou TG, Adler FR, FitzSimmons SC, Cahill BC, Hibbs JR, Marshall BC. Predictive 5-year survivorship model of cystic fibrosis. *Am J Epidemiol* 2001; **153**(4): 345–52.

108. Aurora P, Wade A, Whitmore P, Whitehead B. A model for predicting life expectancy of children with cystic fibrosis. *Eur Respir J* 2000; **16**(6): 1056–60.

109. Dasenbrook EC, Checkley W, Merlo CA, Konstan MW, Lechtzin N, Boyle MP. Association between respiratory tract methicillin-resistant staphylococcus aureus and survival in cystic fibrosis. *JAMA* 2010; **303**(23): 2386–92.

110. Buzzetti R, Alicandro G, Minicucci L, Notarnicola S, Furnari ML, Giordano G et al. Validation of a predictive survival model in Italian patients with cystic fibrosis. *J Cyst Fibros* 2012; **11**(1): 24–9.

111. Hayllar KM, Williams SG, Wise AE, Pouria S, Lombard M, Hodson ME et al. A prognostic model for the prediction of survival in cystic fibrosis. *Thorax* 1997; **52**(4): 313–7. [Epub 1997/04/01].

112. Mayer-Hamblett N, Rosenfeld M, Emerson J, Goss CH, Aitken ML. Developing cystic fibrosis lung transplant referral criteria using predictors of 2-year mortality. *Am J Resp Crit Care* 2002; **166**(12): 1550–5.

113. Viviani L, Bossi A, Assael BM. Absence of a gender gap in survival. An analysis of the Italian registry for cystic fibrosis in the paediatric age. *J Cyst Fibros* 2011; **10**(5): 313–7.

I wish I could meet and talk to others my age who also suffer from CF. This is because they would be going through the same thing as me and we could share experiences. Having CF means that when I am at the Brompton Hospital I am separated from other kids and I am put in a room on my own; I can't meet or talk to any of them. I used to get annoyed by this as I thought it would be great to talk to others, but as I have gotten older my parents have told me everything about the condition and have told me that meeting other children with CF could be a risk to me and them.

I understand that CF will shorten my life, but that's okay! I have known this from a young age, and I feel this has helped me to grow up even more. I may be 15, but I know what I want to do when I'm older and how if I want a family I need to do it sooner rather than later due to my condition. A couple of years ago, I asked what the risks were of my children getting CF. The doctor gave me a thorough explanation, which has given me a much larger knowledge on passing down CF throughout generations.

I try not to let CF affect me every day, and to me it doesn't. But the things I do (nebulizer, tablets, and eating more salt) have just become a routine for me. I make sure I live life to the fullest and take every opportunity as I know that my life will be shorter, but doing this enables me to have a good but perhaps shorter life. My friends and family are a big support and treat me just like everybody else, and to me I am just like any other 15-year-old girl.

WELL CYSTIC FIBROSIS ADULT

KEVIN PASSEY

INTRODUCTION

I am 53 years old and have CF. I have been happily married for 27 years. I run my own computer software company, and I live in a beautiful part of West Sussex. I was diagnosed with CF at the age of 9 months. I have been a patient at the Royal Brompton Hospital in London for many years and work as their CF advocate.

I have a very busy and hardworking business life, with clients all over the world; I am extremely lucky to have a great social life, going on many holidays including skiing and golfing.

CF is a very important part of my day-to-day living; however, I do not let it get me down or rule my life. I do hope that by writing this I will give other CF sufferers, their parents, and loved ones determination; hope; and above all a sense of normality, which is so important to me.

DIAGNOSIS

I was diagnosed with CF when I was 9 months old. At this time, not very much was known about the disease and

specialist centers did not even exist; I just went to the local hospital chest clinic.

When I was a newborn, my mother tells me that she would constantly take me to the doctors because she knew I was unwell, suffering from chest infections, and my nappies would be full of, what she describes as, "melted butter." However, nobody would believe her; she was told she was suffering from postnatal depression, and even my father thought this might be true and she was told to have a holiday and everything would be fine. The holiday was cut short as I became very unwell, and this time she wasn't going to take no for an answer. She took me back to our GP; he took one look at me and an ambulance was called. Finally, they were taking her seriously.

After many tests I was diagnosed with CF, and both my mother and father were told that they were lucky I had lived to 9 months without any treatment and that I would never get any better and would never become a teenager. The best they could hope for was that I would live to between 5- and 8-years-old.

EARLY YEARS

Once on medication for my condition, the early years were pretty uneventful from what I can remember. I went to school as normal, and I didn't really miss out on any activities. I probably got more colds than my friends, and I do remember going into hospital for a nasal polypectomy. I used to go for checkups with my parents, but I wasn't on any long-term antibiotics. I just had to take Pancrex powder with my food. I didn't really understand much about CF and just got on with my schooling. It was when I got into my teenage years that I started to understand a little more.

TEENAGE YEARS

At 15, the polyps had returned and were affecting my breathing so I had another nasal polypectomy. This encouraged me to ask questions about my CF, so my parents started getting information from the CF trust. I went to one of their meetings with my parents, and it was explained that CF sufferers would not live much past 15. I can remember looking at my parents and thinking to myself, that is not great, what is the point of taking any drugs. I was still taking Pancrex for my digestion at the time. I might as well just have a good time and make the most of what little time I had. So that is what I did. During this time I met my girlfriend, and then things really changed. I had found someone that I really liked, and she started to help me take my CF a lot more seriously. At that time, I used to go for checkups every 6 months; but there was no real CF expertise and I can remember on one visit being told that there really was not much they could do for me, that I was fairly well, and to just get on with life. It was at the same visit that they told me, "and by the way you will never father children." I was devastated; I had just found a girlfriend, and she was not going to stay with me after that news. But of course that wasn't the case; we married some 10 years later and have been happily married for the last 27 years.

MARRIED LIFE

I married Jane in May 1985 after a 10-year courtship, I was 25, we had a fabulous wedding, and we honeymooned in Cornwall. Shortly after getting married, I had my final polypectomy.

My early working life saw me traveling all over the world writing software; I loved it, but I felt that I needed new challenges. I had many contacts in the industry so I decided to set up my own company. Jane agreed she would leave the BBC and help me, so KDP Software, Ltd., was established. Our first contract was working for a large stationery company based in Enfield.

We gradually employed more computer programmers and rented some offices in Hatton Garden in the center of London. Business was great, but my health was gradually deteriorating. Commuting from Ruislip to London every day had a huge impact because I picked up infections on the underground, so we decided to sell our first house and buy an apartment in Earls Court so that I could drive to work. However, things still did not improve. I was still not being treated for my CF, I would cough most of the day and night, and my weight dropped to below nine stone. After a trip to my local GP, the turning point came. I was referred to the adult CF unit at the Royal Brompton Hospital, and I finally started to receive the treatment that I so badly needed.

However, this brought new challenges for me; how did I fit the whole new drugs regime into my busy working schedules. I was traveling all over the country at this time and employing 10 programmers, all working on different projects. It was not going to be easy.

But this was the best thing that could have ever happened to me. I started to take Creon; I was given daily oral antibiotics and numerous vitamins. I really started to take my health seriously; this was now more important than anything else. Jane used to help me morning and night with physio, and things changed dramatically. I barely coughed at all, and my weight increased to 12 stone. I had more energy, and life returned to some normality.

In hindsight, I think I had just got used to feeling so unwell and thought this was a normal; after all, I did suffer from CF and I think this is one big issue with CF sufferers that really needs to be addressed.

My physio regime became much easier with the introduction of the flutter, which I make sure I do at least once a day. Now I don't need to call upon my wife so much to complete that part of my health care.

However, further new challenges were to come. On a routine visit to the hospital, I asked my consultant about becoming a father. Jane and I both love children and wondered what the chances were of me fathering my own. I had been told there was no chance that men with CF could father children, but I thought there was no harm in asking.

We were referred to Prof. Winston's clinic at Hammersmith Hospital, and I became the first CF male to undergo epididymal aspiration. We underwent five IVF procedures using the ICSI technique, we achieved 16 embryos, all girls. We were over the moon and so were the consultants; maybe CF men could father children after all. However, it was not meant to be. We lost them all, and I think this was probably a very low point in both of our lives.

However, we decided we could not let this get us down. We only wanted our own children. We couldn't have them, so we put our heart and soul into our business.

As life progressed and I got older, it was felt that maybe my regimen should change with the introduction of nebulized antibiotics. I have been lucky enough not to need IV antibiotics on a regular basis; in fact, I have only ever needed them once.

I think at the time, when it was suggested that I do nebulized antibiotics, I felt my health was on a downward spiral, what next. I gradually got used to the idea, and it is very much a part of my daily life; so I started to nebulize rhDNase once, in the morning, and Promixin twice, once in the morning and last thing at night. Then much more recently, I started Tobi on alternate months. This seems to be working very well, as I rarely get chest infections.

Diet is an extremely important part of keeping well with CF; but fortunately this has never been an issue for me since I got married, as my wife insists I eat a very healthy diet and luckily for me she is an extremely good cook. Of course, eating the odd curry or kebab can't go amiss and I probably drink a little too much beer, but nobody is perfect!

Living with CF and being married of course had its challenges, but then life is one big challenge with or without CF. I think keeping positive, doing plenty of exercise, and keeping active is very important and key to staying well. I ride a mountain bike, and it certainly makes a difference to my breathing.

LIFE AT 53

On November 25, 2012, I will be 53, and life is pretty good. I have a successful business, a lovely home, and a very happy marriage. We try and get a skiing holiday each year and I play golf as much as I can. We also have a West Highland white terrier who requires a lot of walking, which of course keeps us both very active.

So how did I get here with CF? If I am honest, I have never let it get me down. I have always been optimistic, and I am lucky that all my family and friends have never treated me any differently to the rest of our family and friends.

I don't dwell on the illness even if it does take me quite a while to get out in the morning, because of the time it takes to do physio and nebulizing, but this is key to a long and healthy life. Also helpful is taking all the advice the consultants at Brompton give and making sure I give them the correct feedback, not just telling them what I think they want to hear, going for regular checkups and trying to exercise as much as possible. Most importantly, I try to maintain 100% compliance with my drug and vitamin regime; this is not always possible, but it is something that I think has made a big impact on my quality of life. My physio in the morning is something I feel is very important, much like going out in the morning without brushing your teeth, you just wouldn't miss it.

In summary, I get on with my life and I am looking forward to the future with a very positive attitude.

CYSTIC FIBROSIS PATIENT WITH SEVERE CLINICAL COURSE

EMILY HOYLE

On the outside, people with CF look completely normal most of the time. However, on the inside it is a completely different story. In some ways, this is a blessing and in some a curse. It means we can live almost normal lives in some respects. But on the other hand, we do not always get the "attention" we require, for example, a seat on a train or bus; no one will move for you as you look "fine." On the flip side, we can walk into a room and be treated like everyone else and momentarily forget everything we are dealing with. CF is a personal and sometimes embarrassing topic.

MY STORY

As a child, growing up with CF was relatively simple. I did my daily nebulizers, physiotherapy, and cocktail of medication, but I was well protected from the harsh reality of what it meant to have CF and so blissfully grew up just thinking that my life was like everyone else's plus a few drugs. However, when I was 11 I discovered the life expectancy for CF sufferers. My brother, who also has CF, was told he was infertile. I decided on hearing this news that I didn't want any shocks myself so asked the doctor what surprises he had in store for me. I was not prepared for the answer. The average life expectancy for someone with CF when I was told was thirties. So, at the tender age of 11 I grew up. I realized that if I was to die in my thirties there would be a long decline for many years beforehand, which was a lot to stomach.

I didn't discuss it with my friends (as I didn't think that they would be able to empathize with me); I did not want to upset my parents with my fears, as I also realized that I was likely to die before them and I could only imagine the devastation for them. So I decided then that life just went on and I had to do everything possible to maximize my chances.

While at university, my health deteriorated. I would frequently get stopped in the street and be told to stop smoking, having never smoked a cigarette in my life. Over my finals, I spent 2 months in hospital. Following those

2 months in hospital, I spent 8 months at home recuperating. I was completely reliant on my parents again. I couldn't even manage the walk to my bedroom; I waited another 2 months until I was fit enough for that.

Being 21 with long lines up my arm for IVs and on high doses of steroids meant that I lost all self-confidence and despite my school reputation became very insecure and unsure around men. The side effects of the drugs (particularly the steroids) took their toll and my entire body changed shape; my stomach and face swelled up, which made me dread any invitation to a 21st or any other party. On top of this, I was in constant fear of another relapse.

As time continued and my health strengthened, I managed to complete my physics degree; get a job; move to London; and even get a boyfriend, John.

After 2 years, he took me to India and proposed. My young fears of thinking that no one would even sleep with me due to CF were definitely completely unfounded. I couldn't believe how lucky I was. But did he know what he was really in for? Well, he soon learnt. Only 3 weeks after we got engaged, my long feared relapse came. On Christmas Day 2007, I fell ill. The next day I was in hospital again, which was where I remained for the following 5 weeks. I was on all the tubes and drugs that I was on 3 years earlier. I couldn't believe it. I didn't know whether to plan my funeral or my wedding.

My body started to change again and I started to not even want a wedding if I was going to look like I did last time. The support I received from my new fiancé shocked me into fighting again. He promised me that we were getting married even if I came up the isle in a wheel chair attached to oxygen, and if we needed to postpone our wedding day that was fine too. He spent every day he could with me and made me more and more determined to be myself again. And I did it! I had the wedding of my dreams.

After a few years of marital bliss, the thought of children started to enter my head; maybe I should say our heads. These ideas were shattered as the winter came and I got swine flu. A week later, my lungs "shut down." It was happening all over again, although this time it was worse. After weeks of lying in bed trying to recover, I slipped a disk by coughing and had sciatica and couldn't move my right foot, which really stopped any progress. My recovery was the hardest to date and I temporarily developed CF-related diabetes.

For 4 of the 7 weeks I was in hospital, I couldn't leave the room due to swine flu risks. Anyone who came into my isolation room had to wear gowns, gloves, and a mask, so not only did I not see even a human face for 4 weeks but when I did eventually leave my room I felt dizzy and faint as my eyes had not focused beyond the realms of my four walls. I had to start looking out the window more so that I could get used to the idea of the outside world.

The symptom of CF that I believe is the most universally hated is the clogging of the lungs with thick sticky mucus. I can't describe how hard it is to actually produce the mucus. It can cause me to break into a sweat, vomit (from refluxes), and pull muscles. Physiotherapy and all the other daily requirements just to keep patients functioning can quite literally take all day.

Somehow I recovered from swine flu and the diabetes stopped as it was steroid induced, but I could feel that something else was not right. My lung function had improved back up to FEV_1 of 48% and FVC of 100%, but I could feel a block in my left upper lobe despite there being no signs on x-rays, computed tomography (CT) scans, or blood tests. I then started to cough small black dots. Over the months, these black balls (sometimes in sputum sometimes on their own) became bigger. Then one morning, I coughed up one the size of a pea. I caught this one in a sputum pot and took it straight to the hospital as I had an appointment that day. It turned out to be a ball of fungus called scedosporium. After many consultations, I was told that there was a sign of a fungal ball in my CT scan from back when I had swine flu. Well if this ball was still there, it was probably bigger now as what I was coughing up was bigger and I wasn't feeling better. I had a few large hemoptysis as well, where I had coughed up about a half to a pint of blood so I was definitely not improving but was doing my best to stay healthy.

Six months post swine flu, my lung function plummeted and I knew that this time I was not going to get better. I don't know if it was mind over matter or if I just knew my own body. Either way, I was going to fight every step of the way. This to me meant doing all my drugs and saying yes to every test, new drug, and whatever the doctors suggested; it meant doing my physio everyday and asking to go to the gym (even if on oxygen and being wheel-chaired there) and getting on an exercise bike everyday, which I did (and had done since I first got seriously ill 7 years prior).

I spent 3 weeks in hospital and managed to "escape" for my grandfather's funeral, at which I somehow managed to play the saxophone (sitting down) despite the fact that I could tell I needed oxygen. I had to lie down throughout his reception afterward. But I managed his request that I play at his funeral, so I was happy with that.

Two days later, I was due to be a bridesmaid and I managed it. My mother got me ready as I was so breathless I could not bath myself. I had help up and down the aisle by holding another bridesmaid's arm. I struggled to walk to the loo, but I was determined to be at my best friend's wedding. A few days later, I was in hospital with a mixture of relief and disappointment. Damn—I was on oxygen again, never to come off it. The block in my left lung was getting more and more uncomfortable. I still hoped I would improve like last time.

I went into hospital on August 11 and stayed there till December 24. In November, a new drug was going to be tried on me as I was a very "odd" case suffering from an allergic reaction to scedosporium (like ABPA), but my weight was good and the rest of me "worked." If this didn't work, then transplant may be an option. At the time, transplant seemed so terminal. I knew the odds and couldn't believe I was already there. But I knew as things stood that was where I was heading. The drug was monthly, so I knew it was going to take time if I was to recover. But there was still hope and that was the main thing; there must always be hope.

After a few weeks, I remember saying to myself as I did my daily hike up the stairs to bed, "God, please give me a pair of new lungs." I knew then I needed a transplant. My body couldn't cope anymore. I wanted the relief of being looked after in hospital and that's never a good sign. Patients, I think, will all try and push it as long as possible, but we all know how much easier it is once we get into hospital and are looked after. In April, I became a permanent resident in hospital. It was then decided that I should be assessed for transplant. I was never certain how sure the previous two talks of transplant had been as the doctors clearly found it difficult to break it to me as well. I always liked the doctors who would come and sit down and look at me at my level and talk to me as an equal and not as an idiotic patient. I am an expert in my own body and have dealt with CF for longer than some of them have been alive. By the time I was told I would be assessed, I was relieved. I could tell I was declining fast and I felt there was, at last, hope again. Not everyone sees it like this, but this is the only way to look at it. It is a chance to live again.

In May, I had a night where I nearly died. An enormous fungal plug blocked my airways and I couldn't breathe. The nurses all rushed in as I called the normal call bell. I saw the concern in their faces as they called more help and ITU. Suddenly, this huge "pebble" came flying out of my mouth, but there was no relief. I just had to concentrate on every breath. The doctor called my husband who came in and saw me on NIV struggling to breathe. Seeing his face was horrid and I couldn't talk, but he just held my hand and begged me not to leave him and that he loved me. He was in tears and I was helpless. My mother came rushing down in the car from Cambridge to London and arrived later once things were calming down. ITU decided not to take me but considered ventilating me at one point. That shocked me as I knew that if I was ventilated I wasn't coming back. At least that's how I felt, despite what I was told.

My consultant came to see me first thing and looked very concerned and later told me the next few days were touch and go and I was moved to a high dependency room. I was very quickly assessed for transplant. I heard of a guy not getting on the list because he did not weigh enough. I felt like that would be a death sentence, so I begged, hoped, and prayed that I would get on the list. At the time, this seemed like the biggest, most important challenge. I could be prodded, poked, whatever (and I was), I just wanted to get on that list. I was told on June 15, 2012 that I was going to be accepted. There were celebrations all round. I knew the odds, but at last I was on the list; I had done all I could. Now I just had to stay alive and hope that I got that call.

While waiting for a transplant, my friends and family kept me going. It was never spelt out to me how ill I was until I asked. The fungal plugs were getting bigger and more frequent and it was getting harder and harder to breathe through. I knew I didn't have long left. I was giving myself until September in my head.

Days after my birthday in late July, I had my hardest fungal plug and thank goodness the physio was there to talk me through it and talk me through the breathing. I think it saved my life. I realized that I was a scary sight even for doctors. I just didn't want to be the next death on the ward; I wanted to be a success.

A week after my birthday, the nurse walked into my room and said "Emily." I knew immediately by her smile what was coming. It was the call. Then she said that Harefield had some possible lungs. This was it. Mum and a friend were with me. They grabbed each other as my phone rang. And the conversation is a bit of a blur, but all I remember saying is "yes, please" a lot. Then it was all systems go. I paid my credit card bills as I knew that if anything went wrong I had to be prepared. I declared on Facebook I was off to Harefield as I had promised my friends I would. Everything got thrown into a bag. My favorite junior doctor came and said goodbye and good luck with a huge grin on his face. The nurses hugged me goodbye. They had all become my friends over the last year. I could feel their emotions, but mine was excitement and relief as that week I had been getting worse. This was it; please don't be a false call. It was 6 weeks since I had been put on the list, so I knew that statistically it could be a false call.

My only problem was that my husband had gone away after much persuasion to take a break. So he was in Africa. He had decided to go to an island off the coast of Kenya just for the night, and obviously it was that night! I finally got hold of him and he wanted to know whether to fly back. If this was just a false call, he could come back for nothing. So I decided that he should stay put.

As I arrived at Harefield Hospital, the transplant coordinator told me she had "high hopes for these lungs." I was washed, with my mother's help, in pink chlorhexidine from head to toe and waited to hear if it was going to go ahead. Although you have thought about every aspect of what it means to have a transplant, and that someone has to die for you to live, it is still difficult at the time wishing that when the ventilator is turned off the person dies quick enough for you to get their organs. I had a nonbreathing donor, that's all I knew. I was told at 01:15 that the operation would go ahead. I had been kept informed every step of the way and felt in safe hands. I knew I did not have much left in me and was so happy to hear it was finally happening.

I called my husband who was so upset he wasn't there, but then again saying goodbye to him was hard enough on the phone let alone doing it face to face. For that reason, I was glad it was only my mother on that night. She had kept me alive, and this was her achievement as much as my own and my husband's and all the other supporters I had had physically and emotionally. I hugged her and told her she was the best mother I could ever hope for; she was my rock.

I woke up feeling groggy but with no NIV, which I had been using since that night in May. I was annoyed that no one was with me; I had woken up Thursday evening at 8:30 pm, which is after visiting hours. I then chatted all night, high as a kite, poor nurses. Friday morning came and in came Mum and Dad with huge grins. All was well. Then my mother-in-law came in and we all just held hands. My husband was on his way and arrived what felt like minutes later. My vocal chords were damaged, and I couldn't talk properly for weeks/months, lucky John.

Later on, I got extremely frustrated with the lack of communication I had with the doctors. I feel it is essential for doctors to communicate every step of the way with patients. It helps with panic attacks as everyone panics when they get that ill. I definitely panicked before my transplant at times, but the doctors always made me feel better like no one else could. They are the ones with the ability to prescribe medication and make decisions. So it is them who can change things. They are playing God. The lack of communication made me wonder how I was doing and what was going to happen. The weekly ward round is very impersonal; it always has been and a patient will never (I have never heard of one) open up in front of a room full of strangers, half of whom you have never seen and to whom you are just another statistic, or so it feels. The time the consultant came and sat in a chair for 5 minutes made all the difference to my stay and I could relax and then finally ask all my questions. I always kept a list of questions.

My husband cried the first time I walked outside, and suddenly the idea of a normal life crept on me as I got stronger and started to walk, shower, and climb stairs, none of which I had done in months/years without help.

I finally was allowed to say hello to home again. A place I had said goodbye to, thinking it was unlikely I would ever see it again. Then it was home sweet home. I was suddenly down to two very quick nebulizers every day, but compared to what I was on that was (and is) nothing and I have time in the day!

The best thing I noticed was the mornings. I could now spring out of bed and have energy straight away, instead of feeling all the rubbish in my lungs and not being able to move. I can walk my dog, watch Harry (my little brother) play Rugby, and do things I hadn't in ages. Everything was new again and exciting. Lung function was increasing all the time, and I couldn't believe it. I saw my lungs increasing in size on the x-rays. Hospital visits decreased very quickly over the following months, and suddenly I had a life again.

The only sad part is that I can't be around my other bro Ed, the one with CF and so can't see him, but thank God for Skype. I did see him the other day, but we both wore masks.

I keep pinching myself; this has all actually happened. I feel like I have won the lottery. There is not anything that can prepare you for some of the torture you are put through, but, wow, it is worth it and who knows what the future now holds. It's like my grandmother always said, whatever happens, "Life goes on."

RUPERT AND FRANCES PEARCE GOULD

BEGINNING

In 1984, our daughter Emily was born. Within 2 to 3 days, she was breast-feeding voraciously on demand. This was followed almost immediately by an explosive movement of lime green stools. Despite this, we were sent home and told that babies sometimes produced green stools and not to worry.

At the 6-weeks checkup, our competent GP referred Emily to a pediatric clinic at the Westminster Hospital, where she was diagnosed with CF using the sweat test. We were asked if there was a history of similar problems in either family and Rupert recalled his younger brother died at 18 months, of "pneumonia." He spoke to his mother and it became apparent that, whereas death was from pneumonia, in fact his younger brother suffered from CF.

Emily was referred to the Brompton Hospital where the consultant gave us an honest, blunt talk on CF and the prognosis, followed by the fact that treatments were improving every day and that with luck and good management she could survive beyond 21 years. Twenty-one years seemed a long way away and yet such a short life.

The talk helped us look to the future with reality and determination, and we were determined that we would do everything to ensure Emily would live as long and as normally as possible. In short, we had a mission in life! We were visited by a family friend (an adult CF consultant) who talked at length with both of us and gave us a greater sense of optimism for the future. His visit and talk was both comforting and reassuring.

Exhausted from all the feeds, Frances set about mixing pancreatic powder (pre-Creon pills) with a bit of expressed milk, which was spooned into Emily's mouth.

We also had to start the routine of physiotherapy on the lungs—postural drainage and gently percussing her chest with cupped hands. We taught grandparents and, later on, au pairs how to do the physio twice a day. Later on, she would tell us how to do it most effectively and with the least discomfort.

Tiredness and anxiety were constant feelings in those early days, no less so than when Emily was admitted to hospital at 5 months with *Pseudomonas* for a course of IV antibiotics. The existence of a CF nurse specialist to refer to in the hospital was a great help: someone who was always around, to form a relationship with, and to whom we could voice any concerns.

We were enjoying Emily, and we would have liked a family of more than one but realized that there was a one in four chance of having another CF child. At this point, the CF gene had not been isolated, but an early form of antenatal diagnosis was on offer if we wanted to take the risk.

CLOCK STRIKES TWICE

So we decided to try for a second child. Antenatal diagnosis gave us the all clear, which was a relief, and our son Edward was almost born early (in the Majestic Wine car park) some 22 months after Emily.

Unfortunately, within 3 days of his birth Frances was certain that Edward was suffering from CF as he had the same explosive green stools. This was confirmed by the Brompton Hospital a few days later with a sweat test (no DNA test in 1986), and he started taking Creon with his feed straight away, to good effect.

After the initial shock, we decided that we had no choice but to resolve to bring our two CF children up as normally as possible and give them the best chance of survival that we could.

So now we had two children only 22 months apart both with CF. (For the record, some 10 years later we had a third child—screening was better, and he does not have CF.) Having two was not quite double the problem, but it certainly created a strain and there was no way of shortening the time taken to complete the daily routine of physiotherapy and nebulizers.

FAMILY AND FRIENDS

Through the Cystic Fibrosis Trust, we met others who had the same problem, many of whom are still friends today despite having their own trials and tribulations. This was an amazing sense of comfort, and we are eternally grateful to them for all their words of guidance and advice and we were able to build on their experiences and their own optimism for the future.

We had great support from the family. Of course, on Rupert's side we had two "grandparents" who were both carriers and had experience of a child with CF, albeit very briefly. On the other, only one grandparent is a carrier and with a rare mutation.

ADOLESCENCE

When do children grow up? It was our CF nurse Jackie who spotted Edward, aged 15 with a school friend in the pediatric clinic, reading an adult male magazine while younger children with CF were running around with toys and watching Walt Disney. Jackie announced, with amusement, that it was high time for him to move to the adult clinic and join his sister.

At 11 years of age, Emily decided to keep her condition a secret at her new school and instructed Frances not to tell anyone that she had CF. On her first day there, Frances disobeyed her and quietly slipped a pot of Creon pills into the hands of her form mistress should the day arrive when she may forget to bring them into school. That day inevitably arrived, and she was forgiven for letting her teacher know by which time she had selectively told her closer friends about her condition. The same happened when Emily went away to school in the sixth form and her housemistress organized for her to have a separate room to keep all her medication and nebulizers. Only the matron and very close friends knew about her condition. She even kept it from a serious boyfriend for over a year and then consulted with Rupert about whether she ought to tell him.

Edward, on the other hand, was more laid back about his CF and didn't seem to mind people knowing about it. However, that attitude belied the fact that as a teenager he became angry and frustrated with the daily routine of physiotherapy and nebulizers leading to the occasional outburst at school. He was not as open with us about his condition and thought about it a lot more and was no doubt considering the reality of a shortened life expectancy. We think he bottled things up more… If he asked a question about his condition, he only wanted a direct answer and then switched off if we tried to elaborate; he wanted facts. So different from Emily, who wanted to talk about everything.

At this stage, the CF patient has a changing attitude to life. In particular, girls become sensitive of their changing bodies and Dad's offer of physio may well be rejected. Nothing we believe to do with Dad but all to do with the changing body and maturing attitude.

Boys have their own issue, and one has to judge when is the best time to tell him that his fertility has been affected by CF and that he may be sterile.

We were amazed at how much Edward did understand. The consultant who was helping to explain to Edward that he would be sterile was knocked back a bit when at 10 years of age Edward asked, "Good—does that mean that I do not have to use condoms?"

Both our children went on to university, and living away from home was a major point of transition to adulthood. Flatmates and so on were helpful, but they had normal lives and their socializing was indeed a distraction to maintaining a good regime. It seems that all young adults test their bodies, and in this respect a CF adolescent is no different. However, in our case there were other telltale signs that they had overdone it, but we had to learn the art of judgment as to when to say something and when to let them find out for themselves.

Just before her finals at Bristol University, Emily had her first bad bout of flu leading to 3 months in hospital on oxygen and with her resistance being low she caught a secondary virus in hospital. Our lives became geared toward daily visiting at the Brompton Hospital and juggling with two other children (by then, we had another son of 8 years, who does not suffer from CF). During Emily's stay in Brompton, we were reminded of the seriousness of her disease when she had one or two frightening moments and we wondered whether she would ever get better.

She recovered and Bristol University agreed to postpone her finals to the following year. In the meantime, she found a good job in PR based in London. Following her finals, she decided to move to Abu Dhabi to be with her boyfriend (who she went on to marry).

Edward went off to university and managed to keep quite well, playing a lot of sport and bicycling to lectures.

By this time, the adult CF child is in control and we had to remember that Mum and Dad cannot continue to monitor their children and are not in control. So our advice is to ensure that good friends and colleagues have your mobile phone number so that if there is an emergency you can respond and get help. In fact, we were called upon and had to leap into action to provide the support, comfort, and warmth plus of course good food and so on.

When they move away from home, they are beginning to understand the limitations and probably now know their bodies better than their parents. That telling comment from Emily to Rupert "how do you know what it is like—you don't have CF?"

ADULTHOOD

Moving on from university means that the real world is looming and today the future even for CF patients is opening up much more so than when our children were born.

Emily is now happily married. This was a joyous occasion, but one does wonder whether they have chosen a partner who will stay with them on the journey through the most difficult part of their lives. At this stage, our children looked perfectly normal, but explaining the ticking time bomb to a potential partner and what that may entail needs a lot of support. Luckily, Emily chose well and has a fantastic marriage with a loving husband who fully understands the issues and is very supportive.

Another bout of illness followed while she was first engaged and was home for Christmas (winter time is never good). Yet again, there followed 3 months in hospital with a worried fiancé John who flew back to England from Abu Dhabi to see her. The support was needed not just for Emily but reassurance and optimism was needed for John. We worried that he may find it difficult to accept the downside of her disease; at the time, we thought it was perhaps a good thing that he understood what he was taking on. It was a great relief that he still wanted to marry her despite the difficulties that lay ahead.

Emily's decline coincided with a bout of swine flu at the same time as their much loved maternal grandfather was dying. Frances was pulled in all directions, and it was difficult for her to give the two other children (one with CF) much attention.

Edward was fit enough to be able to run the London Marathon and we all went to support him. We were so proud of him. He then went on to do a triathlon, the Great North British Swim, and a Cardiff Half Marathon.

In adulthood, key issues start to emerge. Are CF patients going to have normal careers? Will they get married? Will they have children? All of this with a limited life expectancy hanging over them.

We have always considered that our CF children are the same as any other child and therefore a purpose in life is important. What that purpose is will depend on the individual.

TRANSPLANT

Just as her maternal grandfather died, Emily went into hospital and stayed there for much of the following year culminating in being accepted on the lung transplant list in June 2012. Transplant had not been something we had talked about until the numerous antifungal drugs were failing to make any impact. We had always considered it as a last ditch treatment; but we found ourselves wanting a transplant for Emily more than anything else, especially as it dawned on us that the clinicians were running out of pharmaceutical remedies.

As she was being assessed for transplant, we began to come to terms with the fact that time could be running out. For us, it was a relief that a decision had been made after months of struggling with treatments that were unable to stop the onslaught of fungus in her lungs. For friends, it was a shock as they either didn't realize she was so ill or had been in denial about it.

Keeping positive and keeping going was all that mattered. As time moved on and her condition deteriorated Frances had to have conversations any mother would hope never to have with her daughter, but she needed to be able to discuss what might happen should she not survive. It was hard for both of us, but at the same time she never gave up hope of having a transplant.

For Rupert, there were the pragmatic concerns of what about John, and what about wills, and so on. Emily was, as ever, down to earth and took it all head on. In fact, at times she seemed to be comfortable in hospital and had small parties of friends in her room. This was interspersed with regular visits to the prayer sessions on Sunday.

Her determination to get on the transplant list was apparent in the way she badgered the doctors to book all the medical tests and assessments required, to be accepted on the transplant list. We didn't want to do anything but support her and be there for her whenever John couldn't be.

Following a frightening episode when Emily's airways became blocked with a plug of mucous, preventing her from breathing, we all took turns to spend the night in her room so that she would never be alone. Frances will always remember the late evenings walking Emily through the ward carrying her oxygen for her and chatting to the nurses. Rupert had some lovely evenings trying to beat Emily at backgammon, and John spent many nights with her after work. Like so many in the ward, she was struggling to breathe; it was a worrying time for all of us.

Both John and Rupert had full-time jobs to juggle with and mix with spending evenings, if not all night, with her. Fortunately, Emily was self-driven and always determined and always cheerful, accepting what life was throwing at her.

Edward visited occasionally but was extremely careful and wore a mask to protect himself as well as Emily. Her younger brother Harry visited when he could, as he was away at school. Support from John and a devoted group of friends helped us through this time with moments of fun and humor. We bought her a Dyson fan during the summer, which was a lot quieter at night. Sharing the care with John made it easier, although he needed support as well. He was trying to keep a job going and spending time with Emily.

When the call for a transplant finally came, Emily was relieved and excited. Edward was more openly worried the night of the transplant and called Frances several times during the operation clearly frightened. She had to reassure him that the operation itself had a very high success rate. For him, the experience must have been frightening, as he contemplated his own future and the fear of losing the only person in the family who really understood his condition, could give him good advice, and understand exactly how he felt.

It was probably easier for Frances as she was totally involved in traveling with Emily in the ambulance to Harefield and sharing the excitement and the anticipation with her. Phone calls to close family had to be made, especially to John, who was abroad with his father having a well-earned break, and Rupert, who was in the middle of a difficult meeting. None of us imagined that a match would be found after only 6 weeks on the transplant list. Emily was the most optimistic of us all.

Fortunately, there was a sense of calm and some humor as Frances helped her to prepare for theater and waited to hear whether the donor's lungs were good enough for transplant. There was a sense of excitement as Frances accompanied her to theater. She confesses to having shed a tear as she hugged Emily when she said goodbye in the theater; her parting words were, "I will see you in ITU in a few hours." Rupert had no choice but to snatch some sleep for the challenge of Thursday morning whatever that would entail, and who knew?

As we walked into ITU to see Emily looking beautiful and calm on a ventilator, there was a huge sense of relief that she had reached this stage and gratitude to the poor donor and their family and all the medical effort that had got us to this point. This must have been reflected in the many e-mail texts sent and telephone calls we made over the next few weeks. John set up a Facebook page so that the many well-wishers were kept informed as access to Emily was restricted.

Our outlook changed as Emily made a good recovery over the next few weeks despite a brief setback when she contracted pneumonia. Rupert visibly relaxed more and enjoyed visiting her in hospital, watching more of the Olympics than intended.

Although we saw very little of Edward over this period (as he was not allowed to come and visit Emily), we spoke to him often. We often worried about how he coped with the year when she became so ill and he was not able to visit much, but luckily he had a very supportive girlfriend; we encouraged him to take time off and do some traveling while he was well enough. We are sure that at that time he considered this his last possible time for long-distance travel as he had seen the difficulty Emily had had with travel. Although we worried about him as he traveled through the Far East on his way to Australia and New Zealand, it was good to receive pictures of them on their travels in exotic places and a relief to learn that the bug he caught in Cambodia was totally normal (according to the Australian doctor) and easily treatable.

CONCLUSION

We feel like we have traveled an enormously long way with our two CF children and that we have arrived at a new plateau; hopefully, not even half way. Emily with her new lungs and many more years of life. Edward healthy and still running half marathons but spending half his day keeping fit.

The journey continues with optimism but not without difficulties ahead. We have learned to stand back and give them their independence when they are well but be there for them when we are needed. We only have to look back to those months at the Brompton Hospital to realize how lucky we have been and how grateful we are to all who have helped our two CF adult children on their journey.

PART 2

Basic science for the clinician

Table 4.1 (*Continued*) Most common *CFTR* mutations in the world and their geographical distribution

Legacy name	New nomenclature (cDNA name)	Frequency (%) in the general population[a]	Population with the highest prevalence (frequency in specific population)
R117H	c.350G>A	0.3	European derived
R1162X	c.3484C>T	0.3	Italian, Latin American
R347P	c.1040G>C	0.2	European derived
3849+10kbC>T	c.3717+12191C>T	0.2	Southern European, Middle Eastern
I507del	c.1519_1521delATC	0.2	European derived
394delTT	c.262_263delTT	—	Nordic, Finnish (10%–30%)
G85E	c.254G>A	—	Southern European
R560T	c.1679G>C	—	Northern Irish
A455E	c.1364C>A	—	Dutch (2.6%), North Eastern Quebec (8%)
1078delT	c.948delT	—	French Brittany (5.7%)
2789+5G>A	c.2657+5G>A	—	Spanish
3659delC	c.3528delC	—	Scandinavian (5.4)
R334W	c.1000C>T	—	Southern European, Latin American (2.4%)
1898+1G>T	c.1766+1G>T	—	English (1%–5.5%) European
711+1G>T	c.579+1G>T	—	French, French-Canadian
2183AA>G	c.2051_2052delAAinsG	—	Italian
3905insT	c.3773_3774insT	—	Swiss, Amish, Acadian (6%–17%)
S549N	c.1646G>A	—	Indian, Latin American
2184delA	c.2052delA	—	European derived
Q359K/T360K	c.[1075C>A;1079C>A]	—	Jewish-Georgian (87.5%)
M1101K	c.3302T>A	—	Canadian-Hutterite (69%)
Y122X	c.366T>A	—	French, Reunion Island (48%)
1898+5G>T	c.1766+5G>T	—	Chinese, Taiwan (30%)
3120+1G>T	c.2988G>A	—	African (12%–46%), African-American (11%)
I148T	c.443T>C	—	French-Canadian (9.1%)
1898+5G>T	c.1766+5G>T	—	East Asian—Taiwan (30%)
CFTRdele2,3	c.54-5940_273+10250del21kb	—	Eastern and Western Slavic (1.1%–6.4%)

Source: CF Genetic Analysis Consortium, *Hum Mutat* (4):167–177, 1994.

[a] Frequency is based on the CF mutation database and listed only on reaching > 0.1%. The geographic location (or ethnic group) with the highest prevalence is indicated for some of the mutations.

Some mutations reach a higher frequency in specific populations, due to a founder effect; for example, 48% of all alleles in Ashkenazi Jews in Israel (p.Trp1282X) and 24% in the French Reunion Island (p.Tyr122X). Although most *CFTR* mutations have been associated with European-derived populations, *CFTR* mutations have also been identified in African and East Asian populations, such as *c.2988+1G>A* (legacy name: 3120+1 G>A), which accounts for 46% of African CF alleles and 13% of African-American CF alleles and is the most common after p.Phe508del in this second population.

The different mutations have been divided into five major classes according to their effect on CFTR function[37]

(Table 4.2): defective protein production (class I), defective protein processing (class II), defective protein regulation (class III), defective protein conductance (class IV), and reduced amounts of functional CFTR protein (class V). However, it must be pointed out that these classes are not mutually exclusive and, therefore, a mutation can combine two defects, i.e., be classified as classes II and III as *F508del*. Class I, II, and III mutations have been associated with typical severe multiorgan disease on the basis of clinical studies. In contrast, class IV and V mutations seem to confer sufficient functional CFTR to result in a mild phenotype. This classification based on structure–function is suitable for mutation-targeted therapy as new compounds dedicated to treat the basic defect are now under development. An additional class was previously proposed (class VI), which is associated with a decreased stability of the CFTR protein and/or an increased turnover at the apical cell membrane. This latter class has been poorly investigated as it is difficult to assess, and class VI has been renamed class V following the reclassification by Welsh (2001). However, both class V and VI mutations lead to a reduced amount of functional CFTR protein.

CLASS I: MUTATIONS ALTERING THE PRODUCTION OF THE PROTEIN AND READTHROUGH THERAPY

These mutations result in the total or partial absence of the protein (Table 4.2, Figure 4.3). This class includes (1) nonsense mutations producing an in-frame premature termination codon (PTC)—UAA, UAG, or UGA—and (2) frameshifts or mutations at the invariant dinucleotide splice junctions resulting in the introduction of a PTC. There are two separate molecular mechanisms whereby CFTR protein does not reach the apical cell membrane. In the first, the great majority of the cases, the nonsense-mediated mRNA decay (NMD) pathway degrades the abnormal mRNA containing PTC.[38,39] But in the case of mRNA translation a truncated protein is synthesized, which is unstable and degraded rapidly in the cytoplasm. This results in the absence of expression of the CFTR protein.

However, some PTCs are more "permissive" than others because of differences in the level of mRNA and the possible "readthrough" of PTC, leading to residual CFTR function.[40] The goal of suppression therapy is to reduce the

"proofreading ability" of the ribosome and induce low levels of misreading at PTCs. If enough PTCs are recoded into sense-codons, enough full-length, functional protein may then be restored to provide a therapeutic benefit.

The best characterized drugs active against PTCs are aminoglycosides. Pilot clinical trials have provided proof-of-concept studies indicating readthrough efficiency. CF adults treated topically with gentamicin drops in the nose demonstrated restoration of CFTR-dependent Cl⁻ secretion and protein expression.[41] Intravenous gentamicin also yielded similar results. Interestingly, this was associated with a decrease in mean sweat chloride concentrations and improvement in respiratory status, irrespective of the gentamicin sensitivity of the bacteria present in sputum.[42]

PTC124 was identified by PTC Therapeutics, Inc., by screening a library of 800,000 low-molecular-weight compounds. Significantly, PTC124 (trade name Ataluren) was found to suppress nonsense mutations better than aminoglycosides without nephro- or ototoxic side effects and with no effect on normal termination codons. Phase II clinical trials of PTC124 demonstrated mixed results. While studies in France and Israel found that PTC124 treatment restored CFTR function, an American study did not observe any significant increase in CFTR function.[43–45] This might be due not only to heterogeneity of practice among different study sites but also to variable responses among genotypes according to the level of residual mRNA.[40] This is supported by the Israeli phase II study that showed a correlation between Cl⁻ transport modification and the level of increase in CFTR transcript after gentamicin nasal application. A double-blind, placebo-controlled phase III study across 11 countries comparing Ataluren ($n = 116$) to placebo ($n = 116$) in CF patients with nonsense mutations

Table 4.2 Classification of *CFTR* mutations

Class	Effect on CFTR protein	Functional CFTR	*CFTR* apical expression	Examples of mutations	Potential therapy
I	Defective production	No	No	G542X, W1282X, R553X, R1162X, E822X, 1717-1G>A, 711+1G>T, 621+1G>T	Readthrough therapy (ataluren), NMD inhibitors
II	Impaired processing	No	No	F508del, N1303K, I507del, R1066C, S549R, G85E	Correctors (Lumacaftor), proteostasis strategy
III	Defective regulation	No	Yes	G178R, G551D, G551S, R560T, V520F, G970R, G1244E, S1255P, G1349D	Potentiators (ivacaftor)
IV	Defective conductance	Reduced	Yes	R117H, R334W, R347P, R1070W	Potentiators (ivacaftor)
V	Reduced amount	Reduced	Reduced	3272-26A>G, 3849+10kbC>T, A455E, D565G	NMD inhibitors, splicing modulators

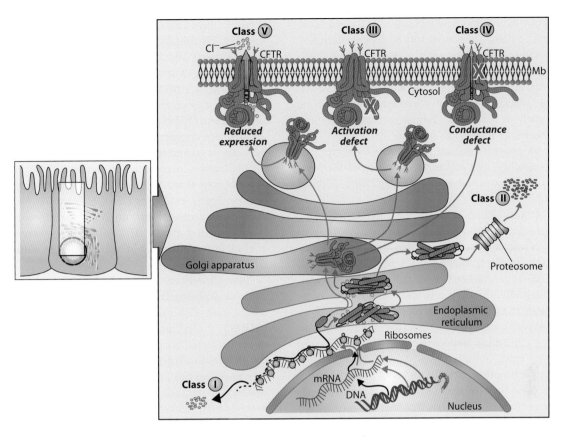

Figure 4.3 Cystic fibrosis transmembrane conductance regulator mutation classes.

is now under evaluation. The primary end point, the relative change from baseline in percentage of predicted forced expiratory volume in one second (FEV_1) at 48 weeks, does not show a significant modification, although there is a positive trend favoring Ataluren (−2.5% change on Ataluren vs. −5.5% change on placebo; $p = .124$).[46] Neither sweat test nor nasal potential difference showed a modification between the two groups of treatment. However, a positive treatment effect is seen in the patients not receiving chronic inhaled antibiotics at baseline (−0.2% change on Ataluren vs. −6.9% change on placebo; $p = .008$), whereas patients with any inhaled aminoglycosides do not demonstrate any significant effect of the drug. This may be related to antagonism between the aminoglycoside molecule and Ataluren for the PTC suppression effect.

Other novel molecules are undergoing in vitro studies, including NMD inhibitors such as amlexanox,[47] a drug used for decades for oral mucosal conditions, and also novel readthrough molecules, such as NB124.[48] However, a lot of issues for this targeted therapy aiming at overcoming PTC still need to be resolved before implementation in routine therapies, among which, very importantly, is their impact on normal stop termination codon and their potential to modify expression of other genes. Nevertheless, this therapeutic concept, which modulates the translation termination process, has led to high hopes for treating genetic disorders due to nonsense mutations, far beyond the field of CF. Indeed, this has already been studied in Duchenne muscular dystrophy, heritable pulmonary arterial hypertension, hemophilia, and metabolic diseases such as phenylketonuria or methylmalonic aciduria.

CLASS II: MUTATIONS ALTERING THE CELLULAR PROCESSING OF THE PROTEIN AND CORRECTOR THERAPIES

Class II mutations are associated with defective protein processing (Table 4.2, Figure 4.3). The major mutation *F508del* is the main example of this class. Almost 100% of the newly synthesized F508del-CFTR is degraded due to improper folding. The misfolded protein is retained in the ER, retrotranslocated in the cytoplasm to be degraded by the ubiquitin/proteasome pathway.[9,10] In this case, the protein is either absent or present in a very small quantity at the plasma membrane. F508del leads to energetic and kinetic instability of NBD1.[49] Moreover, this mutation impairs assembly of the interface between NBD1 and MSD1/MSD2, namely, the fourth cytoplasmic loop (CL4), and thus destabilizes also the conformation of MSD1, MSD2, and NBD2.[50,51] Therefore, correction of both NBD1 energetics and interface instability is required to restore F508del processing.[11,52]

Some small molecules, named CFTR correctors, have been reported to promote the rescue to native folding, therefore allowing the protein to evade ER quality control, enhance surface expression, and increase CFTR-dependent Cl⁻ transport. To date, some correctors have been identified by high-throughput screening such as benzo[c]quinolizinium (MPB) compounds and Corr4a.[53-56]

Vertex Pharmaceuticals, Inc., has engaged a research program to identify F508del correctors. Quinazoline derivatives such as VRT-422 and its medicinal chemistry optimized hit (VRT-325) or pyrazole derivative (VRT-532) behave as pharmacological chaperones by increasing maturation, stability, and cell-surface density of F508del-CFTR in human bronchial epithelial cells from *F508del* homozygotes.[57-59]

VX-809 (trade name Lumacaftor; Vertex Pharmaceuticals) promotes F508del-CFTR conformational maturation and can restore up to 15% of non-CF channel activity in primary respiratory epithelia.[60,61] VX-809 does not seem to stabilize NBD1 but rather to restore its interaction with the fourth intracellular loop (CL4), and therefore the cooperative folding of CFTR, an interpretation supported by computational docking.[62] In vivo bioactivity studies showed a small, dose-dependent improvement in CFTR function in sweat gland epithelium, but they showed no significant change in CFTR function either in the nasal or in the rectal epithelium and no improvement in lung function.[63] A pharmacokinetic optimized derivative, VX-661, less sensitive to CYP3A inducers, is under evaluation.

However, it must be pointed out that all these correctors have a ceiling efficacy in restoring chloride conductance of approximately 10%–15% non-CF human primary epithelia.[53,61] The challenge for therapy discovery for the *F508del* mutation is now to design molecules based on three-dimensional structural information providing precise molecular targets. Computational docking and biophysical studies will design in silico structure-targeted molecules to "complement" the defects due to F508del and counteract both the NBD1 folding defect and misassembly with other domains of the protein.[64] Undoubtedly, this is a new area of research for discovery.

CLASS III: MUTATIONS DISTURBING THE REGULATION OF THE CL⁻ CHANNEL AND POTENTIATOR THERAPIES

These mutations are frequently located in the ATP-binding domain (NBD1 and 2) and are thus referred to as gating mutations (Table 4.2, Figure 4.3). The *G551D* mutation is the most prevalent gating mutation and accounts for 1/25 CF patients. It is caused by substitution of the amino acid glycine by aspartate at position 551 in NBD1 at a crucial point interfacing with NBD2.[65] It abolishes ATP-dependent gating, resulting in an open probability that is approximately 100-fold lower than that of wild-type channels.

Potentiators normalize this defective CFTR Cl⁻ channel gating. One of the first identified CFTR potentiators were molecules belonging to phytoestrogens such as genistein and isoflavone. The most promising one is VX-770, ivacaftor (trade name Kalydeco; Vertex Pharmaceuticals), which has

been developed by testing its activity on the *G551D* mutation. VX-770 specifically targets the *G551D* gating mutation by increasing the channel open probability and therefore the flow of ions transported through the channel.[65] Preclinical in vitro investigations showed improvement in hydration and increased ciliary motion of CF airway epithelium. Phase II clinical studies demonstrated significant within-subject improvements in channel functioning in both the nasal and the sweat gland epithelium, i.e., trend to normalization in sweat chloride and NPD.[66] Moreover, in some treated subjects, the sweat Cl⁻ levels decreased below the diagnostic cutoff for CF of 60 mmol/L. Very interestingly, measures of lung function also showed significant improvements. Phase III clinical trials investigated the efficacy of ivacaftor in adults and children with the *G551D CFTR* mutation.

Two 48-week randomized, double-blind, and placebo-controlled phase III trials were conducted in adolescents/adults with FEV₁ of 40%–90% of the predicted normal (STRIVE study)[67] and in children with FEV₁ of 40%–105% of the predicted normal (ENVISION study).[68] At the end of the 48-week study period, patients were offered the opportunity to rollover to an optional open-label study (PERSIST), designed to monitor the long-term impact of ivacaftor treatment over 96 weeks.[69] In the STRIVE study, at week 24 the percentage of predicted FEV₁ showed a statistically significant treatment effect of 10.6% points ($p < .001$). This ivacaftor-dependent improvement was noted as early as 15 days and was maintained throughout the study, with a treatment effect through week 48.[67] Nearly 75% of ivacaftor-treated adults had a mean improvement of 5% points. Very interestingly, improvements in patients with poor pulmonary function were similar to those in patients with only mild functional impairment. Similar patterns of data were observed for the risk of pulmonary exacerbation (reduced by 55%; $p = .001$) and weight gain (treatment effect, 2.7 kg; $p < .001$). Sweat chloride levels demonstrated a rapid and sustained response compared to placebo with a reduction of 48 mmol/L sweat chloride in comparison with placebo. This effect was seen as early as day 15 and maintained through week 48.

A similar pattern was observed in the ENVISION study. Interim results from the first 12 weeks of PERSIST show that the patients who switched from placebo to ivacaftor showed an improvement in FEV₁ similar to that reported in STRIVE, thus further supporting the beneficial effect of ivacaftor.[69] New patients are now being monitored in the phase IV GOAL study and demonstrate a similar range of improvement as in the phase III study, as assessed by changes in FEV₁, sweat chloride, and body weight. Very interestingly, study in preschool children with "silent lung disease" as assessed by normal initial FEV₁ (2–5 years) also demonstrated a significant improvement in FEV₁ (+11% at day 15 and +7% at day 28) and FEF25-75 (+15% at day 15 and +29% at day 29) and lung clearance index.[68] These remarkable results show for the first time that molecular transformation, i.e., increase in the channel open probability and epithelial CFTR function rescue, can translate into outstanding clinical improvements, obvious from the second week of treatment, even in patients who are asymptomatic.

Ivacaftor also potentiates gating mutations other than *G551D*. Clinical benefit is now under evaluation in patients greater than 6 years with other gating mutations (KONNECTION study).

COMBINED CFTR DEFECT AND COMBINATION THERAPIES

Mutations may induce several CFTR dysfunctions. For example, F508del-CFTR, if located at the plasma membrane, also presents a gating defect.[70] This may involve impairment in NBD dimerization, dimer stability, and/or conformational coupling between the NBDs and MSDs.[71] Therefore, potentiators aiming at normalizing defective F508del-CFTR Cl− channel gating may potentiate the effect of correctors, which rescue the traffic of the protein to the membrane. More generally, potentiators might also be given to increase the conductance of a protein expressed at the membrane and partially functioning in association with suppression therapies for class I mutations and correctors for class II mutations. This is the rationale for combination therapies.

Considering the disappointing results of VX-809 corrector Lumacaftor alone, Vertex decided to design a combination therapy using both potentiator (ivacaftor) and corrector (Lumacaftor). This was based on in vitro studies showing indeed that ivacaftor increased the open probability of F508del-CFTR by fivefold. A phase II study in *F508del* homozygotes treated with Lumacaftor and ivacaftor for 28 days led to a clinically and statistically significant improvement in FEV_1 (increase in relative percentage predicted by around 9%). It was noted that 25% of the patients had improvements greater than 10% and 55% of the patients greater than 5%. There was also a significant improvement in sweat Cl− concentration, albeit low (not more than 10 mmol/L), in comparison to the increase obtained with VX-809 alone in patients carrying the *G551D* mutation.[72] These findings support the initiation of confirmatory phase III studies with ivacaftor and Lumacaftor in patients homozygous for *F508del* and phase II combinatory study with VX-661, an optimized analogue of VX-809.

These combination therapies might also be theoretically considered for compound heterozygotes. However, this deserves further studies because ivacaftor–Lumacaftor therapy did not improve *F508del* heterozygotes.[72]

CLASS IV: MUTATIONS ALTERING THE CONDUCTION OF THE CL− CHANNEL

These mutations are mostly located within MSDs, which are implicated in forming the pore of the channel (Table 4.2, Figure 4.3). The missense mutations located in these regions produce a protein inserted in the membrane, which retains a cAMP-dependent Cl− channel residual activity. Alleles in this class are typically associated with a pancreatic sufficient phenotype.

The *R117H* mutation has been fully characterized. It is a missense mutation replacing arginine by histidine at residue 117, at the external end of TMD2. This mutant is correctly processed and generates cAMP-regulated apical Cl− currents. However, patch-clamp analysis demonstrated a 75% reduction in channel open probability, with alteration in Cl− and HCO_3^- conductance, although both defects are milder than in F508del.[73,74] Because those channels display a residual function with normal regulation, therapies aiming at increasing their activity are efficient.

In vitro studies have shown that Cl− transport of proteins carrying such mutations are increased by VX770, *R117H* being one of the most responsive mutations.[75] Therefore, Vertex Pharmaceuticals is now undertaking clinical trials aiming to study sufficient pancreatic patients with a sweat Cl− less than 85 mmol/L, indicating a residual CFTR function (Table 4.2). A trial in *R117H* patients (with FEV_1 between 40% and 90%) has just begun (KONDUKT study). As patients carrying these mutations are rare, studies in single patients (N of 1 design) carrying other mutations with residual function are considered.

CLASS V: MUTATIONS REDUCING THE AMOUNT OF FUNCTIONAL CFTR PROTEIN

Most of these mutations affect pre-mRNA splicing (Table 4.2, Figure 4.3). These splice site mutations can induce complete or partial exclusion of the exon, and also production of normal mRNA. This process is called alternative splicing. Such mutations will produce either a reduced amount of normal protein (class V mutation) or generate a novel exon sequence and then be classified as class I because they may result in missense, silent, or even nonsense mutations and produce aberrant CFTR. Classically, these mutations are located in the introns close to the splice sites, but a growing number of them have been identified in exons due to the disruption of exonic splicing enhancer motif. Because direct RNA analysis is not routinely performed, it is likely that the number of mutations potentially causing splicing defects is underestimated.

Most of these mutations lead to residual CFTR function. This is, for example, the case for *3849+10kbC>T*, a point mutation in intron 19, which reduces mRNA splicing efficiency to 8% of normal and leads to a mild phenotype with a normal sweat test. But the most frequent and well studied is the deleted transcript of exon 9 (9-). The presence or absence of this exon is correlated with a polymorphism of sequences in the intron 8 located near the acceptor splice site (polyT tract). This polypyrimidine sequence encompasses 5, 7, or 9 thymidines (5T, 7T, or 9T). Whereas 7T or 9T ensures a normal to 90% of normal splicing, 5T allows no more than 10%–40% of normal mRNA, the remaining 60%–90% of mRNA 9- being unable to produce a functional CFTR.[76]

Indeed, the 5T allele by itself has been associated with male infertility due to congenital bilateral absence of the vas deferens (CBAVD), with or without mild or atypical symptoms of CF.[77] Since then, the region has been extended to the adjacent dinucleotide repeats (TG tract), which encompasses different TG repeats (TG11, TG12, or TG13). A longer TG tract (12 or 13) in conjunction with a shorter polyT tract (5T) is more likely to harbor an exon 9- mRNA and exhibit an abnormal phenotype.[78,79]

Interestingly, the phenotypic consequences of the class IV *R117H* mutation are modulated in *cis* by the 5/7/9T polypyrimidine tract in intron 8. R117H/7T is associated with milder forms of CF such as CBAVD, and most of the time even absence of symptoms. In a multicenter French study, the penetrance of classical CF for [R117H;7T]+[F508del] was estimated at 0.03% and that of severe CF in adulthood at 0.06%. Bronchiectasis was observed in 4% of the patients, while respiratory symptoms were quite frequent but generally moderate and nonspecific.[80] [R117H;5T]+[F508del] patients have elevated sweat chloride and clinical CF, which in some cases is severe.[81] R117H-5T is more frequent in Australian and UK populations and the northwestern area of France.[80]

Class V mutations can be targeted by NMD inhibitors, or splicing modulators such as antisense oligonucleotide approach. They might also be improved by ivacaftor. However, the difficulty to predict the efficiency from in vitro studies makes implementation of targeted therapies for this mutation class very challenging.

CLASSIFICATION OF CFTR MUTATIONS BASED ON CLINICAL DESCRIPTION

CFTR mutations can be classed into four groups according to their clinical consequences[36]:

1. Mutations that cause CF disease
2. Mutations that result in a CFTR-related disorder (CFTR-RD)
3. Mutations with no known clinical consequence
4. Mutations of unproved or uncertain clinical relevance

Groups 1 and 2 overlap as some mutations may be associated with different presentations, from isolated CBAVD to CF with sufficient pancreatic function but fully expressed lung disease, as described for D1152H. This is also the case for R117H. In compound heterozygosity with a CF-causing mutation, R117H-5T usually results in pancreatic sufficient CF, whereas R117H-7T should be considered principally as a CFTR-RD-associated mutation with reduced penetrance or may result in no disease at all.[36,80] Moreover, other factors such as progression of the disease with age, environment, and modifier genes can also take a part in the clinical heterogeneity of patients carrying these large-spectrum mutations.

CFTR-RDs are single-organ diseases, whose pathophysiology may be attributed to CFTR defects.[82] The best-studied CFTR-RDs are CBAVD, recurrent acute or chronic pancreatitis, and disseminated bronchiectasis. About 80%–90% of men with CBAVD carry at least one *CFTR* mutation[77] and 50%–60% have two *CFTR* mutations.[83] For this last case, usually one is CF causing (*F508del* in 20%–40% of the cases) and the other is a CFTR-RD-associated mutation (including the 5T variant in about 35% of the patients).[84] *R117H* is also frequently reported (about 30%) in these patients, usually in association with the 7T variant.[85] Among the patients presenting with chronic pancreatitis, the frequency of a single mutation in *CFTR* is 11-fold greater than expected. About 30% carry one *CFTR* mutation and 10%–15% are compound heterozygotes, *F508del* being the most common severe mutation in association with the T5 variant, *R117H-T7, L206W, D1152H, R1070Q, R347H, R334W,* and *2789+5G>A.*[86,87] *CFTR* mutations are found in 10%–50% of series of patients with idiopathic bronchiectasis.[88] However, it must be pointed out that the pathogenic potential of many of the sequence variations identified in these patients is not known. It is therefore not clear whether *CFTR*-related bronchiectasis in these cases is a single-organ manifestation of CF or a condition where *CFTR* mutations play the role of a modifier deleterious gene, acting with an environmental contribution. A prevalence of *CFTR* mutations higher than expected in the general population has also been reported in rhinosinusitis, allergic bronchopulmonary aspergillosis, and sclerosing cholangitis. However, to assess the association between *CFTR* mutations and these disorders is often difficult, because these clinical entities may have other non-CFTR-related etiologies.

Clearly, the aforementioned patients lack the criteria of definition of classical CF, i.e., two CF-causing *CFTR* mutations (according to CFTR-2 database) and/or a sweat chloride above 60 mmol/L.[36,82] Most of these patients have intermediate sweat tests between 30 and 60 mmol/L. Careful monitoring of these patients and ancillary tests may help establish a diagnosis of CF by revealing a second organ disease phenotype, such as pancreatic insufficiency (fecal pancreatic elastase), CBAVD in males, and lung or sinus involvement. Extended DNA analysis sometimes identifies a second mutation involved. However, these tests are available in only a few centers because they require high-technology devices and trained staff. CFTR bioassay tests (nasal potential difference, intestinal ion channel measurements from rectal biopsies in Ussing chamber) may clarify the diagnostic status if they clearly indicate CFTR dysfunction.[89] However, reference values and validation studies for these bioassays are still lacking, which make them difficult to use in routine assessment. Moreover, this functional evaluation may differ according to the tissues, leading to discordant conclusions, according to the tests. This reflects the reality of differential expression of *CFTR* and sensitivity to the level of CFTR defect according to the tissues. Algorithms for a structured diagnostic process have been proposed.[90,91]

Such a dilemma in the diagnostic process is now made more complex by newborn screening because preclinical features at this time, i.e., elevated immunoreactive trypsinogen (IRT), may substitute for later clinical symptoms. At least 2% of infants with hypertrypsinemia (IRT above the 99th percentile) have sweat Cl⁻ levels in the intermediate range (between 30 and 59 mmol/L) and no or one CF-causing mutation. This is clearly a very difficult situation as some babies may remain asymptomatic or develop extremely mild phenotypes that would never be noted clinically as part of the CF spectrum. Conversely, others will turn out to have symptoms consistent with CF or develop CFTR-RD. The diagnosis may remain inconclusive in these situations when extensive genetic studies identify genetic variations with an unclear pathogenic potential or detect mutations associated with a wide spectrum of phenotypes. As bioassays are very challenging in this population, these diagnostic dilemmas are rarely sorted out.[92]

FUTURE PROSPECTS: PROTEOSTASIS STRATEGY TO MODULATE NORMAL CHAPERONES AND IMPEDE ER DEGRADATION

Modulation of the protein quality control system represents a complementary approach to rescue defects in CFTR class II mutants, as occurring for F508del-CFTR. Molecular chaperone complexes sense the CFTR folding state and assist folding or ubiquitination-dependent ERAD, intracellular trafficking machinery, and degradation in the plasma membrane[93] (Figure 4.3). Therapies modulating the activity of molecular chaperones, such as Hsp70 and Hsp90, might, for example, rescue F508del expression. Pharmacological proteostasis regulators already clinically available have been previously tested yielding to indecisive results, including inhibitors of Hsc70 mRNA such as 4-phenylbutryate used for erythrocyte urea cycle disorder;[94] sarcoplasmic/ER calcium pump inhibitors such as cucurmin, thapsigargin, verapamil, and diltiazem[95]; inhibitors of the catalytic activity of the proteasome such as bortezomib used in multiple myeloma; α-glucosidase inhibitors such as miglustat, used in Gaucher lysosomal storage disease[96]; and phosphodiesterase type 5 inhibitors such as sildenafil,[97] used in pulmonary hypertension. Glafenine, an anthranilic acid derivative with analgesic properties, also corrects the misprocessing of CFTR in vitro to approximately 40% of that observed for wild-type CFTR.[98]

Recently, mechanisms for proteostasis regulation have been individualized and may have therapeutic applications. Downregulation of Aha1, an Hsp90 cochaperone ATPase regulator, modulates Hsp90-dependent CFTR protein folding in the ER and rescues F508del at the cell surface.[99,100] Reduction of the acetylation level of histones increases the level of COPII components available for recruitment of F508del-CFTR to exit from ER to the Golgi apparatus. They increase F508del-CFTR expression, trafficking, and activity.[101] Very interestingly, many histone deacetylase inhibitors are drugs already used in treating numerous diseases such as resveratrol, 4-phenylbutryate, valproic acid, and suberoylanilide hydroxamic acid, a compound already approved by the US Food and Drug Administration for lymphoma.

This strategy targeting multiple facets of F508del-CFTR trafficking and degradation could be combined with correctors, which improve CFTR folding. This is clearly a novel approach that might lead to outstanding results far beyond CF. However, as proteostasis regulators also modify the trafficking of other proteins, cautious evaluation of these side effects has to be done.

CONCLUSION

Better understanding of mutation mechanisms and consequences thanks to new genetic tools has provided precise molecular targets and a new pathway for therapeutic strategy. This is a considerable progress. The exciting clinical results of ivacaftor in patients with the *G551D* mutation demonstrate for the first time the clinical efficiency of mutation-targeted therapy. We now know that improving CFTR function at the molecular level results in improvement in lung function and impacts on the daily life of patients and likely on their survival. It is anticipated that the next years will herald an era where therapeutic choices will be driven by personalized genetic information.

Future prospects are to develop corrector and potentiator combinations that achieve near wild-type processing and function. Further studies will be needed to assess the effect of combination therapy in *F508del* heterozygous patients. Before considering prescription of such treatment in newborns with the dream that targeting the basic disease prevents organ damage, long-term efficacy and, above all, long-term tolerance have to be determined. This is clearly one of the most important challenges of mutation-targeted therapeutic strategy.

UPDATE

Clinical benefit of ivacaftor has also been documented in patients >6 years with eight other gating mutations in a similar range as for *G551D*.[102] In patients 6 years and older carrying the *R117H* mutation on at least one allele, ivacaftor treatment yielded to a significant improvement (9.1%) only in the patients over 18 years (Company press release). However, for the whole population, the treatment effect was at the limit of significance. Ongoing studies in patients carrying other mutations with residual function will help to decide who will benefit from this personalized therapy.

The marginal clinical effect of corrector potency of VX-809 (lumacaftor, Vertex Pharmaceuticals) argued for a combination therapy with ivacaftor. A complex Phase II randomized, multiple dose, placebo controlled, double blind, study in F508del homozygotes confirmed the potential benefit[103] and supported 2 enormous ongoing confirmatory phase III studies with ivacaftor and lumacaftor in 1000 patients homozygous for F508del patients. Statistically significant improvements in lung function were observed across each combination dose group compared to placebo, reaching 5.6% (p<0.0001) (Company press release). There were statistically significant decrease in the rates of pulmonary exacerbations compared to those who received placebo up to 39 percent. There were also statistically significant improvements in body mass index compared to placebo and in the proportion of patients with a 5 percent or greater relative improvement in percent predicted FEV_1 compared to placebo. These combination therapies might also be theoretically considered for compound heterozygotes. However, this deserves further studies because the ivacaftor-lumacaftor therapy did not improve F508del heterozygotes. Further development of VX-661, an optimized derivative of VX-809 less sensitive to Cytochrome P4503A (CYP3A) metabolism also includes a study in F508del homozygotes and compound heterozygotes. All these studies are a step forward to personalized therapies.

ACKNOWLEDGMENT

We strongly acknowledge Jean Pierre Laigneau, INSERM, IFR94, University of Paris–Descartes, Paris, France for the illustrations.

REFERENCES

1. Andersen DH. Cystic fibrosis of the pancreas and its relation to celiac disease. *Am J Dis Child* 1938; **56**: 344–99.
2. Tsui LC, Buchwald M, Barker D, Braman JC, Knowlton R, Schumm JW et al. Cystic fibrosis locus defined by a genetically linked polymorphic DNA marker. *Science* 1985 Nov 29; **230**(4729): 1054–7.
3. Kerem BS, Buchanan JA, Durie P, Corey ML, Levison H, Rommens JM et al. DNA marker haplotype association with pancreatic sufficiency in cystic fibrosis. *Am J Hum Genet* 1989 Jun; **44**(6): 827–34.
4. Riordan JR, Rommens JM, Kerem B, Alon N, Rozmahel R, Grzelczak Z et al. Identification of the cystic fibrosis gene: Cloning and characterization of complementary DNA. *Science* 1989 Sep 8; **245**(4922): 1066–73.
5. Ostedgaard LS, Baldursson O, Vermeer DW, Welsh MJ, Robertson AD. A functional R domain from cystic fibrosis transmembrane conductance regulator is predominantly unstructured in solution. *Proc Natl Acad Sci USA* 2000 May 9; **97**(10): 5657–62.
6. Vergani P, Nairn AC, Gadsby DC. On the mechanism of MgATP-dependent gating of CFTR Cl- channels. *J Gen Physiol* 2003 Jan; **121**(1): 17–36.
7. Lukacs GL, Mohamed A, Kartner N, Chang XB, Riordan JR, Grinstein S. Conformational maturation of CFTR but not its mutant counterpart (delta F508) occurs in the endoplasmic reticulum and requires ATP. *EMBO J* 1994 Dec 15; **13**(24): 6076–86.
8. Ward CL, Kopito RR. Intracellular turnover of cystic fibrosis transmembrane conductance regulator. Inefficient processing and rapid degradation of wild-type and mutant proteins. *J Biol Chem* 1994 Oct 14; **269**(41): 25710–8.
9. Jensen TJ, Loo MA, Pind S, Williams DB, Goldberg AL, Riordan JR. Multiple proteolytic systems, including the proteasome, contribute to CFTR processing. *Cell* 1995 Oct 6; **83**(1): 129–35.
10. Ward CL, Omura S, Kopito RR. Degradation of CFTR by the ubiquitin-proteasome pathway. *Cell* 1995 Oct 6; **83**(1): 121–7.
11. Rabeh WM, Bossard F, Xu H, Okiyoneda T, Bagdany M, Mulvihill CM et al. Correction of both NBD1 energetics and domain interface is required to restore DeltaF508 CFTR folding and function. *Cell* 2012 Jan 20; **148**(1–2): 150–63.
12. Thibodeau PH, Richardson JM, 3rd, Wang W, Millen L, Watson J, Mendoza JL et al. The cystic fibrosis-causing mutation deltaF508 affects multiple steps in cystic fibrosis transmembrane conductance regulator biogenesis. *J Biol Chem* 2010 Nov 12; **285**(46): 35825–35.
13. Wang S, Yue H, Derin RB, Guggino WB, Li M. Accessory protein facilitated CFTR-CFTR interaction, a molecular mechanism to potentiate the chloride channel activity. *Cell* 2000 Sep 29; **103**(1): 169–79.
14. Raghuram V, Mak DO, Foskett JK. Regulation of cystic fibrosis transmembrane conductance regulator single-channel gating by bivalent PDZ-domain-mediated interaction. *Proc Natl Acad Sci USA* 2001 Jan 30; **98**(3): 1300–5.
15. Bertrand CA, Frizzell RA. The role of regulated CFTR trafficking in epithelial secretion. *Am J Physiol Cell Physiol* 2003 Jul; **285**(1): C1–18.
16. Sharma M, Pampinella F, Nemes C, Benharouga M, So J, Du K et al. Misfolding diverts CFTR from recycling to degradation: Quality control at early endosomes. *J Cell Biol* 2004 Mar 15; **164**(6): 923–33.
17. Gentzsch M, Chang XB, Cui L, Wu Y, Ozols VV, Choudhury A et al. Endocytic trafficking routes of wild type and DeltaF508 cystic fibrosis transmembrane conductance regulator. *Mol Biol Cell* 2004 Jun; **15**(6): 2684–96.
18. Okiyoneda T, Barriere H, Bagdany M, Rabeh WM, Du K, Hohfeld J et al. Peripheral protein quality control removes unfolded CFTR from the plasma membrane. *Science* 2010 Aug 13; **329**(5993): 805–10.

5

Underlying concepts of the pathophysiology of cystic fibrosis in the sweat gland, GI tract, and lung

RICHARD C. BOUCHER

INTRODUCTION

Although the genetics of cystic fibrosis (CF) are complex, the syndrome of CF generally reflects a loss of function of the gene product of the cystic fibrosis transmembrane regulator (*CFTR*) gene, i.e., the CFTR protein.[1] The CFTR protein appears to function in all tissues affected by CF as a cAMP-regulated anion channel. Typically, the CFTR anion channels conducts Cl^- ion with an efficiency of approximately fourfold greater than the bicarbonate ion.[2] Further, as the name cystic fibrosis transmembrane regulator implies, the CFTR protein may have regulatory effects on other ion transport proteins associated with it in the plasma membrane of epithelial cells.

The syndrome of CF has been broadly characterized as a disease involving bodily epithelia. Consequently, anion and other ion transport processes have been heavily studied in epithelial tissues affected by CF, including the sweat duct, gastrointestinal (GI) tract, the reproductive system, and the respiratory system. Thus, CF had been considered an "epithelial disease." However, more recent data emerging from molecular studies and studies of animal models of CF have suggested that *CFTR* may be expressed in nonepithelial cells, including smooth muscle cells, neuronal cells, and immune cells.[3] The levels of *CFTR* expression in these cell types appear to be lower than epithelial cells, but CFTR function and dysfunction in these cell types may contribute to the syndrome of CF.

An important concept is that the various bodily epithelia that express *CFTR* exhibit quite different physiologies. For example, epithelia that express *CFTR* can, as a part of their normal function, regulate ionic composition but not volume (liquid) transport, but also mediate isotonic volume secretion, or isotonic volume absorption. Thus, the consequences of the loss of CFTR on epithelial function are quite diverse, and at first reflection, somewhat confusing. However, with a better understanding of the role of CFTR in the normal functioning of various epithelia, it has become easier to understand how the loss of CFTR function produces the broad syndrome of CF. In this chapter, we will focus on the consequences of the loss of CFTR function in epithelia/organs based on the differing organ physiologies, with an emphasis on the lung because more than 95% of patients with CF die of chronic pulmonary infection and its consequences.

ORGANS AFFECTED BY CHANGES IN LUMINAL LIQUID ION COMPOSITION IN CF

The classic diagnostic hallmark of CF is the raised sweat Cl^- (and Na^+) values measured by the pilocarpine-stimulated sweat test. The inability to extract Na^+ and Cl^- from sweat of CF subjects can lead to a syndrome of volume dehydration and an inability to thermoregulate in hot environments, leading to a predisposition to heat prostration. Interestingly, because the volume of sweat secretion in CF subjects is approximately 90% that of normal subjects (see Figure 5.1), and because there is no mucin secretion in the sweat gland, there is no obstruction of the sweat duct in CF. The absence of ductal obstruction likely counts for the absence of ductal atresia as seen in the vas deferens, the absence of fibrosis as seen in pancreatic disease, and the absence of infection as seen in the lung.

The sweat gland exhibits the classic acinar secretion and ductal modification physiology of a secretory gland[4–6] (Figure 5.1). With respect to acinar secretion, the sweat gland acinus (coil) secretes Cl^- via electrochemical gradients generated by the activities of the basolateral Na^+-K^+-ATPase pump and basolateral K^+ channels. Transcellular Cl^- secretion is generated via the activities of basolateral Na^+-K^+-$2Cl^-$ cotransporter in series with apical membrane Cl^- channels. Importantly, it appears that CFTR Cl^- channels constitute the minority of Cl^- channels in the apical membrane of the sweat gland acinus. Thus, it is likely that calcium-activated Cl^- channels, perhaps members of the TMEM16 family, mediate the cholinergically stimulated (e.g., pilocarpine) Cl^- secretion that accounts for approximately 90% of Cl^- and volume secretion of the normal sweat acinus. The smaller component, approximately 10% of Cl^- secretion and volume flow, is mediated by cAMP signaling and, ultimately, the CFTR Cl^- channel. Although CF can be diagnosed by the absence of a cAMP-mediated Cl^- secretory flow, it is important to recognize that the non-CFTR-mediated Cl^- and volume flow dominates the sweat acinar secretion and, hence, accounts for the largely preserved volume secretion rates of the CF sweat gland.[6,7]

The normal sweat ductal epithelium is designed to reabsorb Na^+ and Cl^-, but not water from the primary secretion generated by the acinus, to produce a hypotonic liquid for transport onto the skin surface.[4] This physiology is important to (1) preserve salt in the vascular compartment, so blood pressure may be maintained under thermal stresses and (2) to deliver a dilute watery solution onto the skin surface for evaporative loss and thermal regulation. It is important to note that the driving forces for Cl^- in the sweat duct are for entry from the luminal sweat into the cell, i.e., absorption, which may in part reflect the absence of a Na^+-K^+-$2Cl^-$ co-transporter on the basolateral membrane with concomitantly low intracellular Cl^- activities. In parallel, Na^+ is also absorbed from the luminal sweat into the cell "down" a lumen to the cell electrochemical Na^+ gradient through the epithelial Na^+ channel (ENaC). Note, it is important for there to be coordinate absorption of Na^+ and Cl^- from ductal sweat and, interestingly, there have been no reports of reciprocal regulation of CFTR activation and ENaC inhibition in the sweat duct as has been noted in the airways (see Figure 5.3).

In CF, there is an absence of the CFTR protein in the apical ductal membrane. Because it appears that CFTR is the dominant Cl^- channel in the apical membrane of ductal cells, the absence of a pathway for Cl^- entry from the apical solution/lumen to the cell abolishes the capacity for ductal Cl^- absorption.[4] Na^+ absorption is slowed secondarily, e.g., by changes in electrochemical gradients for Na^+ entry. The establishment of high transepithelial differences due to the loss of CFTR Cl^- conductance in the apical membrane also recycles any absorbed Na^+ back into the luminal solution via the paracellular path. Thus, the CF sweat duct is unable to absorb Cl^- or Na^+ and, hence, a high Na^+ Cl^- solution, more or less as produced by the secretory coil, is secreted onto the skin. There are also abnormalities in bicarbonate absorption that can produce changes in CF sweat pH concentrations.[4] Note, that the sweat Na^+ Cl^- concentrations are dependent on the rate of flow through the sweat gland duct. Accordingly, most clinical sweat Cl^- is obtained after maximal stimulation of sweat duct with the pilocarpine (cholinergic) iontophoresis technique.

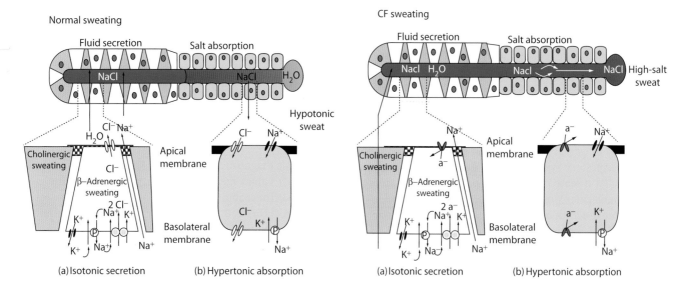

Figure 5.1 Physiology of sweat gland. (a) Normal gland. The gland acinus (upper left) secretes an isotonic fluid from two cell types: (1) a cholinergically regulated cell type (blue) and a β adrenergically regulated cell type (white, and in blow-up, below). In the sweat duct (upper right), NaCl, but not water, is absorbed by sweat ductal cells (right, and in blow-up, below), producing a hypotonic sweat. (b) CF Gland. The sweat gland acinus exhibits normal cholinergically regulated isotonic secretion (accounting for ~90% of total secretion), but defective β adrenergic anion (a) secretion due to the absence of the apical membrane CFTR Cl^- channel (see blow-up). In the CF sweat duct, the absence of an apical membrane CFTR Cl^- channel blocks Cl^- (and other anion) absorption (see blow-up), producing a high NaCl sweat.

ORGANS AFFECTED BY REDUCED LUMINAL VOLUME/VOLUME SECRETION, INCREASED MUCIN CONCENTRATIONS, AND INTRALUMINAL OBSTRUCTION

The GI tract of CF patients is broadly characterized by a failure to secrete Cl⁻ ions to generate sufficient osmotically driven liquid flow to adequately hydrate secreted mucins and mediate normal luminal volume transit. There are some important distinctions, however, between the pathogenesis of CF GI disease, particularly in the pancreas versus the intestines, gallbladder, and probably liver.

The pancreas exhibits a distinct architecture of secretion as compared to sweat glands or salivary glands, i.e., secretory acini and secretory ducts that modify the Na⁺-Cl⁻-rich secretion to produce a NaHCO$_3$-rich fluid secretion (Figure 5.2). There are other critically important differences between the function of the sweat gland and the pancreatic gland. For example, a major function of the pancreatic acinus is to secrete digestive enzymes into the acinar lumen that ultimately will facilitate the digestion of food in the intestinal tract. It appears that there is coordinated vesicle-modulated enzyme secretion and isotonic volume secretion in the acinus that occurs via non-CFTR-dependent Cl⁻ channels, i.e., likely calcium-activated Cl⁻ channels (CaCCs).[8] Although still controversial mechanistically, the pancreatic ducts are designed to secrete bicarbonate-rich isotonic fluid into the pancreatic lumens to further dilute

the pancreatic enzymes and speed the delivery of enzymes from the pancreatic gland to the intestinal lumen.

Importantly, the pancreatic ducts also alkalinize the luminal solution and eventually aid neutralization of the acid gastric contents in duodenum and promote the activity of pancreatic enzymes important for food ingestion. CFTR is richly expressed in pancreatic ducts/ductules. In the pancreatic duct, CFTR functions to secrete Cl⁻, which is then exchanged by functionally coupled apical membrane Cl⁻ bicarbonate exchanger, to produce net bicarbonate secretion.[9] Recent studies indicate that CFTR may have significant bicarbonate permeability,[10] but whether this occurs under physiological conditions needs to be settled. Intracellular bicarbonate is provided by basolateral Na⁺ bicarbonate contransporter, or from carbonic anhydrase–catalyzed CO$_2$ hydration and removal of protons by Na⁺/H exchanger or proton pumps. Indeed, the pancreatic duct can secrete bicarbonate to produce pancreatic "juice" bicarbonate concentrations in excess of 60–150 mM normally. Pancreatic ducts also express calcium-activated Cl⁻ channels, TMEM16a, and significant regulation by purinergic signaling (see Figure 5.3). Nevertheless, these alternative pathways may not be able to rescue secretion in CF.[8,11]

In CF, it is likely that the absence of CFTR Cl⁻ channels in the pancreatic duct has two major consequences.[12,13] First, the inability to secrete anions greatly reduces the ability to secrete sufficient volume into the ducts to dilute pancreatic enzymes and mucins and promote volume transport through the ducts to the duodenal lumen. Second, it is likely that the luminal contents of the pancreatic juice in CF are more acidic than normal due to the failure to generate HCO$_3$ secretion. A consequence of both these defects is that mucin

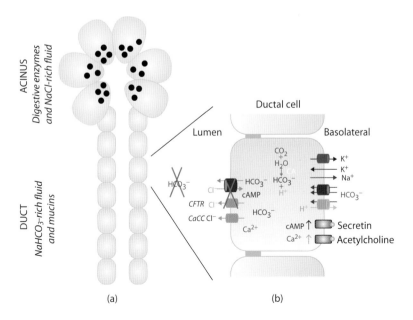

(a) (b)

Figure 5.2 (a) Schematic of intact pancreatic acinus and ductal region, depicting digestive enzymes and fluid secretion of the acinus and modification of that fluid by the duct. (b) Model for ion transport properties of ductal cell. Basolateral barrier contains transport pathways to move HCO$_3$⁻ and Cl⁻ into the cell utilizing gradients generated by the Na⁺-K-ATPase and K⁺ channels. On lumen, CFTR and CaCC channels to mediate Cl⁻ secretion that is exchanged for HCO$_3$⁻ by a luminal exchanger. In CF, luminal Cl⁻ secretion is limited and, hence, secretion of HCO$_3$⁻ is limited, producing luminal dehydration, acidification, and disease.

concentration increases and obstructs the pancreatic ducts, and the failure of pancreatic enzymes to move through the ducts produces "autodigestion" of the pancreatic ducts and retrogradely acini, resulting in loss of pancreatic acinar function. A "bystander" effect of this autodigestion is damage to β cells, which may reduce β cell numbers, and ultimately lead to the increased prevalence of diabetes in CF patients as they age.[14,15] This is actually referred to as pancreatogenic diabetes (type 3c) and may be difficult to detect as the hormonal and metabolic picture is more complex as other islet cells are also destroyed.[16]

In the small intestine, and likely gallbladder and hepatic ducts, the CFTR Cl^- channel is normally responsible for secreting Cl^- and HCO^-_3 into lumens. Consequently, the absence of the CFTR Cl^- channel function in CF leads to a reduction of volume in the lumens of the small intestine, gallbladder, and hepatic ducts.[17,18] This failure to adequately hydrate the lumens of these epithelial structures produces an increased concentration of mucins, perhaps pH-dependent abnormalities in mucin maturation and function,[19,20] and slowing of clearance of luminal contents from the orifices of these organs. In the small intestine, mucins that are concentrated collect between the villi of the small intestine, contributing to failure to adequately absorb nutrients and, perhaps, contributing to a failure to secrete antimicrobial peptides, with resultant bacterial overgrowth in the CF intestine.[21] In the most severe forms, obstruction of gut lumens—meconium ileus—is experienced at birth and the distal intestinal meconium ileus syndrome (DIOS) presents in adults.[22] In the gallbladder, increased mucin concentrations due to decreased volume secretion likely leads to an increased propensity to the formation of gallstones and chronic cholecystitis.[23–27] Finally, in the liver, ductal obstruction can lead to chronic cholestasis inflammation, and ultimately cirrhosis in a small fraction of CF patients.[28–30]

Similar pathophysiologies relate to the reproductive tract in CF. For example, it is likely the vas deferens exerts normally a volume secretory function that moves mucins and proteins through the vas deferens lumens.[31] In CF, the absence of the ability to secrete Cl^- (and volume) into the vas deferens lumen produces a chronic failure to maintain luminal patency and, ultimately the vas deferens becomes atretic, leading to infertility that characterizes more than 99% of male patients with CF. Similarly, the failure to adequately secrete volume via CFTR mechanisms in the oviducts contributes to a reduction in fertility in CF females.[31]

ORGANS AFFECTED BY DECREASED VOLUME, INCREASED MUCIN CONCENTRATIONS, OBSTRUCTION, AND INFECTION

Specific regions of the respiratory tract are affected by the CF constellation of dehydrated surfaces, mucus obstruction, and infection. Typically, the respiratory regions affected in CF are the sinuses in the upper airways and the bronchial airways in the lower lung. The unifying theme for the chronic infection in CF airways is that it represents a "vulnerability" to infection by environmental agents that do not typically produce chronic infections in normal individuals. There are multiple hypotheses linking ion transport abnormalities mediated by CFTR dysfunction to this failure of "host defense" against common environmental agents. These hypotheses can be organized in terms of the normal "multilayering" of innate defense mechanisms that are utilized to keep the lung in a near-sterile state.

ABNORMALITIES OF ANTIMICROBIAL KILLING BY THE AIRWAY SURFACE LIQUIDS THAT LINE SINUS AND BRONCHIAL TREE REGION

The airway secretions are rich in a broad spectrum of antimicrobial proteins, e.g., lactoferrin, lysozyme, antimicrobial peptides, e.g., α/β defensins, LLC-37, and reactive oxygen species that can kill and/or suppress microbial growth for periods. Several scenarios predict a problem with antimicrobial defenses by airway surface liquid (ASL) in CF. First, and probably simplest, is that submucosal glands secrete large quantities of these antimicrobial activities. In CF, gland ducts can be obstructed by mucus due to a reduction in acinar volume secretion and/or inappropriate ductal volume absorption, with a concomitant failure to secrete antimicrobial agents onto airway surfaces.[32,33] Thus, there may be an "obstructive" failure to secrete antimicrobial materials onto airway surfaces. Second, the absence of CFTR dysfunction in the lumen lining epithelial cells produces a failure to secrete bicarbonate onto the airway surface, which produces approximately 0.3–0.5 pH acidification of CF ASL.[34] Recent studies have suggested that this acidification can produce a functional failure of as of yet unidentified antimicrobial peptides to produce short-term killing of bacteria in the CF pig.[35]

It is likely that short-term killing/suppression of bacteria by antimicrobial substances in ASL is important in host defenses. However, it is also likely that this defense mechanism ultimately needs to be complemented by the clearance of bacteria from the lung. Note, the lung is continually exposed to bacteria via inhalation from environmental sources and very likely microaspirations that occur nightly. The notion that ultimately clearance is required to rid the lung of aspirated and/or inhaled bacteria was suggested by the studies of Ganz et al., these investigators noted that antimicrobial activities could suppress bacterial growth for approximately 18 hours in nasal ASL, but after this time, bacteria were selected that were resistant to antimicrobial factors and exhibited exponential growth patterns in normal nasal ASL.[36] Thus, bacterial suppression by antimicrobial factors may be effective for 12–18 hours, but clearance of the remaining/"stunned" bacteria must be accomplished within that time frame to maintain normal lung sterility. Viewed another way, bacteria mutate at a rate for the ability of host phagocytes to clear the airway lumen of infectious agents. For example, host neutrophils normally penetrate, capture, and kill bacteria trapped within normal mucus by moving through the approximately 10-μm mesh to reach intramucus bacteria. In contrast, the mesh size is too small for neutrophils to penetrate mucus to capture and kill chronically infecting bacteria imbedded in CF mucus. This phenomenon has two consequences. First, it greatly limits the ability of the host to clear bacterial infection. Second, the persistent bacterial infection of mucus produces high concentrations of neutrophil chemotaxis agents, drawing neutrophils into the lumen with a persistent "futile" attempt to penetrate the mucin and clear bacteria. This failure to clear the mucus of bacteria produces a persistently high number of neutrophils in the CF lung, e.g., approximately 20 billion at any given point in time, neutrophils that are highly activated and release antimicrobial substances, including elastase. It is the persistent release of active mediators, including elastase, by "frustrated"/activated neutrophils that leads to the airway wall damage that produces the bronchiectasis that ultimately is fatal for CF patients.[33,97]

SUMMARY

In general, CF is a disease caused by epithelial electrolyte transport disturbances in multiple organs. As a general rule, the nature of the electrolyte disturbance can be best analyzed in terms of defective anion transport. The role of anion transport, i.e., to perturb composition or volume, varies on a function of the normal physiology of the affected epithelium and will determine the CF phenotype. With respect to volume regulatory epithelia, CF disease is best analyzed in terms of the interaction of the hydration of the luminal surface and the concentrations of the molecules that "need to be hydrated," i.e., mucins. A critical observation has been that the properties of mucins that cause them to adhere to epithelial surface and block lumens are related to their osmotic pressure, which is a function of the mucin concentration to the third power. Hence, relatively small changes in hydration can produce large changes in mucus adhesive/blocking properties. In particular, in the lung, obstruction of airways with mucins/mucus produces the nidus for the persistent infection and inflammation airway wall damage that characterizes CF. Thus, therapies designed to restore luminal hydration, reduce mucin concentrations, and restore fluid flow are logical for treatment of CF disease. Ultimately, this goal can be best achieved by restoration of mutant CFTR function.

REFERENCES

1. Davis PB. Cystic fibrosis since 1938. *Am J Respir Crit Care Med* 2006; **173**: 475–82.

2. Hug MJ, Clarke LL, Gray MA. How to measure CFTR-dependent bicarbonate transport: From single channels to the intact epithelium. *Methods Mol Biol* 2011; **741**: 489–509.

3. Reznikov LR, Dong Q, Chen JH et al. CFTR-deficient pigs display peripheral nervous system defects at birth. *Proc Natl Acad Sci USA* 2013; **110**(8): 3083–8.

4. Quinton PM. Cystic fibrosis: A disease in electrolyte transport. *FASEB J* 1990; **4**: 2709–17.

5. Sato K, Sato F. Role of calcium in cholinergic and adrenergic mechanisms of eccrine sweat gland secretion. *Am J Physiol* 1981; **241**: C113–C120.

6. Sato K, Sato F. Defective beta adrenergic response of cystic fibrosis sweat glands in vivo and *in vitro*. *J Clin Invest* 1984; **73**: 1763–71.

7. Quinton P, Molyneux L, Ip W et al. Beta-adrenergic sweat secretion as a diagnostic test for cystic fibrosis. *Am J Respir Crit Care Med* 2012; **186**: 732–9.

8. Wilschanski M, Novak I. The CF of Exocrine Pancreas. *Cold Spring Harb Perspect Med* 2013; **3**(5): a009746.

9. Novak I, Greger R. Properties of the luminal membrane of isolated perfused rat pancreatic ducts. Effect of cyclic AMP and blockers of chloride transport. *Pflugers Arch* 1988; **411**: 546–53.

10. Park HW, x Nam JH, Kim JY et al. Dynamic regulation of CFTR bicarbonate permeability by [Cl⁻]i and its role in pancreatic bicarbonate secretion. *Gastroenterology* 2010; **139**: 620–31.

11. Wang J, Haanes KA, Novak I. Purinergic regulation of CFTR and Ca2+-activated Cl⁻ channels and K⁺ channels in human pancreatic duct epithelium. *Am J Physiol Cell Physiol* 2013; **304**(7): C673–84.

12. Ooi CY, Durie PR. Cystic fibrosis transmembrane conductance regulator (CFTR) gene mutations in pancreatitis. *J Cyst Fibros* 2012; **11**: 355–62.

13. Ooi CY, Dorfman R, Cipolli M et al. Type of CFTR mutation determines risk of pancreatitis in patients with cystic fibrosis. *Gastroenterology* 2011; **140**: 153–61.

14. Dashiff C, Suzuki-Crumly J, Kracke B, Britton L, Moreland E. Cystic fibrosis-related diabetes in older adolescents: Parental support and self-management. *J Spec Pediatr Nurs* 2013; **18**: 42–53.

15. Konrad K, Thon A, Fritsch M et al. Comparison of Cystic Fibrosis-Related Diabetes With Type 1 Diabetes Based on a German/Austrian Pediatric Diabetes Registry. *Diabetes Care* 2012; **36**(4): 879–86.

16. Andersen DK. The practical importance of recognizing pancreatogenic or type 3c diabetes. *Diabetes Metab Res Rev* 2012; **28**: 326–8.

17. Borowitz D, Durie PR, Clarke LL et al. Gastrointestinal outcomes and confounders in cystic fibrosis. *J Pediatr Gastroenterol Nutr* 2005; **41**: 273–85.

18. Simpson JE, Gawenis LR, Walker NM, Boyle KT, Clarke LL. Chloride conductance of CFTR facilitates basal Cl⁻/. *Am J Physiol Gastrointest Liver Physiol* 2005; **288**: G1241–G51.

19. Quinton PM. Role of epithelial HCO3(-) transport in mucin secretion: Lessons from cystic fibrosis. *Am J Physiol Cell Physiol* 2010; **299**: C1222–33.

20. Chen EY, Yang N, Quinton PM, Chin WC. A new role for bicarbonate in mucus formation. *Am J.Physiol Lung Cell Mol Physiol* 2010; **299**: L542–L9.

21. Bradford EM, Sartor MA, Gawenis LR, Clarke LL, Shull GE. Reduced NHE3-mediated Na$^+$ absorption increases survival and decreases the incidence of intestinal obstructions in cystic fibrosis mice. *Am J Physiol Gastrointest Liver Physiol* 2009; **296**: G886–G98.

22. Sun L, Rommens JM, Corvol H et al. Multiple apical plasma membrane constituents are associated with susceptibility to meconium ileus in individuals with cystic fibrosis. *Nat Genet* 2012; **44**(5): 562–9.

23. Uc A, Giriyappa R, Meyerholz DK et al. Pancreatic and biliary secretion are both altered in cystic fibrosis pigs. *Am J Physiol Gastrointest Liver Physiol* 2012; **303**: G961–G8.

24. Freudenberg F, Leonard MR, Liu SA, Glickman JN, Carey MC. Pathophysiological preconditions promoting mixed "black" pigment plus cholesterol gallstones in a DeltaF508 mouse model of cystic fibrosis. *Am J Physiol Gastrointest Liver Physiol* 2010; **299**: G205–G24.

25. Lambou-Gianoukos S, Heller SJ. Lithogenesis and bile metabolism. *Surg Clin North Am* 2008; **88**: 1175–94, vii.

26. Sanders NN, Eijsink VG, van den Pangaart PS et al. Mucolytic activity of bacterial and human chitinases. *Biochim Biophys Acta* 2007; **1770**: 839–46.

27. Curry MP, Hegarty JE. The gallbladder and biliary tract in cystic fibrosis. *Curr Gastroenterol Rep* 2005; **7**: 147–53.

28. Rowland M, Gallagher CG, O'Laoide R et al. Outcome in cystic fibrosis liver disease. *Am J Gastroenterol* 2011; **106**: 104–9.

29. Rowland M, Bourke B. Liver disease in cystic fibrosis. *Curr Opin Pulm Med* 2011; **17**: 461–6.

30. Moyer K, BalistreriW. Hepatobiliary disease in patients with cystic fibrosis. *Curr Opin Gastroenterol* 2009; **25**: 272–8.

31. Chan LN, Tsang LL, Rowlands DK, Rochelle LG, Boucher RC, Liu CQ, Chan HC. Distribution and regulation of ENaC subunit and CFTR mRNA expression in murine female reproductive tract. *J Membr Biol* 2002; **185**: 165–76.

32. Ballard ST, Spadafora D. Fluid secretion by submucosal glands of the tracheobronchial airways. *Respir Physiol Neurobiol* 2007; **159**: 271–7.

33. Wine JJ, Joo NS. Submucosal glands and airway defense. *Proc Am Thorac Soc* 2004; **1**: 47–53.

34. Coakley RD, Grubb BR, Paradiso AM, Gatzy JT, Johnson LG, Boucher RC. Abnormal surface liquid pH regulation by cultured cystic fibrosis bronchial epithelium. *Proc Natl Acad Sci USA* 2003; **100**: 16083–8.

35. Pezzulo AA, Tang XX, Hoegger MJ et al. Reduced airway surface pH impairs bacterial killing in the porcine cystic fibrosis lung. *Nature* 2012; **487**: 109–13.

36. Ganz T. Defensins: Antimicrobial peptides of innate immunity. *Nat Rev Immunol* 2003; **3**: 710–20.

37. Deriy LV, Gomez EA, Zhang G et al. Disease-causing mutations in the cystic fibrosis transmembrane conductance regulator determine the functional responses of alveolar macrophages. *J Biol Chem* 2009; **284**: 35926–38.

38. Stick SM, Brennan S, Murray C et al. Bronchiectasis in infants and preschool children diagnosed with cystic fibrosis after newborn screening. *J Pediatr* 2009; **155**: 623–8.

39. Mott LS, Park J, Murray CP et al. Progression of early structural lung disease in young children with cystic fibrosis assessed using CT. *Thorax* 2012; **67**: 509–16.

40. Donaldson SH, Bennett WD, Zeman KL, Knowles MR, Tarran R, Boucher RC. Mucus clearance and lung function in cystic fibrosis with hypertonic saline. *N Engl J Med* 2006; **354**: 241–50.

41. Noone PG, Bennett WD, Regnis JA et al. Effect of aerosolized uridine-5'-triphosphate on airway clearance with cough in patients with primary ciliary dyskinesia. *Am J Respir Crit Care Med* 1999; **160**: 144–9.

42. Noone PG, Leigh MW, Sannuti A et al. Primary ciliary dyskinesia: Diagnostic and phenotypic features. *Am J Respir Crit Care Med* 2004; **169**: 459–67.

43. Boucher RC. Airway surface dehydration in cystic fibrosis: Pathogenesis and therapy. *Annu Rev Med* 2007; **58**: 157–70.

44. Tarran R, Button B, Picher M et al. Normal and cystic fibrosis airway surface liquid homeostasis: The effects of phasic shear stress and viral infections. *J Biol Chem* 2005; **280**: 35751–9.

45. Rossier BC, Stutts MJ. Activation of the epithelial sodium channel (ENaC) by serine proteases. *Annu Rev Physiol* 2009; **71**: 361–79.

46. Myerburg MM, McKenna EE, Luke CJ, Frizzell RA, Kleyman TR, Pilewski JM. Prostasin expression is regulated by airway surface liquid volume and is increased in cystic fibrosis. *Am J Physiol Lung Cell Mol Physiol* 2008; **294**: L932–L41.

47. Myerburg MM, Harvey PR, Heidrich EM, Pilewski JM, Butterworth MB. Acute regulation of the epithelial sodium channel in airway epithelia by proteases and trafficking. *Am J Respir Cell Mol Biol* 2010; **43**: 712–9.

48. Tong Z, Illek B, Bhagwandin VJ, Verghese GM, Caughey GH. Prostasin, a membrane-anchored serine peptidase, regulates sodium currents in JME/CF15 cells, a cystic fibrosis airway epithelial cell line. *Am J Physiol* 2004; **87**: L928–L35.

49. Nimishakavi S, Besprozvannaya M, Raymond WW, Craik CS, Gruenert DC, Caughey GH. Activity and inhibition of prostasin and matriptase on apical and basolateral surfaces of human airway epithelial cells. *Am J Physiol Lung Cell Mol Physiol* 2012; **303**: L97–106.

50. Boucher RC. Human airway ion transport (Part 2). *Am J Respir Crit Care Med* 1994; **150**: 581–93.

51. Gaillard EA, Kota P, Gentzsch M, Dokholyan NV, Stutts MJ, Tarran R. Regulation of the epithelial Na$^+$ channel and airway surface liquid volume by serine proteases. *Pflugers Arch* 2010; **460**: 1–17.

52. Alli AA, Bao HF, Alli AA et al. Phosphatidylinositol phosphate-dependent regulation of Xenopus ENaC by MARCKS protein. *Am J Physiol Renal Physiol* 2012; **303**: F800–F11.

53. Ma HP, Saxena S, Warnock DG. Anionic phospholipids regulate native and expressed epithelial sodium channel (ENaC). *J Biol Chem* 2002; **277**: 7641–4.

54. Mason SJ, Paradiso AM, Boucher RC. Regulation of transepithelial ion transport and intracellular calcium by extracellular adenosine triphosphate in human normal and cystic fibrosis airway epithelium. *Br J Pharmacol* 1991; **103**: 1649–56.

55. Namkung W, Finkbeiner WE, Verkman AS. CFTR-adenylyl cyclase I association responsible for UTP activation of CFTR in well-differentiated primary human bronchial cell cultures. *Mol Biol Cell* 2010; **21**: 2639–48.

56. Randell SH, Boucher RC, the University of North Carolina Virtual Lung Group. Effective mucus clearance is essential for respiratory health. *Am J Respir Cell Mol Biol* 2006; **35**: 20–28.

57. Lazarowski ER, Tarran R, Grubb BR, van Heusden VA, Okada S, Boucher RC. Nucleotide release provides a mechanism for airway surface liquid homeostasis. *J Biol Chem* 2004; **279**: 36855–64.

58. Stutts MJ, Canessa CM, Olsen JC et al. CFTR as a cAMP-dependent regulator of sodium channels. *Science* 1995; **269**: 847–50.

59. Chen JH, Stoltz DA, Karp PH et al. Loss of anion transport without increased sodium absorption characterizes newborn porcine cystic fibrosis airway epithelia. *Cell* 2010; **143**: 911–23.

60. Rogan MP, Reznikov LR, Pezzulo AA et al. Pigs and humans with cystic fibrosis have reduced insulin-like growth factor 1 (IGF1) levels at birth. *Proc Natl Acad Sci USA* 2010; **107**: 20571–5.

61. Boucher RC, Stutts MJ, Knowles MR, Cantley L, Gatzy JT. Na$^+$ transport in cystic fibrosis respiratory epithelia. Abnormal basal rate and response to adenylate cyclase activation. *J Clin Invest* 1986; **78**: 1245–52.

62. Cotton CU, Stutts MJ, Knowles MR, Gatzy JT, Boucher RC. Abnormal apical cell membrane in cystic fibrosis respiratory epithelium. An in vitro electrophysiologic analysis. *J Clin Invest* 1987; **79**: 80–5.

63. Stutts MJ, Knowles MR, Gatzy JT, Boucher RC. Oxygen consumption and ouabain binding sites in cystic fibrosis nasal epithelium. *Pediatr Res* 1986; **20**: 1316–20.

64. Willumsen NJ, Boucher RC. Sodium transport and intracellular sodium activity in cultured human nasal epithelium. *Am J Physiol* 1991; **261**: C319–C31.

65. Willumsen NJ, Boucher. Transcellular sodium transport in cultured cystic fibrosis human nasal epithelium. *Am J Physiol* 1991; **261**: C332–C41.

66. Chinet TC, Fullton JM, Yankaskas JW, Boucher JR, Stutts MJ. Sodium-permeable channels in the apical membrane of human nasal epithelial cells. *Am J Physiol* 1993; **265**: C1050–C60.

67. O'Donoghue DL, Dua V, Moss GW, Vergani P. Increased apical Na$^+$ permeability in cystic fibrosis is supported by a quantitative model of epithelial ion transport. *J Physiol* 2013; **591**: 3681–92.

68. Gentzsch M, Dang H, Dang Y et al. The cystic fibrosis transmembrane conductance regulator impedes proteolytic stimulation of the epithelial Na$^+$ channel. *J Biol Chem* 2010; **285**: 32227–32.

69. Button B, Picher M, Boucher RC. Differential effects of cyclic and constant stress on ATP release and mucociliary transport by human airway epithelia. *J Physiol (Lond.)* 2007; **580**: 577–92.

70. Rand S, Prasad SA. Exercise as part of a cystic fibrosis therapeutic routine. *Expert Rev Respir Med* 2012; **6**: 341–51.

71. Holland AE, Button BM. Physiotherapy for cystic fibrosis in Australia: Knowledge and acceptance of the consensus statement recommendations. *Respirology* 2012; **18**(4): 652–6.

72. Button B, Cai LH, Ehre C et al. A periciliary brush promotes the lung health by separating the mucus layer from airway epithelia. *Science* 2012; **337**: 937–41.

73. Kesimer M, Ehre C, Burns KA, Davis CW, Sheehan JK, Pickles RJ. Molecular organization of the mucins and glycocalyx underlying mucus transport over mucosal surfaces of the airways. *Mucosal Immunol* 2012; **6**(2): 379–92.

74. Goralski JL, Boucher RC, Button B. Osmolytes and ion transport modulators: New strategies for airway surface rehydration. *Curr Opin Pharmacol* 2010; **10**(3): 294–9.

75. Peterson-Carmichael SL, Harris WT, Goel R et al. Association of lower airway inflammation with physiologic findings in young children with cystic fibrosis. *Pediatr Pulmonol* 2009; **44**: 503–11.

76. Bhattacharyya S, Balakathiresan NS, Dalgard C et al. Elevated miR-155 promotes inflammation in cystic fibrosis by driving hyperexpression of interleukin-8. *J Biol Chem* 2011; **286**: 11604–15.

77. Livraghi-Butrico A, Kelly EJ, Klem ER et al. Mucus clearance, MyD88-dependent and MyD88-independent immunity modulate lung susceptibility to spontaneous bacterial infection and inflammation. *Mucosal Immunol* 2012; **5**: 397–408.

78. Mall M, Grubb BR, Harkema JR, O'Neal WK, Boucher RC. Increased airway epithelial Na$^+$ absorption produces cystic fibrosis-like lung disease in mice. *Nat Med* 2004; **10**: 487–93.

79. Mall MA, Harkema JR, Trojanek JB et al. Development of chronic bronchitis and emphysema in beta-epithelial Na$^+$ channel-overexpressing mice. *Am J Respir Crit Care Med* 2008; **177**: 730–42.

80. Wielputz MO, Eichinger M, Zhou Z et al. In vivo monitoring of cystic fibrosis-like lung disease in mice by volumetric computed tomography. *Eur Respir J* 2011; **38**: 1060–70.

81. Livraghi-Butrico A, Grubb AB, Kelly EJ et al. Genetically determined heterogeneity of lung disease in a mouse model of airway mucus obstruction. *Physiol Genomics* 2012; **44**: 470–84.

82. Livraghi A, Grubb BR, Hudson EJ et al. Airway and lung pathology due to mucosal surface dehydration in β-epithelial Na+ channel-overexpressing mice: Role of TNF-α and IL-4Rα signaling, influence of neonatal development, and limited efficacy of glucocorticoid treatment. *J Immunol* 2009; **182**: 4357–67.

83. Worlitzsch D, Tarran R, Ulrich M et al. Effects of reduced mucus oxygen concentration in airway Pseudomonas infections of cystic fibrosis patients. *J Clin Invest* 2002; **109**: 317–25.

84. Van LA, Eltzschig HK. Role of pulmonary adenosine during hypoxia: extracellular generation, signaling and metabolism by surface adenosine deaminase/CD26. *Expert Opin Biol Ther* 2007; **7**: 1437–47.

85. Koeppen M, Eckle T, Eltzschig HK. Interplay of hypoxia and A2B adenosine receptors in tissue protection. *Adv Pharmacol* 2011; **61**: 145–86.

86. Grenz A, Homann D, Eltzschig HK. Extracellular adenosine: a safety signal that dampens hypoxia-induced inflammation during ischemia. *Antioxid Redox Signal* 2011; **15**: 2221–34.

87. Eltzschig HK, Thompson LF, Karhausen J et al. Endogenous adenosine produced during hypoxia attenuates neutrophil accumulation: Coordination by extracellular nucleotide metabolism. *Blood* 2004; **104**: 3986–92.

88. Yoon SS, Coakley R, Lau GW et al. Anaerobic killing of mucoid Pseudomonas aeruginosa by acidified nitrite derivatives under cystic fibrosis airway conditions. *J Clin Invest* 116: 436–46.

89. Tunney MM, Field TR, Moriarty TF et al. Detection of anaerobic bacteria in high numbers in sputum from patients with cystic fibrosis. *Am J Respir Crit Care Med* 2008; **177**: 995–1001.

90. Tunney MM, Klem EM, Fodor AA et al. Use of culture and molecular analysis to determine the effect of antibiotic treatment on microbial community diversity and abundance during exacerbation in patients with cystic fibrosis. *Thorax* 2011; **66**: 579–84.

91. Fodor AA, Klem ER, Gilpin DF, Elborn JS, Boucher RC, Tunney MM, Wolfgang MC. The adult cystic fibrosis airway microbiota is stable over time and infection type, and highly resilient to antibiotic treatment of exacerbations. *PLoS One* 2012; **7**: e45001.

92. Bartlett JG. Anaerobic bacterial infection of the lung. *Anaerobe* 2012; **18**: 235–9.

93. Bartlett JG. The role of anaerobic bacteria in lung abscess. *Clin Infect Dis* 2005; **40**: 923–5.

94. Singh PK, Parsek MR, Greenberg EP, Welsh MJ. A component of innate immunity prevents bacterial biofilm development. *Nature* 2002; **417**: 552–5.

95. Matsui H, Wagner VE, Hill DB et al. A physical linkage between CF airway surface dehydration and *P. aeruginosa* biofilms. *Proc Natl Acad Sci USA* 2006; **103**: 18131–6.

96. Kavanaugh NL, Ribbeck K. Selected antimicrobial essential oils eradicate Pseudomonas spp. and *Staphylococcus aureus* biofilms. *Appl Environ Microbiol* 2012; **78**: 4057–61.

97. Vandivier RW, Fadok VA, Hoffmann PR et al. Elastase-mediated phosphatidylserine receptor cleavage impairs apoptotic cell clearance in cystic fibrosis and bronchiectasis. *J Clin Invest* 2002; **109**: 661–70.

6

What have we learned from animal models?

UTA GRIESENBACH AND ERIC W.F.W. ALTON

CYSTIC FIBROSIS MOUSE MODELS

A couple of years after the cloning of the human cystic fibrosis transmembrane conductance regulator gene (CFTR), the first cystic fibrosis (CF) mouse had been generated[1] using molecular techniques to "knockout" *Cftr* expression. Today, a large number of CF mouse models are available (see later). CF knockout mice do not spontaneously develop CF-like lung disease, but have been useful to highlight a number of important points including (1) showing a strong correlation between residual *Cftr* expression and survival based on gut disease, (2) highlighting the importance of strain differences and thereby the potential effect of modifier genes, and more recently (3) allowing the dissection of Cftr effects in individual tissues and cell types using the conditional Cftr knock-in and knockout mouse models.

STANDARD EMBRYONIC STEM CELL TECHNOLOGY IS USED TO GENERATE CF KNOCKOUT MICE

To generate CF mouse models, the *Cftr* locus is modified in mouse embryonic stem (ES) cells using a well-established method based on interaction (homologous recombination) between an exogenous piece of DNA (the targeting vector) and a specific region within the *Cftr* gene. An appropriate target cell clone is then identified using molecular biology techniques, expanded and injected into early mouse blastocysts (Figure 6.1a). The blastocysts are reimplanted into female recipients and contribute to the developing embryo. Importantly, blastocysts and ES cells are derived from mice with different coat colors, and chimeric offsprings can easily be recognized (Figure 6.1b) and used for subsequent breeding steps to generate homozygote CF mice.

GUT DISEASE SEVERITY IS VARIABLE

Since cloning of the *CFTR* gene in 1989, a large number of Cftr-modified mice has been generated by either attempting to abolish Cftr mRNA expression ("null" animals) or by introducing a naturally occurring mutation such as ΔF508, G551D, or R117H.[2] Most of these animals suffer from intestinal disease (the most pronounced phenotype in CF mice, see below for more detailed description) often leading to premature death. However, gut disease severity varies and this provides valuable information.

1. In some Cftr "null" mice, the targeting strategy did not "knockout" Cftr mRNA completely (leaky mutations), but lead to retention of approximately 2%,[3] 5%,[4] or 10%[5] of residual CFTR function. Importantly, there was a strong correlation between gut disease severity and survival, and the amount of residual Cftr expression (Table 6.1). These data indicate that a low level (~5%) of residual Cftr expression (in each cell) significantly ameliorates CF gut disease, thereby providing a benchmark for the development of new treatments such as gene therapy, assuming that the results of gene therapy in the gut predict that in other organs.
2. The first nucleotide-binding fold, which includes amino acid 508, is very well conserved between mouse and man. However, mice carrying the ΔF508 mutation (Cftr[tm1Eur]) only have mild gut disease implying that in mice the mutant ΔF508 protein retains sufficient activity to ameliorate intestinal disease.[2,6]
3. Mice carrying the "mild" mutation R117H, which is associated with mild pancreatic disease in man, also had milder intestinal disease[7] thereby replicating the human genotype–phenotype correlation.

85

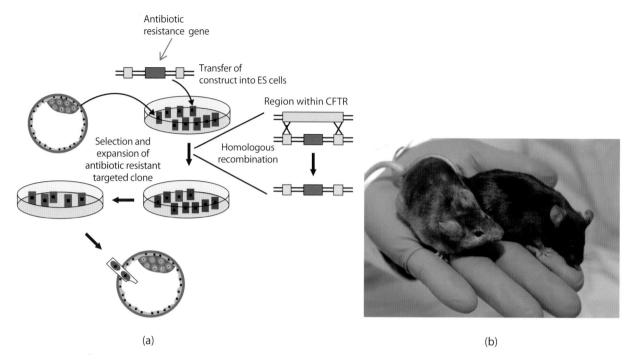

(a) (b)

Figure 6.1 Generation of CF knockout mice. (a) The murine *Cftr* locus is modified in mouse embryonic stem (ES) cells using a well-established method based on homologous recombination between an exogenous piece of DNA (the targeting vector, generally carrying a selectable marker such as the neomycin-resistance gene to help with selective amplification of modified cells) and a specific region within the *Cftr* gene. An appropriate target cell clone is then identified using molecular biology techniques, expanded and injected into early mouse blastocysts. The blastocysts are reimplanted into female recipients and contribute to the developing embryo. (b) Blastocysts and ES cells are derived from mice with different coat colors and chimeric off-spring (multicolored mouse in the left of the picture) can easily be recognized and used for subsequent breeding steps to generate homozygote CF mice.

Table 6.1 Comparison of residual Cftr expression and survival in different strains of CF knockout mice

Mouse strain	Residual Cftr expression (%)	Survival to maturity (%)	Reference
Cftr[tm1Unc]/Cftr[tm1Unc]	0	<5	1
Cftr[tm1Bay]/Cftr[tm1Bay]	2	~40	3
Cftr[tm1Bay]/Cftr[tm1Hgu]	5	~100	4
Cftr[tm1Hgu]/Cftr[tm1Hgu]	10	~100	5

CF MICE REPLICATE THE CF PHENOTYPE IN SOME ORGANS, BUT NOT IN OTHERS

As mentioned above, intestinal disease caused by mucus obstruction followed by perforation and peritonitis is the most prominent phenotype in CF mice and the leading cause of premature mortality in these animals. In general, the bioelectric properties in the gut (cAMP-mediated chloride secretion) correlate with the amount of residual Cftr function and it has therefore been suggested that the occurrence of gut disease in mice also reflects a defect in ion and water transport.[2]

Rozmahel et al. showed that gut disease severity had a genetic component by comparing survival and demonstrating differences in different strains of mice, carrying the same CF mutation.[8] The group identified a locus on mouse chromosome 7 that may be implicated. This study was followed by human studies aimed at identifying modifier genes implicated in the occurrence of meconium ileus (MI)[9–11]; and has recently led to identification of several potential loci in genome-wide association study.[11]

In contrast to man, mice do not develop significant pancreatic disease, possibly due to an overall lower expression of Cftr in murine pancreas, and/or the presence of alternative calcium-mediated chloride channels,[12] which can substitute for Cftr-mediated chloride secretion. However, despite unimpaired exocrine pancreatic function, ΔF508 mice have less adipose tissue due to altered hepatic lipogenesis when compared to their non-CF littermates.[13] The authors suggest that the latter is independent of malabsorption, and may partly explain why pancreatic enzyme replacement therapy is unable to completely restore normal body mass in CF patients. In contrast to man, male CF mice do have a normal vas deferens and are therefore fertile. Studies in CF mice also indicated delayed puberty[14] and showed that sperm transport in female mice was impaired.[15] In addition,

60. McKeon DJ, Condliffe AM, Cowburn AS et al. Prolonged survival of neutrophils from patients with Delta F508 CFTR mutations. *Thorax* 2008; **63**(7): 660–1.

61. Moriceau S, Kantari C, Mocek J et al. Coronin-1 is associated with neutrophil survival and is cleaved during apoptosis: Potential implication in neutrophils from cystic fibrosis patients. *J Immunol* 2009; **182**(11): 7254–63.

62. Moriceau S, Lenoir G, Witko-Sarsat V. In cystic fibrosis homozygotes and heterozygotes, neutrophil apoptosis is delayed and modulated by diamide or roscovitine: Evidence for an innate neutrophil disturbance. *J Innate Immun* 2010; **2**(3): 260–6.

63. Keel M, Ungethum U, Steckholzer U et al. Interleukin-10 counterregulates proinflammatory cytokine-induced inhibition of neutrophil apoptosis during severe sepsis. *Blood* 1997; **90**(9): 3356–63.

64. Mercer-Jones MA, Heinzelmann M, Peyton JC, Wickel D, Cook M, Cheadle WG. Inhibition of neutrophil migration at the site of infection increases remote organ neutrophil sequestration and injury. *Shock* 1997; **8**(3): 193–9.

65. Jungas T, Motta I, Duffieux F, Fanen P, Stoven V, Ojcius DM. Glutathione levels and BAX activation during apoptosis due to oxidative stress in cells expressing wild-type and mutant cystic fibrosis transmembrane conductance regulator. *J Biol Chem* 2002; **277**(31): 27912–8.

66. Bianchi SM, Prince LR, McPhillips K et al. Impairment of apoptotic cell engulfment by pyocyanin, a toxic metabolite of *Pseudomonas aeruginosa*. *Am J Respir Crit Care Med* 2008; **177**(1): 35–43.

67. Sagel SD, Chmiel JF, Konstan MW. Sputum biomarkers of inflammation in cystic fibrosis lung disease. *Proc Am Thorac Soc* 2007; **4**(4): 406–17.

68. Greene CM. How can we target pulmonary inflammation in cystic fibrosis? *Open Respir Med J* 2010; **4**: 18–9.

69. Bergin DA, Greene CM, Sterchi EE et al. Activation of the epidermal growth factor receptor (EGFR) by a novel metalloprotease pathway. *J Biol Chem* 2008; **283**(46): 31736–44.

70. Bergsson G, Reeves EP, McNally P et al. LL-37 complexation with glycosaminoglycans in cystic fibrosis lungs inhibits antimicrobial activity, which can be restored by hypertonic saline. *J Immunol* 2009; **183**(1): 543–51.

71. Roum JH, Buhl R, McElvaney NG, Borok Z, Crystal RG. Systemic deficiency of glutathione in cystic fibrosis. *J Appl Physiol* 1993; **75**(6): 2419–24.

72. Kelly E, Greene CM, McElvaney NG. Targeting neutrophil elastase in cystic fibrosis. *Expert Opin Ther Targets* 2008; **12**(2): 145–57.

73. Geraghty P, Rogan MP, Greene CM et al. Neutrophil elastase up-regulates cathepsin B and matrix metalloprotease-2 expression. *J Immunol* 2007; **178**(9): 5871–8.

74. Weldon S, McNally P, McElvaney NG et al. Decreased levels of secretory leucoprotease inhibitor in the pseudomonas-infected cystic fibrosis lung are due to neutrophil elastase degradation. *J Immunol* 2009; **183**(12): 8148–56.

75. Brinkmann V, Reichard U, Goosmann C et al. Neutrophil extracellular traps kill bacteria. *Science* 2004; **303**(5663): 1532–5.

76. Buchanan JT, Simpson AJ, Aziz RK et al. DNase expression allows the pathogen group A Streptococcus to escape killing in neutrophil extracellular traps. *Curr Biol* 2006; **16**(4): 396–400.

77. Wartha F, Beiter K, Albiger B et al. Capsule and D-alanylated lipoteichoic acids protect *Streptococcus pneumoniae* against neutrophil extracellular traps. *Cell Microbiol* 2007; **9**(5): 1162–71.

78. Witko-Sarsat V, Halbwachs-Mecarelli L, Schuster A et al. Proteinase 3, a potent secretagogue in airways, is present in cystic fibrosis sputum. *Am J Respir Cell Mol Biol* 1999; **20**(4): 729–36.

79. Goldstein W, Doring G. Lysosomal enzymes from polymorphonuclear leukocytes and proteinase inhibitors in patients with cystic fibrosis. *Am Rev Respir Dis* 1986; **134**(1): 49–56.

80. Ferry G, Lonchampt M, Pennel L, de Nanteuil G, Canet E, Tucker GC. Activation of MMP-9 by neutrophil elastase in an in vivo model of acute lung injury. *FEBS Lett* 1997; **402**(2–3): 111–5.

81. Imai K, Yokohama Y, Nakanishi I et al. Matrix metalloproteinase 7 (matrilysin) from human rectal carcinoma cells. Activation of the precursor, interaction with other matrix metalloproteinases and enzymic properties. *J Biol Chem* 1995; **270**(12): 6691–7.

82. Shamamian P, Schwartz JD, Pocock BJ et al. Activation of progelatinase A (MMP-2) by neutrophil elastase, cathepsin G, and proteinase-3: A role for inflammatory cells in tumor invasion and angiogenesis. *J Cell Physiol* 2001; **189**(2): 197–206.

83. Dalet-Fumeron V, Guinec N, Pagano M. In vitro activation of pro-cathepsin B by three serine proteinases: Leucocyte elastase, cathepsin G, and the urokinase-type plasminogen activator. *FEBS Lett* 1993; **332**(3): 251–4.

84. Kohri K, Ueki IF, Nadel JA. Neutrophil elastase induces mucin production by ligand-dependent epidermal growth factor receptor activation. *Am J Physiol Lung Cell Mol Physiol* 2002; **283**(3): L531–40.

85. Devaney JM, Greene CM, Taggart CC, Carroll TP, O'Neill SJ, McElvaney NG. Neutrophil elastase up-regulates interleukin-8 via toll-like receptor 4. *FEBS Lett* 2003; **544**(1–3): 129–32.

86. Nakamura H, Yoshimura K, McElvaney NG, Crystal RG. Neutrophil elastase in respiratory epithelial lining fluid of individuals with cystic fibrosis induces interleukin-8 gene expression in a human bronchial epithelial cell line. *J Clin Invest* 1992; **89**(5): 1478–84.

87. Shao MX, Nadel JA. Dual oxidase 1-dependent MUC5AC mucin expression in cultured human airway epithelial cells. *Proc Natl Acad Sci USA* 2005; **102**(3): 767–72.

88. Shao MX, Nadel JA. Neutrophil elastase induces MUC5AC mucin production in human airway epithelial cells via a cascade involving protein kinase C, reactive oxygen species, and TNF-alpha-converting enzyme. *J Immunol* 2005; **175**(6): 4009–16.

89. Walsh DE, Greene CM, Carroll TP et al. Interleukin-8 up-regulation by neutrophil elastase is mediated by MyD88/IRAK/TRAF-6 in human bronchial epithelium. *J Biol Chem* 2001; **276**(38): 35494–9.

90. Cooley J, Takayama TK, Shapiro SD, Schechter NM, Remold-O'Donnell E. The serpin MNEI inhibits elastase-like and chymotrypsin-like serine proteases through efficient reactions at two active sites. *Biochemistry* 2001; **40**(51): 15762–70.

91. Rawlings ND, Tolle DP, Barrett AJ. Evolutionary families of peptidase inhibitors. *Biochem J* 2004; **378**(Pt 3): 705–16.

92. Huovila AP, Turner AJ, Pelto-Huikko M, Karkkainen I, Ortiz RM. Shedding light on ADAM metalloproteinases. *Trends Biochem Sci* 2005; **30**(7): 413–22.

93. Travis J, Owen M, George P et al. Isolation and properties of recombinant DNA produced variants of human alpha 1-proteinase inhibitor. *J Biol Chem* 1985; **260**(7): 4384–9.

94. Rogers J, Kalsheker N, Wallis S et al. The isolation of a clone for human alpha 1-antitrypsin and the detection of alpha 1-antitrypsin in mRNA from liver and leukocytes. *Biochem Biophys Res Commun* 1983; **116**(2): 375–82.

95. Molmenti EP, Perlmutter DH, Rubin DC. Cell-specific expression of alpha 1-antitrypsin in human intestinal epithelium. *J Clin Invest* 1993; **92**(4): 2022–34.

96. Cichy J, Potempa J, Travis J. Biosynthesis of alpha1-proteinase inhibitor by human lung-derived epithelial cells. *J Biol Chem* 1997; **272**(13): 8250–5.

97. Hu C, Perlmutter DH. Cell-specific involvement of HNF-1beta in alpha(1)-antitrypsin gene expression in human respiratory epithelial cells. *Am J Physiol Lung Cell Mol Physiol* 2002; **282**(4): L757–65.

98. Mason DY, Cramer EM, Masse JM, Crystal R, Bassot JM, Breton-Gorius J. Alpha 1-antitrypsin is present within the primary granules of human polymorphonuclear leukocytes. *Am J Pathol* 1991; **139**(3): 623–8.

99. Mulgrew AT, Taggart CC, Lawless MW et al. Z alpha1-antitrypsin polymerizes in the lung and acts as a neutrophil chemoattractant. *Chest* 2004; **125**(5): 1952–7.

100. Venembre P, Boutten A, Seta N et al. Secretion of alpha 1-antitrypsin by alveolar epithelial cells. *FEBS Lett* 1994; **346**(2–3): 171–4.

101. Bergin DA, Reeves EP, Meleady P et al. alpha-1 Antitrypsin regulates human neutrophil chemotaxis induced by soluble immune complexes and IL-8. *J Clin Invest* 2010; **120**(12): 4236–50.

102. Churg A, Wang RD, Xie C, Wright JL. alpha-1-Antitrypsin ameliorates cigarette smoke-induced emphysema in the mouse. *Am J Respir Crit Care Med* 2003; **168**(2): 199–207.

103. Daemen MA, Heemskerk VH, van't Veer C et al. Functional protection by acute phase proteins alpha(1)-acid glycoprotein and alpha(1)-antitrypsin against ischemia/reperfusion injury by preventing apoptosis and inflammation. *Circulation* 2000; **102**(12): 1420–6.

104. Ikari Y, Mulvihill E, Schwartz SM. alpha 1-Proteinase inhibitor, alpha 1-antichymotrypsin, and alpha 2-macroglobulin are the antiapoptotic factors of vascular smooth muscle cells. *J Biol Chem* 2001; **276**(15): 11798–803.

105. Ikebe N, Akaike T, Miyamoto Y et al. Protective effect of S-nitrosylated alpha(1)-protease inhibitor on hepatic ischemia-reperfusion injury. *J Pharmacol Exp Ther* 2000; **295**(3): 904–11.

106. Johnson DA, Barrett AJ, Mason RW. Cathepsin L inactivates alpha 1-proteinase inhibitor by cleavage in the reactive site region. *J Biol Chem* 1986; **261**(31): 14748–51.

107. Morihara K, Tsuzuki H, Harada M, Iwata T. Purification of human plasma alpha 1-proteinase inhibitor and its inactivation by *Pseudomonas aeruginosa* elastase. *J Biochem* 1984; **95**(3): 795–804.

108. Doumas S, Kolokotronis A, Stefanopoulos P. Anti-inflammatory and antimicrobial roles of secretory leukocyte protease inhibitor. *Infect Immun* 2005; **73**(3): 1271–4.

109. Mc Elvaney NG, Crystal RG (Eds). *The Lung*. New York, NY: Lippincott-Raven; 1997

110. Wiedow O, Harder J, Bartels J, Streit V, Christophers E. Antileukoprotease in human skin: An antibiotic peptide constitutively produced by keratinocytes. *Biochem Biophys Res Commun* 1998; **248**(3): 904–9.

111. Williams SE, Brown TI, Roghanian A, Sallenave JM. SLPI and elafin: One glove, many fingers. *Clin Sci (Lond)* 2006; **110**(1): 21–35.

112. Zhang Y, DeWitt DL, McNeely TB, Wahl SM, Wahl LM. Secretory leukocyte protease inhibitor suppresses the production of monocyte prostaglandin H synthase-2, prostaglandin E2, and matrix metalloproteinases. *J Clin Invest* 1997; **99**(5): 894–900.

113. Geraghty P, Greene CM, O'Mahony M, O'Neill SJ, Taggart CC, McElvaney NG. Secretory leucocyte protease inhibitor inhibits interferon-gamma-induced cathepsin S expression. *J Biol Chem* 2007; **282**(46): 33389–95.

114. Ding A, Thieblemont N, Zhu J, Jin F, Zhang J, Wright S. Secretory leukocyte protease inhibitor interferes with uptake of lipopolysaccharide by macrophages. *Infect Immun* 1999; **67**(9): 4485–9.

115. Jin FY, Nathan C, Radzioch D, Ding A. Secretory leukocyte protease inhibitor: A macrophage product induced by and antagonistic to bacterial lipopolysaccharide. *Cell* 1997; **88**(3): 417–26.

116. McNeely TB, Shugars DC, Rosendahl M, Tucker C, Eisenberg SP, Wahl SM. Inhibition of human immunodeficiency virus type 1 infectivity by secretory leukocyte protease inhibitor occurs prior to viral reverse transcription. *Blood* 1997; **90**(3): 1141–9.

117. Greene CM, McElvaney NG, O'Neill SJ, Taggart CC. Secretory leucoprotease inhibitor impairs Toll-like receptor 2- and 4-mediated responses in monocytic cells. *Infect Immun* 2004; **72**(6): 3684–7.

118. Taggart CC, Greene CM, McElvaney NG, O'Neill S. Secretory leucoprotease inhibitor prevents lipopolysaccharide-induced IkappaBalpha degradation without affecting phosphorylation or ubiquitination. *J Biol Chem* 2002; **277**(37): 33648–53.

119. Sagel SD, Wagner BD, Anthony MM, Emmett P, Zemanick ET. Sputum biomarkers of inflammation and lung function decline in children with cystic fibrosis. *Am J Respir Crit Care Med* 2012; **186**(9): 857–65.

120. Zani ML, Tanga A, Saidi A et al. SLPI and trappin-2 as therapeutic agents to target airway serine proteases in inflammatory lung diseases: Current and future directions. *Biochem Soc Trans* 2011; **39**(5): 1441–6.

121. Alkemade JA, Molhuizen HO, Ponec M et al. SKALP/elafin is an inducible proteinase inhibitor in human epidermal keratinocytes. *J Cell Sci* 1994; **107** (Pt 8): 2335–42.

122. Nonomura K, Yamanishi K, Yasuno H, Nara K, Hirose S. Up-regulation of elafin/SKALP gene expression in psoriatic epidermis. *J Invest Dermatol* 1994; **103**(1): 88–91.

123. Pfundt R, van Ruissen F, van Vlijmen-Willems IM et al. Constitutive and inducible expression of SKALP/elafin provides anti-elastase defense in human epithelia. *J Clin Invest* 1996; **98**(6): 1389–99.

124. Sallenave JM, Shulmann J, Crossley J, Jordana M, Gauldie J. Regulation of secretory leukocyte proteinase inhibitor (SLPI) and elastase-specific inhibitor (ESI/elafin) in human airway epithelial cells by cytokines and neutrophilic enzymes. *Am J Respir Cell Mol Biol* 1994; **11**(6): 733–41.

125. van Wetering S, van der Linden AC, van Sterkenburg MA et al. Regulation of SLPI and elafin release from bronchial epithelial cells by neutrophil defensins. *Am J Physiol Lung Cell Mol Physiol* 2000; **278**(1): L51–8.

126. Hochstrasser K, Albrecht GJ, Schonberger OL, Rasche B, Lempart K. An elastase-specific inhibitor from human bronchial mucus. Isolation and characterization. *Hoppe Seylers Z Physiol Chem* 1981; **362**(10): 1369–75.

127. Wiedow O, Luademann J, Utecht B. Elafin is a potent inhibitor of proteinase 3. *Biochem Biophys Res Commun* 1991; **174**(1): 6–10.

128. Reid PT, Marsden ME, Cunningham GA, Haslett C, Sallenave JM. Human neutrophil elastase regulates the expression and secretion of elafin (elastase-specific inhibitor) in type II alveolar epithelial cells. *FEBS Lett* 1999; **457**(1): 33–7.

129. Simpson AJ, Cunningham GA, Porteous DJ, Haslett C, Sallenave JM. Regulation of adenovirus-mediated elafin transgene expression by bacterial lipopolysaccharide. *Hum Gene Ther* 2001; **12**(11): 1395–406.

130. Simpson AJ, Maxwell AI, Govan JR, Haslett C, Sallenave JM. Elafin (elastase-specific inhibitor) has anti-microbial activity against gram-positive and gram-negative respiratory pathogens. *FEBS Lett* 1999; **452**(3): 309–13.

131. Guyot N, Butler MW, McNally P et al. Elafin, an elastase-specific inhibitor, is cleaved by its cognate enzyme neutrophil elastase in sputum from individuals with cystic fibrosis. *J Biol Chem* 2008; **283**(47): 32377–85.

132. Jin F, Nathan CF, Radzioch D, Ding A. Lipopolysaccharide-related stimuli induce expression of the secretory leukocyte protease inhibitor, a macrophage-derived lipopolysaccharide inhibitor. *Infect Immun* 1998; **66**(6): 2447–52.

133. Guyot N, Zani ML, Berger P, Dallet-Choisy S, Moreau T. Proteolytic susceptibility of the serine protease inhibitor trappin-2 (pre-elafin): Evidence for tryptase-mediated generation of elafin. *Biol Chem* 2005; **386**(4): 391–9.

134. Butler MW, Robertson I, Greene CM, O'Neill SJ, Taggart CC, McElvaney NG. Elafin prevents lipopolysaccharide-induced AP-1 and NF-kappaB activation via an effect on the ubiquitin-proteasome pathway. *J Biol Chem* 2006; **281**(46): 34730–5.

135. Rogan MP, Geraghty P, Greene CM, O'Neill SJ, Taggart CC, McElvaney NG. Antimicrobial proteins and polypeptides in pulmonary innate defence. *Respir Res* 2006; **7**: 29.

136. Ganz T. Defensins: Antimicrobial peptides of innate immunity. *Nat Rev Immunol* 2003; **3**(9): 710–20.

137. Smith JJ, Travis SM, Greenberg EP, Welsh MJ. Cystic fibrosis airway epithelia fail to kill bacteria because of abnormal airway surface fluid. *Cell* 1996; **85**(2): 229–36.

138. Goldman MJ, Anderson GM, Stolzenberg ED, Kari UP, Zasloff M, Wilson JM. Human beta-defensin-1 is a salt-sensitive antibiotic in lung that is inactivated in cystic fibrosis. *Cell* 1997; **88**(4): 553–60.

139. Bals R, Weiner DJ, Meegalla RL, Accurso F, Wilson JM. Salt-independent abnormality of antimicrobial activity in cystic fibrosis airway surface fluid. *Am J Respir Cell Mol Biol* 2001; **25**(1): 21–5.

140. Taggart CC, Greene CM, Smith SG et al. Inactivation of human beta-defensins 2 and 3 by elastolytic cathepsins. *J Immunol* 2003; **171**(2): 931–7.

141. Felgentreff K, Beisswenger C, Griese M, Gulder T, Bringmann G, Bals R. The antimicrobial peptide cathelicidin interacts with airway mucus. *Peptides* 2006; **27**(12): 3100–6.

142. Chen CI, Schaller-Bals S, Paul KP, Wahn U, Bals R. Beta-defensins and LL-37 in bronchoalveolar lavage fluid of patients with cystic fibrosis. *J Cyst Fibro* 2004; **3**(1): 45–50.

143. Yim S, Dhawan P, Ragunath C, Christakos S, Diamond G. Induction of cathelicidin in normal and CF bronchial epithelial cells by 1,25-dihydroxyvitamin D(3). *J Cyst Fibro* 2007; **6**(6): 403–10.

144. Weiner DJ, Bucki R, Janmey PA. The antimicrobial activity of the cathelicidin LL37 is inhibited by F-actin bundles and restored by gelsolin. *Am J Respir Cell Mol Biol* 2003; **28**(6): 738–45.

145. Bucki R, Byfield FJ, Janmey PA. Release of the antimicrobial peptide LL-37 from DNA/F-actin bundles in cystic fibrosis sputum. *Eur Respir J.* 2007; **29**(4): 624–32.

146. Reeves EP, Bergin DA, Murray MA, McElvaney NG. The involvement of glycosaminoglycans in airway disease associated with cystic fibrosis. ScientificWorldJournal 2011; **11**: 959–71.

147. Reeves EP, Williamson M, O'Neill SJ, Greally P, McElvaney NG. Nebulized hypertonic saline decreases IL-8 in sputum of patients with cystic fibrosis. *Am J Respir Crit Care Med* 2011; **183**(11): 1517–23.

148. Singh PK, Parsek MR, Greenberg EP, Welsh MJ. A component of innate immunity prevents bacterial biofilm development. *Nature* 2002; **417**(6888): 552–5.

149. Travis SM, Conway BA, Zabner J et al. Activity of abundant antimicrobials of the human airway. *Am J Respir Cell Mol Biol* 1999; **20**(5): 872–9.

150. Harmsen MC, Swart PJ, de Bethune MP et al. Antiviral effects of plasma and milk proteins: Lactoferrin shows potent activity against both human immunodeficiency virus and human cytomegalovirus replication in vitro. *J Infect Dis* 1995; **172**(2): 380–8.

151. Beljaars L, van der Strate BW, Bakker HI et al. Inhibition of cytomegalovirus infection by lactoferrin in vitro and in vivo. *Antiviral Res* 2004; **63**(3): 197–208.

152. Shin K, Wakabayashi H, Yamauchi K et al. Effects of orally administered bovine lactoferrin and lactoperoxidase on influenza virus infection in mice. *J Med Microbiol* 2005; **54**(Pt 8): 717–23.

153. Soukka T, Tenovuo J, Lenander-Lumikari M. Fungicidal effect of human lactoferrin against *Candida albicans*. *FEMS Microbiol Lett* 1992; **69**(3): 223–8.

154. Baveye S, Elass E, Mazurier J, Spik G, Legrand D. Lactoferrin: A multifunctional glycoprotein involved in the modulation of the inflammatory process. *Clin Chem Lab Med* 1999; **37**(3): 281–6.

155. Conneely OM. Antiinflammatory activities of lactoferrin. *J Am Coll Nutr* 2001; **20**(Suppl 5): 389S–95S.

156. Baveye S, Elass E, Fernig DG, Blanquart C, Mazurier J, Legrand D. Human lactoferrin interacts with soluble CD14 and inhibits expression of endothelial adhesion molecules, E-selectin and ICAM-1, induced by the CD14-lipopolysaccharide complex. *Infect Immun* 2000; **68**(12): 6519–25.

157. Britigan BE, Lewis TS, Waldschmidt M, McCormick ML, Krieg AM. Lactoferrin binds CpG-containing oligonucleotides and inhibits their immunostimulatory effects on human B cells. *J Immunol* 2001; **167**(5): 2921–8.

158. Rogan MP, Taggart CC, Greene CM, Murphy PG, O'Neill SJ, McElvaney NG. Loss of microbicidal activity and increased formation of biofilm due to decreased lactoferrin activity in patients with cystic fibrosis. *J Infect Dis* 2004; **190**(7): 1245–53.

159. Fett JW, Strydom DJ, Lobb RR et al. Lysozyme: A major secretory product of a human colon carcinoma cell line. *Biochemistry* 1985; **24**(4): 965–75.

160. Skerrett SJ, Liggitt HD, Hajjar AM, Wilson CB. Cutting edge: Myeloid differentiation factor 88 is essential for pulmonary host defense against *Pseudomonas aeruginosa* but not *Staphylococcus aureus*. *J Immunol* 2004; **172**(6): 3377–81.

161. Cheung DO, Halsey K, Speert DP. Role of pulmonary alveolar macrophages in defense of the lung against *Pseudomonas aeruginosa*. *Infect Immun* 2000; **68**(8): 4585–92.

162. Ojielo CI, Cooke K, Mancuso P et al. Defective phagocytosis and clearance of *Pseudomonas aeruginosa* in the lung following bone marrow transplantation. *J Immunol* 2003; **171**(8): 4416–24.

163. Hauschildt S, Kleine B. Bacterial stimulators of macrophages. *Int Rev Cytol* 1995; **161**: 263–331.

164. Bruscia EM, Zhang PX, Ferreira E et al. Macrophages directly contribute to the exaggerated inflammatory response in cystic fibrosis transmembrane conductance regulator -/- mice. *Am J Respir Cell Mol Biol* 2009; **40**(3): 295–304.

165. Tan HL, Regamey N, Brown S, Bush A, Lloyd CM, Davies JC. The Th17 pathway in cystic fibrosis lung disease. *Am J Respir Crit Care Med* 2011; **184**(2): 252–8.

166. Tiringer K, Treis A, Fucik P et al. A Th17- and Th2-skewed cytokine profile in cystic fibrosis lungs represents a potential risk factor for *Pseudomonas aeruginosa* infection. *Am J Respir Crit Care Med* 2013; **187**(6): 621–9.

167. Iannitti RG, Carvalho A, Cunha C, De Luca A, Giovannini G, Casagrande A, et al. Th17/Treg imbalance in murine cystic fibrosis is linked to indoleamine 2,3-dioxygenase deficiency but corrected by kynurenines. *Am J Respir Crit Care Med.* 2013; **187**(6): 609–20. doi: 10.1164/rccm.201207-1346OC. Epub 2013 Jan 10.

168. Bals R, Wang X, Wu Z et al. Human beta-defensin 2 is a salt-sensitive peptide antibiotic expressed in human lung. *J Clin Invest* 1998; **102**(5): 874–80.

169. Tager AM, Wu J, Vermeulen MW. The effect of chloride concentration on human neutrophil functions: Potential relevance to cystic fibrosis. *Am J Respir Cell Mol Biol* 1998; **19**(4): 643–52.

170. Song Z, Wu H, Ciofu O et al. *Pseudomonas aeruginosa* alginate is refractory to Th1 immune response and impedes host immune clearance in a mouse model of acute lung infection. *J Med Microbiol* 2003; **52**(Pt 9): 731–40.

171. Chotirmall SH, Smith SG, Gunaratnam C et al. Effect of estrogen on pseudomonas mucoidy and exacerbations in cystic fibrosis. *N Engl J Med* 2012; **366**(21): 1978–86.

172. Sibley CD, Parkins MD, Rabin HR, Duan K, Norgaard JC, Surette MG. A polymicrobial perspective of pulmonary infections exposes an enigmatic pathogen in cystic fibrosis patients. *Proc Natl Acad SciUSA* 2008; **105**(39): 15070–5.

173. Goldstein EJ, Citron DM, Goldman RJ. National hospital survey of anaerobic culture and susceptibility testing methods: Results and recommendations for improvement. *J Clin Microbiol* 1992; **30**(6): 1529–34.

174. Zemanick ET, Wagner BD, Sagel SD, Stevens MJ, Accurso FJ, Harris JK. Reliability of quantitative real-time PCR for bacterial detection in cystic fibrosis airway specimens. *PloS one* 2010; **5**(11): e15101.

175. Eley BM, Cox SW. Proteolytic and hydrolytic enzymes from putative periodontal pathogens: Characterization, molecular genetics, effects on host defenses and tissues and detection in gingival crevice fluid. *Periodontol* 2000; **31**(1): 105–24.

176. Ruoff KL, Ferraro MJ. Hydrolytic enzymes of "*Streptococcus milleri*". *J Clin Microbiol* 1987; **25**(9): 1645–7.

177. Tayebjee MH, Tan KT, Macfadyen RJ, Lip GYH. Abnormal circulating levels of metalloprotease 9 and its tissue inhibitor 1 in angiographically proven peripheral arterial disease: Relationship to disease severity. *J Intern Med* 2005; **257**(1): 110–6.

178. Jie Bao G, Kari K, Tervahartiala T, Sorsa T, Meurman JH. Proteolytic activities of oral bacteria on prommp-9 and the effect of synthetic proteinase inhibitors. *Open Dent J* 2008; **2**: 96–102.

179. Krauss JL, Potempa J, Lambris JD, Hajishengallis G. Complementary Tolls in the periodontium: How periodontal bacteria modify complement and Toll-like receptor responses to prevail in the host. *Periodontol* 2000; **52**: 141–62.

180. Potempa M, Potempa J, Kantyka T et al. Interpain A, a cysteine proteinase from *Prevotella intermedia*, inhibits complement by degrading complement factor C3. *PLoS Pathog* 2009; **5**(2): e1000316.

181. Kikkert R, Laine ML, Aarden LA, Van Winkelhoff AJ. Activation of toll-like receptors 2 and 4 by gram-negative periodontal bacteria. *Oral Microbiol Immunology* 2007; **22**(3): 145–51.

182. Mirmonsef P, Zariffard MR, Gilbert D, Makinde H, Landay AL, Spear GT. Short-chain fatty acids induce pro-inflammatory cytokine production alone and in combination with toll-like receptor ligands. *Am J Reprod Immunol* 2012; **67**(5): 391–400.

183. van Ewijk BE, Wolfs TFW, Aerts PC et al. RSV mediates *Pseudomonas aeruginosa* binding to cystic fibrosis and normal epithelial cells. *Pediatr Res* 2007; **61**(4): 398–403.

184. Oliver B, Lim S, Wark P et al. Rhinovirus exposure impairs immune responses to bacterial products in human alveolar macrophages. *Thorax* 2008; **63**: 519–25.

185. Petersen NT, Hoiby N, Mordhorst CH, Lind K, Flensborg EW, Bruun B. Respiratory infections in cystic fibrosis patients caused by virus, chlamydia and mycoplasma—Possible synergism with *Pseudomonas aeruginosa*. *Acta Paediatr Scand* 1981; **70**(5): 623–8.

186. Collinson J, Nicholson K, Cancio E et al. Effects of upper respiratory tract infections in patients with cystic fibrosis. *Thorax* 1996; **51**(11): 1115–2.

187. Armstrong DS, Grimwood K, Carlin JB et al. Lower airway inflammation in infants and young children with cystic fibrosis. *Am J Respir Crit Care Med* 1997; **156**(4): 1197–204.

188. Mastronarde JG, Monick MM, Hunninghake GW. Oxidant tone regulates IL-8 production in epithelium infected with respiratory syncytial virus. *Am J Respir Cell Mol Biol* 1995; **13**(2): 237–44.

189. Kurt-Jones EA, Popova L, Kwinn L et al. Pattern recognition receptors TLR4 and CD 14 mediate response to respiratory syncytial virus. *Nature Immunol* 2000; **1**(5): 398–401.

190. Vareille M, Kieninger E, Alves MP et al. Impaired type I and type III interferon induction and rhinovirus control in human cystic fibrosis airway epithelial cells. *Thorax* 2012; **67**(6): 517–25.

191. Latge JP. *Aspergillus fumigatus* and aspergillosis. *Clin Microbiol Rev* 1999; **12**(2): 310–50.

192. Rementeria A, Lopez-Molina N, Ludwig A et al. Genes and molecules involved in *Aspergillus fumigatus* virulence. *Rev Iberoam Micol* 2005; **22**(1): 1–23.

193. Clark IA, Gray KM, Rockett EJ et al. Increased lymphotoxin in human malarial serum, and the ability of this cytokine to increase plasma interleukin-6 and cause hypoglycaemia in mice: Implications for malarial pathology. *Trans R Soc Trop Med Hyg* 1992; **86**(6): 602–7.

194. Akira S, Uematsu S, Takeuchi O. Pathogen recognition and innate immunity. *Cell* 2006; **124**(4): 783–801.

195. Netea MG, Warris A, Van der Meer JW et al. *Aspergillus fumigatus* evades immune recognition during germination through loss of toll-like receptor-4-mediated signal transduction. *J Infect Dis* 2003; **188**(2): 320–6.

196. Chai LY, Vonk AG, Kullberg BJ et al. *Aspergillus fumigatus* cell wall components differentially modulate host TLR2 and TLR4 responses. *Microbes Infect* 2011; **13**(2): 151–9.

197. Shoham S, Levitz SM. The immune response to fungal infections. *Br J Haematol* 2005; **129**(5): 569–82.

198. Wang JE, Warris A, Ellingsen EA et al. Involvement of CD14 and toll-like receptors in activation of human monocytes by *Aspergillus fumigatus* hyphae. *Infect Immun* 2001; **69**(4): 2402–6.

199. Ramaprakash H, Ito T, Standiford TJ, Kunkel SL, Hogaboam CM. Toll-like receptor 9 modulates immune responses to *Aspergillus fumigatus* conidia in immunodeficient and allergic mice. *Infect Immun* 2009; **77**(1): 108–19.

200. Ramirez-Ortiz ZG, Specht CA, Wang JP et al. Toll-like receptor 9-dependent immune activation by unmethylated CpG motifs in *Aspergillus fumigatus* DNA. *Infect Immun* 2008; **76**(5): 2123–9.

201. Carvalho A, Pasqualotto AC, Pitzurra L, Romani L, Denning DW, Rodrigues F. Polymorphisms in toll-like receptor genes and susceptibility to pulmonary aspergillosis. *J Infect Dis* 2008; **197**(4): 618–21.

202. Novak N, Yu CF, Bussmann C et al. Putative association of a TLR9 promoter polymorphism with atopic eczema. *Allergy* 2007; **62**(7): 766–72.

203. Salvenmoser S, Seidler MJ, Dalpke A, Muller FM. Effects of caspofungin, *Candida albicans* and *Aspergillus fumigatus* on toll-like receptor 9 of GM-CSF-stimulated PMNs. *FEMS Immunol Med Microbiol* 2010; **60**(1): 74–7.

204. Balloy V, Chignard M. The innate immune response to *Aspergillus fumigatus*. *Microbes Infect* 2009; **11**(12): 919–27.

205. Steele C, Rapaka RR, Metz A et al. The beta-glucan receptor dectin-1 recognizes specific morphologies of *Aspergillus fumigatus*. *PLoS Pathog* 2005; **1**(4): e42.

206. Latge JP. Tasting the fungal cell wall. *Cell Microbiol* 2010; **12**(7): 863–72.

207. Brown GD, Gordon S. Immune recognition. A new receptor for beta-glucans. *Nature* 2001; **413**(6851): 36–7.

208. Gantner BN, Simmons RM, Canavera SJ, Akira S, Underhill DM. Collaborative induction of inflammatory responses by dectin-1 and toll-like receptor 2. *J Exp Med* 2003; **197**(9): 1107–17.

209. Werner JL, Metz AE, Horn D et al. Requisite role for the dectin-1 beta-glucan receptor in pulmonary defense against *Aspergillus fumigatus*. *J Immunol* 2009; **182**(8): 4938–46.

210. Bellocchio S, Bozza S, Montagnoli C et al. Immunity to *Aspergillus fumigatus*: The basis for immunotherapy and vaccination. *Med Mycol* 2005; **43**(Suppl 1): S181–8.

211. Mehrad B, Strieter RM, Standiford TJ. Role of TNF-alpha in pulmonary host defense in murine invasive aspergillosis. *J Immunol* 1999; **162**(3): 1633–40.

212. Mehrad B, Wiekowski M, Morrison BE et al. Transient lung-specific expression of the chemokine KC improves outcome in invasive aspergillosis. *Am J Respir Crit Care Med* 2002; **166**(9): 1263–8.

213. Rivera A, Van Epps HL, Hohl TM, Rizzuto G, Pamer EG. Distinct CD4+-T-cell responses to live and heat-inactivated *Aspergillus fumigatus* conidia. *Infect Immun* 2005; **73**(11): 7170–9.

214. Bellocchio S, Montagnoli C, Bozza S et al. The contribution of the toll-like/IL-1 receptor superfamily to innate and adaptive immunity to fungal pathogens in vivo. *J Immunol* 2004; **172**(5): 3059–69.

215. Zelante T, De Luca A, Bonifazi P et al. IL-23 and the Th17 pathway promote inflammation and impair antifungal immune resistance. *Eur J Immunol* 2007; **37**(10): 2695–706.

216. Coughlan CA, Chotirmall SH, Renwick J et al. The effect of *Aspergillus fumigatus* infection on vitamin D receptor expression in cystic fibrosis. *Am J Respir Crit Care Med* 2012; **186**(10): 999–1007.

217. Chotirmall SH, O'Donoghue E, Bennett K, Gunaratnam C, O'Neill SJ, McElvaney NG. Sputum *Candida albicans* presages FEV decline and hospital-treated exacerbations in cystic fibrosis. *Chest* 2010; **138**(5): 1186–95.

218. Bulawa CE, Miller DW, Henry LK, Becker JM. Attenuated virulence of chitin-deficient mutants of *Candida albicans*. *Proc Natl Acad Sci USA* 1995; **92**(23): 10570–4.

219. Buurman ET, Westwater C, Hube B, Brown AJ, Odds FC, Gow NA. Molecular analysis of CaMnt1p, a mannosyl transferase important for adhesion and virulence of *Candida albicans*. *Proc Natl Acad Sci USA* 1998; **95**(13): 7670–5.

220. Lussier M, Sdicu AM, Shahinian S, Bussey H. The *Candida albicans* KRE9 gene is required for cell wall beta-1,6-glucan synthesis and is essential for growth on glucose. *Proc Natl Acad Sci USA* 1998; **95**(17): 9825–30.

221. Csank C, Schroppel K, Leberer E et al. Roles of the *Candida albicans* mitogen-activated protein kinase homolog, Cek1p, in hyphal development and systemic candidiasis. *Infect Immun* 1998; **66**(6): 2713–21.

222. Masuoka J. Surface glycans of *Candida albicans* and other pathogenic fungi: Physiological roles, clinical uses, and experimental challenges. *Clin Microbiol Rev* 2004; **17**(2): 281–310.

223. Timpel C, Strahl-Bolsinger S, Ziegelbauer K, Ernst JF. Multiple functions of Pmt1p-mediated protein O-mannosylation in the fungal pathogen *Candida albicans*. *J Biol Chem* 1998; **273**(33): 20837–46.

224. Cutler JE. N-glycosylation of yeast, with emphasis on *Candida albicans*. *Med Mycol* 2001; **39**(Suppl 1): 75–86.

225. Ernst JF, Prill SK. O-glycosylation. *Med Mycol* 2001; **39**(Suppl 1): 67–74.

226. Marr KA, Balajee SA, Hawn TR et al. Differential role of MyD88 in macrophage-mediated responses to opportunistic fungal pathogens. *Infect Immun* 2003; **71**(9): 5280–6.

227. Underhill DM, Gantner B. Integration of Toll-like receptor and phagocytic signaling for tailored immunity. *Microbes Infect* 2004; **6**(15): 1368–73.

228. Underhill DM, Ozinsky A. Phagocytosis of microbes: Complexity in action. *Annu Rev Immunol* 2002; **20**: 825–52.

229. Underhill DM, Ozinsky A, Hajjar AM et al. The toll-like receptor 2 is recruited to macrophage phagosomes and discriminates between pathogens. *Nature* 1999; **401**(6755): 811–5.

230. Kilpatrick DC. Mannan-binding lectin: Clinical significance and applications.*Biochim Biophys Acta* 2002; **1572**(2–3): 401–13.

231. Brouwer N, Dolman KM, van Houdt M, Sta M, Roos D, Kuijpers TW. Mannose-binding lectin (MBL) facilitates opsonophagocytosis of yeasts but not of bacteria despite MBL binding. *J Immunol* 2008; **180**(6): 4124–32.

232. Lee SJ, Gonzalez-Aseguinolaza G, Nussenzweig MC. Disseminated candidiasis and hepatic malarial infection in mannose-binding-lectin-A-deficient mice. *Mol Cell Biol* 2002; **22**(23): 8199–203.

233. Brown GD. Dectin-1: A signalling non-TLR pattern-recognition receptor. *Nat Rev Immunol* 2006; **6**(1): 33–43.

234. Brown GD, Herre J, Williams DL, Willment JA, Marshall AS, Gordon S. Dectin-1 mediates the biological effects of beta-glucans. *J Exp Med* 2003; **197**(9): 1119–24.

235. Ghosh S, Howe N, Volk K, Tati S, Nickerson KW, Petro TM. *Candida albicans* cell wall components and farnesol stimulate the expression of both inflammatory and regulatory cytokines in the murine RAW264.7 macrophage cell line. *FEMS Immunol Med Microbiol* 2010; **60**(1): 63–73.

236. McGreal EP, Rosas M, Brown GD et al. The carbohydrate-recognition domain of Dectin-2 is a C-type lectin with specificity for high mannose. *Glycobiology* 2006; **16**(5): 422–30.

237. Sato K, Yang XL, Yudate T et al. Dectin-2 is a pattern recognition receptor for fungi that couples with the Fc receptor gamma chain to induce innate immune responses. *J Biol Chem* 2006; **281**(50): 38854–66.

238. Jouault T, El Abed-El Behi M, Martinez-Esparza M et al. Specific recognition of *Candida albicans* by macrophages requires galectin-3 to discriminate *Saccharomyces cerevisiae* and needs association with TLR2 for signaling. *J Immunol* 2006; **177**(7): 4679–87.

239. Cambi A, Gijzen K, de Vries IJ et al. The C-type lectin DC-SIGN (CD209) is an antigen-uptake receptor for *Candida albicans* on dendritic cells. *Eur J Immunol* 2003; **33**(2): 532–8.

240. Paats MS, Bergen IM, Bakker M et al. Cytokines in nasal lavages and plasma and their correlation with clinical parameters in cystic fibrosis. *J Cyst Fibros* 2013; **12**(6): 623–9.

241. Karp CL, Flick LM, Park KW et al. Defective lipoxin-mediated anti-inflammatory activity in the cystic fibrosis airway. *Nature Immunol* 2004; **5**(4): 388–92.

242. Verriere V, Higgins G, Al-Alawi M et al. Lipoxin A4 stimulates calcium-activated chloride currents and increases airway surface liquid height in normal and cystic fibrosis airway epithelia. *PloS One* 2012; **7**(5): e37746.

8

CFTR and interactions with modifier genes and the environment: Genotype–phenotype correlations and modifier genes

NICHOLAS J. SIMMONDS, R.J. DARRAH, AND M.L. DRUMM

INTRODUCTION

Since the discovery of the cystic fibrosis transmembrane conductance regulator (*CFTR*) gene in 1989, over 1900 mutations have been reported, although the contribution of many to disease is still unclear.[1,2] It was anticipated that different mutations would correlate with different degrees of disease phenotypes and explain the wide spectrum of disease, but this has been only partially realized as only a small proportion of mutations correlate strongly with specific phenotypes, such as pancreatic status.[3] Poor correlation between *CFTR* genotype and disease phenotype is most evidenced by the wide variation in pulmonary manifestations, which is particularly important as at least 90% of CF morbidity and mortality relates to pulmonary disease. For example, two individuals homozygous for the most common mutation, *F508del*, may have very disparate lung function and much worse prognosis as forced expiratory volume in 1 second (FEV$_1$) is closely linked to survival.[4]

Disease variability and lack of genotype–phenotype correlation indicate that other factors must contribute to phenotype variation; these are generally recognized as a combination of genetic, environmental, and stochastic influences. Because the DNA sequence of any two unrelated individuals is approximately 99.9% identical, variants (or polymorphisms) in the remaining 0.1% must be sufficient to alter protein structure and function, thus affecting the severity of disease expression and response to treatment. Polymorphisms, not contained within *CFTR*, are termed "gene modifiers" and include single-base nucleotide substitutions (also termed single nucleotide polymorphisms [SNPs]); small-scale, multibase deletions or insertions; and repeat variations (also termed short tandem repeats). These are more common than mutations in the general population and, alone, are not enough

to cause disease. As a result of the International HapMap Project—a multicountry collaboration to fully sequence the whole human genome—at least 10 million SNPs are thought to exist.[5] Early evidence for gene modifiers in CF came from *CFTR* knockout mice, demonstrating a locus on chromosome 7, distinct from *CFTR*, as a risk factor for intestinal obstruction.[6] Further evidence emerged from twin and sibling studies, confirming that monozygotic twins have a significantly higher concordance in severity of lung disease than dizygotic twins, suggesting that even when *CFTR* mutations are identical and the environment is the same other genes can influence phenotype.[7]

Studies of heritability allow us to better understand the impact of gene modifiers on disease expression by quantitatively measuring the relative contribution of genetic (i.e., heritability) versus environmental factors. CF twin studies have demonstrated a heritability estimate of 0.54–1.0 for lung disease and 0.76 for persistent *Pseudomonas aeruginosa* infection, in contrast to diabetes and meconium ileus, which are almost exclusively genetically influenced (i.e., heritability estimate of ~1.0).[8,9] Interestingly, distal intestinal obstruction syndrome, which shares some pathological features to meconium ileus but occurs later in life, carries virtually no genetic risk.[10]

The focus of this chapter is on modifying genes not contained within *CFTR*; however, it is recognized that there are still many unanswered questions about variances within CFTR itself. Although over 1900 variances are now recognized, only 190 of these have been fully analyzed, of which 122 are currently classified as disease-causing mutations.[11] Of the remaining variances, there is variable penetrance and disease potential—some cause CF some of the time, some cause a "mild" form of CF (termed CFTR-related disorder), and some have no effect or association with CF. There is even the possibility that a second mutation may favorably modify the effects of another. An example of this variability is the polypyrimidine tract of the intron 8 acceptor splice site, of which there are three common alleles—(T)5, (T)7, and (T)9, denoting 5, 7, and 9 thymidines, respectively. The (T)5 variant when inherited *in trans* with another disease-causing mutation has a much greater potential for disease than the others, which are usually regarded as "normal" variants.[12]

EVOLUTION OF MODIFIER STUDIES

Economics has played a large role in the strategies used to identify modifying genes and loci, with early studies utilizing single, small cohorts of subjects (some just a few dozen) without validation in subsequent populations, which would today be considered an essential prerequisite of a good study. Rapid improvements in genotyping technology and the consequent drops in cost have allowed more recent studies to focus on statistical power and have incorporated hundreds and thousands of subjects. While this should increase the robustness of the studies, it also introduces some logistical issues as early studies mostly utilized "in-house" genotyping assays, developed for a handful of variants in a gene or genes of interest, while commercial platforms use completely different criteria, such as allele frequency and genomic coverage, in their choice of variants. Thus, although one would hope to utilize the smaller, earlier studies as discovery, or hypothesis-generating, data sets, with the more recent studies being useful for both validation of the earlier surveys and discovery of new loci, it has not been so simple, as often the two do not probe the same variants, or even correlated (linked) variants of the same gene.

Some of the earlier studies alluded to here were carried out even before there was evidence of genetic involvement of disease phenotypic variation. Once heritability was established, solidifying the concept that genetic variation contributes to the clinical heterogeneity observed in CF, it was reasonable to make the investments needed to search for the genes or loci responsible for the heterogeneity. Financial constraints limited most early studies to focus on a limited number of "candidate" genes and their variants. These genes were chosen because they encoded products that were involved in some physiologic process believed to be involved in CF pathophysiology. For example, the exuberant inflammatory response of CF airways and its apparent role in destruction of the lung led to the examination of inflammation-related genes as potential modifiers. In one of the earliest CF lung disease modifier studies, Hull and Thompson genotyped 53 CF patients for variants in the genes encoding tumor necrosis factor-α (TNFα) and glutathione-S-transferase M1 (GSTM1) and examined these variants for correlations with lung function and body weight.[13] Shortly afterward, innate defense processes were investigated as another CF-relevant trait and variants in the gene encoding the serum antimicrobial protein mannose-binding lectin-2 (MBL2) were assessed for association with lung function and survival of

149 CF patients.[14] Unlike the high allele frequencies of TNFα and GSTM1, the MBL2 variants are rare, requiring a greater number of subjects to find multiple individuals with each of the various genotypes.

These early studies pioneered the gene modifier field, showing nominal associations that have not held up in subsequent, larger cohort studies and thus are likely artifacts of small sample sizes.[15,16] Importantly, as is typically true of fields in their infancy, these studies identified the difficulties and limitations of such studies, including small sample sizes, variants with low allele frequencies, and the use of cross-sectional phenotypic data for a trait that changes over time, paving the way for future studies.

As a consequence of realizing these limitations, larger patient cohorts were attained by consortium efforts and longitudinal pulmonary phenotypes were developed for use in these studies.[15,17] The first of the consortium studies examined 1306 CF subjects from the United States and Canada (808 in the original analysis and 498 in a replication) for associations with a panel of 16 variants across 10 candidate genes and found two variants in one gene, *TGFβ1*, encoding transforming growth factor β1, associated with lung disease severity.[15]

As these studies progressed, the cost of genotyping dropped dramatically and patients continued to be enrolled. It therefore became feasible to carry out genome-wide association studies (GWAS), sampling hundreds of thousands of polymorphisms representing nearly all the genes of the genome to look for associations between common variants and magnitude of disease-related phenotypes.[16,18]

The current frontier for genetics and the search for modifiers involve genomic sequencing, which has the potential to capture all variations. It is estimated that one of every 200–300 nucleotides is variable in the three-billion-nucleotide human genome, and thus sampling even hundreds of thousands of polymorphisms probes only a small fraction of the variation. A first step toward whole genome sequencing, a process referred to as exome sequencing, examining the protein coding portion of the genome, has been carried out and identified *DCTN4* (encodes for dynactin 4, a subunit of the dynactin protein complex involved in intracellular movement along microtubules) as a potential disease modifier, tracking with the age at which patients become infected by *P. aeruginosa*.[19] Similar to array-based SNP genotyping, sequencing costs continue to drop and thus it is expected that soon these types of association studies will incorporate whole genome sequencing.

SPECIFIC GENE MODIFIERS OF CYSTIC FIBROSIS

The search for gene modifiers of CF has been progressing steadily as gene analysis technology has developed from the candidate-gene approach to linkage analyses, exome sequencing, and GWAS. Many of the observed associations are listed in Table 8.1 and discussed in the following

Table 8.1 Genetic modifiers of CF disease phenotypes

Gene	Name	Location	Cystic fibrosis phenotype				
			Lung function	*P. aeruginosa* acquisition/ infection	Meconium ileus/ intestinal obstruction	Liver disease	Diabetes
ADIPOR2	Adiponectin receptor 2	12p31.31			GWAS Possible effect		
APIP	APAF1-interacting protein	11p13	GWAS Possible effect				
DCTN4	Dynactin 4 protein	5q33.1		Exome sequencing Possible effect			
EHF	Ets homologous factor	11p12	GWAS Possible effect				
IFRD1	Interferon-related developmental regulator 1	7q31.1	GWAS Possible effect				
IL8	Interleukin 8	4q13-q21	Candidate Possible effect				
IL1β	Interleukin 1β	2q14	Candidate Possible effect				
MBL2	Mannose-binding lectin 2	10q11.2	Candidate Probable effect	Candidate Probable effect			
MSRA	Methionine sulfoxide reductase A	8p23.1			Candidate Probable effect		
SERPINA1	Serpin peptidase inhibitor, clade A, member 1	14q32.1	Candidate No effect	Candidate Likely no effect		Candidate Possible effect	
SLC26A9	Solute carrier family 26, member 9	1q32.1			GWAS Possible effect		
SLC6A14	Solute carrier family 6, member 14	Xq23			GWAS Possible effect		
TCF7L2	Transcription factor 7-like 2	10q25.3					Candidate Probable effect
TGFβ1	Transforming growth factor β1	19q13.1	Candidate Probable effect	Candidate No effect		Candidate Likely no effect	

Note: For each CF phenotype, the study type is given with the strength of association based on the following: probable effect: association observed in ≥3 independent populations with $n \geq 1000$ in total; possible effect: association observed in ≥2 independent populations with $n \geq 500$ in total (with the exception of exome sequencing); likely no effect: no association observed in ≥2 independent populations with $n \geq 500$ in total; no effect: no association observed in ≥3 independent populations with $n \geq 1000$ in total.

want to be stronger and more muscular.[122–124] In one study of 54 adolescents, with CF, 44.8% of women with a BMI less than the 50th percentile reported desiring a smaller body size or were content with their current size, compared to only 8% of men.[125] These gender-related differences in attitude toward body image are most notable in adolescents and adults, but can be found in younger children as well.[126] Furthermore, these attitudinal differences lead to behavior differences. Regular exercise is beneficial to CF patients,[127,128] and men are more aerobically fit[128] and are almost three times more likely than women to exercise regularly.[121] Furthermore, perception of self as underweight is associated with greater use of nutritional supplements,[124] and men eat better and more frequently than women.[121,124]

STRESS AND MENTAL HEALTH

Stress appears to have a negative impact on the course of some diseases by impairing immune function.[47,129] Of greater potential importance for children with CF, however, is that parental experience of stress may lead to impaired personal and family function,[130] which would have a direct and specific effect on adherence and other aspects of disease self-management.

Excessive stress in caregivers can lead to depression, dysfunctional behaviors (including drug and alcohol abuse), and physical illness. A significant proportion of mothers of children with CF show depressive symptoms soon after diagnosis of their child, independent of the degree of the child's illness,[131] and many parents continue to report significant psychological distress years afterward.[132] Studies by Patterson et al.[130,133] in the early 1990s suggested that stress and family dysfunction lead to decreased adherence and worse disease outcomes, and recent studies have shown the prevalence of anxiety and depression in patients with CF as well as parents to be as high as 30%, significantly elevated compared with the general population.[134] Depression, in particular, is associated with an increased likelihood of nonadherence and of worse health outcomes including quality of life and lung function.[135–139]

DIFFERENCES IN THE USE OF MEDICAL TREATMENT AS A CAUSE OF VARIABILITY IN CF OUTCOMES

Improvements in preservation of lung function and prolongation of life in the current generation of people with CF are attributable to the development of new therapies and also to increased knowledge regarding the optimal and proactive use of medications and treatments that have been available to patients for some time. Although the relative contribution of individual therapies cannot be clearly demarcated, it is likely that they are all synergistic.

DIFFERENCES IN PROVISION OF EVIDENCE-BASED CARE

The CF Foundation in the United States, the CF Trust in the United Kingdom, and their counterparts elsewhere have developed consensus guidelines and fostered a network of knowledgeable CF care providers, ensuring the general availability and dissemination of medical expertise and promoting a focused research agenda.[140–144] Although not all CF patients choose to attend designated CF care centers, the relative advantage of center-based care can be measured (even though this is made difficult by the presumed tendency for sicker patients to obtain care at accredited centers).[145,146]

Despite efforts to identify optimal CF care and ensure that it is provided in a consistent manner, significant variation in practice patterns[147] and disease outcomes[2,148] can be found, even when comparisons are adjusted for case mix.[149] In particular, reports from the Epidemiologic Study of Cystic Fibrosis (ESCF) show that care centers whose patients had better than average pulmonary function monitored their patients more actively and prescribed more IV antibiotics.[150,151]

Although some practice variations among CF care centers may reflect differences in scientific opinion among CF specialty physicians, variability in the implementation of consensus guidelines and evidence-based treatment approaches are often inadvertent. The care of patients with a chronic disease such as CF involves a complex series of decisions whose realization requires detailed follow through by an interdisciplinary healthcare team over a long period of time. This type of care is best rendered within a system that is flexible and customizable while incorporating multicomponent strategies to ensure that all steps in the process of care are supported and carried out correctly,[152] allowing knowledgeable practitioners to consistently provide the care they identify as appropriate to all of their patients.[149]

In recognition of the benefit of systematic approaches to care, the CF Foundation has organized quality improvement training initiatives for CF care teams in the United States, reconfigured its patient registry to make it a useful tool to track relevant patient- and center-based data, and promoted benchmarking activities.[153] Similar efforts have been adopted in Europe, especially in Germany.[154,155] These efforts have met with mixed results, but there have been a number of reported successes. For example, by developing a standardized approach to nutritional assessment and treatment, one large American CF program was able to improve the median BMI of its pediatric patients over a 15-month period from 35.2 to 42.0 percentile, increasing the percentage of patients with BMI >50th percentile by 11.8%.[156] Similar improvements in lung function have been reported following the institution of an algorithm for diagnosis and treatment of pulmonary exacerbations.[157]

PATIENT ADHERENCE TO PRESCRIBED MEDICAL REGIMENS

The high rate of nonadherence to CF treatment recommendations makes this an important consideration when examining reasons for variations in disease outcome.[103–105] Significant difficulties in the accurate measurement of adherence exist, so any conclusions must be drawn with caution.[158] Recent studies using pharmacy refill records demonstrate the unsurprising association between adherence (measured as medication possession) and lung function.[159,160]

Knowledge about CF[161,162] and specifically an understanding of the treatment regimen and its rationale seem to be important prerequisites for adherence.[163–165] Good family function[130,133] predicts better adherence; on the other hand, family stress is associated with nonadherence,[166] and as noted earlier, the effect of depression on disease outcomes is primarily mediated by its effect on adherence.[137]

CONCLUSION

Although CF is a classic Mendelian autosomal recessive disease, caused by alterations of the *CFTR* gene, its expression is influenced by a host of complex interactions with other genes and with an environment that consists not only of specific biologic and physical effectors but also a pervasive social and cultural setting that has major implications for health. Furthermore, the disease course is modified by healthcare interventions whose impact depends on both the clinical expertise of knowledgeable providers and also on the success of a complex delivery system that currently delivers results with uneven success. For any individual with CF, these three influences interact in varying ways (Figure 9.2), so it is of little wonder that overall, there is a significant unpredictability regarding eventual outcome.

REFERENCES

1. FitzSimmons SC. The changing epidemiology of cystic fibrosis. *J Pediatr* 1993; **122**: 1–9
2. Cystic Fibrosis Foundation. *Cystic Fibrosis Foundation Patient Registry, 2003 Annual Data Report.* Bethesda, MD: Cystic Fibrosis Foundation; 2004.
3. Kosorok MR, Zeng L, West SE, et al. Acceleration of lung disease in children with cystic fibrosis after *Pseudomonas aeruginosa* acquisition. *Pediatr Pulmonol* 2001; **32**(4): 277–87.
4. Nixon GM, Armstrong DS, Carzino R, et al. Clinical outcome after early *Pseudomonas aeruginosa* infection in cystic fibrosis. *J Pediatr* 2001; **138**(5): 699–704.
5. Emerson J, Rosenfeld M, McNamara S, et al. *Pseudomonas aeruginosa* and other predictors of mortality and morbidity in young children with cystic fibrosis. *Pediatr Pulmonol* 2002; **34**(2): 91–100.
6. Li Z, Kosorok MR, Farrell PM, et al. Longitudinal development of mucoid *Pseudomonas aeruginosa* infection and lung disease progression in children with cystic fibrosis. *JAMA* 2005; **293**(5): 581–8.
7. Pillarisetti N, Williamson E, Linnane B, et al. Infection, inflammation, and lung function decline in infants with cystic fibrosis. *Am J Respir Crit Care Med* 2011; **184**(1): 75–81.
8. Stick SM, Brennan S, Murray C, et al. Bronchiectasis in infants and preschool children diagnosed with cystic fibrosis after newborn screening. *J Pediatr* 2009; **155**(5): 623–8.
9. Demko CA, Byard PJ, Davis PB. Gender differences in cystic fibrosis: *Pseudomonas aeruginosa* infection. *J Clin Epidemiol* 1995; **48**(8): 1041–9.
10. Maselli JH, Sontag MK, Norris JM, et al. Risk factors for initial acquisition of *Pseudomonas aeruginosa* in children with cystic fibrosis identified by newborn screening. *Pediatr Pulmonol* 2003; **35**(4): 257–62.
11. Stutman HR, Lieberman JM, Nussbaum E, et al. Antibiotic prophylaxis in infants and young children with cystic fibrosis: A randomized controlled trial. *J Pediatr* 2002; **140**(3): 299–305.
12. Ratjen F, Comes G, Paul K, et al. Effect of continuous antistaphylococcal therapy on the rate of *P. aeruginosa* acquisition in patients with cystic fibrosis. *Pediatr Pulmonol* 2001; **31**(1): 13–6.
13. Jones AM, Dodd ME, Doherty CJ, et al. Increased treatment requirements of patients with cystic fibrosis who harbour a highly transmissible strain of *Pseudomonas aeruginosa*. *Thorax* 2002; **57**(11): 924–5.
14. Tummler B, Koopmann U, Grothues D, et al. Nosocomial acquisition of *Pseudomonas aeruginosa* by cystic fibrosis patients. *J Clin Microbiol* 1991; **29**(6): 1265–7.
15. Kosorok MR, Jalaluddin M, Farrell PM, et al. Comprehensive analysis of risk factors for acquisition of *Pseudomonas aeruginosa* in young children with cystic fibrosis. *Pediatr Pulmonol* 1998; **26**(2): 81–8.
16. Hoiby N, Pedersen SS. Estimated risk of cross-infection with *Pseudomonas aeruginosa* in Danish cystic fibrosis patients. *Acta Paediatr Scand* 1989; **78**(3): 395–404.
17. Pedersen SS, Jensen T, Pressler T, et al. Does centralized treatment of cystic fibrosis increase the risk of *Pseudomonas aeruginosa* infection? *Acta Paediatr Scand* 1986; **75**(5): 840–5.
18. Kerem E, Corey M, Stein R, et al. Risk factors for *Pseudomonas aeruginosa* colonization in cystic fibrosis patients. *Pediatr Infect Dis J* 1990; **9**(7): 494–8.
19. Armstrong D, Grimwood K, Carlin JB, et al. Severe viral respiratory infections in infants with cystic fibrosis. *Pediatr Pulmonol* 1998; **26**(6): 371–9.

20. LiPuma JJ. Burkholderia cepacia. Management issues and new insights. *Clin Chest Med* 1998; **19**(3): 473–86, vi.

21. Corey M, Farewell V. Determinants of mortality from cystic fibrosis in Canada, 1970-1989. *Am J Epidemiol* 1996; **143**(10): 1007–17.

22. Ledson MJ, Gallagher MJ, Jackson M, et al. Outcome of *Burkholderia cepacia* colonisation in an adult cystic fibrosis centre. *Thorax* 2002; **57**(2): 142–5.

23. McCloskey M, McCaughan J, Redmond AO, et al. Clinical outcome after acquisition of Burkholderia cepacia in patients with cystic fibrosis. *Ir J Med Sci* 2001; **170**(1): 28–31.

24. Muhdi K, Edenborough FP, Gumery L, et al. Outcome for patients colonised with Burkholderia cepacia in a Birmingham adult cystic fibrosis clinic and the end of an epidemic. *Thorax* 1996; **51**(4): 374–7.

25. Lewin LO, Byard PJ, Davis PB. Effect of *Pseudomonas cepacia* colonization on survival and pulmonary function of cystic fibrosis patients. *J Clin Epidemiol* 1990; **43**(2): 125–31.

26. Chen JS, Witzmann KA, Spilker T, et al. Endemicity and inter-city spread of *Burkholderia cepacia* genomovar III in cystic fibrosis. *J Pediatr* 2001; **139**(5): 643–9.

27. Govan JR, Brown PH, Maddison J, et al. Evidence for transmission of *Pseudomonas cepacia* by social contact in cystic fibrosis. *Lancet* 1993; **342**(8862): 15–9.

28. Dasenbrook EC, Checkley W, Merlo CA, et al. Association between respiratory tract methicillin-resistant Staphylococcus aureus and survival in cystic fibrosis. *JAMA* 2010; **303**(23): 2386–92.

29. Vanderhelst E, De Meirleir L, Verbanck S, et al. Prevalence and impact on FEV(1) decline of chronic methicillin-resistant *Staphylococcus aureus* (MRSA) colonization in patients with cystic fibrosis. A single-center, case control study of 165 patients. *J Cyst Fibros* 2012; **11**(1): 2–7.

30. Olivier KN, Group NTMiCS. The natural history of non-tuberculous mycobacteria in patients with cystic fibrosis. *Paediatr Respir Rev* 2004; **5** (Suppl A): S213–6.

31. Esther CR Jr., Esserman DA, Gilligan P, et al. Chronic *Mycobacterium abscessus* infection and lung function decline in cystic fibrosis. *J Cyst Fibros* 2010; **9**(2): 117–23.

32. Fillaux J, Bremont F, Murris M, et al. Assessment of Aspergillus sensitization or persistent carriage as a factor in lung function impairment in cystic fibrosis patients. *Scand J Infect Dis* 2012; **44**(11): 842–7.

33. Hansen CR. *Stenotrophomonas maltophilia*: To be or not to be a cystic fibrosis pathogen. *Curr Opin Pulm Med* 2012; **18**(6): 628–31.

34. De Baets F, Schelstraete P, Van Daele S, et al. *Achromobacter xylosoxidans* in cystic fibrosis: Prevalence and clinical relevance. *J Cyst Fibros* 2007; **6**(1): 75–8.

35. Wang EE, Prober CG, Manson B, et al. Association of respiratory viral infections with pulmonary deterioration in patients with cystic fibrosis. *N Engl J Med* 1984; **311**(26): 1653–8.

36. Smyth AR, Smyth RL, Tong CY, et al. Effect of respiratory virus infections including rhinovirus on clinical status in cystic fibrosis. *Arch Disease Childhood* 1995; **73**(2): 117–20.

37. Hiatt PW, Grace SC, Kozinetz CA, et al. Effects of viral lower respiratory tract infection on lung function in infants with cystic fibrosis. *Pediatrics* 1999; **103**(3): 619–26.

38. Collinson J, Nicholson KG, Cancio E, et al. Effects of upper respiratory tract infections in patients with cystic fibrosis. *Thorax* 1996; **51**(11): 1115–22.

39. Colasurdo GN, Fullmer JJ, Elidemir O, et al. Respiratory syncytial virus infection in a murine model of cystic fibrosis. *J Med Virol* 2006; **78**(5): 651–8.

40. Borowitz D, Robinson KA, Rosenfeld M, et al. Cystic Fibrosis Foundation evidence-based guidelines for management of infants with cystic fibrosis. *J Pediatr* 2009; **155** (6 Suppl 1): S73–93.

41. Borowitz D. The interrelationship of nutrition and pulmonary function in patients with cystic fibrosis. *Curr Opin Pulm Med* 1996; **2**(6): 457–61.

42. Schoni MH, Casaulta-Aebischer C. Nutrition and lung function in cystic fibrosis patients: Review. *Clin Nutr* 2000; **19**(2): 79–85.

43. Steinkamp G, von der Hardt H. Improvement of nutritional status and lung function after long-term nocturnal gastrostomy feedings in cystic fibrosis. *J Pediatr* 1994; **124**(2): 244–9.

44. Steinkamp G, Wiedemann B. Relationship between nutritional status and lung function in cystic fibrosis: Cross sectional and longitudinal analyses from the German CF quality assurance (CFQA) project. *Thorax* 2002; **57**(7): 596–601.

45. Konstan MW, Butler SM, Wohl ME, et al. Growth and nutritional indexes in early life predict pulmonary function in cystic fibrosis. *J Pediatr* 2003; **142**(6): 624–30.

46. Lai HJ, Shoff SM, Farrell PM. Recovery of birth weight z score within 2 years of diagnosis is positively associated with pulmonary status at 6 years of age in children with cystic fibrosis. *Pediatrics* 2009; **123**(2): 714–22.

47. Bor DH, Epstein PR. Pathogenesis of respiratory infection in the disadvantaged. *Semin Respir Infect* 1991; **6**: 194–203.

48. James WP, Nelson M, Ralph A, et al. Socioeconomic determinants of health. The contribution of nutrition to inequalities in health. *BMJ* 1997; **314**(7093): 1545–9.

49. Stoddard JJ, Miller T. Impact of parental smoking on the prevalence of wheezing respiratory illness in children. *Am J Epidemiol* 1995; **141**: 96–102.

50. Tager IB, Ngo L, Hanrahan JP. Maternal smoking during pregnancy. *Am J Respir Crit Care Med* 1995; **152**: 977–83.

51. Eisner MD, Klein J, Hammond SK, et al. Directly measured second hand smoke exposure and asthma health outcomes. *Thorax* 2005; **60**(10): 814–21.

52. Rubin BK. Exposure of children with cystic fibrosis to environmental tobacco smoke. *N Engl J Med* 1990; **323**(12): 782–8.

53. Smyth A, O'Hea U, Williams G, et al. Passive smoking and impaired lung function in cystic fibrosis. Arch Disease Child 1994; **71**(4): 353–4.

54. Kovesi T, Corey M, Levison H. Passive smoking and lung function in cystic fibrosis. *Am Rev Respir Disease* 1993; **148**(5): 1266–71.

55. Campbell PW 3rd, Parker RA, Roberts BT, et al. Association of poor clinical status and heavy exposure to tobacco smoke in patients with cystic fibrosis who are homozygous for the F508 deletion. *J Pediatr* 1992; **120**(2 Pt 1): 261–4.

56. Gilljam H, Stenlund C, Ericsson-Hollsing A, et al. Passive smoking in cystic fibrosis. *Respir Med* 1990; 84(4): 289–91.

57. Collaco JM, Vanscoy L, Bremer L, et al. Interactions between secondhand smoke and genes that affect cystic fibrosis lung disease. *JAMA* 2008; **299**(4): 417–24.

58. King K, Martynenko M, Bergman MH, et al. Family composition and children's exposure to adult smokers in their homes. *Pediatrics* 2009; **123**(4): e559–64.

59. Rosenfeld M, Emerson J, McNamara S, et al. Risk factors for age at initial Pseudomonas acquisition in the cystic fibrosis epic observational cohort. *J Cyst Fibros* 2012; **11**(5): 446–53.

60. Gauderman WJ, Avol E, Gilliland F, et al. The effect of air pollution on lung development from 10 to 18 years of age. *N Engl J Med* 2004; **351**(11): 1057–67.

61. Pope CA, 3rd, Thun MJ, Namboodiri MM, et al. Particulate air pollution as a predictor of mortality in a prospective study of US adults. *Am J Respir Crit Care Med* 1995; **151**(3 Pt 1): 669–74.

62. Goeminne P, Kiciński M, Vermeulen F, et al. Impact of air pollution on cystic fibrosis pulmonary exacerbations: A case-crossover analysis. *Chest* 2013; **143**(4): 946–54.

63. Collaco JM, McGready J, Green DM, et al. Effect of temperature on cystic fibrosis lung disease and infections: A replicated cohort study. PLoS ONE 2011; **6**(11): e27784.

64. Goldhagen J, Remo R, Bryant T 3rd, et al. The health status of southern children: A neglected regional disparity. *Pediatrics* 2005; **116**(6): e746–53.

65. Kim S, Quinton HB, Schechter MS. The association of CF outcomes with state child health index. *Pediatr Pulmonol* 2011; **46** (Suppl 34): 364.

66. Marmot M. Social determinants of health: From observation to policy. *Med J Aust* 2000; **172**(8): 379–82.

67. Taylor-Robinson D, Schechter MS. Health inequalities and cystic fibrosis. *BMJ* 2011; **343**: d4818.

68. Reijneveld SA. The impact of individual and area characteristics on urban socioeconomic differences in health and smoking. *Int J Epidemiol* 1998; **27**(1): 33–40.

69. Gazmararian JA, Adams MM, Pamuk ER. Associations between measures of socioeconomic status and maternal health behavior. *Am J Prev Med* 1996; **12**(2): 108–15.

70. Pincus T, Esther R, DeWalt DA, et al. Social conditions and self-management are more powerful determinants of health than access to care. *Ann Intern Med* 1998; **129**(5): 406–11.

71. Schmitzberger R, Rhomberg K, Buchele H, et al. Effects of air pollution on the respiratory tract of children. *Pediatr Pulmonol* 1993; **15**(2): 68–74.

72. Apter AJ, Reisine ST, Affleck G, et al. Adherence with twice-daily dosing of inhaled steroids. Socioeconomic and health-belief differences. *Am J Respir Crit Care Med* 1998; **157**(6 Pt 1): 1810–7.

73. Jolly DL, Nolan T, Moller J, et al. The impact of poverty and disadvantage on child health. *J Paediatr Child Health* 1991; **27**(4): 203–17.

74. Mackenbach JP, Kunst AE, Cavelaars AE, et al. Socioeconomic inequalities in morbidity and mortality in western Europe. The EU Working Group on Socioeconomic Inequalities in Health. *Lancet* 1997; **349**(9): 1655–9.

75. Krieger N, Williams DR, Moss NE. Measuring social class in US public health research: Concepts, methodologies, and guidelines. *Ann Rev Pub Health* 1997; **18**: 341–78.

76. Kawachi I, Kennedy BP. Income inequality and health: Pathways and mechanisms. *Health Serv Res* 1999; **34**(1 Pt 2): 215–27.

77. Davey Smith G, Hart C, Hole D, et al. Education and occupational social class: Which is the more important indicator of mortality risk? *J Epidemiol Commun Health* 1998; **52**(3): 153–60.

78. Fein O. The influence of social class on health status: American and British research on health inequalities. *J Gen Intern Med* 1995; **10**(10): 577–86.

79. Zill N. Parental schooling and children's health. *Public Health Reports* 1996; **111**(1): 34–43.

80. Britton J. Effects of social class, sex, and region of residence on age at death from cystic fibrosis. *BMJ* 1989; **298**: 483–7.

81. Barr HL, Britton JR, Smyth AR, et al. The association between socioeconomic status and gender with median age at death from cystic fibrosis in England and Wales: 1959 to 2008. *BMJ* 2011; **343**: d4662.

82. Taylor-Robinson DC, Smyth RL, Diggle PJ, et al. The effect of social deprivation on clinical outcomes and the use of treatments in the UK cystic fibrosis population: A longitudinal study. *Lancet Respir Med* 2013; **1**(2): 121–8.

83. Schechter MS, Shelton BJ, Margolis PA, et al. The association of socioeconomic status with outcomes in cystic fibrosis patients in the United States. *Am J Respir Crit Care Med* 2001; **163**: 1331–7.

84. O'Connor GT, Quinton HB, Kahn R, et al. Case-mix adjustment for evaluation of mortality in cystic fibrosis. *Pediatr Pulmonol* 2002; **33**(2): 99–105.

85. O'Connor GT, Quinton HB, Kneeland T, et al. Median household income and mortality rate in cystic fibrosis. *Pediatrics* 2003; **111**(4 Pt 1): e333–9.

86. Stephenson A, Hux J, Tullis E, et al. Socioeconomic status and risk of hospitalization among individuals with cystic fibrosis in Ontario, Canada. *Pediatr Pulmonol* 2011; **46**(4): 376–84.

87. Anthony H, Paxton S, Bines J, et al. Psychosocial predictors of adherence to nutritional recommendations and growth outcomes in children with cystic fibrosis. *J Psychosom Res* 1999; **47**(6): 623–34.

88. Haire-Joshu D, Morgan G, Fisher JEB. Determinants of cigarette smoking. *Clin Chest Med* 1991; **4**: 711–24.

89. Nelson DE, Emont SL, Brackbill RM, et al. Cigarette smoking prevalence by occupation in the United States. A comparison between 1978 to 1980 and 1987 to 1990. *J Occup Med* 1994; **36**(5): 516–25.

90. Schechter MS, Emerson J, Rosenfeld M. The relationship of socioeconomic status and environmental tobacco smoke exposure with disease outcomes in the EPIC observational cohort. *Pediatr Pulmonol* 2012; **47** (Suppl 35): 379.

91. Wheeler BW, Ben-Shlomo Y. Environmental equity, air quality, socioeconomic status, and respiratory health: A linkage analysis of routine data from the Health Survey for England. *J Epidemiol Community Health* 2005; **59**(11): 948–54.

92. Goss CH, Newsom SA, Schildcrout JS, et al. Effect of ambient air pollution on pulmonary exacerbations and lung function in cystic fibrosis. *Am J Respir Crit Care Med* 2004; **169**(7): 816–21.

93. Szanton SL, Gill JM, Allen JK. Allostatic load: A mechanism of socioeconomic health disparities? *Biol Res Nurs* 2005; **7**(1): 7–15.

94. Schechter MS, Cruz I, Blackwell LS, et al. Risk factors for anxiety and depression in cystic fibrosis. *Pediatr Pulmonol* 2010 (Suppl 33) (45): 109–10.

95. Halfon NaPN. Childhood asthma and poverty; differential impacts and utilization of health services. Pediatrics 1993; **91**: 56–61.

96. Finkelstein JA, Brown RW, Schneider LC, et al. Quality of care for preschool children with asthma: The role of social factors and practice setting. *Pediatrics* 1995; **95**: 389–94.

97. Weiss KB, Gergen PJ, Crain EF. Inner-city asthma. The epidemiology of an emerging US public health concern. *Chest* 1992; **101** (6 Suppl): 362S–7S.

98. Schechter MS, Silva SJ, Morgan WJ, et al. Association of socioeconomic status with outpatient monitoring and the use of chronic CF therapies. *Pediatr Pulmonol* 2005; **28** (Suppl): 330.

99. Schechter MS, Pasta D, Morgan WJ, et al. Socioeconomic status and the likelihood of antibiotic treatment for pulmonary exacerbations. *Pediatr Pulmonol* 2005: **28** (Suppl): 331.

100. Henley LD, Hill ID. Errors, gaps, and misconceptions in the disease-related knowledge of cystic fibrosis patients and their families. *Pediatrics* 1990; **85**: 1008–14.

101. Henley LD, Hill ID. Global and specific disease-related information needs of cystic fibrosis patients and their families. *Pediatrics* 1990; **85**(6): 1015–21.

102. Quon BS, Psoter K, Mayer-Hamblett N, et al. Disparities in access to lung transplantation for cystic fibrosis patients by socioeconomic status. *Am J Respir Crit Care Med* 2012; **186**(10): 1008–13.

103. Abbott J, Dodd M, Webb AK. Health perceptions and treatment adherence in adults with cystic fibrosis. *Thorax* 1996; **51**(12): 1233–8.

104. Conway SP, Pond MN, Hamnett T, et al. Compliance with treatment in adult patients with cystic fibrosis. *Thorax* 1996; **51**(1): 29–33.

105. Quittner AL, Espelage DL, Ievers-Landis C, et al. Measuring adherence to medical treatments in childhood chronic illness: Considering multiple methods and sources of information. *J Clin Psychol Med Settings* 2000; **7**(1): 41–54.

106. DiMatteo MR. Enhancing patient adherence to medical recommendations. *JAMA* 1994; **271**: 79–82.

107. Braun L. Race, ethnicity, and health: Can genetics explain disparities? *Perspect Biol Med* 2002; **45**(2): 159–74.

108. Hamosh A, FitzSimmons SC, Macek M Jr., et al. Comparison of the clinical manifestation of cystic fibrosis in black and white patients. *J Pediatr* 1998; **132**: 255–9.

109. Watts KD, Seshadri R, Sullivan C, et al. Increased prevalence of risk factors for morbidity and mortality in the US Hispanic CF population. *Pediatr Pulmonol* 2009; **44**(6): 594–601.

110. Oliver MN, Muntaner C. Researching health inequities among African Americans: The imperative to understand social class. *Int J Health Serv* 2005; **35**(3): 485–98.

111. LaVeist TA. Disentangling race and socioeconomic status: A key to understanding health inequalities. *J Urban Health* 2005; **82** (2 Suppl 3): iii26–34.

112. Rosenfeld M, Davis R, FitzSimmons S, et al. Gender gap in cystic fibrosis mortality. *Am J Epidemiol* 1997; **145**(9): 794–803.

113. Dodge JA, Lewis PA, Stanton M, et al. Cystic fibrosis mortality and survival in the UK: 1947-2003. *Eur Respir J* 2007; **29**(3): 522–6.

114. Jackson AD, Daly L, Jackson AL, et al. Validation and use of a parametric model for projecting cystic fibrosis survivorship beyond observed data: A birth cohort analysis. *Thorax* 2011; **66**(8): 674–9.

115. Olesen HV, Pressler T, Hjelte L, et al. Gender differences in the Scandinavian cystic fibrosis population. *Pediatr Pulmonol* 2010; **45**(10): 959–65.

116. Viviani L, Bossi A, Assael BM. Absence of a gender gap in survival. An analysis of the Italian registry for cystic fibrosis in the paediatric age. *J Cyst Fibros* 2011; **10**(5): 313–7.

117. Verma N, Bush A, Buchdahl R. Is there still a gender gap in cystic fibrosis? *Chest* 2005; **128**(4): 2824–34.

118. Coakley RD, Sun H, Clunes LA, et al. 17Beta-estradiol inhibits Ca2+-dependent homeostasis of airway surface liquid volume in human cystic fibrosis airway epithelia. *J Clin Invest* 2008; **118**(12): 4025–35.

119. Chotirmall SH, Greene CM, Oglesby IK, et al. 17Beta-estradiol inhibits IL-8 in cystic fibrosis by up-regulating secretory leucoprotease inhibitor. *Am J Respir Crit Care Med* 2010; **182**(1): 62–72.

120. Stallings VA. Gender, death and cystic fibrosis: Is energy expenditure a component? *J Pediatr* 2003; **142**(1): 4–6.

121. Willis E, Miller R, Wyn J. Gendered embodiment and survival for young people with cystic fibrosis. *Soc Sci Med* 2001; **53**(9): 1163–74.

122. Abbott J, Conway S, Etherington C, et al. Perceived body image and eating behavior in young adults with cystic fibrosis and their healthy peers. *J Behav Med* 2000; **23**(6): 501–17.

123. Anthony H, Paxton S, Catto-Smith A, et al. Physiological and psychosocial contributors to malnutrition in children with cystic fibrosis: Review. *Clin Nutr* 1999; **18**(6): 327–35.

124. Walters S. Sex differences in weight perception and nutritional behaviour in adults with cystic fibrosis. *J Hum Nutr Diet* 2001; **14**(2): 83–91.

125. Simon SL, Duncan CL, Horky SC, et al. Body satisfaction, nutritional adherence, and quality of life in youth with cystic fibrosis. *Pediatr Pulmonol* 2011; **46**(11): 1085–92.

126. Truby H, Paxton AS. Body image and dieting behavior in cystic fibrosis. *Pediatrics* 2001; **107**(6): E92.

127. Nixon PA, Orenstein DM, Kelsey SF, et al. The prognostic value of exercise testing in patients with cystic fibrosis. *N Engl J Med* 1992; **327**(25): 1785–8.

128. Orenstein DM, Nixon PA. Exercise performance and breathing patterns in cystic fibrosis: Male-female differences and influence of resting pulmonary function. *Pediatr Pulmonol* 1991; **10**(2): 101–5.

129. Busse WW, Kiecolt-Glaser JK, Coe C, et al. NHLBI Workshop summary. Stress and asthma. *Am J Respir Crit Care Med* 1995; **151**(1): 249–52.

130. Patterson JM, Budd J, Goetz D, et al. Family correlates of a 10-year pulmonary health trend in cystic fibrosis. *Pediatrics* 1993; **91**: 383–9.

131. Quittner AL, DiGirolamo AM, Michel M, et al. Parental response to cystic fibrosis: A contextual analysis of the diagnosis phase. *J Pediatr Psychol* 1992; **17**(6): 683–704.

132. Thompson RJ, Gustafson KE, Hamlett KW, et al. Psychological adjustment of children with cystic fibrosis: The role of child cognitive processes and maternal adjustment. *J Pediatr Psychol* 1992; **17**: 741–55.

133. Patterson JM, McCubbin HI, Warwick WJ. The impact of family functioning on health changes in children with cystic fibrosis. *Soc Sci Med* 1990; **31**(2): 159–64.

134. Besier T, Born A, Henrich G, et al. Anxiety, depression, and life satisfaction in parents caring for children with cystic fibrosis. *Pediatr Pulmonol* 2011; **46**(7): 672–82.

135. Besier T, Goldbeck L. Anxiety and depression in adolescents with CF and their caregivers. *J Cyst Fibros* 2011; **10**(6): 435–42.

136. Yohannes AM, Willgoss TG, Fatoye FA, et al. Relationship between anxiety, depression, and quality of life in adult patients with cystic fibrosis. *Respir Care* 2012; **57**(4): 550–6.

137. Smith BA, Modi AC, Quittner AL, et al. Depressive symptoms in children with cystic fibrosis and parents and its effects on adherence to airway clearance. *Pediatr Pulmonol* 2010; **45**(8): 756–63.

138. Goldbeck L, Besier T, Hinz A, et al. Prevalence of symptoms of anxiety and depression in German patients with cystic fibrosis. *Chest* 2010; **138**(4): 929–36.

139. Cruz I, Marciel KK, Quittner AL, et al. Anxiety and depression in cystic fibrosis. *Semin Respir Crit Care Med* 2009; **30**(5): 569–78.

140. Borowitz D, Baker RD, Stallings V. Consensus report on nutrition for pediatric patients with cystic fibrosis. *J Pediatr Gastroenterol Nutr* 2002; **35**(3): 246–59.

141. Cystic Fibrosis Foundation Center Committee and Guidelines Subcommittee. Cystic Fibrosis Foundation guidelines for patient services, evaluation, and monitoring in cystic fibrosis centers. *Am J Dis Child* 1990; **144**(12): 1311–2.

142. Committee CPGfCF. *Clinical Practice Guidelines for Cystic Fibrosis.* Bethesda, MD: Cystic Fibrosis Foundation; 1997.

143. Aris RM, Merkel PA, Bachrach LK, et al. Guide to bone health and disease in cystic fibrosis. *J Clin Endocrinol Metab* 2005; **90**(3): 1888–96.

144. Yankaskas JR, Marshall BC, Sufian B, et al. Cystic fibrosis adult care: Consensus conference report. *Chest* 2004; **125** (1 Suppl): 1S–39S.

145. Collins CE, MacDonald-Wicks L, Rowe S, et al. Normal growth in cystic fibrosis associated with a specialised centre. *Arch Dis Child* 1999; **81**(3): 241–6.

146. Mahadeva R, Webb K, Westerbeek RC, et al. Clinical outcome in relation to care in centres specialising in cystic fibrosis: Cross sectional study. *BMJ* 1998; **316**(7147): 1771–5.

147. Konstan MW, Butler SM, Schidlow DV, et al. Patterns of medical practice in cystic fibrosis: Part I. Evaluation and monitoring of health status of patients. Investigators and Coordinators of the Epidemiologic Study of Cystic Fibrosis. *Pediatr Pulmonol* 1999; **28**(4): 242–7.

148. Stern M, Wiedemann B, Wenzlaff P. From registry to quality management: The German Cystic Fibrosis Quality Assessment project 1995 2006. *Eur Respir J* 2008; **31**(1): 29–35.

149. Schechter MS. Demographic and center-related characteristics associated with low weight in pediatric cf patients. *Pediatr Pulmonol* 2002; (Suppl 22) (34): 156–7.

150. Johnson C, Butler SM, Konstan MW, et al. Factors influencing outcomes in cystic fibrosis: A center-based analysis. *Chest* 2003; **123**(1): 20–7.

151. Padman R, McColley SA, Miller DP, et al. Infant care patterns at epidemiologic study of cystic fibrosis sites that achieve superior childhood lung function. *Pediatrics* 2007; **119**(3): e531–7.

152. Berwick DM. Continuous improvement as an ideal in health care. *N Engl J Med* 1989; **320**(1): 53–6.

153. Schechter MS, Gutierrez HH. Improving the quality of care for patients with cystic fibrosis. *Curr Opin Pediatr* 2010; **22**(3): 296–301.

154. Stern M. The use of a cystic fibrosis patient registry to assess outcomes and improve cystic fibrosis care in Germany. *Curr Opin Pulm Med* 2011; **17**(6): 473–7.

155. Stern M, Niemann N, Wiedemann B, et al. Benchmarking improves quality in cystic fibrosis care: A pilot project involving 12 centres. *Int J Qual Health Care* 2011; **23**(3): 349–56.

156. Leonard A, Davis E, Rosenstein BJ, et al. Description of a standardized nutrition classification plan and its relation to nutritional outcomes in children with cystic fibrosis. *J Pediatr Psychol* 2009; **35**(1): 116–23.

157. Kraynack NC, McBride JT. Improving care at cystic fibrosis centers through quality improvement. *Semin Respir Crit Care Med* 2009; **30**(5): 547–58.

158. Greenberg RN. Overview of patient compliance with medication dosing: A literature review. *Clin Ther* 1984; **6**(5): 592–9.

159. Eakin MN, Bilderback A, Boyle MP, et al. Longitudinal association between medication adherence and lung health in people with cystic fibrosis. *J Cyst Fibros* 2011; **10**(4): 258–64.

160. Briesacher BA, Quittner AL, Saiman L, et al. Adherence with tobramycin inhaled solution and health care utilization. *BMC Pulm Med* 2011; **11**: 5.

161. Koocher GP, McGrath ML, Gudas LJ. Typologies of nonadherence in cystic fibrosis. *J Dev Behav Pediatr* 1990; **11**(6): 353–8.

162. Gudas LJ, Koocher GP, Wypij D. Perceptions of medical compliance in children and adolescents with cystic fibrosis. *J Dev Behav Pediatr* 1991; **12**(4): 236–42.

163. Ievers CE, Brown RT, Drotar D, et al. Knowledge of physician prescriptions and adherence to treatment among children with cystic fibrosis and their mothers. *J Dev Behav Pediatr* 1999; **20**(5): 335–43.

164. Lask B. Non-adherence to treatment in cystic fibrosis. *J Royal Soc Med* 1994; **87** (Suppl 21): 25–7.

165. Quittner AL, Drotar D, Ievers-Landis C, et al. Adherence to medical teatments in adolescents with cystic fibrosis: The development and evaluation of family-based interventions. In: Drotar D (ed). *Promoting Adherence to Medical Treatment in Childhood Chronic Illness: Concepts, Methods, and Interventions*. Mahwah, NJ: Erlbaum Associates; 2000.

166. Eddy ME, Carter BD, Kronenberger WG, et al. Parent relationships and compliance in cystic fibrosis. *J Pediatr Health Care* 1998; **12**(4): 196–202.

Diagnostic aspects of cystic fibrosis

Diagnosis of the symptomatic patient

COLIN WALLIS AND NICHOLAS J. SIMMONDS

INTRODUCTION

Making the diagnosis of cystic fibrosis (CF) has lifelong implications and repercussions for the affected individual and their family. The diagnosis needs to be made accurately and as early as possible. A late diagnosis is often preceded by a history of hospital visits, family anguish, anger and guilt, and a delay in the initiation of early treatment that may have an impact on long-term outcome. Equally disturbing is a small but increasing experience of the child or adult, diagnosed with CF, whom on review—often years later—is found to have been misdiagnosed.[1]

The introduction of newborn screening (NBS) in many countries, where the prevalence of CF is high, has completely changed the challenges of diagnosis in CF. It is now more common for a pediatrician to be facing a family of an outwardly healthy newborn child with a diagnostic label of CF made on screening information rather than clinical presentation. These aspects are dealt with in the forthcoming chapter.

However, all clinicians dealing with CF will also need to be aware of the child or adult who has escaped diagnosis through the screening process (which will never be perfect) and presents clinically or through family screening. This may be because of birth in a nonscreening area or prior to the introduction of screening, a technical error with the screening process, or a false negative screening test. Awareness of atypical forms is important for this group of children and adults and this chapter focuses on the clinical spectrum of CF disease at diagnosis and the tests available for confirmation.

In most cases, making the diagnosis is easy. An individual has suggestive clinical symptoms or a family history and a positive sweat test confirms the suspicions of CF. A triad of clinical features based on recurrent chest infections, pancreatic insufficiency, and failure to thrive was established in the 1960s and has been a useful phenotypic benchmark for a CF diagnosis for nearly 40 years.[2] The sweat test remains a very useful discriminator between those with and those without CF. But even before the identification of the CF gene, there were reported cases of "sweat test negative CF," and the concept of a broader phenotypic range had been promulgated.[3]

It was always hoped that the discovery of the gene for CF and its disease-causing mutations would provide diagnostic certainty. Two mutations within the *CFTR* gene would mean CF; normal genes would exclude the diagnosis. But it has not worked out that simply. Indeed, in the two decades since the discovery of the CF gene, the situation is probably even more confusing and the number of "atypical" or "unusual" cases is growing.[4,5] The phenotype for an individual with two *CFTR* mutations can range from completely normal to a classical CF phenotype.

Labels are defining and the diagnosis of classical CF carries with it important implications. Failure to identify and label a patient with CF could lead to delays in effective therapies. But inappropriate categorization of a patient with an atypical form of CF leads to an unnecessary burden of therapies and lifestyle restrictions. When considering the diagnosis of CF, clinicians must be aware of the expanding phenotype for this condition and the subclassification of CF into "classical," atypical, or CFTR-related disorders,[6,7] and more recently an unavoidable consequence of the screening process—a screen-positive child with potentially two CF genes who has no evidence of disease and may not even have evidence of CFTR dysfunction.

PRESENTING CLINICAL FEATURES

A Cystic Fibrosis Foundation (CFF) Consensus Panel (USA) synthesized diagnostic criteria for CF, based on the presence of one or more characteristic clinical features or a history of CF in a sibling, or a positive NBS test, plus laboratory evidence of a CFTR abnormality.[8] The key features are summarized in Figure 10.1. The basic premise of the consensus statement is that CF is a clinical and not a genetic diagnosis although acknowledging that genetic testing may have a role in sorting out atypical clinical situations. Any such document must be considered a work in progress to accommodate new developments and acknowledged shortcomings.[9]

The majority of children with CF in areas which do not screen present with a history of bulky offensive fatty stools, failure to thrive, and recurrent chest infections[10]; 10%–15% will present with meconium ileus shortly after birth. The range of clinical features suspicious of CF is listed in Table 10.1. The spectrum of presenting features is wide and vigilance is required to prevent missed diagnostic opportunities—especially in ethnic groups where CF is less common or in children who are considered "too healthy." The presenting features can vary with the age at time of clinical presentation as indicated in Table 10.2. In the days before widespread neonatal screening, approximately 90% of children with access to modern health care were diagnosed with CF by the age of 1 year.[11] In atypical cases however, the diagnosis is often delayed into adulthood. This latter group is often pancreatic sufficient with a milder (but not necessarily absent) pulmonary phenotype.

In addition to suspicious clinical features, a clinician may need to confirm the diagnosis of CF in other settings: (1) postnatal confirmation may be required when an antenatal test has proven suspicious but not confirmatory for CF; (2) a postnatal screening program may have identified a child as high risk for CF; and (3) an individual may be under investigation following the diagnosis of CF in a family member.

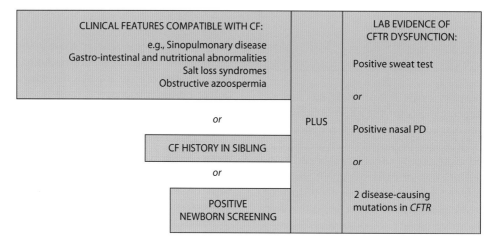

Figure 10.1 Diagnostic criteria for cystic fibrosis (CF). (From Rosenstein BJ, Cutting GR, *J Pediatr* 1998; 132: 589–95. With permission.)

Table 10.1 Clinical features consistent with a CF diagnosis

Sinopulmonary disease:		Chronic cough or sputum production
		Wheeze
		Finger clubbing
		Nasal polyposis or chronic sinusitis
		Culture of characteristic CF organism
		e.g., *P. aeruginosa* or nontuberculous mycobacteria in sputum, staphylococcal empyema
Gastrointestinal signs:		
	Intestinal	Meconium ileus, rectal prolapse, DIOS
	Pancreatic	Pancreatic insufficiency, pancreatitis
	Hepatic	Focal biliary cirrhosis, portal hypertension
		Prolonged neonatal jaundice
Nutritional and salt loss sequelae		Failure to thrive
		Acute salt loss
		Pseudo-Bartter syndrome, chronic metabolic alkalosis
		Hypoproteinemia–edema syndrome
		Kwashiorkor-like disease with skin changes
		Vitamin K deficiency, which may present with bleeding in the newborn period
Obstructive azoospermia		Bilateral absence of the vas deferens

CF, cystic fibrosis; DIOS, distal intestinal obstructive syndrome.

Table 10.2 Clinical features of CF at diagnosis in unscreened populations grouped according to age and approximate order of frequency

0–2 years

- Failure to thrive
- Steatorrhea
- Recurrent chest infections including bronchiolitis/bronchitis
- Meconium ileus
- Rectal prolapse
- Edema/hypoproteinemia/"kwashiorkor" skin changes
- Severe pneumonia/empyema
- Salt depletion syndrome
- Prolonged neonatal jaundice
- Vitamin K deficiency with bleeding diathesis

3–16 years

- Recurrent chest infections or "asthma"
- Clubbing and "idiopathic" bronchiectasis
- Steatorrhea
- Nasal polyps and sinusitis
- Chronic intestinal obstruction, intussusception
- Heat exhaustion with hyponatremia
- CF diagnosis in a relative

Adulthood (often atypical CF)

- Azoospermia/congenital absence of the vas deferens
- Bronchiectasis
- Chronic sinusitis
- Acute or chronic pancreatitis
- Allergic bronchopulmonary aspergillosis
- Focal biliary cirrhosis
- Abnormal glucose tolerance
- Portal hypertension
- Cholestasis/gall stones

Source: Reproduced and adapted from Wallis C. Diagnosis and presentation of cystic fibrosis. In: Chernick V, Boat T, Wilmott R, Bush A (Eds). *Kendig's Disorders of the Respiratory Tract in Children.* 7th ed. Philadelphia, PA: Saunders Elsevier; 2006. pp. 866–72. With permission.

A clinical suspicion for the diagnosis of CF can be supported by a number of confirmatory tests and investigations.

CONFIRMATORY TESTS

THE SWEAT TEST

The sweat test was first described in 1959 and remains the gold standard for the diagnosis of CF.[12] In the majority (98% in the US CFF Registry) of CF patients with typical features and identified *CFTR* mutations, the sweat test is diagnostic. In atypical forms, sweat chloride levels may fall into the intermediate range and there are rare examples of patients with CF, confirmed on genetic testing, who have a normal sweat test.[13,14] There are a number of other rare conditions (sometimes single case reports) that have been associated with a positive sweat test, but these are usually clearly distinguishable by their clinical features. Examples are listed in Table 10.3. The commonest cause of a false positive sweat test is operator inexperience, followed by dry eczematous skin in the patient.

The standard sweat test (Gibson and Cooke technique) requires skill and care and should be undertaken by accredited laboratories. Localized sweating is stimulated by the iontophoresis of pilocarpine into the skin and collected at a standardized rate. Guidelines for sweat testing procedures and precautions are published and testing should be carried out by experienced personnel using standardized methodologies in facilities with a regular throughput.[15–17]

Patient selection

Sweat tests can be reliably performed after 2 weeks of age in infants greater than 3 kg who are normally hydrated and without significant systemic illness. During the first

Table 10.3 Examples of non-CF causes of a positive sweat test

- Adrenal insufficiency or stress
- Anorexia nervosa
- Autonomic dysfunction
- Ectodermal dysplasia
- Eczema
- Fucosidosis
- G6PD deficiency
- Glycogen storage disease type 1
- Hypoparathyroidism
- Hypothyroidism
- Malnutrition from various causes including HIV infection
- Nephrogenic diabetes insipidus
- Nephrosis
- Pseudohypoaldosteronism
- Progressive familial intrahepatic cholestasis

G6PD, glucose-6-phosphate dehydrogenase; HIV, human immunodeficiency syndrome.

24 hours after birth in term infants, sweat electrolyte values may be transiently elevated.[18] After the first week a decline in the levels occurs and an elevated value can be used to confirm a diagnosis of CF.[19] In a retrospective review of sweat tests in preterm and full-term infants, adequate sweat collection could be obtained in infants ≥36 weeks who weighed >2 kg and were greater than 3 days postnatal age (Figure 10.2).[20] Children who are systemically unwell, edematous, or on corticosteroids should have their testing delayed. Normal adolescents and adults tend to have higher sweat chloride levels (up to 60 mmol/L) and therefore borderline values in this age group may not reflect CF.

Sweat collection

The flexor surface of the forearm is the preferred site although other sites may be considered if the arms are eczematous or otherwise unsuitable. Great care must be taken at all stages of the testing to avoid contamination. Electrodes should be of a suitable size and curvature to fit snugly on the patient's limb.

Sweat is collected on filter paper, gauze, or via Macroduct tubing over a controlled period of time to ensure that the rate of sweating and the total sweat collected are sufficient and standardized.[21,22] During the process of collection, the sweat must be protected from contamination and dehydration. Sweat should be collected for a period between 20 and 30 minutes.

Sweat analysis

The sweat secretion rate, measured as an average rate over the collection period, should not be less than 1 g/m²/min. Chloride is the analyte of choice.[23,24] A sweat chloride

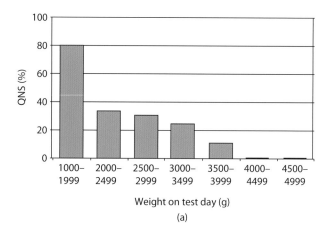

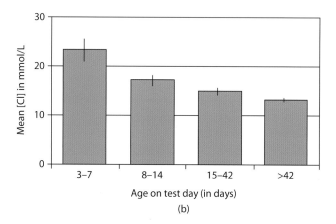

Figure 10.2 (a) Effect of infant weight at time of testing on likelihood of failure of collecting >75 mg sweat (QNS = quantity not sufficient as represented by a percentage failure rate. (b) Mean chloride concentration at different postnatal ages in infants without CF. (From Eng W, Legrys VA, Schechter MS, Laughon MM, Barker PM, *Pediatr Pulmonol* 2005; 40: 64–7. With permission.)

concentration of more than 60 mmol/L is considered positive and levels below 40 mmol/L are likely to be in the normal range, and CF is considered to be unlikely although not excluded.[25] This lower limit has been dropped still further by some authorities as increasing experience shows CFTR-related abnormalities with sweat chloride in the 30–60 mmol/L range. Intermediate levels between 30 and 60 mmol/L may be associated with atypical forms of CF and need to be interpreted with caution.[26,27] Some normal adults can have values in the intermediate range. There is evidence from NBS that initial intermediate or high normal chloride readings may also occur in the affected premature infant or newborn and may need repeating.[28]

Sweat chloride levels greater than 150 mmol/L are not physiological and should be questioned and repeated. A false positive sweat test in the severely malnourished child or the critically ill child in intensive care needs cautious interpretation and follow-up. Case reports also describe a nonsense mutation in the *CFTR* gene associated with

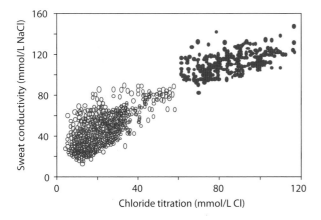

Figure 10.3 Comparison of conductivity method and chloride concentration in sweat of 3834 patients with CF (solid circles) and without CF (empty circles). (From Lezana JL, Vargas MH, Karam-Bechara J, Aldana RS, Furuya ME, *J Cyst Fibros* 2003; 2: 1–7. With permission.)

elevated sweat chloride in the absence of clinical features of CF.[29] The sweat sodium levels are less reliable and should never be used in isolation.

The osmolality of sweat records the total solute concentration in millimoles per kilogram of sweat. The reference ranges for osmolality are wide: children with CF have sweat osmolality values greater than 200 mmol/kg with normal ranges falling between 50 and 150 mmol/kg. Positive and equivocal results (between 150 and 200 mmol/kg) should be followed up by a quantitative analysis of chloride concentration.

Research continues to explore the development of an easier sweat test. Collecting systems such as the nanoduct are achieving credibility and the role of sweat conductivity as a diagnostic tool in CF is also gaining credence.[30,31] Conductivity represents a nonselective measurement of ions and good correlation between the results of sweat chloride concentrations and sweat conductivity have been shown. In one large trial, the best conductivity cut-off value to diagnose CF was ≥90 mmol/L, and the best conductivity cut-off value to exclude CF was <75 mmol/L (Figure 10.3).[32] For conductivity, a provisional upper physiological limit of 170 mmol/L may be used pending further evidence. Currently, many clinicians and laboratories will choose to confirm a positive sweat conductivity result with a formal measurement of chloride concentration.

MUTATION ANALYSIS

The identification of the CF gene in 1989 and the characterization of its protein product (CFTR) held the promise that the diagnostic dilemmas for the condition were over.[33] Two identifiable mutations meant you had the disease. Unfortunately, it has not worked out that simply. Although two disease-causing mutations are very supportive of the diagnosis of CF in the appropriate clinical setting, there are a number of caveats.

First, there are over 1900 different CF gene mutations associated with CF disease as recorded and rising on a website dedicated to this tally (http://www.genet.sickkids.on.ca /cftr). Examples of *CFTR* mutations are listed in Table 10.4. The dominance of the (*F508* mutation is highlighted and present in >70% of CF alleles in Caucasian populations.[10] Confirming the diagnosis of CF based on the presence of two CF-causing mutations is highly specific but not very sensitive. Sensitivity is decreased due to the large number of CF mutations. Most laboratories will only search routinely for the commonest mutations within their geographical region. Customizing mutation panels to match the patient's ethnic background and clinical presentation can enhance the sensitivity of DNA testing in CF. For example, there are CF mutations that occur with increased frequency in specific population groups, such as the Ashkenazi Jewish (*W1282X*) or African (*3120 + 1G → A*) patients, and in patients with specific clinical features, such as pancreatic sufficiency (*R117H* and *A445E*), male fertility (*3849 + 10kbC → T*), or normal concentrations of sweat electrolytes (*3849 + 10kbC → T*).[34,35] Extended analysis of the whole *CFTR* gene by exon sequencing and multiply ligation probe amplification is possible but not routinely available as a first-line investigation.

Second, alterations in the *CFTR* gene designated as CF-causing mutations should fulfill at least one of the criteria as shown in Table 10.5. In addition to the "disease-causing" mutations, there are also recognizable polymorphisms that do not necessarily result in a clinical phenotype but may influence the structure of the final protein product when associated with another mild mutation, such as *R117H*. The thymidine tract in intron 8 is a well-described example, where the 5T allele leads to a substantial reduction in functional protein compared with 9T; 7T is intermediate.[36]

Failure to find two CF mutations from a selective or extended search does not exclude the diagnosis of CF. To exclude a patient with symptoms of CF and a positive sweat test from potentially beneficial treatment because the laboratory cannot detect two CF mutations would clearly be misguided. There are also rare reports of patients with classical CF symptoms and signs and a positive sweat test who do not appear to have any mutations in the *CFTR* gene even with extended genetic analysis involving sequencing all 27 exons and the intron–exon boundaries.[37] These findings suggest that on these rare occasions CF may be caused by mutations within the promotor region of the *CFTR* gene, in one of the introns or even in a distant controlling gene from an unrelated locus.[38]

Finally, although two mutations are very supportive of the diagnosis of CF in the appropriate clinical setting, two alterations in the gene for CFTR does not necessarily mean that the subject will develop classic CF disease.[39] There is evidence of a corrective effect of a second mutation in cis with a disease-causing one, altering the electrolyte imbalance on the cell surface, for example.[40] The

Table 10.4 Common mutations that cause cystic fibrosis listed according to frequency

Traditional name	HGVS[a] nomenclature	Frequency in Caucasians (%)[b]
ΔF508	p.Phe3508del	75.0
G551D	p.Gly551Asp	3.4
G542X	p.gly542X	1.8
R117H	p.arg117His	1.3
621 + 1G → T	c.489 + 1G → T	1.3
1717 − 1G → T	c.1585 − 1G → A	0.6
1898 + 1G → T	c.1766 + 1G → A	0.6
ΔI507	p.Ile507del	0.5
N1303K	p.Asn1303Lys	0.5
R560T	p.arg560Thr	0.4
Q493X	c.1477C → T	0.3
R1162X	p.Arg1162X	0.3
R533X	p.Arg553X	0.3
W1282X	p.Trp1282X	0.3
3659delC	c.3527_3528delC (p.Lys1177Serfs)	0.3
1154insTC	c.1021_1022dup (p.Phe342HisfsX28)	0.3
E60X	p.Glu60X	0.2
G85E	p.Gly85Glu	0.2
P67L	c.200C → T (p.Pro67Leu)	0.2
R347P	p.Arg347Pro	0.2
V520F	p.Val520Phe	0.2
1078delT	c.946_947delT (p.Phe316Leufs)	0.1
2184delA	c.2052_2053delA (p.Lys684Asnfs)	0.1
A455E	p.Ala455Glu	0.1
R334W	p.Arg334Trp	0.1
S549N	p.Ser549Asn	0.1
2789 + 5G → A	c.2657 + 5G → A	0.1
3849 + 10kbC → T	c.3717 + 10kbC → T	0.1
711 + 1G → T	c.579 + 1G → T	0.1

Source: Reproduced and adapted from Wallis C. Diagnosis and presentation of cystic fibrosis. In: Chernick V, Boat T, Wilmott R, Bush A (Eds). *Kendig's Disorders of the Respiratory Tract in Children.* 7th ed. Philadelphia, PA: Saunders Elsevier; 2006. pp. 866–72. With permission.

[a] "New" Human Genome Variation Society nomenclature (http://www.hgvs.org/)
[b] Listed frequency for Caucasian populations. Variations in frequency occur between different ethnic groups and geographic regions.

Table 10.5 Features of a disease-producing mutation in the *CFTR* gene

- A change in the aminoacid sequence that severely affects CFTR synthesis and/or function
- A deletion, insertion, or nonsense mutation, which introduces a premature termination signal (stop mutation)
- Alteration to the first two or last two nucleotides of an intron splice site
- A novel aminoacid sequence that is not a "normal" variant (found in at least 100 carriers within the subject's ethnic background)

clinical phenotype associated with two *CFTR* mutations is far broader than could ever have been anticipated.[41] Examples are listed in Table 10.6 and the importance of these atypical forms of CF are discussed further below. The CFTR2 (http://www.cftr2.org) website is a useful resource designed to provide information about specific CF mutations to patients, researchers, and the general public. For each mutation included in the database, the website provides information about: (1) disease status, i.e., if the mutation is disease causing or not (or of varying clinical consequence) and (2) clinical characteristics—the average lung function, pancreatic status, and *Pseudomonas aeruginosa* infection rates in patients in the CFTR2 database with the specified mutation.

Table 10.6 The range of clinical phenotypes associated with two mutations in the CF gene

1. Classical CF

- Sinopulmonary disease with pancreatic insufficiency, gastrointestinal and nutritional consequences, high sweat chloride concentration, and male infertility
- As above but pancreatic sufficient

2. Atypical CF (nonclassic)

- Sinopulmonary disease and male fertility with a normal sweat test
- Severe sinusitis and congenial bilateral absence of the vas deferens
- Male infertility only
- Recurrent idiopathic pancreatitis
- Allergic bronchopulmonary aspergillosis
- Sclerosing cholangitis
- Salt-losing syndromes

3. No clinical features at time of assessment

- With positive sweat test
- With normal or intermediate sweat test

CF PHENOTYPES

There are four major contributing factors that influence the path from genotype to end organ involvement and an individual's eventual phenotype:

1. *The severity of the individual CFTR mutations.* "Mild" mutations may cause milder phenotypic effects, but when there is a mixture of mild and severe mutations the final impact is unpredictable. Similarly, coexistent polymorphisms hitchhiking within the *CFTR* gene may influence the final protein product. Pancreatic phenotype can sometimes be predicted by genotype and pancreatic insufficiency is almost invariably associated with two "severe" mutations. The correlation between genotype and phenotype for a pulmonary phenotype is not reliably predictive and the course of lung disease in CF is especially vulnerable to environmental and modifier genes.[42] Sometimes, mild mutations may have a dominant effect on severe mutations with a "corrective" effect. This beneficial impact can produce pancreatic sufficiency, for example, although a similar positive effect on lung function is less predictable.
2. *Modifying genes.* Genes lying elsewhere in the genome have significant influence on the behavior of the CFTR protein.[43] These genes and their protein products can correct or exacerbate influencing pathological processes such as the biochemistry of the cell surface liquid, the innate and acquired immunity of the lungs, and may even influence the predisposition to meconium ileus.[44] Each individual with CF is likely to have an immense orchestra of modifying genes and proteins

unique to themselves and influential on their clinical outcome.[45]
3. *Environmental factors.* The environment in which an individual with CF lives and grows has central bearing on the outcome of their disease.[46] Treatment and adherence to therapy, socioeconomic circumstances and diet, exposure to infections such as *P. aeruginosa* or viral infections in infancy can produce a sustained negative influence on the clinical course.[47]
4. *The passage of time.* CF is not necessarily an all or nothing disease. A clinical phenotype can emerge with time especially in some of the atypical forms and regular reviews of the CF classification may be required. Effective therapies and adherence to treatment can help stall the disease progression. Patients with documented pancreatic sufficiency in childhood can become pancreatic insufficient in later life. Some but not all patients with CF will develop diabetes, liver disease, and osteoporosis.

CLASSIFICATION OF CF PHENOTYPES

There is lack of consensus between the US[48] and European[49] CF societies on the exact diagnostic terminologies for the phenotypic forms of CF although the principles remain similar.[50,51] Broadly speaking, four groups can be considered.

CLASSICAL CF

The diagnosis of classical CF needs to be made early and confidently. No racial group is exempt and children of ethnic minorities or mixed heritage are at greatest risk of a delayed or missed diagnosis. The clinical features of recurrent chest infections, malabsorption with pancreatic insufficiency in the majority (but not all), or an infant presenting with meconium ileus, rectal prolapse, or unexplained malnutrition requires investigation. Although pancreatic insufficiency is present in around 85% of classical CF patients, pancreatic sufficient patients are not necessarily excluded from the classical CF category. A positive sweat test and/or two *CFTR* mutations is diagnostic. Appropriate therapy should be introduced without delay. Common causes for a delayed diagnosis include failure to consider the diagnosis because the patient looks "too healthy"; substandard sweat test methodology or misinterpretation of an inadequate sample of sweat; and the failure to repeat a previously borderline sweat test in the face of ongoing clinical concerns.

ATYPICAL (NONCLASSIC) CF

There is a growing group of children and adults who do not present with the full spectrum of clinical features associated with classical CF. The terms "equivocal CF" or "variant CF" have also been used to describe these atypical forms. There may be limited end organ involvement. Sweat testing can be normal, equivocal, or positive and CFTR analysis may reveal one, two, or no mutations depending on the sophistication of analysis. In patients with atypical CF who have two identified *CFTR* mutations, one is usually a "mild" mutation resulting in partial CFTR expression and function. Examples of such conditions are included in Table 10.6 and often represent the mildest end of the CF spectrum. On the basis of registry data, approximately 2% of individuals who fulfill the criteria for the diagnosis of CF fall in the atypical category. It is very likely, however, that this is an underrepresentation as it is probable that many of these atypical cases are undiagnosed or present for the first time in adult life.[52–54]

Recent reviews have recognized that it is inappropriate to label individuals with these atypical forms as having classical CF.[5,54] Both the diagnostic labeling and medical management needs to be tailored to the patient's individual phenotype and requirements. The introduction of arduous therapies aimed at the patient with classical CF does not seem appropriate or beneficial. The negative connotations of a CF label can be avoided with a more considered approach to diagnostic categorization, embracing subcategorization and accepting the atypical forms of CF. It is not necessarily a license for complacency, as with time, classical clinical features of CF can emerge and require action.

CFTR-RELATED DISORDERS

CFTR-related disorders (or CFTR dysfunction) is a term coined to describe subjects with a clinical entity associated with CFTR dysfunction that does not fulfill the diagnostic criteria for CF.[55] These single-organ CF-like conditions carry a higher incidence of *CFTR* mutations than could be expected by chance but have no other indicators of either classical or atypical CF. CFTR-related disorders appear to be influenced by CFTR dysfunction but are under greatest influence from non-*CFTR* genes and environmental influences. These authors fully acknowledge that the distinction of CFTR-related disorders from atypical CF is not clear-cut—especially in pediatrics where the emergence of the full phenotype may occur with time. Diagnostic algorithms for the investigation of these disorders have been proposed.[55] Three main clinical entities illustrate this phenotype:

1. Congenital bilateral absence of the vas deferens
2. Acute recurrent or chronic pancreatitis
3. Disseminated bronchiectasis

SCREENED POSITIVE PATIENTS WITH HYPERTRYPSINOGENEMIA AND AN INCONCLUSIVE DIAGNOSIS (CFSPID)

CFTR-related metabolic syndrome

This fourth category of CF phenotype has arisen as a result of the wide introduction of NBS for CF. NBS infants with hypertrypsinogenemia are being identified with two *CFTR* mutations (one of which may not be characterized as "disease causing") or one identified mutation and an equivocal sweat test who do not fit the criteria for a CF diagnosis. There is no evidence of end organ CF disease, at least on standard clinical work-ups; whether subtle abnormalities would be detected by bronchoscopy, high-resolution computed tomography (CT) or lung clearance index (LCI) is as yet undetermined, and it is an open question how far investigations should be pushed to "exclude" end organ function. The clumsy name—"CFTR-related metabolic syndrome"—(designed more to satisfy certain countries' billing and coding requirements than on linguistic merit) has been suggested for this group.[56] Although recognized previously and described as "pre-CF,"[7] the prevalence may now be as much as 1 in 10 newborn screened babies (CFF data 2011—Dr. C. Ren, pers. comm.) and is an increasingly common and unavoidable consequence of NBS. There is the potential that clinical features will emerge with time but there is insufficient clinical or biochemical evidence to label the carrier of the gene mutations with a disease. A recent consensus document by Munck et al. is referenced and discussed in the next chapter on screening. Herein they consider the designation CFSPID—"cystic fibrosis screen positive, inconclusive diagnosis"—and divide this group into two: 1) those with a normal sweat chloride and one or two mutations, and 2) those with an intermediate sweat chloride and one or no *CFTR* mutations. Management options are proposed. Nasal potential difference (PD) measurement may have some role in assessing the *CFTR* function further and is discussed in more detail later in this chapter.[57] Most clinicians would advise a program of careful surveillance, including repeating the sweat test at a year.[58] Therapy is reserved for early end organ changes, although how invasively these should be sought is unclear.[59] The role of prophylactic therapy such as physiotherapy or antibiotics is unclear.

ADULT PRESENTATION

Individuals with milder phenotypes may present in adulthood. They usually have atypical CF and may present with single-organ involvement and normal nutritional status.[52,60] For this reason, they may present to a variety of medical specialists depending on the end organ most affected, including infertility, gastroenterology, and otorhinolaryngology clinics. They may also have been under a general respiratory clinic with "idiopathic" bronchiectasis and undergone some or no CF specific investigations as, traditionally, general adult respiratory physicians were less aware of the wide spectrum of CF disease. Even if CF investigations are initiated in this setting, the diagnosis can be delayed as interpretation may be limited or tests not completed (e.g., with extended CFTR analysis). This is compounded by the considerable diagnostic challenge of these patients, even in the hands of experts, as they are more likely than classical CF to have an equivocal or even normal sweat chloride and only one or even no identifiable *CFTR* mutation.[61] In this situation, other techniques, such as nasal PD measurement and extended gene analysis, can improve the diagnostic yield, but even then a small number of patients are left without a secure diagnosis.[49,62] As routine CFTR genotyping detects mutations that are common to the specific population of the region that it serves (e.g., in the United Kingdom, most laboratories test for 50 mutations, detecting 85%–90% of alleles in white Britons), mutations of patients presenting in adulthood with atypical features may be missed as they are proportionately more likely to have rare mutations. Extended CFTR analysis, therefore, should be performed, but on rare occasions it too will fail to identify two mutations.[63] Measuring CFTR function by nasal PD has particular utility when adults present with possible CF as it can improve diagnostic yields and, in most cases, discriminate diagnostic subgroups, although the precise diagnostic thresholds are yet to be fully determined.[50]

Irrespective of the precise terminology and age of presentation, if evidence of abnormal CFTR function exists and compatible symptoms are present, it is appropriate to follow-up these patients in a setting with CF expertise as there is potential for progression (e.g., of bronchiectasis) and other CFTR-related complications. Genetic counseling and family/partner screening should also be initiated, if indicated.

ADDITIONAL SUPPORTIVE INVESTIGATIONS IN ATYPICAL PRESENTATIONS

Occasionally, a clinician faces difficulties establishing the label of CF. The commonest situation is the patient with clinical features partially consistent with CF but a nondiagnostic sweat test and only one identified CF mutation. Further evaluation is required to determine whether the patient is a carrier for CF or has an atypical form. It is equally important to ensure that an alternative diagnosis has been excluded. Part of the differential diagnosis will include conditions such as immunodeficiency, Shwachman–Diamond syndrome, primary ciliary dyskinesia, and allergic disease. It is also recognized that molecular abnormalities other than CFTR dysfunction can masquerade as atypical CF.[64]

The following ancillary testing is suggested, tailoring these additional supportive investigations to the clinical picture.

FURTHER ASSESSMENT OF CFTR DYSFUNCTION

Nasal PD measurement

Nasal PD measurement takes advantage of the two main components of CFTR-mediated ion transport in the respiratory tract: Cl^- secretion and $Na+$ absorption. In CF, the lack of functional CFTR in the apical membrane results in defective Cl^- secretion, coupled with $Na+$ hyperabsorption owing to unregulated (and open) epithelial sodium channels. Water follows $Na+$ hyperabsorption and with an ineffective compensatory flow mechanism in the opposite direction, depletion of the airway surface liquid rapidly ensues. Nasal PD measures the voltage created by Cl^- and $Na+$ as they move across the epithelium.

Nasal PD is measured by placing an exploring electrode on the surface of the respiratory epithelium (most commonly on the floor of the nose or under the inferior turbinate) and a reference electrode into the subcutaneous tissue of the forearm or over an area of abraded skin (Figure 10.4 and Video 10.1).[65] The abnormalities of ion

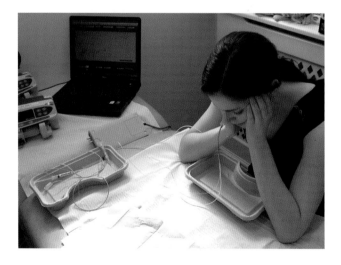

Figure 10.4 Patient undergoing nasal potential difference (PD) measurement as part of the diagnostic work-up for possible CF. An exploring nasal electrode (within the catheter) and reference (skin) electrode are positioned as shown. Perfusing solutions pass through the catheter onto the nasal mucosa and into the catching bowl. A real-time readout of PD (millivolt) is displayed during the procedure.

transport in CF produce a number of differences in PD measurements when compared to normal nasal mucosal measurements (Figure 10.5). Specifically, in CF there is a more negative basal PD in keeping with Na^+ hyperabsorption; a greater change in PD (becoming less negative) occurs after the application of amiloride to the nasal epithelium; there is little or no response to perfusion of the mucosa with a Cl^- free solution (passive Cl^- secretion) or

the addition of the cyclic adenosine monophosphate agonist, isoprenaline, which activates normal CFTR. A typical result for CF and normal nasal PD is shown in Figure 10.4. The total Cl^- secretory response is the most sensitive discriminator between CF and non-CF epithelia.

The technique has evolved over many years and although originally used as a research tool, it now has wider recognition in the clinical arena.[66-68] The test requires an experienced operator and considerable cooperation from the subject, with careful placement of the nasal electrode. Perfusion rate and the duration of the perfusion are important variables. Results may be difficult to interpret in the presence of allergic or infectious rhinitis and nasal polyps. Adaptations of the technique have allowed measurements in newborns while asleep using an extremely low flow rate.[69]

Its utility in the diagnosis of difficult or possible CF cases has been highlighted in recent publications,[50,70] and there is evidence that it correlates with specific disease manifestations and severity.[71-74] In one study of 208 patients classified as having CFTR-related disorders, 35 were reclassified as either having atypical CF (19 patients of whom 15 had azoospermia) or "unlikely CF" (16 patients) on the basis of their nasal PD.[50] Currently it is not widely available, but with ongoing technical refinements and standardization, it is likely to become a more integral component of the diagnostic work-up in the future.

ASSESSMENT OF END ORGAN EFFECTS

Detailed structural imaging of the lung parenchyma

Modern CT technology using high-resolution scans can demonstrate early structural changes to the small airways that are not readily visible on plain radiographic films.[75] In addition to assessing bronchial wall thickening and dilation in the smallest of bronchioles, the presence of air trapping representing early changes to the bronchioles may be visible on expiratory images.[76]

Evaluation of the paranasal sinuses

The sinuses are highly sensitive to altered CFTR function. Plain radiographs, CT imaging, and MRI views of the sinuses can show opacification and the presence of polyps. It would be very unusual in older children and adults with CF to have normal sinus imaging on CT scanning.

Pancreatic function testing

Pancreatic insufficiency is usually clinically evident but further testing can be helpful in selected cases. Previously, pancreatic function testing required sophisticated technology with invasive sampling techniques and stimulation protocols. As an alternative, prolonged timed stool collections for fecal fat analysis have been suggested but remain unpopular with patients and laboratories. The quantification of fecal

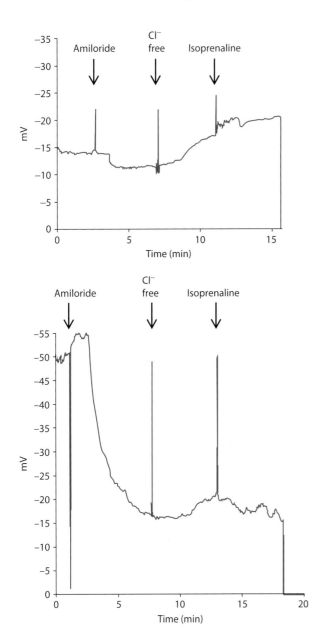

Figure 10.5 Nasal PD measurement in a healthy subject (top) and patient with classic CF (bottom). In a healthy person, the baseline PD is less negative and increases by a small amount in the presence of amiloride, followed by a large negative change in the presence of zero chloride and isoprenaline, reflecting hyperpolarization from chloride secretion. In contrast to CF, where a more negative basal PD is present, with a greater change in the presence of amiloride, followed by minimal, or no, chloride secretion.

by a particularly virulent course, high fevers, bacteremia, rapid deterioration in lung function, and early death. This syndrome is not limited to *B. cenocepacia* and has been described with other species of *Burkholderia* including *Burkholderia dolosa, B. multivorans, and B. cepacia*.[30-33] However, it should be noted that a particular species does not predict outcomes. Patients harboring the same species can have markedly different courses; some remain stable, whereas others deteriorate. The molecular strategies used to distinguish *Burkholderia* spp. are described further in Chapter 14.

STENOTROPHOMONAS MALTOPHILIA

This intrinsically multi-drug-resistant gram-negative bacillus is a well-known hospital-acquired pathogen in non-CF patients and is isolated with increasing frequency from the respiratory tract of CF patients. In 2011, the overall prevalence of this organism in CF patients in the United States was 14% (range 0%–28.6% in individual centers).[15] Transient colonization also appears to be common.[34] Increased use of antibiotics may be a potential risk factor for acquisition of *Stenotrophomonas maltophilia*.[35]

The pathogenic role of *Stenotrophomonas maltophilia* in CF is unclear. Case–control studies have not shown that *Stenotrophomonas maltophilia* has a significant impact on lung function or mortality.[36,37] In contrast, the 5-year survival of patients with severe lung function at initial isolation of *Stenotrophomonas maltophilia* was lower compared to patients without *Stenotrophomonas maltophilia*.[34] Most recently, chronic *Stenotrophomonas maltophilia* infection was shown to be associated with severe pulmonary exacerbations[38] and a threefold increased risk of death or lung transplantation.[39] However, such epidemiologic studies may not be able to distinguish if *Stenotrophomonas maltophilia* is a marker of severe lung disease or a cause of progressive lung disease.

ACHROMOBACTER XYLOSOXIDANS

The clinical significance of *Achromobacter* in CF also remains unclear. *Achromobacter* spp. are detected from 6.2% of CF patients in the United States[15] and from 17.5% of patients in a French CF center.[40] However, the reported prevalence of *Achromobacter* is most likely an underestimate as core laboratories have found higher rates compared to laboratories serving as CF centers in the United States.[41] This is likely due to misidentification; *Achromobacter* spp. are frequently misidentified as other non-lactose-fermenting gram-negative bacilli using commercial systems. In addition, *P. aeruginosa*, *Burkholderia* spp., and *Stenotrophomonas maltophilia* may be misidentified as *Achromobacter* spp.[42]

Recent work using multilocus sequence typing (MLST) analysis has revealed that *Achromobacter* consists of at least 7 species and 14 recently described genomovars of which most have been detected in CF patients.[28]

Achromobacter xylosoxidans accounted for 42% of strains and *Achromobacter ruhlandii* accounted for 23.5% of strains isolated from CF patients.[27] Similar observations were made in Denmark as *Achromobacter xylosoxidans* and *Achromobacter ruhlandii* represented 64% and 7% of *Achromobacter* strains, respectively.[43]

Although an association between *Achromobacter xylosoxidans* and decline in lung function has been described,[44] the clinical impact of *Achromobacter* spp. is difficult to assess as these microorganisms are cultured from older patients with more advanced lung disease concomitantly infected with other CF pathogens.[45]

MOLDS

ASPERGILLUS SPP.

Aspergillus spp. are often recovered from CF respiratory tract specimens, and *Aspergillus fumigatus* is the most common species. In the United States, 15% of patients had positive cultures for this mold in 2011 including 10.5% of those greater than 18 years old and 20.4% of those greater than or equal to 18 years old. Both oral and aerosolized antimicrobial agents have been shown to be risk factors for colonization with *Aspergillus* spp.[46,47] Colonization with *Aspergillus* has not been shown to adversely affect lung function[47] but was associated with an increased risk of pulmonary exacerbations.[48]

Allergic pulmonary aspergillosis (APBA) is diagnosed in 2%–10% of CF patients and can be associated with a dramatic loss of lung function.[49,50] However, diagnosing ABPA can be very difficult due to the complex diagnostic criteria for APBA in CF, confusion regarding these criteria, and limited recognition of ABPA by providers.[51] This immunologically mediated syndrome is marked by elevated IgE response, specific antibodies to *Aspergillus fumigatus*, peripheral eosinophilia, and reactive airway disease (see Chapter 16).

SCEDOSPORIUM SPP.

Scedosporium spp. can be isolated from the lungs of 0.7% of CF patients;[15] however, higher rates have been described in a single center in which 8.6% of patients were colonized/infected with *Scedosporium apiospermum* over 5 years.[52] At present, the clinical significance of this mold in CF is unclear, but following lung transplantation it has caused death due to disseminated disease.[53,54] Furthermore, *Scedosporium apiospermum* has been associated with ABPA.[55]

OTHER YEASTS AND MOLDS

Candida species are commonly recovered from cultures of the respiratory tract of CF patients. In the United States, 16%

of patients grew *Candida* from respiratory tract specimens in 2011.[15] The pathogenic role of *Candida* remains unclear, but recent work has focused on the inflammatory potential of *Candida* spp. in CF.[56] In a single-center study, *Candida* was associated with exacerbations and decline in lung function.[57] Vulvovaginal candidiasis, posttransplant candidiasis, and candidemia associated with central venous catheters have all been described in CF patients.[56]

NONTUBERCULOUS MYCOBACTERIA

Since the early 1990s, there has been an increasing appreciation that nontuberculous mycobacteria (NTMs) are pathogens in CF patients. It has been difficult to establish the overall prevalence and incidence of NTMs in CF due to a lack of standardized surveillance strategies, the complexity of microbiologic processing (see later), and geographic diversity of specific NTM species. Most recently, *Mycobacterium abscessus* has been found to consist of three subspecies: *Mycobacterium bolletii*, *Mycobacterium massiliense*, and *M. abscessus*.[58] Whereas *Mycobacterium avium* complex (MAC) appears to be most common in the United States,[59] *Mycobacterium simiae* is most common in Israeli CF patients[60] and *M. abscessus* is most common in French children with CF.[61] Risk factors for NTMs may include geographic proximity to large bodies of water, ABPA, and steroid therapy.[62]

It can be difficult to determine if NTM is exacerbating CF lung disease. Signs and symptoms of mycobacterial disease are nonspecific and may be consistent with CF pulmonary exacerbations. Patients harboring *M. abscessus* are more likely to fulfill the American Thoracic Society diagnostic criteria for NTM disease than patients harboring MAC.[63] The European and US CF communities are currently collaborating on NTM guidelines, which will provide recommendations for diagnosis and treatment.

VIRUSES

The contribution of respiratory viral pathogens, particularly respiratory syncytial virus and rhinovirus, to CF lung disease has been appreciated for decades.[64-67] As many as 40% of exacerbations may be associated with viral infections. Several recent studies have evaluated the frequency of viral pathogens during pulmonary exacerbations using molecular strategies including multiplex reverse transcription polymerase chain reaction systems. Rhinovirus can be detected in children with CF who were clinically stable as well as in those during exacerbations, but the viral load was 10-fold higher in those having exacerbations.[68] Upper tract symptoms were correlated with viral detection in young children and adolescents.[69]

CLINICAL MICROBIOLOGY AND LABORATORY METHODS

Several national and international societies have published recommendations for processing CF specimens.[70,71] Recommendations from these guidelines are summarized in the following subsections.

OBTAINING CYSTIC FIBROSIS RESPIRATORY SPECIMENS

Respiratory tract specimens from CF patients can include throat swabs, deep oropharyngeal swabs, bronchoalveolar lavage (BAL), spontaneously expectorated sputum, and induced sputum, as well as cultures from the sinuses and those obtained by lung transplantation. All should be labeled "CF Specimen" to ensure appropriate processing as described later. Oropharyngeal cultures are obtained in children too young to expectorate. BAL is generally reserved for research protocols, lung transplant recipients, or patients with atypical courses who cannot produce sputum. While expectorated sputum is considered the ideal specimen, more than or equal to 1.0 mL should be collected to ensure an adequate volume for plating on selective media. The concordance of upper and lower airway specimens has been studied and, overall, upper airway cultures do not always predict lower airway cultures.[72,73] Most recently, induced sputum has been studied in pediatric CF patients and compared with either throat swabs or expectorated sputum; induced, sputum had a higher microbiologic yield than the other specimens.[74] Only lower airway specimens can be used to detect NTMs or to quantify bacterial pathogens in research studies.

TRANSPORTING CYSTIC FIBROSIS SPECIMENS

Specimens must be transported to the appropriate laboratory as soon as possible. However, many CF centers do not have clinical microbiology laboratories on site. If processing is delayed more than 2 hours, specimens should not be frozen but should be stored at 4°C and processed within 24 hours to avoid loss of viable pathogens and overgrowth by others.

IMPROVING DETECTION OF POTENTIAL PATHOGENS IN CYSTIC FIBROSIS RESPIRATORY SPECIMENS

There are no data to support the use of homogenizing agents such as dithiothreitol or the routine performance of Gram staining. However, selective media are critically important to isolate specific pathogens. Current recommendations for selective media and the rationale for use are shown in Table 13.3. Oropharyngeal swabs from nonexpectorating patients should also be plated on selective media. Plates should be incubated in ambient air at 35°C–37°C and

Table 13.3 Selective media for CF respiratory tract specimens

Organism	Recommended media	Comments
Staphylococcus aureus	Mannitol salt agar Columbia/colistin-nalidixic acid agar CHROMagar Staphylococcus aureus selective agar	CF strains may be thymidine deficient due to trimethoprim–sulfamethoxazole use and require mannitol salt agar for growth May appear as small colony variants
H. influenzae	Blood or chocolate agar (supplemented with bacitracin or cefsulodin)	
P. aeruginosa	MacConkey agar	Nonpigmented strains make detection challenging
Burkholderia spp.	OFPBL agar B. cepacia selective agar MAST selective agar Pseudomonas cepacia agar	Inclusion of polymyxin enhances recovery as B. cepacia complex is resistant
Stenotrophomonas maltophilia	MacConkey agar VIA agar DNase agar confirmatory media	Investigational Steno medium agar containing amphotericin, vancomycin, and imipenem improved yield
Achromobacter spp.	MacConkey agar	
Mycobacteria spp.	NALC-NaOH and oxalic acid decontamination step	
Aspergillus spp.	Sabouraud media Molds grow well on OFPBL and blood agar	Aspergillus spp. and other molds do not grow well on Mycosel
Other gram positives	Sheep blood agar supplemented with neomycin and gentamicin (streptococcal selective agar)	
Other gram negatives	MacConkey agar	

Note: OFPBL, oxidative fermentative bacitracin polymyxin B lactose.

examined following overnight incubation and again after 24 hours to detect P. aeruginosa, Staphylococcus aureus, and other gram-negative rods. Plates should be incubated in ambient air at 35°C–37°C for 5 days to detect Burkholderia spp. and for as long as 7 days to detect fungi. Plates should be incubated in 5% CO_2 at 35°C–37°C and examined following overnight incubation and again after 24 hours to detect H. influenzae.

Sputum specimens processed for NTMs should undergo acid fast staining with a fluorochrome technique, e.g., auramine-phenol.[75] To improve detection of NTMs and prevent contamination with P. aeruginosa, sputum specimens from CF patients must be processed differently than such specimens from non-CF patients. A decontamination step with N-acetyl-l-cysteine and sodium hydroxide (NALC-NaOH) is required, followed by 5% oxalic acid.[76] However, in a laboratory proficiency study, failure to detect NTMs occurred at low inoculums, i.e., 10^4 CFU per mL.[77] Chlorhexidine can also be used to decontaminate CF specimens.[78] Specimens should be incubated for 6–8 weeks to accommodate slowly growing mycobacterial species.

ACCURATE IDENTIFICATION OF POTENTIAL PATHOGENS

All non-lactose-fermenting gram-negative rods should be speciated. However, current commercially available assays for speciation rely on biochemical tests that measure metabolic processes. These may fail to accurately speciate gram-negative rods in CF specimens. Thus, molecular identification strategies are required for accurate speciation, particularly for Burkholderia, Pandorea, and Ralstonia species (Table 13.2), as described further in Chapter 14. Such molecular methodologies may be needed for Stenotrophomonas maltophilia, Achromobacter spp., and atypical isolates of P. aeruginosa as well. Collaboration with specialty laboratories or reference laboratories is generally needed to perform molecular identification.

While pigmented and/or mucoid strains of P. aeruginosa are usually correctly identified, misidentification of P. aeruginosa by commercial systems can also occur.[79,80] Molecular methods have proven superior to phenotypic identification.[81]

SUSCEPTIBILITY TESTING

The optimal methodology of antimicrobial susceptibility testing for both mucoid and nonmucoid strains of P. aeruginosa was elucidated. Studies comparing five different methods, a reference microbroth dilution assay, Kirby–Bauer disks, E-tests, and the automated commercial systems Vitek® and Microscan®, found that the agar-based diffusion methods (Kirby Bauer disks and E-test) were most accurate[82,83] as the commercial systems Vitek and Microscan had unacceptably high rates of very major (i.e., false-susceptible) and major (i.e., false-resistant) errors.[84] Thus, the Clinical and Laboratory Standards Institute (CLSI) endorsed the use of antibiotic impregnated disks or reference broth microdilution assays to determine the susceptibility of multi-drug-resistant strains of *P. aeruginosa* isolated from patients with CF.[85]

Susceptibility testing of *Staphylococcus aureus* and *H. influenzae* should be those used for non-CF isolates guided by professional societies, e.g., the CLSI and the European Committee on Antimicrobial Susceptibility Testing. Recommendations for susceptibility testing for NTMs include clarithromycin for MAC and clarithromycin, cefoxitin, amikacin, tigecycline, imipenem, minocycline, moxifloxacin, and linezolid for *M. abscessus* spp.[75]

SYNERGY TESTING

For nearly two decades, there had been a great deal of interest in developing synergy testing to guide treatment of multi-drug-resistant organisms in CF. Two methods of synergy testing were described for CF isolates: the checkerboard method and minimal bactericidal concentration test (MBCT) broth testing.[86,87] Although numerous in vitro combinations were found to be active, clinical correlation with these results was lacking. In a multicenter study of patients undergoing a pulmonary exacerbation, CF patients were randomized to treatment guided by MBCT results or treatment selected by the treating physician.[88] No differences in the primary outcome, time until next pulmonary exacerbation, were found nor were there significant differences in end-of-treatment bacterial density, treatment failures, or improvement in lung function. Thus, the US CF Foundation guidelines have not recommended performing synergy studies to guide treatment.[89]

CONTROVERSIES AND UNANSWERED QUESTIONS

SMALL COLONY VARIANTS

Small colony variant (SCV) *Staphylococcus aureus* has been described for over two decades and are hypermutable, are relatively antibiotic resistant, and appear to evolve within the unique environment of the CF lung.[90] This phenotype appears as small, nonhemolytic, and nonpigmented slowly growing colonies that grow on enriched media (e.g., sheep blood or chocolate agars) and thus is not readily identified as *Staphylococcus aureus*.[91] The clinical significance of SCV strains remains unclear, but such strains are found in older patients with more advanced lung disease who have had substantial exposure to antibiotics, most notably

trimethoprim–sulfamethoxazole. SCVs of *P. aeruginosa*, *B. cenocepacia*, and *Stenotrophomonas maltophilia* have also been described.[92–95] If SCV strains are found to cause worsening lung disease or their detection is necessary to accurately detect specific species, it will be necessary to consistently identify SCVs in clinical microbiology laboratories to provide appropriate treatment strategies.

SUSCEPTIBILITY TESTING

Although susceptibility testing is currently recommended for CF isolates, there is controversy about the relative usefulness and cost-effectiveness of susceptibility testing.[96–98] This is because susceptibility testing is not clearly correlated with treatment outcomes; patients frequently clinically improve when treated with agents to which their organisms are resistant in vitro or fail to improve when treated with agents to which their organisms are susceptible. The reasons for this are multifactorial. CF pathogens grow in biofilms, as previously described, and isolates grown in laboratories are grown planktonically in liquid media. Multiple morphotypes of *P. aeruginosa* are present within the CF lung, which have varying susceptibility profiles, and it is unclear which morphotype is associated with clinical worsening. However, susceptibility testing is useful epidemiologically as resistance to certain agents, e.g., ceftazidime and meropenem, unmasked patient-to-patient transmission of epidemic *Pseudomonas* strains.[99,100] Furthermore, it is crucial to monitor methicillin and vancomycin resistance among *Staphylococcus aureus* strains due to the infection control implications of such organisms.

BIOFILM SUSCEPTIBILITY TESTING

One of the more intriguing concepts in susceptibility testing is the potential role of susceptibility testing of bacteria grown in biofilms. Bacteria growing in a biofilm are in stationary phase and do not express antibiotic targets expressed by bacteria growing in log phase.[8] Thus, the minimal inhibitory concentration (MIC) of log-phase bacteria are often much lower than the MIC of stationary-phase bacteria.[101] In a study assessing the clinical relevance of biofilm susceptibility testing, the change in sputum density of *P. aeruginosa* was similar among subjects treated using conventional susceptibility testing versus biofilm susceptibility testing.[101] A recent Cochrane review concluded that the current evidence is insufficient to recommend biofilm susceptibility testing be used to guide therapy for *P. aeruginosa*.[102]

BREAKPOINTS FOR AEROSOLIZED ANTIBIOTICS

Current susceptibility breakpoints are irrelevant for aerosolized antibiotics as much higher concentrations of active drug are delivered to the lung, which can overcome many mechanisms of resistance.[103] There are no data to support a breakpoint for aerosolized tobramycin, colistin, or aztreonam.

DETECTION OF SPECIFIC PATHOGENS

Certain bacterial species, such as *P. aeruginosa*, and members of the *B. cepacia* complex, are associated with poor clinical prognosis when present in lower airway secretions from CF patients. Detecting their presence in airway samples provides important information that guides treatment. A range of culture-independent methodologies can be used for detection of these and other pathogens, with varying degrees of sophistication.

PCR-based detection assays

In their simplest form, PCR-based assays can detect the presence of a bacterial species in nucleic acids extracted from respiratory samples. PCR assays typically take advantage of regions of DNA that may be conserved within members of the same species, but which are divergent or not present in other species. Specific primers can be devised for these regions. When used in a PCR reaction, these primers amplify this region specifically if it is present in the DNA extracts from clinical samples. The resulting products, or "amplicons," are detected either by fluorescent gel electrophoresis or by the production of fluorescent reporters generated during amplification. Verification that the target region from the species in question has been amplified is indirectly assessed by size or probe specificity in fluorescent reporter-based assays.

The use of such PCR assays to detect specific bacterial species has several advantages over culture-based microbiology. First, the need for incubation of cultures is removed, making these approaches markedly more rapid and overcoming the problem of detecting bacterial populations that have refractory growth in vitro. Second, DNA extraction and PCR amplification can be automated, thus reducing the labor burden and increasing standardization. Third, being based on DNA sequence rather than phenotypes, the potential for species misidentification is greatly reduced.

Specific PCR assays have been developed to detect a range of bacterial species of interest in the context of CF respiratory infections, with performance comparing favorably with culture-based detection. For example, the ability of conventional culture and a PCR-based assay to detect *B. cenocepacia* was compared in the analysis of more than 6000 respiratory CF samples collected at the Prague Cystic Fibrosis Centre over a period spanning more than 10 years.[22] This study found that *B. cenocepacia* detection by PCR preceded detection by culture in a substantial number of patients (more than 30% of all *B. cenocepacia*–positive patients), with this early detection allowing measures to limit transmission between patients to be implemented more rapidly.

Quantitative PCR

Quantitative (q) or real-time PCR assays extend the analysis previously. These assays are based on the detection of a signal during the amplification process. The signal generated is proportionate to the number of template sequences present and can be calibrated to the signal observed for DNA standards extracted from known numbers of bacterial cells (Figure 14.2). As such, this extends PCR from the detection to the quantification of pathogens.

Although analogous to culture-based colony count determination, q-PCR has advantages. Many of these relate to those outlined for PCR in terms of time and labor saving, as well as the lack of reliance on phenotypic information. Again, the accuracy and flexibility of q-PCR assays has led to their rapid expansion in their use to detect pathogens in CF respiratory samples. Examples of q-PCR assays for the detection of bacterial respiratory pathogens are shown in Table 14.1.

Multiplex q-PCR

By using different reporter systems, it is possible to extend q-PCR assays to include several distinct targets within the same PCR reaction. This process is known as "multiplexing" and allows the rapid detection and quantification of a panel of pathogens of interest.

Multiplex assays can further reduce the time and cost of pathogen detection by removing the need for panels of parallel reactions. This same need to provide inexpensive, rapid data is driving further innovation toward assays combining sample preparation and analysis within a single reaction vessel. Several assays are commercially available and validated for diagnostic use, primarily for the detection of atypical bacterial species and respiratory viruses. A comparison of the performance of six such systems in the analysis of respiratory secretions is described by Pillet et al.[30]

High-resolution melt analysis

An alternative to species-specific amplification is to perform PCR using conditions that allow the amplification of DNA targets from a broader range of bacteria. Amplified regions corresponding to individual species or strains are then differentiated on the basis of the target-specific temperature at which each amplicon "melts," a factor determined by their sequence. This approach, known as high-resolution melt (HRM) analysis, has the advantage of allowing a single assay to be performed for a set of pathogens while retaining the ability to distinguish between them.

HRM assays have been developed to detect and differentiate a range of bacterial species considered of clinical importance in CF, including nontuberculous mycobacteria (NTM)[31] and clonal *P. aeruginosa* isolates.[32]

BACTERIAL COMMUNITY CHARACTERIZATION

Concepts

In contrast to standard, selective diagnostic microbiology, culture-independent analytical techniques have emerged to detect the presence of DNA-based signatures that are

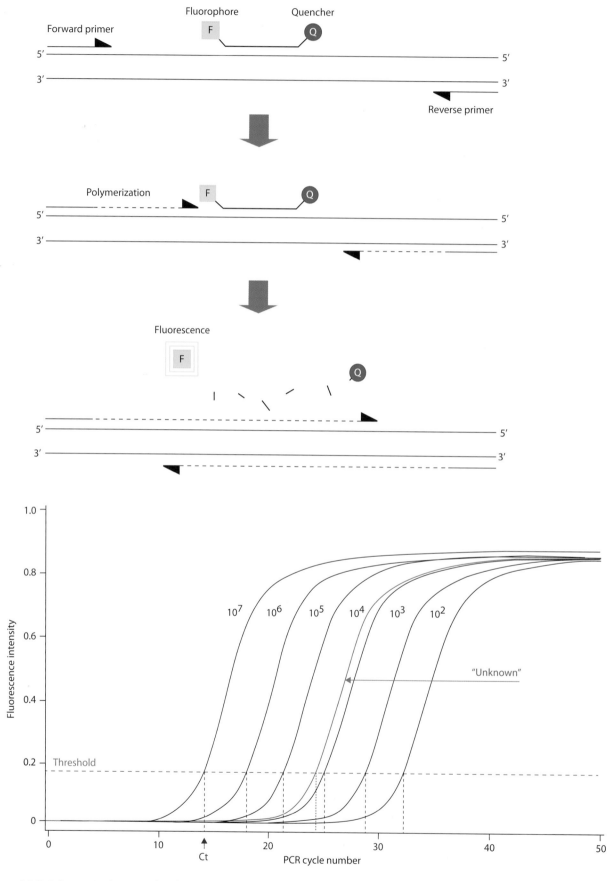

Figure 14.2 Schematic showing the distribution of nine hypervariable regions within the *16S ribosomal RNA* gene, which make it suitable for discriminatory PCR-based assays across a wide range of bacterial species.

26. Kais M, Spindler C, Kalin M, Ortqvist A, Giske CG. Quantitative detection of *Streptococcus pneumoniae*, *Haemophilus influenzae*, and *Moraxella catarrhalis* in lower respiratory tract samples by real-time PCR. *Diagn Microbiol Infect Dis* 2006; **55**: 169–78.

27. Meyler KL, Meehan M, Bennett D, Cunney R, Cafferkey M. Development of a diagnostic real-time polymerase chain reaction assay for the detection of invasive *Haemophilus influenzae* in clinical samples. *Diagn Microbiol Infect Dis* 2012; **74**: 356–62. doi: 10.1016/j.diagmicrobio.2012.08.018.

28. Olson AB, Sibley CD, SchmidtL, Wilcox MA, Surette MG, Corbett CR. Development of real-time PCR assays for detection of the *Streptococcus milleri* group from cystic fibrosis clinical specimens by targeting the cpn60 and 16S rRNA genes. *J Clin Microbiol* 2010; **48**: 1150–60.

29. Park H, Kim C, Park KH, Chang CL. Development and evaluation of triplex PCR for direct detection of mycobacteria in respiratory specimens. *J Appl Microbiol* 2006; **100**: 161–7.

30. Pillet S, Lardeux M, Dina J et al. Comparative evaluation of six commercialized multiplex PCR kits for the diagnosis of respiratory infections. *PLoS One* 2013; **8**: e72174.

31. Perng CL, Chen HY, Chiueh TS, Wang WY, Huang CT, Sun JR. Identification of non-tuberculous mycobacteria by real-time PCR coupled with a high-resolution melting system. *J Med Microbiol* 2012; **61**: 944–51.

32. Anuj SN, Whiley DM, Kidd TJ et al. Rapid single-nucleotide polymorphism-based identification of clonal *Pseudomonas aeruginosa* isolates from patients with cystic fibrosis by the use of real-time PCR and high-resolution melting curve analysis. *Clin Microbiol Infect* 2011; **17**: 1403–8.

33. Rogers GB, Marsh P, Stressmann AF et al. The exclusion of dead bacterial cells is essential for accurate molecular analysis of clinical samples. *Clin Microbiol Infect* 2010; **16**: 1656–8.

34. Rogers GB, Hoffman LR, Whiteley M, Daniels TW, Carroll MP, Bruce KD. Revealing the dynamics of polymicrobial infections: Implications for antibiotic therapy. *Trends Microbiol* 2010; **18**: 357–64.

35. Stressmann FA, Rogers GB, van der Gast CJ et al. Long-term cultivation-independent microbial diversity analysis demonstrates that bacterial communities infecting the adult cystic fibrosis lung show stability and resilience. *Thorax* 2012; **67**: 867–73.

36. Rogers GB, Carroll MP, Serisier DJ, Hockey PM, Jones G, Bruce KD. Characterization of bacterial community diversity in cystic fibrosis lung infections by use of 16S ribosomal DNA terminal restriction fragment length polymorphism profiling. *J Clin Microbiol* 2004; **42**: 5176–83.

37. Petrosino JF, Highlander S, Luna RA, Gibbs RA, Versalovic J. Metagenomic pyrosequencing and microbial identification. *Clin Chem* 2009; **55**: 856–66.

38. Delhaes L, Monchy S, Fréalle E et al. The airway microbiota in cystic fibrosis: A complex fungal and bacterial community—implications for therapeutic management. *PLoS One* 2012; **7**: e36313.

39. Rogers GB, Shaw D, Marsh RL, Carroll MP, Serisier DJ, Bruce KD. Respiratory microbiota: Addressing clinical questions, informing clinical practice. *Thorax* 2015; **70**: 74–81.

40. Novais RC, Thorstenson YR. The evolution of pyrosequencing for microbiology: From genes to genomes. *J Microbiol Methods* 2011; **86**: 1–7.

41. DeSantis TZ, Brodie EL, Moberg JP, Zubieta IX, Piceno YM, Andersen GL. High-density universal 16S rRNA microarray analysis reveals broader diversity than typical clone library when sampling the environment. *Microb Ecol* 2007; **53**: 371–83.

42. Cox MJ, Allgaier M, Taylor B et al. Airway microbiota and pathogen abundance in age-stratified cystic fibrosis patients. *PLoS One* 2010; **5**: e11044.

43. van der Gast CJ, Walker AW, Stressmann FA et al. Partitioning core and satellite taxa from within cystic fibrosis lung bacterial communities. *ISME J* 2011; **5**: 780–91.

44. Tunney MM, Klem ER, Fodor AA et al. Use of culture and molecular analysis to determine the effect of antibiotic treatment on microbial community diversity and abundance during exacerbation in patients with cystic fibrosis. *Thorax* 2011; **66**: 579–84.

45. Zhao J, Schloss PD, Kalikin LM et al. Decade-long bacterial community dynamics in cystic fibrosis airways. *Proc Natl Acad Sci USA* 2012; **109**: 5809–14.

46. Klepac-Ceraj V, Lemon KP, Martin TR et al. Relationship between cystic fibrosis respiratory tract bacterial communities and age, genotype, antibiotics and *Pseudomonas aeruginosa*. *Environ Microbiol* 2010; **12**: 1293–303.

47. Goddard AF, Staudinger BJ, Dowd SE et al. Direct sampling of cystic fibrosis lungs indicates that DNA-based analyses of upper-airway specimens can misrepresent lung microbiota. *Proc Natl Acad Sci USA* 2012; **109**: 13769–74.

48. Rogers GB, Hoffman LR, Carroll MP, Bruce KD. Interpreting infective microbiota: The importance of an ecological perspective. *Trends Microbiol* 2013; **21**: 271–6.

49. Pressler T, Bohmova C, Conway S et al. Chronic *Pseudomonas aeruginosa* infection definition: EuroCareCF Working Group report. *J Cyst Fibros* 2011; **10**(Suppl 2): S75–8.

50. Rogers GB, Cuthbertson L, Hoffman LR et al. Reducing bias in bacterial community analysis of lower respiratory infections. *ISME J* 2013; **7**: 697–706.

15

Infection control

ANDREW M. JONES

INTRODUCTION

The acquisition of a new pathogen for patients with cystic fibrosis (CF) can adversely influence the progression of their lung disease and ultimately their survival. Strains of some of the typical CF bacterial pathogens are transmissible between patients with CF. A high standard of infection control practice is therefore essential in CF clinical care and requires close collaboration between CF, microbiology, and infection control teams. Components of infection control practice in CF, in addition to standard universal precautions, include measures to prevent patient-to-patient transfer of pathogens and a program of advice and education for patients, carers, and staff, with the success of these policies continually assessed by a program of microbiological surveillance.

CROSS-INFECTION

There are a number of pathogens that have been responsible for outbreaks of infection among patients with CF (Table 15.1), often with evidence of patient-to-patient spread.[1] Therefore, in addition to standard infection control precautions, a policy of cohort segregation and patient isolation has become established into clinical practice at CF centers.

BURKHOLDERIA CEPACIA COMPLEX (BCC)

Outbreaks of infection with epidemic strains of *Burkholderia cenocepacia* were first identified at CF centers in the late 1980s and early 1990s.[2] Several strains of *B. cenocepacia* were associated with large cross-infection outbreaks and one strain, known as "*B. cenocepacia* strain ET-12," spread among patients in several countries.[3,4] The infected patients suffered from an increased morbidity

and reduced survival.[5] In many countries, they were also excluded from lung transplantation programs due to an association with poor post-transplant outcomes.[6,7] Strict cohort segregation policies were introduced at CF centers to contain spread.[1] These measures were also applied to social gatherings and meetings. This had profound effects on the support and functioning of the CF community, with infected patients banned from group activity and educational events. Although two DNA "markers" ("*Burkholderia cepacia* epidemic strain marker" and "cable pilus") were initially identified to be associated with epidemic *B. cenocepacia* strains, it was later shown that these were not accurate indicators of transmissibility.[8] Subsequently it was recognized that some *B. cenocepacia* strains could replace other BCC, sometimes referred to as "superinfection."[9] This too was often associated with a marked clinical deterioration of the patients and therefore the initial cohort segregation policies were further extended to isolate patients individually or segregate by strain of organism.

The success of these infection control measures has resulted in a marked decline in the number of cases and changed the distribution of BCC species responsible for infections in patients with CF.[1] The majority of new isolations are due to acquisition of sporadic environmental strains than through cross-infection.[10] Although cases of new infection with sporadic strains of *B. cenocepacia* are occasionally encountered, this is less common than some of the other BCC species. In many centers, the prevalence of other species of the BCC, in particular *Burkholderia multivorans*, now outnumbers those of *B. cenocepacia*. Figure 15.1 demonstrates the changing incidence and prevalence of BCC infection at the Manchester Adult CF Centre over the past three decades. There was a marked increase in incidence of BCC infection in the years 1992 to 1994, which was later found to be due to the emergence and spread of epidemic *B. cenocepacia* infection among patients at the center. Cohort segregation and isolation measures were subsequently introduced for all patients with BCC infection. Patients with BCC infection were seen on a different day to other CF patients for their outpatient appointments and were housed as inpatients in single rooms on a respiratory ward away from the main CF facility. If patients needed to attend the radiology or any other department in the hospital, the staff phoned ahead to ensure that there is no other CF patient in the department. The success of these measures has been tracked through a program of microbiological surveillance, with identification and strain typing of all *Burkholderia* species. This has demonstrated that while new infections are encountered, these are due to sporadic environmental strains and the spread of epidemic *B. cenocepacia* has been curtailed.

Cross-infection outbreaks, however, have also been reported with other BCC species, including *B. multivorans*,[11,12] *Burkholderia pyrrocinia*,[13] and *Burkholderia dolosa*.[14] Spread with these species has been mainly confined among patients at single CF centers, rather than at a national or international level. The relative virulence of the other BCC species is less clear, although the outbreak of *B. dolosa* infection at a CF centre in Boston was

associated with an accelerated fall in lung function decline and an increase in mortality.

Other non-BCC *Burkholderia* species can also infect patients with CF. The most commonly encountered is *Burkholderia gladioli*, but cases of melioidosis due to *Burkholderia pseudomallei* infection have been reported in patients with CF who have visited subtropical regions of Southeast Asia and Northern Australia.[15] It has, therefore, been recommended that people with CF planning to travel to subtropical countries where *B. pseudomallei* infection is endemic should be advised to avoid visiting rural areas during the rainy season.

PSEUDOMONAS AERUGINOSA

P. aeruginosa cross-infection outbreaks have been reported at specialist CF centers in Europe, Australia, and Canada.[16–23] Some strains have infected patients at a number of centers within a country, whereas others seem relatively confined to small numbers of unrelated patients attending individual CF centers. One particular strain, the Liverpool Epidemic Strain, has been isolated from patients at a number of CF centers both in the United Kingdom[24] and Canada.[16]

Some reports have suggested that infection with some transmissible strains of *P. aeruginosa* may be associated with increased treatment requirements,[25] an accelerated fall in lung function[26] or even excess mortality.[27] The true clinical impact of cross-infection for patients already chronically infected with other sporadic strains remains unresolved. Isolates of some transmissible strains have been noted to exhibit unusual phenotypic features, including multiresistance to antipseudomonal antibiotics. However, none of the phenotypic features are reliably

Table 15.1 Pathogens associated with reported outbreaks of infection at CF centers

Pseudomonas aeruginosa
Burkholderia cenocepacia
Burkholderia dolosa
Burkholderia multivorans
Burkholderia pyrrocinia
Methicillin-resistant *Staphylococcus aureus*
Pandoraea apista
Achromobacter xylosoxidans
Mycobacterium abscessus

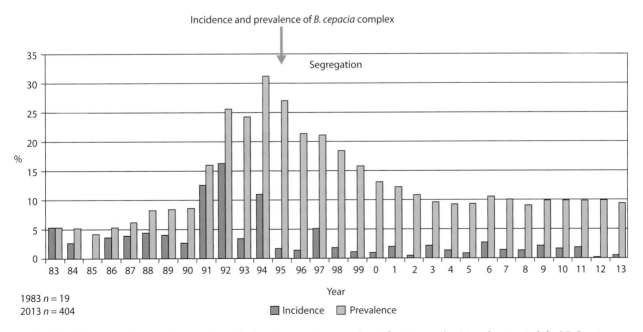

Figure 15.1 Incidence and prevalence of *Burkholderia cepacia* complex infection at the Manchester Adult CF Centre.

diagnostic and while some transmissible *P. aeruginosa* may have a tendency to exhibit a multiresistant phenotype, a spectrum of antibiogram patterns are encountered with both transmissible and sporadic strains.[1] The identification of a transmissible strain rests on a combination of genotyping of individual bacterial isolates, knowledge of the prevalence of individual strains in the local environment, and the epidemiological details of the patients who harbor any shared strain.

There are several observations that support patient-to-patient transmission as the most likely mode of spread. First, studies during cross-infection outbreaks have failed to isolate the transmissible strains from the inanimate environment of the CF centers; the only reservoirs found have been the patients themselves.[28,29] Second, airborne dissemination of transmissible strains by infected patients has been demonstrated.[28-30] Finally, those CF centers that have instigated cohort segregation and isolation measures for patients infected with transmissible *P. aeruginosa* have reported a subsequent decreasing incidence of infection.[19,31]

There is preliminary evidence that transmissible strains may also have a greater ability than sporadic strains to defy the eradication therapies used by CF teams, either through an increased predisposition to display a multiresistant phenotype during the initial stages of infection and/or potentially other as yet undefined properties. Of five cases of new *P. aeruginosa* infection among previously *P. aeruginosa*-naive patients at the Manchester Adult CF Centre, four failed to eradicate the pathogen despite aggressive antibiotic treatment.[32] It is, therefore, essential to segregate those patients free of *P. aeruginosa* infection from others who harbor transmissible strains.

OTHER EMERGING GRAM-NEGATIVE PATHOGENS

There are a number of Gram-negative organisms, such as *Stenotrophomonas maltophilia*, *Inquilinos limosus*, *Pandoraea apista*, *Achromobacter xylosoxidans*, that generally exhibit a low prevalence of infection among patients with CF. At present, there have not been any large-scale cross-infection outbreaks reported with these organisms; however, clusters of patients at CF centers with shared strains of *A. xylosoxidans*, potentially as a result of cross-infection, have been reported.[33]

METHICILLIN-RESISTANT *STAPHYLOCOCCUS AUREUS* (MRSA)

In the past decade, there has been an increase in MRSA infection rates in patients with CF. The prevalence of MRSA infection varies between CF centers and between countries. The 2012 UK CF Trust Registry figures show a prevalence of 3.3%, whereas the 2012 US CF Foundation Registry reports a prevalence of 26.5% for MRSA. Although the majority of infections within the CF population are with healthcare-associated MRSA strains, community-acquired MRSA rates are increasingly encountered in patients at CF centers in some countries, including the United States.[34,35] Factors that have been associated with increased risk of acquisition of MRSA infection include prolonged or repeated inpatient admissions, failure to isolate cases, careers in healthcare, and working as or living with a healthcare professional.[36-38]

NONTUBERCULOUS MYCOBACTERIA

Unlike *Mycobacterium tuberculosis*, patient-to-patient spread of nontuberculous mycobacteria was thought to be extremely rare or even nonexistent. However, this assumption has recently been challenged following two reported outbreaks of *Mycobacterium abscessus* cross-infection at the CF Centers in Seattle[39] and Papworth.[40] Although the mechanism of transmission of infection is at present unclear, these initial findings highlight a potential need to further revise cohort segregation policies.

RESPIRATORY VIRUSES

Many of the exacerbations experienced by patients with CF are associated with respiratory viruses.[41] Infection control policies at CF centers should include measures to minimize potential risk of spread of respiratory viruses both among patients and to staff. When caring for a patient with a respiratory viral infection, gloves, aprons, and masks should be worn by staff, particularly during close contact with a patient while they are undertaking nebulization therapy or practicing airway clearance.

IMPLICATIONS OF CROSS-INFECTION CONTROL

HEALTHCARE FACILITIES

To minimize the potential for nosocomial transmission of infection, the CF healthcare facilities should be maintained to a high standard and standard infection control precautions should be in place. Handwashing should be practiced by all staff before and after contact with each patient. Spirometry, airway clearance, and nebulization should be performed in the patient's own room. If more detailed respiratory function testing is required, this should be carried out in a well-ventilated room. All respiratory secretions should be stored in a pot with a closed lid. Wherever possible, equipment should be single patient use and patients should be encouraged to bring their own equipment into hospital for personal use; all equipment should be cleaned and decontaminated according to the manufacturer's instructions.

The design of CF centers needs to enable patients to be accommodated with comfort and dignity while maintaining a high quality of clinical care and minimizing the risk of cross-infection. All inpatients should have their own single room with en-suite facilities (Figures 15.2 and 15.3). Measures should be taken to counteract the potential boredom and isolation for patients during prolonged inpatients stays, including frequent contact with staff, family, and peers who do not have CF, and access to the Internet and other means of communication. Inpatients should be provided with the means to exercise daily. Group exercise sessions for CF patients present a risk of cross-infection, therefore exercise should be conducted on an individual basis in the patient's own room

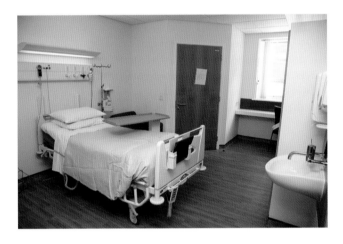

Figure 15.2 Photograph of a single en-suite inpatient room.

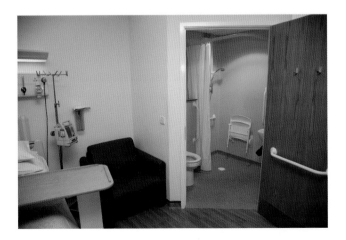

Figure 15.3 Photograph of a single en-suite inpatient room.

or if a gym or exercise room is used then it should be ensured that the air exchange in the facility is optimized and that the timing of the sessions should be such that there is a time interval of 30 minutes between patients and a hierarchy for timing of sessions with those infected with pathogens that carry greatest risk of transmission being allocated access later in the day.

At large specialist centers, patients are often segregated into cohorts for outpatient clinics according to the dominant pathogen that they harbor, and then individually isolated. In CF outpatient clinics, there should be an adequate number of rooms and an appointment system that allows patients to be placed directly in a room and avoids patients waiting together. Consideration needs to be given to the possibility of cross-infection if patients with CF meet in other departments within hospitals, such as pharmacy and radiology. Measures can be taken to minimize the possibility, such as the dispensing of medication by a pharmacist directly to the patients in their own outpatient room, and close communication between CF and radiology departments to stagger appointments for patients with CF who require radiological examinations and priority processing for CF patients when they arrive in the department. As the number of pathogens associated with potential cross-infection continues to increase, the future design of new build CF centers should consider the provision of negative pressure rooms in both inpatient and outpatient facilities.

ERADICATION OF EARLY INFECTION

Aggressive antibiotic therapies to eradicate early infection are important tools in the armory of CF clinical teams in preventing the development of chronic infection with bacterial pathogens.[42,43] For those patients who become culture-negative, there is then the question of whether the infection is merely suppressed or if it has been truly eradicated? In those CF centers where cohort segregation is part of infection control practice, a decision must be made where to place the patient until it is established if infection has been cleared. Many centers apply a guideline of a minimum of 6–12 months of negative cultures before the patient is considered clear of infection.

RISKS TO NON-CF PATIENTS

Although transmission of pathogens can occur between patients with CF, the risk of person-to-person spread of pathogens from CF patients to other patients where standard infection control precautions are in place is very low. Outbreaks of BCC infection have been reported in intensive care units; however in most cases, theses were unrelated to CF patients and contamination of the environment or medical solutions by BCC has been thought to be the primary source. Two case reports have documented cross-infection with a transmissible *P. aeruginosa* strain from patients with

CF to patients with non-CF bronchiectasis. One reported spread to another close family member,[44] while another reported transmission from a CF patient to another patient with non-CF bronchiectasis following a group exercise session.[45] Although caution should be exercised, given the high prevalence of *P. aeruginosa* infection in CF, cross-infection from CF to other patients at present still seems to be a relatively uncommon occurrence. Infection control guidelines do not advocate the wearing of face masks by patients with CF within hospital facilities; there is no evidence to support such a practice and this can unnecessarily stigmatize patients.

EDUCATION AND ADVICE FOR PATIENTS, CARERS, AND STAFF

The potential for acquisition of a pathogen whether through environmental exposure or as a result of cross-infection is a topic of considerable anxiety for many patients and their carers. Surveys show that the majority of patients and carers support the implementation of strict cross-infection measures, including patient segregation, despite the adverse effects on peer support and communal activities.[46,47] Although studies have shown airborne dissemination of CF pathogens, the infective load for transmission of an organism is unknown, and it is not possible to accurately quantify the risk of cross-infection in any particular setting. However, it can be assumed that some situations will confer a greater risk of cross-infection between patients, such as prolonged exposure in confined environments or episodes involving physical contact. Holiday camps and other social gatherings for patients with CF are now discouraged. A continual program of education in all aspects of infection control practice for patients, carers, and staff is important in ensuring high standards are continually maintained. This should include an explanation of details of local infection control practice, both for all patients and their carers when they move to a new center and as part of the local induction of new staff, and presentation of the results of regular infection control audits to all CF center staff. The considerable benefits of specialist center care with an experienced CF multidisciplinary team against any potential small risk for cross-infection should be highlighted. Even during a cross-infection outbreak at the Copenhagen CF Centre, patients who attended the unit had better outcomes than those who received their care elsewhere.[48]

Carers in healthcare will involve increased exposure to healthcare-associated pathogens; infection with MRSA is more frequently encountered in patients with CF who work in healthcare professions.[36,42] Those patients considering a career in healthcare should be suitably counseled to make an informed decision. Similarly, the discussion should include the implications for their career if a healthcare professional with CF subsequently acquires infection with a pathogen that poses a risk to other patients.

OUTSIDE THE HOSPITAL

Most CF infections are due to sporadic strains of pathogens that are acquired from the environment. However, the actual risk of acquisition of new infection at any one time is very low. Any risk must be balanced against the benefit of undertaking recreational activities. There are very few situations that present a significant risk, although caution should be exercised in use of hot tubs as this has occasionally been associated with acquisition of *P. aeruginosa* infection. People with CF planning to travel to subtropical countries where *B. pseudomallei* infection is endemic should be discouraged from visiting rural areas of subtropical countries during the rainy season. *Aspergillus fumigatus* is fairly ubiquitous, but certain environments such as compost heaps, rotting vegetation, and damp buildings can be particularity heavily contaminated. Certain activities including renovation work in old damp buildings, mucking out horses, and digging in compost may therefore involve heavy exposure and should be avoided.

Infection control in CF is a subject that will continuously present challenges and ethical dilemmas for which often there are no straightforward solutions or right or wrong answers, for example, when more than one patient enrolls in the same school class or college course. Each situation must be addressed on an individual case basis, but a satisfactory resolution is easier to accomplish if patients and carers, their CF teams, and representatives from their place of work/study work agree to engage in open discussion together to find an acceptable solution.

MICROBIOLOGICAL SURVEILLANCE

Microbiological surveillance is key component in infection control, both to allow the prompt initiation of eradication therapy in early infection and to evaluate the success of cross-infection control measures. There should be regular meetings between the CF, microbiology, and infection control teams. Rates of infection with individual organisms should be closely monitored, and strain typing of pathogens should be performed in suspected outbreaks of infection. For pathogens with relatively low prevalence (<10%) among CF patients, strain typing of an isolate from each patient can be performed, but for pathogens with a higher prevalence, such as *P. aeruginosa*, isolates from a representative number of patients (approximately 50 per center) should be genotyped to see if shared strains are present. Isolates from all cases of new infections with pathogens that have been associated with cross-infection outbreaks (Table 15.1) should be genotyped to evaluate if this represents either a strain shared with other patients at the center or acquisition of a unique strain. It should be noted that the finding of a shared strain between patients may not always imply patient-to-patient spread; this information should be evaluated in combination with the known prevalence of any strain in the environment and the epidemiology of the cases.

REFERENCES

1. Govan JR, Brown AR, Jones AM. Evolving epidemiology of Pseudomonas aeruginosa and the Burkholderia cepacia complex in cystic fibrosis lung infection. *Future Microbiol* 2007; **2**: 153–64.

2. Isles A, Maclusky I, Corey M, Gold R, et al. Pseudomonas cepacia infection in cystic fibrosis: An emerging problem. *J Pediatr* 1984; **104**: 206–10.

3. Govan JR, Brown PH, Maddison J, Doherty CJ, et al. Evidence for transmission of Pseudomonas cepacia by social contact in cystic fibrosis. *Lancet* 1993; **342**: 15–9.

4. LiPuma JJ, Dasen SE, Nielson DW, Stern RC, et al. Person-to-person transmission of Pseudomonas cepacia between patients with cystic fibrosis. *Lancet* 1990; **336**: 1094–6.

5. Jones AM, Dodd ME, Govan JR, Barcus V, et al. Burkholderia cenocepacia and Burkholderia multivorans: Influence on survival in cystic fibrosis. *Thorax* 2004; **59**: 948–51.

6. Alexander BD, Petzold EW, Reller LB, Palmer SM, et al. Survival after lung transplantation of cystic fibrosis patients infected with Burkholderia cepacia complex. *Am J Transplant* 2008; **8**: 1025–30.

7. De Soyza A, Meachery G, Hester KL, Nicholson A, et al. Lung transplantation for patients with cystic fibrosis and Burkholderia cepacia complex infection: A single-center experience. *J Heart Lung Transplant* 2010; **29**: 1395–404.

8. LiPuma JJ, Spilker T, Gill LH, Campbell PW 3rd, et al. Disproportionate distribution of Burkholderia cepacia complex species and transmissibility markers in cystic fibrosis. *Am J Respir Crit Care Med* 2001; **164**: 92–6.

9. Ledson MJ, Gallagher MJ, Corkill JE, Hart CA, et al. Cross infection between cystic fibrosis patients colonised with Burkholderia cepacia. *Thorax* 1998; **53**: 432–6.

10. France MW, Dodd ME, Govan JR, Doherty CJ, et al. The changing epidemiology of Burkholderia species infection at an adult cystic fibrosis centre. *J Cyst Fibros* 2008; **7**: 368–72.

11. Biddick R, Spilker T, Martin A, LiPuma JJ. Evidence of transmission of Burkholderia cepacia, Burkholderia multivorans and Burkholderia dolosa among persons with cystic fibrosis. *FEMS Microbiol Lett* 2003; **228**: 57–62.

12. Whiteford ML, Wilkinson JD, McColl JH, Conlon FM, et al. Outcome of Burkholderia (Pseudomonas) cepacia colonisation in children with cystic fibrosis following a hospital outbreak. *Thorax* 1995; **50**: 1194–8.

13. Campana S, Taccetti G, Ravenni N, Favari F, et al. Transmission of Burkholderia cepacia complex: Evidence for new epidemic clones infecting cystic fibrosis patients in Italy. *J Clin Microbiol* 2005; **43**: 5136–42.

14. Kalish LA, Waltz DA, Dovey M, Potter-Bynoe G, et al. Impact of Burkholderia dolosa on lung function and survival in cystic fibrosis. *Am J Respir Crit Care Med* 2006; **173**: 421–5.

15. O'Carroll MR, Kidd TJ, Coulter C, Smith HV, et al. Burkholderia pseudomallei: Another emerging pathogen in cystic fibrosis. *Thorax* 2003; **58**: 1087–91.

16. Aaron SD, Vandemheen KL, Ramotar K, Giesbrecht-Lewis T, et al. Infection with transmissible strains of Pseudomonas aeruginosa and clinical outcomes in adults with cystic fibrosis. *JAMA* 2010; **304**: 2145–53.

17. Armstrong D, Bell S, Robinson M, Bye P, et al. Evidence for spread of a clonal strain of Pseudomonas aeruginosa among cystic fibrosis clinics. *J Clin Microbiol* 2003; **41**: 2266–7.

18. Denton M, Kerr K, Mooney L, Keer V, et al. Transmission of colistin-resistant Pseudomonas aeruginosa between patients attending a pediatric cystic fibrosis center. *Pediatr Pulmonol* 2002; **34**: 257–61.

19. Jones AM, Dodd ME, Govan JR, Doherty CJ, et al. Prospective surveillance for Pseudomonas aeruginosa cross-infection at a cystic fibrosis center. *Am J Respir Crit Care Med* 2005; **171**: 257–60.

20. Jones AM, Webb AK, Govan JR, Hart CA, et al. Pseudomonas aeruginosa cross-infection in cystic fibrosis. *Lancet* 2002; **359**: 527–8.

21. Kidd TJ, Ramsay KA, Hu H, Marks GB, et al. Shared Pseudomonas aeruginosa genotypes are common in Australian cystic fibrosis centres. *Eur Respir J* 2012; **41**: 1091–100.

22. McCallum SJ, Corkill J, Gallagher M, Ledson MJ, et al. Superinfection with a transmissible strain of Pseudomonas aeruginosa in adults with cystic fibrosis chronically colonised by P. aeruginosa. *Lancet* 2001; **358**: 558–60.

23. Pitt TL. Cross infection of cystic fibrosis patients with Pseudomonas aeruginosa. *Thorax* 2002; **57**: 921.

24. Scott FW, Pitt TL. Identification and characterization of transmissible Pseudomonas aeruginosa strains in cystic fibrosis patients in England and Wales. *J Med Microbiol* 2004; **53**: 609–15.

25. Jones AM, Dodd ME, Doherty CJ, Govan JR, et al. Increased treatment requirements of patients with cystic fibrosis who harbour a highly transmissible strain of Pseudomonas aeruginosa. *Thorax* 2002; **57**: 924–5.

26. Al-Aloul M, Crawley J, Winstanley C, Hart CA, et al. Increased morbidity associated with chronic infection by an epidemic Pseudomonas aeruginosa strain in CF patients. *Thorax* 2004; **59**: 334–6.

27. Nixon GM, Armstrong DS, Carzino R, Carlin JB, et al. Clinical outcome after early Pseudomonas aeruginosa infection in cystic fibrosis. *J Pediatr* 2001; **138**: 699–704.

28. Jones AM, Govan JR, Doherty CJ, Dodd ME, et al. Identification of airborne dissemination of epidemic multiresistant strains of Pseudomonas aeruginosa at a CF centre during a cross infection outbreak. *Thorax* 2003; **58**: 525–7.

29. Panagea S, Winstanley C, Walshaw MJ, Ledson MJ, et al. Environmental contamination with an epidemic strain of Pseudomonas aeruginosa in a Liverpool cystic fibrosis centre, and study of its survival on dry surfaces. *J Hosp Infect* 2005; **59**: 102–7.

30. Wainwright CE, France MW, O'Rourke P, Anuj S, et al. Cough-generated aerosols of Pseudomonas aeruginosa and other Gram-negative bacteria from patients with cystic fibrosis. *Thorax* 2009; **64**: 926–31.

31. Griffiths AL, Jamsen K, Carlin JB, Grimwood K, et al. Effects of segregation on an epidemic Pseudomonas aeruginosa strain in a cystic fibrosis clinic. *Am J Respir Crit Care Med* 2005; **171**: 1020–5.

32. Gilchrist FJ, France M, Bright-Thomas R, Doherty C, et al. Can transmissible strains of Pseudomonas aeruginosa be successfully eradicated? *Eur Respir J* 2011; **38**: 1483–6.

33. Hansen CR, Pressler T, Ridderberg W, Johansen HK, et al. Achromobacter species in cystic fibrosis: Cross-infection caused by indirect patient-to-patient contact. *J Cyst Fibros* 2013; **12**: 609–15.

34. Elizur A, Orscheln RC, Ferkol TW, Atkinson JJ, et al. Panton-Valentine Leukocidin-positive methicillin-resistant Staphylococcus aureus lung infection in patients with cystic fibrosis. *Chest* 2007, **131**: 1718–25.

35. Goodrich JS, Sutton-Shields TN, Kerr A, Wedd JP, et al. Prevalence of community-associated methicillin-resistant Staphylococcus aureus in patients with cystic fibrosis. *J Clin Microbiol* 2009; **47**: 1231–3.

36. Downey DG, Kidd TJ, Coulter C, Bell SC. MRSA eradication in a health care worker with cystic fibrosis: Re-emergence or re-infection? *J Cyst Fibros* 2005; **4**: 205–7.

37. Givney R, Vickery A, Holliday A, Pegler M, et al. Methicillin-resistant Staphylococcus aureus in a cystic fibrosis unit. *J Hosp Infect* 1997; **35**: 27–36.

38. Nadesalingam K, Conway SP, Denton M. Risk factors for acquisition of methicillin-resistant Staphylococcus aureus (MRSA) by patients with cystic fibrosis. *J Cyst Fibros* 2005; **4**: 49–52.

39. Aitken ML, Limaye A, Pottinger P, Whimbey E, et al. Respiratory outbreak of Mycobacterium abscessus subspecies massiliense in a lung transplant and cystic fibrosis center. *Am J Respir Crit Care Med* 2012; **185**: 231–2.

40. Bryant JM, Grogono DM, Greaves D, Foweraker J, et al. Whole-genome sequencing to identify transmission of Mycobacterium abscessus between patients with cystic fibrosis: A retrospective cohort study. *Lancet* 2013; **381**: 1551–60.

41. Flight WG, Bright-Thomas RJ, Tilston P, Mutton KJ, et al. Incidence and clinical impact of respiratory viruses in adults with cystic fibrosis. *Thorax* 2013.

42. Doe SJ, McSorley A, Isalska B, Kearns AM, et al. Patient segregation and aggressive antibiotic eradication therapy can control methicillin-resistant Staphylococcus aureus at large cystic fibrosis centres. *J Cyst Fibros* 2010; **9**: 104–9.

43. Taccetti G, Campana S, Festini F, Mascherini M, et al. Early eradication therapy against Pseudomonas aeruginosa in cystic fibrosis patients. *Eur Respir J* 2005; **26**: 458–61.

44. McCallum SJ, Gallagher MJ, Corkill JE, Hart CA, et al. Spread of an epidemic Pseudomonas aeruginosa strain from a patient with cystic fibrosis (CF) to non-CF relatives. *Thorax* 2002; **57**: 559–60.

45. Robinson P, Carzino R, Armstrong D, Olinsky A. Pseudomonas cross-infection from cystic fibrosis patients to non-cystic fibrosis patients: Implications for inpatient care of respiratory patients. *J Clin Microbiol* 2003; **41**: 5741.

46. Griffiths AL, Armstrong D, Carzino R, Robinson P. Cystic fibrosis patients and families support cross-infection measures. *Eur Respir J* 2004; **24**: 449–52.

47. Waine DJ, Whitehouse J, Honeybourne D. Cross-infection in cystic fibrosis: The knowledge and behaviour of adult patients. *J Cyst Fibros* 2007; **6**: 262–6.

48. Zimakoff J, Hoiby N, Rosendal K, Guilbert JP. Epidemiology of Pseudomonas aeruginosa infection and the role of contamination of the environment in a cystic fibrosis clinic. *J Hosp Infect* 1983; **4**: 31–40.

FURTHER READING

Cystic Fibrosis Trust. Report of the UK Cystic Fibrosis Trust Control Infection Control Working Group. *The* Burkholderia cepacia *Complex: Suggestions for Prevention and Infection Control*. London, United Kingdom: Cystic Fibrosis Trust; 2004. CF Trust website—www.cftrust.co.uk.

Cystic Fibrosis Trust. Report of the UK Cystic Fibrosis Trust Control Infection Control Working Group. Pseudomonas aeruginosa *Infection in People with Cystic Fibrosis: Suggestions for Prevention and Infection Control*. London, United Kingdom: Cystic Fibrosis Trust; 2004. CF Trust website—www.cftrust.co.uk.

Cystic Fibrosis Trust. Report of the UK Cystic Fibrosis Trust Control Infection Control Working Group. *Methicillin-Resistant* Staphylococcus aureus *(MRSA): Suggestions for Prevention and Infection Control*. London, United Kingdom: Cystic Fibrosis Trust; 2008. CF Trust website—www.cftrust.co.uk.

LiPuma JJ. The changing microbial epidemiology in cystic fibrosis. *Clin Microbiol Rev* 2010; **23**: 299–323.

Saiman L, Siegel J, Cystic Fibrosis Foundation. Infection control recommendations for patients with cystic fibrosis: Microbiology, important pathogens, and infection control practises to prevent patient-to-patient transmission. *Infect Control Hosp Epidemiol* 2003; **24** (5 Suppl): S6–52.

PART 4

Clinical aspects of cystic fibrosis

16

Respiratory disease: Infectious complications

J. STUART ELBORN, IAN M. BALFOUR-LYNN, AND DIANA BILTON

INTRODUCTION

Most people with cystic fibrosis (CF) die from respiratory failure, which is a consequence of progressive lung damage resulting from chronic infection and inflammation. The airways of people with CF are susceptible to initial colonization and subsequent infection by organisms that are not adequately cleared. A host–bacteria relationship is established with airway epithelium and alveolar tissue becoming injured due to the effects of a large number of inflammatory mediators and bacterial products. These include cytokines, bacterial and host defense proteases, and oxygen-derived free radicals. Early in life, *Staphylococcus aureus* is the main organism that infects the airway, but by the end of the second decade *Pseudomonas aeruginosa* is the dominant infecting organism. Nontuberculous mycobacteria are increasingly important pathogens. Aggressive treatment of pulmonary bacterial infection with antibiotics is the most important and effective intervention in the treatment of CF. Respiratory viral infections also play an important role in the early natural history of airway infection. Finally, various species of fungi may cause infection and allergy in the airways.

BACTERIOLOGY

Intermittent and chronic bacterial infection of the airways is a hallmark of the lung disease in CF (Figure 16.1). Infection occurs early in life and is the result of impaired mucociliary clearance and altered immune responses, secondary to reduced or absent CFTR function.[1] Hydration of airways surface liquid is critical to the maintenance of normal mucociliary clearance, and an appropriate state of hydration results from changes in osmotic pressures.[2,3] The

concentration of chloride and sodium is regulated by CFTR and the epithelial sodium channel, but this is deranged in CF.[3] The impairment of mucociliary clearance sets up the conditions for inhaled bacteria to lodge in the airway mucus, and after initial colonization, to chronically infect the airway.[1,3]

In addition to the impairment of mucociliary clearance, abnormalities in the pH of airways surface liquid impairs innate immune responses, which further encourages bacterial persistence.[4] These, and probably other, as yet unidentified impacts of CFTR dysfunction create an environment filled with pathogenic bacteria; these adapt by forming biofilms, and thus resist further attack by the innate and adaptive immune systems. In time, host and bacterial protease responses further inactivate complement, immunoglobulin and cell receptors on neutrophils to impair further the ability to clear bacteria, and patients are left with substantial and persistent infection.[5]

Furthermore, respiratory mucus is an anaerobic environment, and as the mucus layer increases, and mucus plugs develop, the environmental niche within the airway encourages obligate and facultative anaerobes.[6–8] *S. aureus* and *P. aeruginosa*, classic microbial pathogens in CF, are both facultative anaerobes and are able to metabolize in aerobic and anaerobic environments. Recent culture and molecular sequencing data suggest that in addition to these common pathogens, a range of anaerobic and aerobic pathogens are present in the CF airway, indicating complex microbial flora.[9,10] Many of these organisms occur in the upper respiratory tract and are obligate anaerobes and presumably are aspirated from the upper airway into the lungs.[10,11]

There has been increasing interest in the diverse microbiota in the airways in CF and other chronic lung conditions associated with infection. These studies, in general, demonstrate that *Pseudomonas*, *S. aureus*, *Burkholderia cepacia complex*, *Haemophilus influenzae*, *Achromobacter xylosoxidans*, and *Stenotrophomonas maltophilia* are the

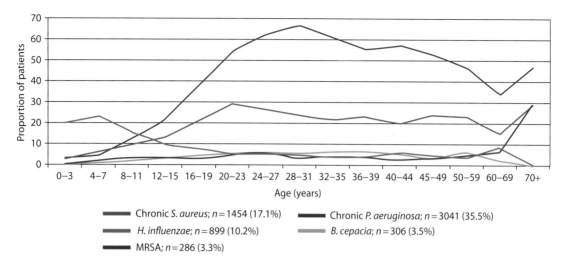

Figure 16.1 UK CF Registry 2012 data for infecting organisms by age. (Available at www.cysticfibrosis.org.uk /media/316760 /Scientific%20Registry%20Review%202012.pdf; accessed May 5, 2015.)

dominant pathogens in the majority of people with CF.[8–11] However, a wide range of other less commonly recognized organisms have been identified. As noted above, many of these are anaerobic bacteria such as *Prevotella* species, *Veillonella* species, and *Rothia* species.[10,11] A wide range of Streptococcal species from the viridans and mitis groups are also present. A full understanding of the importance of these bacteria is not clear, some studies suggest that in CF a narrowing of the diversity of the microbiota is associated with more severe disease. Current and future studies will hopefully determine the importance of this level of diversity and if antibiotic therapy can be appropriately directed to achieve clinical improvement without damaging the community structure of other bacteria present in the airways.[9,10,12]

Infection with microorganisms impacts survival in patients with CF.[12,13] Chronic infection with *P. aeruginosa* and other Gram-negative bacteria are associated with reduced survival compared to patients who are not chronically infected with Gram-negative organisms.[13,14] The reasons for this are not entirely clear and may relate to virulence factors derived from some species versus others. In addition, Methicillin-resistant *Staphylococcus aureus* (MRSA) is associated with a worse survival. Chronic bacterial infection drives at least some pulmonary exacerbations, which are also known to be associated with poorer outcomes in CF (see Chapter 13).

INFECTION CONTROL

The source of bacteria entering and consequently infecting the airways in people with CF is not entirely understood.[12] Gram-negative organisms such as *P. aeruginosa* and *B. cepacia complex* are found in specific environmental niches usually associated with damp environments and often in soil where they may be found around root structures in plants. There is a possibility that sometimes these organisms enter the airways following aerosolization, but

there is strong evidence that in certain situations these bacteria can be passed from person to person.[13,15,16] *B. cenocepacia* ET12 is the archetypal organism known to do this and resulted in major outbreaks in a number of CF centers in the 1980s and early 1990s.[17,18] Since then, further outbreaks have occurred with other members of this complex, and as this organism is associated with increased virulence, it is usually treated with considerable caution.[19] A number of other studies have demonstrated patient to patient spread of *P. aeruginosa*, MRSA,[20–23] and most recently reports from centers in the United Kingdom and United States suggest patient to patient spread of *Mycobacterium abscessus*.[24,25]

These observations have resulted in the implementation of strict infection control measures in CF centers (see Chapter 15).[26] There needs to be good microbial surveillance of prevalent strains of bacteria such as *P. aeruginosa*, *B. cepacia complex* organisms and MRSA. There should also be very strict hygiene precautions, with all people coming into contact with people with CF being aware of the potential for cross infection[26] (see Chapter 15 for further discussion).

SPUTUM PROCESSING AND IDENTIFICATION OF BACTERIA

The surveillance of microbes in the airways of peple with CF is important to determine the correct antibacterial therapy.[27] It is recommended that a respiratory sample should be taken at each hospital visit and at the time of any pulmonary exacerbation. This preferably should be sputum (including induced samples), though a cough swab may be used if a patient cannot expectorate. In younger children, bronchoalveolar lavage is sometimes used, particularly in patients who are not responding to usual therapy. Selected media should be used to enhance the detection of common respiratory pathogens such as *P. aeruginosa*, *B. cepacia complex*, *S. aureus* and *H. influenzae*. If nontuberculous mycobacterium is suspected, then an automated liquid culture system and a solid medium such as Lowenstein Jensen should also be used.[27] The presence of all bacteria should be reported and identified to species level. Methodology for detection of bacteria is further discussed in Chapter 11.

Sensitivity testing should be undertaken for early and intermittent infections but studies in patients with chronic *P. aeruginosa* infection have not demonstrated any benefit from using antimicrobial susceptibility data. In addition, in chronic infection, conventional susceptibility testing is poorly reproducible.

ANTIBACTERIAL CHEMOTHERAPY IN CF

Antimicrobial therapy in CF has a long history, and effective treatment of infection is one of the key advances that have resulted in improved outcomes over the past 50 years. *S. aureus* was identified in 1949 as the predominant pathogen in cultures taken from young children with CF. Subsequently, *P. aeruginosa* was identified as an organism associated with bronchiectasis and chronicity. From the late 1950s, *P. aeruginosa* was reported with increasing frequency from children with CF and the mucoid phenotype for *P. aeruginosa* was first described in 1966. Specific antimicrobial therapy in CF has therefore been directed against these organisms. Over the subsequent decades, a range of other dominant organisms have presented challenges for antibiotic therapy. These include members of the *B. cenocepacia* complex, *S. maltophilia*, *Achromobacter* species, and other Gram-negative infections. Nontuberculous mycobacterial infection is also emerging as a new challenge for antibiotic treatment for people with CF.

ANTIBIOTIC PROPHYLAXIS AND TREATMENT

Staphylococcus aureus

The presence of *S. aureus* in airway secretions from 50% of people with CF has prompted clinicians to consider the use of prophylactic antibiotics to prevent and control Staphylococcal infection in the early years.[28,29] This area of treatment has been, and remains, controversial. In small studies, prophylactic treatment from diagnosis with flucloxacillin has been associated with a reduction in the frequency of Staphylococcal cultures and a reduction in admission to hospital, but no long-term improvements have been demonstrated in lung function.[24,31] These observations were followed up with a clinical trial of cephalexin, a more broad-spectrum antibiotic, which did not demonstrate any clinical efficacy, but there was an increase in the frequency of new infections with *P. aeruginosa*.[28,33] These observations have been supported by a number of registry studies with an association between antibiotic prophylaxis and acquisition of *P. aeruginosa*.[29,32] In a recent updated Cochrane Review, a meta-analysis of 4 studies including 401 patients under the age of seven was reported.[28] In this analysis, no significant increase in the number of isolates

of *P. aeruginosa* was demonstrated between treated and untreated groups from reported studies, though there was a trend toward a lower cumulative isolation rate of *P. aeruginosa* in the patients treated with long-term antibiotics at 2–3 years and a higher isolation rate from 4–6 years. These studies used a range of antibiotics including flucloxacillin, co-trimoxazole, cefadroxil, and cephalexin, and the major benefit was reduced frequency of isolation of *S. aureus* from airways culture. It is unclear what the clinical benefits of simply reducing the frequency of culture of *S. aureus* might be. Further studies in this area are unlikely as most centers now treat young children with CF empirically based on symptoms. In children not responding to standard therapy, a bronchoalveolar lavage may be indicated, but there is no advantage to regular surveillance bronchoscopy.[34]

MRSA

Infection with MRSA has increased in prevalence in hospitals in developed countries and this has been paralleled by similar increases in prevalence in CF patients in some North American and European Centers, although rates are generally higher in the United States than in Europe. A positive culture for MRSA is associated with lower lung function, a higher rate of hospital admission, and increased antibiotic usage.[35] In addition, an association with increased mortality has also been described though the possibility of intrinsic biases in this analysis may have overestimated this effect.[36] MRSA isolates from people with CF tend to reflect the local epidemiology of MRSA.

ANTIBIOTIC THERAPY FOR STAPHYLOCOCCUS AUREUS (MSSA AND MRSA)

S. aureus is a common infecting pathogen in children and adults with CF. It is routinely cultured in clinical laboratories and it is most frequently a methicillin-sensitive organism. Identification of these bacteria in sputum is not always associated with pulmonary symptoms but it is usually treated with a view to eradication.[28] Oral flucloxacillin, dicloxacillin, fusidic acid, co-trimoxazole, and tetracyclines such as minocycline or doxycycline are effective against this organism (but should not be used in children <12 years old).[37] Usually, treatment is continued for at least 14 days, though in individuals with persistent isolation of MSSA longer periods up to 3 months may be justified. In the majority of patients, this organism is cleared from sputum culture but in some there is persistent infection. Treatment may be escalated to intravenous delivery with combinations such as flucloxacillin and aminoglycoside, oral rifampicin or linezolid, and there is some anecdotal support for using inhaled aminoglycosides and vancomycin.

The most effective treatment regimen for MRSA has not been identified.[38] Combinations of two antibiotics including rifampicin, fusidic acid, vancomycin, vibramycin, teicoplanin, co-trimoxazole, and linezolid have all been demonstrated to achieve eradication. For eradication therapy, these should be combined with mupirocin nasal application and chlorhexidine bodywash.[30] There are currently a number of clinical trials underway to determine the most effective regimen.

HAEMOPHILUS INFLUENZAE

H. influenzae, particularly in its non-typeable and non-capsulate forms are common in CF. This organism can persist in biofilms which can be disrupted by azithromycin. However macrolide resistance is common in CF and bronchiectasis. There are relatively few studies investigating the best treatment for *H. influenzae* though up to 40% of patients infected with this organism may demonstrate resistance to a range of antibiotic classes. Suitable antibiotics are co-amoxiclav and doxycycline, and antibiotic sensitivities will be helpful in antibiotic selection.[37]

PSEUDOMONAS AERUGINOSA

P. aeruginosa is commonly isolated from the airways of people with CF particularly as lung disease becomes more prominent and as patients get older.[39,40] In most registries, more than 60% of people with CF isolate *P. aeruginosa* by the third decade in life.[39,40] *P. aeruginosa* has a large genome and has the ability to adapt to the environment of the CF airways despite biophysical and immunological mechanisms which should result in clearance of the organism.[36] In particular, the ability of *P. aeruginosa* to develop a protective biofilm and develop resistance to antibiotics is a key adaptation to the environmental niche of the CF airways.[41] The intrinsic hypermutability of *P. aeruginosa* in genes, and the selection for these in the CF airway is a further mechanism of adaptation. *P. aeruginosa* is therefore well protected against innate immune responses and antibiotics.[41] In contrast to the debate around antibiotic prophylaxis for *S. aureus*, there is currently no evidence for antibiotic prophylaxis against *P. aeruginosa*. There is an ongoing clinical trial using avian derived immunoglobulin Y antibodies. These are gargled to determine if this intervention in the upper airway might prevent lower airways infection.[13] Trials of antipseudomonal vaccines have been disappointing,[42] as has a pilot study of prophylactic nebulized aminoglycosides.[43]

ERADICATION THERAPY

There is a compelling rationale for antibiotic eradication therapy for first and further new episodes of *P. aeruginosa* infection in CF.[13] This approach was championed by the Copenhagen Center who demonstrated in early studies, using a historical comparative cohort that the combination of inhaled colistin and oral ciprofloxacin resulted in approximately an 80% success in eradication.[44] Subsequent studies such as the ELITE and EPIC studies have demonstrated that inhaled tobramycin for 4 weeks is also an effective antibiotic eradication therapy.[45,46] In two small studies, no difference was identified between these two regimens with comparable eradication rates.[47,48]

Eradication therapy is now a recommended part of most guidelines for the treatment of new or repeated infection with *P. aeruginosa*.[12,37] It is less clear what the best treatment for failure to eradicate should be. A recent recommendation from a consensus group was that after two attempts at eradication using inhaled and oral therapy, intravenous antipseudomonal antibiotics should be considered. A clinical trial (Torpedo, http://www.torpedo-cf.org.uk/index.html) comparing colistin/ciprofloxacin and intravenous antibiotics is currently underway in the United Kingdom. Current best practice is that all new isolates of *P. aeruginosa* should initiate an attempt at eradication.

TREATMENT OF CHRONIC *PSEUDOMONAS AERUGINOSA* INFECTION

In around 60% of people with CF, *P. aeruginosa* eventually cannot be eradicated and chronic infection ensues.[12,39,40] When this occurs, the bacteria frequently have a mucoid phenotype and are in a biofilm.[41] This and other important adaptations reduce the effectiveness of innate host defense and make treatment with antibiotics less effective.[49] When chronic infection has developed, treatment with long-term aerosolized antibiotics may be an important and effective intervention. Tobramycin[50,51] and aztreonam lysine[52–54] are therapies approved by most regulators throughout the world. Both of these treatments have demonstrated superiority over placebo for measurements of lung function, quality of life and reduction in pulmonary exacerbations.[12] Colistin is also used in chronic suppressive therapy and its nebulized form has been accepted as a therapy because of its historical use rather than randomized controlled trials. Tobramycin and colistin have recently been developed as dry powder-inhaled antibiotics[51,55,56]; tobramycin as TobiPodhaler® and colistin as Colobreathe®. Both of these drugs have demonstrated noninferiority for key clinical outcomes to tobramycin delivered by nebulizer but exhibited increased cough as a common side effect.[51]

Inhaled nebulized antibiotics have a positive effect on bacterial load, lung function, quality of life and frequency of pulmonary exacerbations.[12] Colistin is given as a continuous twice-daily therapy, while tobramycin is licensed for administration as alternate month therapy. Many patients describe increased symptoms and reduced lung function during the month off tobramycin, resulting in many patients taking two different inhaled antibiotics in monthly cycles. The optimal regimen for combining and sequencing inhaled antibiotic therapy as long-term suppressive therapy has yet to be determined. It is unlikely that a randomized controlled trial will be conducted to allow any further direct comparisons between regimens to answer the question of whether continuous nebulized antibiotics using alternating drugs (tobramycin or aztreonam lysine or colistin) would be superior to the current recommended month on month off regimen.

A number of other inhaled antibiotic therapies against *P. aeruginosa* are in development. Levofloxacin and ciprofloxacin as dry powder inhalers, and ciprofloxacin and amikacin as a liposomal formulation are in various stages of development and may become available in the near future.[57–59] How these drugs will be used in combination is not clear.

TREATING EXACERBATIONS IN PATIENTS WITH CHRONIC *PSEUDOMONAS AERUGINOSA* INFECTION

Pulmonary exacerbations are very significant events in people with CF. They are associated with an increase in pulmonary symptoms, reduction in lung function, systemic symptoms including weight loss, and often evidence of local and systemic inflammation.[60–62] This topic is discussed in depth in Chapter 13. The frequency of pulmonary exacerbations is associated with more rapid decline in lung function and reduced survival. Prevention of pulmonary exacerbations is therefore a key intervention and there is good evidence that long-term suppressive antibiotic therapy, concomitant human DNase (Pulmozyme), oral azithromycin, and inhaled hypertonic saline reduce the time to next exacerbation in clinical trials, and by extrapolation reduce the frequency of these events in people with CF.[60] Correcting CFTR function with ivacaftor also reduces pulmonary exacerbations in patients with at least one G551D mutation.[63] Optimizing long-term treatment to reduce these events and the inflammatory injury they cause to the lungs in people with CF is a critically important intervention.[61]

Optimizing the antibiotic selection and duration of treatment is important in treating pulmonary exacerbations. Around 25% of pulmonary exacerbations result in a failure to return to baseline lung function and/or rapid relapse.[64–66] Selection of antibiotics for treatment of such exacerbations is largely empirical, either intravenously or orally, depending on the severity. Using current techniques to determine in vitro antimicrobial susceptibility, including synergy testing, does not appear to improve the outcomes.[12] This is a particular problem with *P. aeruginosa* as with repeated antibiotic therapy these organisms demonstrate in vitro resistance. However, response to antibiotics does not appear to relate directly to in vitro susceptibility as currently determined in microbiology laboratories.[12] The choice of antibiotics to treat a pulmonary exacerbation, or decision to change antibiotics in a non-responding patient, is determined by both a knowledge of previous combinations of antibiotics which worked well for that patient, and limitations due to previous antibiotic allergy and toxicity. It is not determined by in vitro antimicrobial sensitivity.

There is a good historical and current rationale for the use of a combination of extended-action penicillin plus an aminoglycoside. Conventionally, this therapy has been for 14 days though in a recent registry-based study 10 days may be a sufficient period for the majority of patients.[67] However, this approach has not been subjected to a prospective study.

STENOTROPHOMONAS MALTOPHILIA AND *ACHROMOBACTER* SPECIES

S. maltophilia and *Achromobacter* species are relatively commonly isolated although the prevalence is very variable, with some centers reporting up to 25% prevalence for either organism.[68] The clinical significance of these organisms is hard to determine, though it is clear that individual patients with either of these bacteria as their predominant pathogen can have progressive deterioration in lung function and pulmonary exacerbations. Studies have shown associations with increased exacerbations and poorer outcomes, and these bacteria should be considered significant pathogens.

A range of antibiotics can be useful against these organisms, including tetracyclines, co-trimoxazole, colistin, and piperacillin/tazobactam. There are no eradication studies in the people infected with these bacteria, but it is logical to attempt to clear these organisms if possible. Inhaled colistin and/or oral co-trimoxazole can be used for *S. maltophilia* infection or combinations of the above antibiotics for exacerbations.[12]

Burkholderia cepacia complex strains

Treatment of these organisms is quite problematic. In general, members of this complex have intrinsic antibiotic resistance and *B. cenocepacia*, which historically has been the most common *Burkholderia* in people with CF, is almost universally pan-resistant.[12] There are no long-term antibiotics recommended for treatment of patients with chronic infection, and a recent study of inhaled aztreonam lysine demonstrated no benefit.[69] Intravenous antibiotic treatment is based on a number of studies, which would suggest that tetracycline, co-trimoxazole, chloramphenicol, colistin, ceftazidime, meropenem, and piperacillin/tazobactam combinations may have clinical efficacy.[12,38]

Cepacia syndrome describes rapid deterioration in a patient either when first acquiring *B. cepacia* complex organisms or after many years of chronic infection, sometimes following a precipitating event like a viral infection (Figure 16.2). It has been most commonly associated with *B. cenocepacia* but also occurs with *B. multivorans* infection. There are usually associated signs of sepsis with swinging

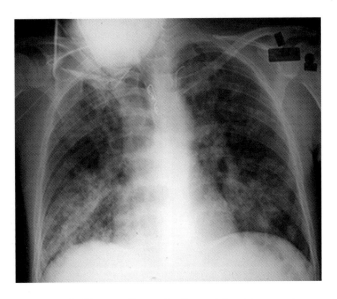

Figure 16.2 Chest radiograph of an adult with cepacia syndrome.

fevers, weight loss, and progressive infiltrates on the chest radiograph.

The syndrome is often fatal despite aggressive antibiotic therapy. It is interesting that there is anecdotal evidence of improvements when immunosuppressive therapy is combined with antibiotic therapy. In particular, the use of cyclosporin and corticosteroids yielded a successful outcome, suggesting that an overexuberant inflammatory response is partly responsible for pulmonary damage.[70]

Nontuberculous mycobacterial (NTM) infection

These are emerging organisms that are currently causing diagnostic and therapeutic challenges.[12,71–73] A number of NTM have been isolated from people with CF, though the predominant groups are the *M. avium complex* (MAC) and *M. abscessus complex* organisms. *M. abscessus* complex infection in CF and other chronic lung conditions is associated with diagnostic difficulties. The diagnosis of NTM infection is problematic as both symptoms and CT scan changes can be similar to those found in CF lung disease itself. The American Thoracic Society (ATS) guidelines can be used to help decide when to initiate treatment.[71] It is most important to ensure regular surveillance for future NTM cultures following a first isolate. A single sputum isolate would not usually be treated. Persistent positive cultures, associated with radiological decline (serial CT scanning may be helpful) and an associated fall in lung function despite appropriate treatment of other pathogens, justifies initiation of specific therapy (Figure 16.3). It is clear that if cultures for usual CF bacteria are negative in the face of declining lung function, then a hard look for NTM species in repeated sputum samples and if necessary bronchoalveolar lavage should be performed to exclude NTM infection. It is recommended that all CF patients producing sputum should have at least an annual culture for NTM species.

Treatment for MAC can follow the ATS guidelines that recommend a three-drug regimen of a macrolide, ethambutol, and rifampicin. Macrolides should never be used as a single agent as this promotes macrolide resistance that yields unfavorable outcomes. Thus, once a first positive culture for MAC is obtained, macrolide therapy for CF should be temporarily suspended while the patient is fully assessed to see if the infection is persistent or whether it is simply a one-off culture. Treatment can be problematic if the patient has concomitant *Aspergillus* infection, as use of the rifamycins renders azole therapy ineffective because of enzyme induction, making it impossible to produce therapeutic levels of azoles. In this situation regular pulses of the antifungal intravenous caspofungin have been used. If treatment for MAC is being initiated because of rapid deterioration, then use of intravenous amikacin is indicated alongside introduction of the oral drugs to gain rapid control. The use of nebulized amikacin for MAC can assist in maintaining control of infection, but lack of trial data has hampered this approach in the United States, even though it is a recognized therapy in the United Kingdom.

Treatment of *M. abscessus* is hampered by its resistance to standard antituberculous agents as well as a wide range of other antimicrobial therapies. *M. abscessus* isolates may appear initially susceptible to macrolides but after extended incubation become resistant. This is due to the presence of an inducible *erm* gene. This gene is absent in the subspecies *bolletii*, hence the reported success rate for treatment is higher than for other *abscessus* subspecies.

Amikacin is the most active agent for treating *M. abscessus* along with tigecycline. In the absence of controlled trials, regimens have been developed by expert consensus and usually involve initial intravenous therapy with a combination of amikacin, and tigecycline or cefoxitin, in addition to imipenem or meropenem, as well as an oral macrolide. The options are to curtail intravenous therapy after 3 weeks and use maintenance therapies including fluoroquinolones, macrolides, and tetracyclines in combination with nebulized amikacin (the European approach); versus continued prolonged use of intravenous amikacin and tigecycline (the US approach.) The basis for recommending nebulized amikacin is to avoid potential ototoxicity resulting from long-term intravenous amikacin.[12] Currently, international guidelines are being developed to help further guide treatment of *M. abscessus*, and it is clear that international collaboration should lead to comparison of the regimens to determine the best therapy.

Emerging data on the subspecies of the *M. abscessus* complex will help us characterize the clinical course and best treatment approach. Recognition of the absent *erm* gene in *M. bolletii* has been informative and we need to determine whether different members of the complex (currently named as *M. massiliense*, *M. bolletii*, and *M. abscessus sensu stricto*) have different clinical effects and different virulence and antibiotic susceptibilities. Further research is required before identification of the subspecies can be used to guide the best treatment regimen.

Other bacterial species

Many other bacterial species are being identified in the airway microbiota in people with CF. Whether treatment

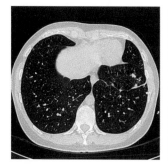
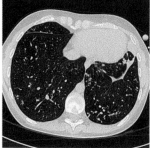

Figure 16.3 CT chest scans of an adult with *M. abscessus* showing progression of the disease (left-hand figure baseline, right-hand figure 6 months later).

is required for organisms such as *Streptococcus* species and anaerobic bacteria such as *Prevotella, Veillonella, Rothia,* and *Actinomyces* species is not clear.[7,8,74] Many of these species are found in lower numbers in the upper airways but are not usually found in lower airways in high numbers. There may be changes in how we perceive treatment with antibiotics over the next few years, as second-generation sequencing provides more insight into the complex microbiota of the airways in people with CF, but antimicrobial therapy will remain the key cornerstone for the modulation of infection and inflammation in CF.

ANTIBIOTIC RESISTANCE

Antibiotic resistance is a considerable problem in bacteria causing infection in the CF airway.[5,41] The competitive environment between microbiota and the enormous amount of antibiotics given to people with CF create conditions where adaptive resistance can easily develop.[41] The CF lung environment is a niche where bacteria encounter stressful conditions that effect gene expression and ultimately the bacterial phenotype. For example, *P. aeruginosa* in the airway environment downregulates the number of metabolic, mobility, and virulence genes, and upregulates membrane permeability and efflux genes.[41] These are adaptive responses to the rather toxic environment within the CF airway. On top of all this, antimicrobial resistance is selected for, with recurrent use of both oral and intravenous antibiotics. Over time, with continuous and repeated antibiotic courses, many patients develop multiresistant *P. aeruginosa*.[75,76] Resistance can also develop in *S. aureus, H. influenzae* and other less commonly isolated bacteria. *B. cepacia complex, A. xylosoxidans* and *S. maltophilia* are inherently resistant to many of the other antibiotics used in CF and this can be further driven by exposure to antibiotics. *B. cepacia* remains almost unique, particularly *B. cenocepacia,* in that it is constitutively resistant to almost all of the antibiotics used in CF.

The implications of bacterial resistance are difficult to unravel. There is wide experience that treatment with intravenous and inhaled antibiotics in patients with evidence of antimicrobial resistance, still results in clinical responses. This may be due to other actions of antibiotics in addition to antimicrobial killing. However, in general, resistance of microorganisms in the CF airway is associated with poorer outcomes, and particularly in those patients who have constitutive resistance to antibiotics, choosing specific antibiotic therapy can be a challenge.[64,77]

ANTIBIOTIC TOXICITY

Antibiotic toxicity is an increasing challenge in CF and particularly relates to the impact of aminoglycosides.[78] Oral antibiotics are generally safe for long-term use, though can predispose patients to infection with *Clostridium difficile* and oral *Candida* infection. Inhaled antibiotics are also generally safe. However, inhaled aminoglycoside serum concentrations should be monitored carefully when used

in conjunction with intravenous treatment as toxicity with this combination has been described.[79] Acute renal failure has been reported following nebulized tobramycin treatment but is a rare event. Dry powder inhaled antibiotics are associated with cough and may, in a small number of patients, cause bronchoconstriction. There is little evidence to support or discourage the use of nebulized inhaled antibiotics during pregnancy. Systemic absorption is low, so drug delivery to the developing baby is small. An assessment of individual risk needs to be made with each patient.

Toxicity is a much greater challenge with intravenous antibiotics and a number of studies have highlighted the risk of renal failure in patients with CF, particularly with gentamicin.[78] This is exacerbated in the presence of concomitant nephrotoxic drugs. Gentamicin should not be used for intravenous therapy and tobramycin is used in preference. All aminoglycosides can cause renal tubular damage and may be worsened by CF-related diabetes, which is a common morbidity. Hearing impairment is also commonly found in individuals with CF who receive aminoglycosides.[79] Some of these side effects may be mitigated by using once-daily rather than three-times-daily tobramycin.[80] Care should also be taken to ensure that other nephrotoxic drugs are not co-prescribed, and that estimated glomerular filtration rate and plasma magnesium are carefully monitored.[81] Some centers undertake an annual pure tone audiogram in individuals receiving frequent courses of aminoglycosides.

ANTIBIOTIC ALLERGY

Allergic reactions to antibiotics are thought to be more common in CF patients than in the general population, though the increased prevalence of allergic reactions may be due to more frequent exposure to antibiotics. Allergic reactions can occur to most of the antibiotics used in CF but are particularly frequent with the β-lactam piperacillin.[82] Interestingly, there is little cross-reactivity between penicillin and other β-lactam antibiotics. Allergic reactions can be investigated with serum and skin prick testing; however, the utility of these in people with CF is unclear.[83] Antibiotic allergies should be clearly documented in patients' notes. Mostly these reactions are T-cell related and a number of reports have indicated that desensitization is possible.[84]

RESPIRATORY VIRUSES

Respiratory viral infections have a significant impact on patients with CF, especially in the autumn (fall) and winter, and respiratory viruses may precipitate up to 40% of chest exacerbations.[85–87] Their effect has probably been underestimated in the past, and this is likely due to difficulties in identifying them, especially from expectorated viscous sputum and thick mucoid airway secretions. It has now been shown that by using molecular techniques (PCR), it is possible to identify most respiratory viruses in the sputum of CF patients.[88] A further small study found that the sensitivity of PCR was greater using sputum compared to nasal swabs in adults with CF.[89] In one study in children, 71 patients had 165 respiratory exacerbations and 46% were positive for viruses in nasal swabs, compared to 17% of nasal swabs when they were asymptomatic; as expected, upper respiratory symptoms were strong predictors for viral detection.[90] Viral pathogens have been shown to be important in adults with respiratory exacerbations, and not just in children.[91,92] In a study of adults with an acute chest exacerbations requiring intravenous antibiotics, those with an accompanying viral infection had a greater fall in lung function, less response to treatment, and a shorter time to their next exacerbation.[93] Viruses implicated in causing infections in CF are the same as those that may affect anyone, namely rhinovirus, respiratory syncytial virus (RSV), parainfluenza virus types 1–4, influenza A and B, human metapneumovirus (hMPV), adenovirus, and coronavirus.[94–97] Human metapneumovirus was initially isolated in 2001, and is a paramyxovirus closely related to RSV[98]; in a study of 7- to 18-year-olds with CF, the infection rates and clinical impact of hMPV were similar to that of RSV.[96]

There is no evidence that infants, children, or adults with CF are more susceptible to viral infections than healthy people, but the impact is greater, and the outcome worse as the lower respiratory tract is affected more often.[85,94,99–101] A number of studies have produced conflicting results over whether the inflammatory response toward respiratory viral infection in nasal and bronchial epithelial cells are exaggerated or not in CF patients. Viral infections may lead to increased frequency and duration of hospitalization for respiratory exacerbations,[102] followed by deterioration in clinical status and lung function,[85,87] which may persist for several months.[100,102] The viruses that have the greatest impact in CF are RSV and influenza. RSV predominates in infants although CF infants have the same number of RSV infections as non-CF infants in any season.[103] In addition to causing acute pulmonary exacerbations and worsening of airway obstruction, RSV can sometimes cause more severe problems, including prolonged hospitalization, persistent hypoxemia, and even a need for mechanical ventilation. Complications can last for several months after the acute infection; one study with a 2-year follow-up found increased respiratory symptoms and worse chest radiograph score in infants who had had RSV.[86] In older children and adults, influenza has the greatest effect, sometimes leading to a significant fall in lung function[104] and deterioration in clinical status;[105] primary influenza pneumonia can also occur.

In March 2009, the first reports of pandemic H1N1 influenza appeared in Mexico, and by July 2009, in their winter, the first reported cases in adults with CF came out of Australia.[106] Despite great initial concerns, most patients in fact had a mild clinical course and were managed with antiviral agents, alongside robust infection-control policies.[106] The European CF Society (A) H1N1 study group reported on 110 cases from 10 countries.[107] Main symptoms were fever, a respiratory exacerbation, and fatigue; and around half required intravenous antibiotics and half required hospitalization. While many were mild, 31% required supplemental oxygen, 5 patients required noninvasive ventilation, and 3 patients with preexisting severe lung disease died.[107] Most regained their baseline lung function 1 month after the infection.

Respiratory viral infections are also associated with onset of secondary bacterial infections, and the first isolation of a particular organism (particularly *P. aeruginosa*) often follows a viral infection.[108,109] One study, in which respiratory viral infections were confirmed on bronchoalveolar lavage (in 52% of infants hospitalized for respiratory disease), found that at 12- to 60-month follow-up, the first isolation of *P. aeruginosa* was more common in the infants who had been hospitalized for respiratory illness than those who were not (35% vs. 6%).[110] The pathophysiology is not well understood, but the association may be due to epithelial damage caused by the viruses with subsequent airway inflammation, as well as impairment of the cough reflex and mucociliary clearance. On the other hand, it may simply be that bacteria were already present in the lungs, but were isolated at the time of increased mucus production and expectoration only because of the viral infection. This is more likely in children as sputum production is often minimal. A recent study has shown that superinfection with rhinovirus in patients already chronically infected with mucoid *P. aeruginosa* disperses the biofilm, thus liberating the planktonic bacteria, which are more pro-inflammatory than those in the biofilm; this increases the chemokine response and possibly contributes to subsequent lower respiratory tract exacerbations.[111]

ANTIVIRAL STRATEGIES

The viruses have relatively short incubation periods (less than a week), and transmission occurs primarily via direct contact (skin or aerosol) with an infected person or something they have recently handled.[26] It is sensible to keep people with obvious upper respiratory tract infections away from CF infants if possible. Droplet infection via the nose and eyes can occur within 3 feet (1 m) with influenza and adenovirus. In hospitalized infants, isolation in a cubicle or cohorting of infected patients is important, but success relies on rapid diagnosis, and a number of techniques are available. Staff must be meticulous with infection precautions, particularly hand-washing.

IMMUNIZATION

A Cochrane systematic review did not find any evidence from randomized studies that influenza immunization is beneficial to patients with CF.[112] However, the immunogenic effect in CF children is similar to normal children[113] and several studies have shown it to be safe.[103] In addition, a small retrospective study found significantly fewer isolations of influenza in nasal swabs in those vaccinated versus those who were not.[113] Consequently, influenza immunization is recommended annually for CF patients aged over 6 months; immunization of immediate family members is also recommended.[103] There is still no licensed vaccine for those aged under 6 months, and children aged 6–35 months require two half-doses 1 month apart. In addition, those aged 3–8 years who are receiving the vaccine for the first time also require two doses 1 month apart, but for succeeding years receive a single dose similarly to adults.[103] There is now a live attenuated intranasal influenza vaccine (Fluenz®) available for those aged 2–18 years. A recent study has shown that the nasal vaccine was as safe as injectable vaccine in children and adolescents with CF.[114] It cannot be used if the child is acutely wheezy on the day or within 7 days; or if the child is on systemic steroids (within 14 days). There may be issues also in the presence of large nasal polyps. Currently, there is no effective RSV vaccine available. Passive immunoprophylaxis with palivizumab (a monoclonal antibody to RSV) may have some benefit in ex-premature babies with chronic lung disease, but so far there are insufficient data to determine its effectiveness in CF infants. The only randomized controlled trial of palivizumab, sponsored by the manufacturers, studied 186 infants over 3 seasons; they failed to find any significant differences to multiple outcomes, although they did demonstrate there were no safety issues (published as an abstract only).[115] The American Academy of Pediatrics does not recommend its use in CF infants due to insufficient data.[116] Nevertheless, some think it a good idea—a survey of North American CF centers, showed that 74% of 83 centers had prescribed it to CF children in their first year, although only 41% considered it as the standard of care for all infants with CF.[117] By contrast, in the United Kingdom only 3/34 (10%) pediatric centers that responded to a survey said they had prescribed palivizumab, to a total of 14 infants.[118]

ANTIVIRAL DRUGS

There may be a role for the neuraminidase inhibitors oral oseltamivir or inhaled zanamivir when used early (ideally within a few hours of onset of symptoms, and at least within 48 hours) in influenza infection, as well as for prophylaxis of nonimmunized patients exposed to influenza.[119] This is most likely to be valuable during an influenza epidemic. The updated 2009 recommendations added (to the 2003 guidance) that zanamivir is now recommended as a treatment option for children aged 5–12 years in "at-risk" groups if influenza is circulating and they can start treatment within 36 hours of first symptoms. Evidence is lacking in CF, but one difficulty is recognizing a chest exacerbation as being due to influenza early enough in the illness for the drug to be effective. Amantadine is not recommended for treatment or prophylaxis of influenza.[119]

Inhaled ribavirin (a nucleotide analogue) is licensed for use in RSV infection but has limited effectiveness and is rarely used in otherwise healthy infants; it is not indicated in CF. There is some evidence that the leukotriene receptor antagonist montelukast reduces respiratory symptoms (particularly cough) for a month post-RSV bronchiolitis, when

given within 7 days of onset of symptoms[120]; other studies did not find this.[121] It may be worthwhile trying in CF infants, although no study in this group has been undertaken.

ANTIBACTERIAL PROPHYLAXIS

When patients have an upper respiratory tract infection (most commonly due to rhinovirus), unless symptoms are trivial, many clinicians advise antibiotic prophylaxis (principally against *H. influenzae*)—for example, with co-amoxiclav for at least 2 weeks.[32] This is not based on trial evidence in CF patients, but is supported by clinical experience and a randomized controlled trial in non-CF patients with common colds. It was found that 5 days of co-amoxiclav benefited 20% of patients whose nasopharyngeal secretions had also grown bacteria (*H. influenzae*, *Moraxella catarrhalis*, or *Streptococcus pneumoniae*).[122] Some centers advocate doubling the dose of the flucloxacillin the child is on for chronic *S. aureus* infection during colds, but that offers no additional benefit against *H. influenzae*.

FUNGAL INFECTIONS

Fungi are widely distributed in the environment, and their spores are the correct particle size (2–4 microns) to facilitate airway deposition. The presence of a perturbed airway surface with inflammation and structural damage makes the CF lung an ideal environment for survival and growth of these organisms.

Aspergillus is, by far, the most common fungus isolated in CF and can cause a variety of lung diseases including airway infection (now termed aspergillus bronchitis), allergic bronchopulmonary aspergillosis (ABPA), aspergilloma and a slowly invasive aspergillosis. Some CF patients may manifest all of these manifestations in their lifetime while others have none and the underlying predisposition for fungal lung disease in CF is not entirely clear, although the aggressive treatments and eradication of *Pseudomonas spp.* has been associated with an increased recognition of fungal problems. Research in interactions between bacteria and fungi in the lung may offer new insights for future management.

While *Aspergillus* is the leading player in CF fungal lung disease, we are now recognizing the significance of other fungal species including *Scedosporium* and *Exophiala*. It appears that both these fungi and probably others can cause the same spectrum of disease as *Aspergillus* species.

ASPERGILLUS BRONCHITIS

Aspergillus has been noted to grow in the airways of CF patients with varied prevalence depending on culture techniques.[123] An apparent increase in overall prevalence may be as a result of more aggressive use of antibiotics, particularly *Pseudomonas* eradication strategies.[124,125] Previously, *Aspergillus*, without evidence of hypersensitivity, was regarded as an innocent bystander but there is increasing evidence that *Aspergillus* in the airways is a cause of accelerated lung function decline.[126] A small pilot eradication study based on this premise was hampered by the use of itraconazole without drug level monitoring, thus not ensuring that those on active drug received effective therapy.[127] Case series have coined the term aspergillus bronchitis,[128] and suggested *Aspergillus* growth in the absence of other pathogens in CF patients, with troublesome coughing and decline in lung function, warrant a trial of antifungal therapy. Aspergillus bronchitis may be better defined with the use of specific IgG antibodies and sputum galactomannan, separating out a group of patients with elevated IgG antibodies in response to airway infection without an IgE response.[129] Clinical trials utilizing these criteria to define phenotypic groups are required to determine the best treatment approach. In the meantime, a CF patient with new symptoms of irritable cough and growth of *Aspergillus* in the absence of any other pathogens or evidence of ABPA may warrant a trial of an antifungal therapy for a month.

ALLERGIC BRONCHOPULMONARY ASPERGILLOSIS

Allergic bronchopulmonary aspergillosis (ABPA) is a hypersensitivity disease of the lung resulting from an overexuberant immune response to aspergillus antigens. It occurs in adult patients with asthma and in all ages of patients with CF. The UK CF registry data from 2012 reported a prevalence overall of 10.3% varying from 7.4% in children under 16 years to 12.5% in the population 16 years and older.

The clinical picture can vary but there is a classic scenario where the patient may present acutely with wheezing, dyspnea, chest pain, and cough productive of plugs of sputum with brown/black flecks. In addition, there may be flu-like symptoms of myalgia and fever. Lung function tests demonstrate increased airflow obstruction and a chest radiograph demonstrates new infiltrates, which characteristically melt away in response to systemic corticosteroid therapy (Figure 16.4).

A more insidious scenario presents more of a diagnostic challenge. In this situation, ABPA may present simply as a slow chronic deterioration in symptoms and lung function with poor response to intravenous antibiotics; and in the presence of an already abnormal chest radiograph, may not be associated with the classic patchy infiltrates. In this setting, a chest CT scan may be more helpful demonstrating proximal bronchiectasis and bronchocentric inflammatory changes.

The diagnosis relies on putting the clinical picture together with evidence of a hypersensitivity reaction to *Aspergillus*. As no single criterion is discriminatory, and the underlying disease in CF complicates disease definition, guidelines have been developed to help define the combination of clinical, radiological, and immunological features that lead to a diagnosis of ABPA in CF.[130]

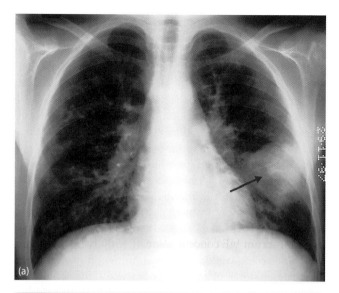

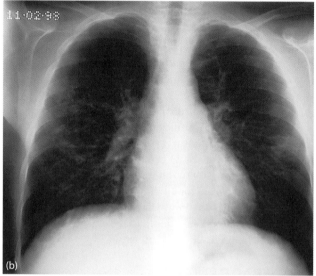

Figure 16.4 Chest radiographs of a child showing **(a)** infiltration due to ABPA (arrow) and **(b)** follow-up 10 weeks later showing considerable improvement after oral corticosteroid therapy.

A "classic case" is defined as follows:

- Acute or subacute clinical deterioration (cough, wheeze, exercise intolerance, exercise-induced asthma, decline in pulmonary function, increased sputum) not attributable to another etiology
- Serum total IgE concentration of >1000 IU/mL (2400 ng/mL), unless the patient is receiving systemic corticosteroids (if so, retest when steroid treatment is discontinued)
- Immediate cutaneous reactivity to *Aspergillus* (prick skin test wheal of 13 mm in diameter with surrounding erythema, while the patient is not being treated with systemic antihistamines) or in vitro presence of serum IgE antibody to *A. fumigatus*

- Precipitating antibodies to *A. fumigatus* or serum IgG antibody to *A. fumigatus* by an in vitro test
- New or recent abnormalities on chest radiography (infiltrates or mucus plugging) or chest CT (bronchiectasis) that have not cleared with antibiotics and standard physiotherapy

Minimum diagnostic criteria[130] were also defined as follows:

- Acute or subacute clinical deterioration (cough, wheeze, exercise intolerance, exercise induced asthma, change in pulmonary function, or increased sputum production) not attributable to another etiology.
- Total serum IgE concentration of >500 IU/mL (1200 ng/mL). If ABPA is suspected and the total IgE level is 200–500 IU/mL, repeat testing in 1–3 months is recommended. If patient is taking corticosteroids, repeat when steroid treatment is discontinued.
- Immediate cutaneous reactivity to *Aspergillus* (prick skin test wheal of 13 mm in diameter with surrounding erythema while the patient is not being treated with systemic antihistamines) or in vitro demonstration of IgE antibody to *A. fumigatus*.
- One of the following:
  a. Precipitins to *A. fumigatus* or in vitro demonstration of IgG antibody to *A. fumigatus*
  b. New or recent abnormalities on chest radiography (infiltrates or mucus plugging) or chest CT (bronchiectasis) that have not cleared with antibiotics and standard physiotherapy

Given the challenges in diagnosis, it is crucial that a CF clinician retains a high index of suspicion and considers investigations for ABPA where there is failure of response to antimicrobial therapy. Furthermore, international guidelines recommend that both children and adults with CF have an annual assessment measurement of serum IgE as a screening tool.

Treatment of ABPA with corticosteroids is recommended to attenuate the inflammatory reaction generated by the immune response to *Aspergillus*. Attenuation of the antigen burden is achieved with the use of antifungal therapy. The aim of therapy is to restore lung function and prevent progression of lung disease, particularly further progression of bronchiectasis, although randomized trial data is lacking.

While oral prednisolone is highly effective, prolonged courses are associated with increased risk of diabetes mellitus, osteoporosis, and impaired growth; thus every effort is made to minimize the exposure to steroids while preventing further lung damage. Antifungals may be beneficial in treatment of ABPA in CF as steroid-sparing agents, in a similar way to their use in ABPA associated with asthma.[131,132]

Itraconazole is poorly absorbed in CF and the liquid formulation is recommended, with regular assessment of levels to ensure appropriate dosing. Voriconazole is better absorbed but like itraconazole has significant drug interactions. Posaconazole has been used as a third line agent. Nebulized antifungal agents have also been used as steroid sparers when oral agents are not tolerated.

The starting dose of oral prednisolone is 0.5–1 mg/kg/day (maximum of 60 mg) for 1 or 2 weeks which then should be converted to the same daily dose but on alternate days for a couple of weeks and then gradually tapered down every 2 weeks as judged by response in terms of lung function and symptoms, as well as an assessment of the IgE.[37] The aim should be to achieve withdrawal of steroids at 2–3 months. Antifungal therapy with the azoles should not be continued beyond 6 months without careful thought because of the cumulative risks of photosensitivity and skin cancer.

For patients with recurrent relapses, or where steroid dependence is a concern, other approaches can be adopted. We have maintained stability with the use of regular courses of intravenous caspofungin. The role of anti-IgE monoclonal antibody therapy with omalizumab is not established in terms of evidence from a randomized controlled trial, but case report data suggests it may be a useful therapy.[133] Use of pulsed intravenous methylprednisolone combined with an oral azole presents another alternative to prolonged oral steroid use.[134]

OTHER FUNGAL SPECIES

Candida albicans is frequently isolated in sputum samples from adults and has in the past been viewed as a contaminant. Oral candidiasis is a recognized complication of prolonged antibiotic therapy in CF and as a result positive sputum cultures for this organism have largely been ignored. Recent data suggest that this assumption may not be true and that *Candida* in sputum samples may be associated with greater decline in lung function and an increase in exacerbations.[135]

The other fungal species that have emerged as potential pathogens in CF are *Scedosporium apiospermum* and *Exophiala dermatitidis*. More work is required to characterize the syndromes associated with these fungal species but we have observed an ABPA-like picture as well as a fungal bronchitis with both these species. Voriconazole appears to be useful in treating both *Scedosporium* and *Exophiala* but it is important to gain specialist advice on susceptibility of the organisms.

REFERENCES

1. Livraghi-Butrico A, Kelly EJ, Wilkinson KJ et al. Loss of CFTR function exacerbates the phenotype of Na+ hyperabsorption in murine airways. *Am J Physiol Lung Cell Mol Physiol* 2013; **304**: L469-80.
2. Button B, Cai LH, Ehre C et al. A periciliary brush promotes the lung health by separating the mucus layer from airway epithelia. *Science* 2012; **337**: 937–41.

3. Boucher RC. Cystic fibrosis: A disease of vulnerability to airway surface dehydration. *Trends Mol Med* 2007; **13**: 231–40.

4. Pezzulo AA, Tang XX, Hoegger MJ et al. Reduced airway surface pH impairs bacterial killing in the porcine cystic fibrosis lung. *Nature* 2012; **487**: 109–13.

5. Cohen TS, Prince A. Cystic fibrosis: A mucosal immunodeficiency syndrome. *Nat Med* 2012; **18**: 509–19.

6. Worlitzsch D, Tarran R, Ulrich M et al. Effects of reduced mucus oxygen concentration in airway Pseudomonas infections of cystic fibrosis patients. *J Clin Invest* 2002; **109**: 317–25.

7. Tunney MM, Field TR, Moriarty TF et al. Detection of anaerobic bacteria in high numbers in sputum from patients with cystic fibrosis. *Am J Respir Crit Care Med* 2008; **177**: 995–1001.

8. Tunney MM, Klem ER, Fodor AA et al. Use of culture and molecular analysis to determine the effect of antibiotic treatment on microbial community diversity and abundance during exacerbation in patients with cystic fibrosis. *Thorax* 2011; **66**: 579–84.

9. Zhao J, Schloss PD, Kalikin LM et al. Decade-long bacterial community dynamics in cystic fibrosis airways. *Proc Natl Acad Sci USA* 2012; **109**: 5809–14.

10. Fodor AA, Klem ER, Gilpin DF et al. The adult cystic fibrosis airway microbiota is stable over time and infection type, and highly resilient to antibiotic treatment of exacerbations. *PLoS One* 2012; **7**: e45001.

11. Stressmann FA, Rogers GB, van der Gast CJ et al. Long-term cultivation-independent microbial diversity analysis demonstrates that bacterial communities infecting the adult cystic fibrosis lung show stability and resilience. *Thorax* 2012; **67**: 867–73.

12. Döring G, Flume P, Heijerman H, Elborn JS; Consensus Study Group. Treatment of lung infection in patients with cystic fibrosis: Current and future strategies. *J Cyst Fibros* 2012; **11**: 461–79.

13. Govan JR, Brown AR, Jones AM. Evolving epidemiology of *Pseudomonas aeruginosa* and the *Burkholderia cepacia* complex in cystic fibrosis lung infection. *Future Microbiol* 2007; **2**: 153–64.

14. Courtney JM, Bradley J, Mccaughan J et al. Predictors of mortality in adults with cystic fibrosis. *Pediatr Pulmonol* 2007; **42**(6): 525–32.

15. Wainwright CE, France MW, O'Rourke P et al. Cough-generated aerosols of *Pseudomonas aeruginosa* and other Gram-negative bacteria from patients with cystic fibrosis. *Thorax* 2009; **64**: 926–31.

16. Clifton IJ, Peckham DG. Defining routes of airborne transmission of *Pseudomonas aeruginosa* in people with cystic fibrosis. *Expert Rev Respir Med* 2010; **4**: 519–29.

17. Govan JR, Brown PH, Maddison J et al. Evidence for transmission of Pseudomonas cepacia by social contact in cystic fibrosis. *Lancet* 1993; **342**: 15–9.

18. Jones AM, Dodd ME, Webb AK. Burkholderia cepacia: Current clinical issues, environmental controversies and ethical dilemmas. *Eur Respir J* 2001; **17**: 295–301.

19. Kalish LA, Waltz DA, Dovey M et al. Impact of Burkholderia dolosa on lung function and survival in cystic fibrosis. *Am J Respir Crit Care Med* 2006; **173**: 421–5.

20. Dasenbrook EC, Checkley W, Merlo CA et al. Association between respiratory tract methicillin-resistant *Staphylococcus aureus* and survival in cystic fibrosis. *JAMA* 2010; **303**: 2386–92.

21. Jones AM, Govan JR, Doherty CJ et al. Spread of a multiresistant strain of Pseudomonas aeruginosa in an adult cystic fibrosis clinic. *Lancet* 2001; **358**: 557–8.

22. Jones AM, Govan JR, Doherty CJ et al. Identification of airborne dissemination of epidemic multiresistant strains of *Pseudomonas aeruginosa* at a CF centre during a cross infection outbreak. *Thorax* 2003; **58**: 525–7.

23. Aaron SD, Vandemheen KL, Ramotar K et al. Infection with transmissible strains of *Pseudomonas aeruginosa* and clinical outcomes in adults with cystic fibrosis. *JAMA* 2010; **304**: 2145–53.

24. Goss CH, Muhlebach MS. Review: *Staphylococcus aureus* and MRSA in cystic fibrosis. *J Cyst Fibros* 2011; **10**: 298–306.

25. Bryant JM, Grogono DM, Greaves D et al. Whole-genome sequencing to identify transmission of Mycobacterium abscessus between patients with cystic fibrosis: A retrospective cohort study. *Lancet* 2013; pii: S0140-6736(13)60632-7. doi: 10.1016/S0140-6736(13)60632-7.

26. Saiman L, Siegel J; Cystic Fibrosis Foundation Consensus Conference on Infection Control Participants. Infection control recommendations for patients with cystic fibrosis: Microbiology, important pathogens, and infection control practices to prevent patient-to-patient transmission. *Am J Infect Control* 2003; **31**(3 Suppl): S1–62.

27. Laboratory standards for processing microbiological samples from people with cystic fibrosis. Report of the UK Cystic Fibrosis Trust Microbiology Laboratory Standards Working Group. 1st Edition, Sept 2010. https://www.cysticfibrosis.org.uk/media/82034/CD_Laboratory_Standards_Sep_10.pdf.

28. Smyth AR, Walters S. Prophylactic anti-staphylococcal antibiotics for cystic fibrosis. Cochrane Database Syst Rev 2012, Issue 12. Art. No.: CD001912. DOI: 10.1002/14651858.CD001912.pub2.

29. Razvi S, Quittell L, Sewall A et al. Respiratory microbiology of patients with cystic fibrosis in the United States, 1995 to 2005. *Chest* 2009; **136**: 1554–60.

30. Jain K, Smyth AR. Current dilemmas in antimicrobial therapy in cystic fibrosis. *Expert Rev Respir Med* 2012; **6**: 407–22.

31. Weaver T, Green MR, Nicholson K et al. Prognosis in cystic fibrosis treated with continuous flucloxacillin from the neonatal period *Arch Dis Child* 1994; **70**: 84–9.

32. Stutman HR, Lieberman JM, Nussbaum E, Marks MI. Antibiotic prophylaxis in infants and young children with cystic fibrosis: A randomized controlled trial. *J Pediatr* 2002; **140**: 29.

33. Ratjen F, Comes G, Paul K et al. Effect of continuous antistaphylococcal therapy on the rate of *P. aeruginosa* acquisition in patients with cystic fibrosis. *Pediatr Pulmonol* 2001; **31**: 13–16.

34. Jain K, Wainwright C, Smyth AR. Bronchoscopy guided antimicrobial therapy for cystic fibrosis. Cochrane Database Syst Rev 2013; **12**: CD009530. doi: 10.1002/14651858.CD009530.pub2.

35. Dasenbrook EC, Merlo CA, Diener-West M et al. Persistent methicillin-resistant *Staphylococcus aureus* and rate of FEV1 decline in cystic fibrosis. *Am J Respir Crit Care Med* 2008; **178**: 814–21.

36. Dasenbrook EC, Checkley W, Merlo CA, Konstan MW, Lechtzin N, Boyle MP. Association between respiratory tract methicillin-resistant *Staphylococcus aureus* and survival in cystic fibrosis. *JAMA* 2010; **303**: 2386–92.

37. Antibiotic treatment for Cystic Fibrosis. Report of the UK Cystic Fibrosis Trust antibiotic Working Group. 3rd edition May 2009. https://www.cysticfibrosis.org.uk/media/82010/CD_Antibiotic_treatment_for_CF_May_09.pdf.

38. Lo DK, Hurley MN, Muhlebach MS, Smyth AR. Interventions for the eradication of methicillin-resistant *Staphylococcus aureus* (MRSA) in people with cystic fibrosis. *Cochrane Database Syst Rev* 2013; **2**: CD009650. doi: 10.1002/14651858.CD009650.pub2.

39. Cystic fibrosis foundation patient registry 2011 annual data report. Bethesda, MD: Cystic Fibrosis Foundation, 2012.

40. Cystic Fibrosis Trust Annual data report, 2011, http://www.cftrust.org.uk/media/82506/CR_Annual_Data_Report_2011_Jan_13.pdf.

41. Folkesson A, Jelsbak L, Yang L et al. Adaptation of *Pseudomonas aeruginosa* to the cystic fibrosis airway: An evolutionary perspective. *Nat Rev Microbiol* 2012; **10**: 841–51.

42. Johansen HK, Gøtzsche PC. Vaccines for preventing infection with *Pseudomonas aeruginosa* in cystic fibrosis. Cochrane Database Syst Rev 2013; **6**: CD001399. doi:10.1002/14651858.CD001399.pub3.

43. Heinzl B, Eber E, Oberwaldner B, Haas G, Zach MS. Effects of inhaled gentamicin prophylaxis on acquisition of *Pseudomonas aeruginosa* in children with cystic fibrosis: A pilot study. *Pediatr Pulmonol* 2002; **33**: 32–7.

44. Valerius NH, Koch C, Høiby N. Prevention of chronic *Pseudomonas aeruginosa* colonisation in cystic fibrosis by early treatment. *Lancet* 1991; **338**: 725–6.

45. Ratjen F, Munck A, Kho P, Angyalosi G; ELITE Study Group. Treatment of early *Pseudomonas aeruginosa* infection in patients with cystic fibrosis: The ELITE trial. *Thorax* 2010; **65**: 286–91.

46. Treggiari MM, Retsch-Bogart G, Mayer-Hamblett N et al. Comparative efficacy and safety of 4 randomized regimens to treat early *Pseudomonas aeruginosa* infection in children with cystic fibrosis. *Arch Pediatr Adolesc Med* 2011; **165**: 847–56.

47. Proesmans M, Vermeulen F, Boulanger L, Verhaegen J, De Boeck K. Comparison of two treatment regimens for eradication of *P. aeruginosa* infection in children with cystic fibrosis. *J Cyst Fibros* 2013; **12**(1): 29–34.

48. Taccetti G, Bianchini E, Cariani L et al. Early antibiotic treatment for *Pseudomonas aeruginosa* eradication in patients with cystic fibrosis: A randomised multicentre study comparing two different protocols. *Thorax* 2012; **67**(10): 853–9.

49. Williams HD, Davies JC. Basic science for the chest physician: *Pseudomonas aeruginosa* and the cystic fibrosis airway. *Thorax* 2012; **67**: 465–7.

50. Ramsey BW, Pepe MS, Quan JM et al. Intermittent administration of inhaled tobramycin in patients with cystic fibrosis. *N Engl J Med* 1999; **340**: 23–30.

51. Parkins MD, Elborn JS. Tobramycin Inhalation Powder™: A novel drug delivery system for treating chronic Pseudomonas aeruginosa infection in cystic fibrosis. *Expert Rev Respir Med* 2011; **5**: 609–22.

52. Oermann CM, McCoy KS, Retsch-Bogart GZ et al. *Pseudomonas aeruginosa* antibiotic susceptibility during long-term use of aztreonam for inhalation solution (AZLI). *J Antimicrob Chemother* 2011; **66**: 2398–404.

53. Assael BM, Pressler T, Bilton D et al. for the AZLI Active Comparator Study Group. Inhaled aztreonam lysine vs. inhaled tobramycin in cystic fibrosis: A comparative efficacy trial. *J Cyst Fibros* 2012; **12**(2): 130–40.

54. Oermann CM, Retsch-Bogart GZ, Quittner AL et al. An 18-month study of the safety and efficacy of repeated courses of inhaled aztreonam lysine in cystic fibrosis. *Pediatr Pulmonol* 2010; **45**: 1121–34.

55. Schuster A, Haliburn C, Döring G et al. Safety, efficacy and convenience of colistimethate sodium dry powder for inhalation (Colobreathe® DPI) in cystic fibrosis patients: A randomised study. *Thorax* 2013; **68**(4): 344–50.

56. Konstan MW, Flume PA, Kappler M et al. Safety, efficacy and convenience of tobramycin inhalation powder in cystic fibrosis patients: The EAGER trial. *J Cyst Fibros* 2011; **10**: 54–61.

57. Hoffman LR, Ramsey BW. Cystic fibrosis therapeutics: The road ahead. *Chest* 2013; **143**: 207–13.

58. Ramsey B, Rowe SM, Borowitz DS et al. Progress in cystic fibrosis and the CF Therapeutics. Development Network. *Thorax* 2012; **67**: 882–90.

59. Ramsey BW, Banks-Schlegel S, Accurso FJ et al. Future directions in early cystic fibrosis lung disease research: An NHLBI workshop report. *Am J Respir Crit Care Med* 2012; **185**: 887–92.

60. Cohen-Cymberknoh M, Shoseyov D, Kerem E. Managing cystic fibrosis: Strategies that increase life expectancy and improve quality of life. *Am J Respir Crit Care Med* 2011; **183**: 1463–71.

61. Stenbit AE, Flume PA. Pulmonary exacerbations in cystic fibrosis. *Curr Opin Pulm Med* 2011; **17**: 442–7.

62. Bilton D, Canny G, Conway S et al. Pulmonary exacerbation: Towards a definition for use in clinical trials. Report from the EuroCare CF Working Group on outcome parameters in clinical trials. *J Cyst Fibros* 2011; **10** Suppl 2: S79–81.

63. Ramsey BW, Davies J, McElvaney NG et al; VX08-770-102 Study Group. A CFTR potentiator in patients with cystic fibrosis and the G551D mutation. *N Engl J Med* 2011; **365**: 1663–72.

64. Parkins MD, Rendall JC, Elborn JS. Incidence and risk factors for pulmonary exacerbation treatment failures in patients with cystic fibrosis chronically infected with *Pseudomonas aeruginosa*. *Chest* 2012; **141**: 485–93.

65. Sanders DB, Bittner RC, Rosenfeld M et al. Failure to recover to baseline pulmonary function after cystic fibrosis pulmonary exacerbation. *Am J Respir Crit Care Med* 2010; **182**: 627–32.

66. Sanders DB, Hoffman LR, Emerson J et al. Return of FEV1 after pulmonary exacerbation in children with cystic fibrosis. *Pediatr Pulmonol* 2010; **45**: 127–34.

67. VanDevanter DR, O'Riordan MA, Blumer JL, Konstan MW. Assessing time to pulmonary function benefit following antibiotic treatment of acute cystic fibrosis exacerbations. *Respir Res* 2010; **11**: 137.

68. Waters V, Yau Y, Prasad S et al. *Stenotrophomonas maltophilia* in cystic fibrosis: Serologic response and effect on lung disease. *Am J Respir Crit Care Med* 2011; **183**: 635–40.

69. Tullis DE, Burns JL, Retsch-Bogart GZ et al. Inhaled aztreonam for chronic Burkholderia infection in cystic fibrosis: A placebo-controlled trial. *J Cyst Fibros* 2014; **13**(3): 296–305.

70. Gilchrist FJ, Webb AK, Bright-Thomas RJ et al. Successful treatment of cepacia syndrome with a combination of intravenous cyclosporine, antibiotics and oral corticosteroids. *J Cyst Fibros* 2012; **11**: 458–60.

71. Griffith DE, Aksamit T, Brown-Elliott BA et al; ATS Mycobacterial Diseases Subcommittee; American Thoracic Society; Infectious Disease Society of America. An official ATS/IDSA statement: Diagnosis, treatment, and prevention of nontuberculous mycobacterial diseases. *Am J Respir Crit Care Med* 2007; **175**: 367–416.

72. Brown-Elliott BA, Nash KA, Wallace RJ Jr. Antimicrobial susceptibility testing, drug resistance mechanisms, and therapy of infections with nontuberculous mycobacteria. *Clin Microbiol Rev* 2012; **25**: 545–82.

73. Waters V, Ratjen F. Antibiotic treatment for nontuberculous mycobacteria lung infection in people with cystic fibrosis. *Cochrane Database Syst Rev.* 2012; **12**: CD010004. doi: 10.1002/14651858.CD010004.pub2.

74. Zhao J, Schloss PD, Kalikin LM et al. Decade-long bacterial community dynamics in cystic fibrosis airways. *Proc Natl Acad Sci U S A.* 2012; **109**(15): 5809–14. doi: pnas.org/cgi/doi/10.1073/pnas.1120577109.

75. Oermann CM, McCoy KS, Retsch-Bogart GZ et al. Pseudomonas aeruginosa antibiotic susceptibility during long-term use of aztreonam for inhalation solution (AZLI). *J Antimicrob Chemother* 2011; **66**: 2398–404.

76. Block JK, Vandemheen KL, Tullis E et al. Predictors of pulmonary exacerbations in patients with cystic fibrosis infected with multi-resistant bacteria. *Thorax* 2006; **61**: 969–74.

77. Aaron SD, Vandemheen KL, Ferris W et al. Combination antibiotic susceptibility testing to treat exacerbations of cystic fibrosis associated with multiresistant bacteria: A randomised, double-blind, controlled clinical trial. *Lancet* 2005; **366**: 463–71.

78. Smyth A, Lewis S, Bertenshaw C et al. A case control study of acute renal failure in cystic fibrosis patients in the United Kingdom. *Thorax* 2008; **63**: 532–5.

79. Smyth A, Tan KH, Hyman-Taylor P et al. Once versus three-times daily regimens of tobramycin treatment for pulmonary exacerbations of cystic fibrosis: The TOPIC study: A randomized controlled trial. *Lancet* 2005; **365**: 573–8.

80. Mulheran M, Hyman-Taylor P, Tan KH et al. Absence of cochleotoxicity measured by standard and high-frequency pure tone audiometry in a trial of once-versus three-times-daily tobramycin in cystic fibrosis patients. *Antimicrob Agents Chemother* 2006; **50**: 2293–9.

81. Scott CS, Retsch-Bogart GZ, Henry MM. Renal failure and vestibular toxicity in an adolescent with cystic fibrosis receiving gentamicin and standard-dose ibuprofen. *Pediatr Pulmonol* 2001; **31**: 314–6.

82. Burrows JA, Nissen LM, Kirkpatrick CM, Bell SC. Beta-lactam allergy in adults with cystic fibrosis. *J Cyst Fibros* 2007; **6**: 297–303.

83. Parmar JS, Nasser S. Antibiotic allergy in cystic fibrosis. *Thorax* 2005; **60**: 517–20.

84. Whitaker P, Naisbitt D, Peckham D. Nonimmediate β-lactam reactions in patients with cystic fibrosis. *Curr Opin Allergy Clin Immunol* 2012; **12**: 369–75.

85. Wang EE, Prober CG, Manson B et al. Association of respiratory viral infections with pulmonary deterioration in patients with cystic fibrosis. *N Engl J Med* 1984; **311**: 1653–8.

86. Abman SH, Ogle JW, Butler-Simon N et al. Role of respiratory syncytial virus in early hospitalizations for respiratory distress of young infants with cystic fibrosis. *J Pediatr* 1988; **113**: 826–30.

87. Smyth AR, Smyth RL, Tong CY et al. Effect of respiratory virus infections including rhinovirus on clinical status in cystic fibrosis. *Arch Dis Child* 1995; **73**: 117–20.

88. Punch G, Syrmis MW, Rose BR et al. Method for detection of respiratory viruses in the sputa of patients with cystic fibrosis. *Eur J Clin Microbiol Infect Dis* 2005; **24**: 54–7.

89. Jones AM, Flight W, Isalska B, et al. Diagnosis of respiratory viral infections in cystic fibrosis by PCR using sputum samples. *Eur Respir J* 2011; **38**: 1486–7.

90. Wat D, Gelder C, Hibbitts S et al. The role of respiratory viruses in cystic fibrosis. *J Cyst Fibros* 2008; **7**: 320–8.

91. Hoek RA, Paats MS, Pas SD, et al. Incidence of viral respiratory pathogens causing exacerbations in adult cystic fibrosis patients. *Scand J Infect Dis* 2013; **45**: 65–9.

92. Flight WG, Bright-Thomas RJ, Tilston P, et al. Incidence and clinical impact of respiratory viruses in adults with cystic fibrosis. *Thorax* 2014; **69**(3): 247–53.

93. Etherington C, Naseer R, Conway SP, et al. The role of respiratory viruses in adult patients with cystic fibrosis receiving intravenous antibiotics for a pulmonary exacerbation. *J Cyst Fibros* 2014; **13**: 49–55.

94. Wat D, Doull I. Respiratory virus infections in cystic fibrosis. *Paediatr Respir Rev* 2003; **4**: 172–7.

95. van Ewijk BE, van der Zalm MM, Wolfs TF, van der Ent CK. Viral respiratory infections in cystic fibrosis. *J Cyst Fibros* 2005; **4** Suppl 2: 31–6.

96. Garcia DF, Hiatt PW, Jewell A et al. Human metapneumovirus and respiratory syncytial virus infections in older children with cystic fibrosis. *Pediatr Pulmonol* 2007; **42**: 66–74.

97. Burns JL, Emerson J, Kuypers J et al. Respiratory viruses in children with cystic fibrosis: Viral detection and clinical findings. *Influenza Other Resp Viruses* 2012; **6**: 218–23.

98. McIntosh K, McAdam AJ. Human metapneumovirus: An important new respiratory virus. *N Engl J Med* 2004; **350**: 431–3.

99. Ramsey BW, Gore EJ, Smith AL et al. The effect of respiratory viral infections on patients with cystic fibrosis. *Am J Dis Child* 1989; **143**: 662–8.

100. Hiatt PW, Grace SC, Kozinetz CA et al. Effects of viral lower respiratory tract infection on lung function in infants with cystic fibrosis. *Pediatrics* 1999; **103**: 619–26.

101. van Ewijk BE, van der Zalm MM, Wolfs TF et al. Prevalence and impact of respiratory viral infections in young children with cystic fibrosis: Prospective cohort study. *Pediatrics* 2008; **122**: 1171–6.

102. Abman SH, Ogle JW, Harbeck RJ et al. Early bacteriologic, immunologic, and clinical courses of young infants with cystic fibrosis identified by neonatal screening. *J Pediatr* 1991; **119**: 211–7.

103. Malfroot A, Adam G, Ciofu O et al. for the European Cystic Fibrosis Society (ECFS) Vaccination Group. Immunisation in the current management of cystic fibrosis patients. *J Cyst Fibros* 2005; **4**: 77–87.

104. Pribble CG, Black PG, Bosso JA, Turner RB. Clinical manifestations of exacerbations of cystic fibrosis associated with nonbacterial infections. *Pediatrics* 1990; **117**: 200–4.

105. Conway SP, Simmonds EJ, Littlewood JM. Acute severe deterioration in cystic fibrosis associated with influenza A virus infection. *Thorax* 1992; **47**: 112–4.

106. France MW, Tai S, Masel PJ et al. The month of July: An early experience with pandemic influenza A (H1N1) in adults with cystic fibrosis. *BMC Pulm Med* 2010; **10**: 8.

107. Viviani L, Assael BM, Kerem E; ECFS (A) H1N1 study group. Impact of the A (H1N1) pandemic influenza (season 2009–2010) on patients with cystic fibrosis. *J Cyst Fibros* 2011; **10**: 370–6.

108. Petersen NT, Høiby N, Mordhorst CH et al. Respiratory infections in cystic fibrosis patients caused by virus, *Chlamydia* and mycoplasma: Possible synergism with *Pseudomonas aeruginosa*. *Acta Paediatr Scand* 1981; **70**: 623–8.

109. Collinson J, Nicholson KG, Cancio E et al. Effects of upper respiratory tract infections in patients with cystic fibrosis. *Thorax* 1996; **51**: 1115–22.

110. Armstrong D, Grimwood K, Carlin JB et al. Severe viral respiratory infections in infants with cystic fibrosis. *Pediatr Pulmonol* 1998; **26**: 371–9.

111. Chattoraj SS, Ganesan S, Jones AM et al. Rhinovirus infection liberates planktonic bacteria from biofilm and increases chemokine responses in cystic fibrosis airway epithelial cells. *Thorax* 2011; **66**: 333–9.

112. Dharmaraj P, Smyth RL. Vaccines for preventing influenza in people with cystic fibrosis. *Cochrane Database Syst Rev* 2009; **4**. Art. No.: CD001753. DOI: 10.1002/14651858.CD001753.pub2.

113. Gruber WC, Campbell PW, Thompson JM et al. Comparison of live attenuated and inactivated influenza vaccines in cystic fibrosis patients and their families: Results of a 3–year study. *J Infect Dis* 1994; **169**: 241–7.

114. Boikos C, De Serres G, Lands LC et al. Safety of live attenuated influenza vaccination in cystic fibrosis. *Pediatr* 2014;134:e983–91.

115. Cohen AH, Boron ML, Dingivan C, Gaithersburg A. Phase IV study of the safety of synagis (Palivizumab) for prophylaxis of respiratory syncytial virus disease in children with cystic fibrosis. *Am Thorac Soc Meeting Abstracts* 2005; **2**: 178.

116. Committee on Infectious Diseases. Modified recommendations for use of Palivizumab for prevention of respiratory syncytial virus infections. *Pediatrics* 2009; **124**: 1694–701.

117. Giusti R. North American synagis prophylaxis survey. *Pediatr Pulmonol* 2009; **44**: 96–8.

118. McCormack J, Southern KW. A national survey of Palivizumab for infants with cystic fibrosis. *Pediatr Pulmonol* 2006; Suppl 29: 360.

119. National Institute for Clinical Excellence. Amantadine, oseltamivir and zanamivir for the treatment of influenza. Review of NICE technology appraisal guidance 58. NICE technology appraisal guidance 168, 2009. Available at www.nice.org.uk.

120. Bisgaard H for the Study Group on Montelukast and Respiratory Syncytial Virus. A randomized trial of montelukast in respiratory syncytial virus post-bronchiolitis. *Am J Respir Crit Care Med* 2003; **167**: 379–83.

121. Bisgaard H, Flores-Nunez A, Goh A et al. Study of montelukast for the treatment of respiratory symptoms of post-respiratory syncytial virus bronchiolitis in children. *Am J Respir Crit Care Med* 2008; **178**: 854–60.

122. Kaiser L, Lew D, Hirschel B et al. Effects of antibiotic treatment in the subset of common-cold patients who have bacteria in nasopharyngeal secretions. *Lancet* 1996; **347**: 1507–10.

123. Borman AM, Palmer MD, Delhaes L et al. Lack of standardization in the procedures for mycological examination of sputum samples from CF patients: A possible cause for variations in the prevalence of filamentous fungi. *Med Mycol* 2010; **48** Suppl 1: S88–97.

124. Jubin V, Ranque S, Stremier Le Bel N et al. Risk factors for Aspergillus colonization and allergic bronchopulmonary aspergillosis in children with cystic fibrosis. *Pediatr Pulmonol* 2010; **45**: 764–71.

125. Bargon J, Dauletbaev N, Köhler B et al. Prophylactic antibiotic therapy is associated with an increased prevalence of *Aspergillus* colonization in adult cystic fibrosis patients. *Respir Med* 1999; **93**: 835–8.

126. Amin R, Dupois A, Aaron SD et al. The effect of chronic infection with *Aspergillus fumigatus* on lung function and hospitalizations in cystic fibrosis patients. *Chest* 2010; **137**: 171–6.

127. Aaron SD, Vandemheen KL, Freitag et al. Treatment of *Aspergillus fumigatus* in patients with cystic fibrosis: A randomised placebo-controlled pilot study. *PloS One* 2012; **7**: e36077.

128. Shoseyov D, Brownlee KG, Conway SP et al. *Aspergillus* bronchitis in cystic fibrosis. *Chest* 2006; **130**: 222–6.

129. Baxter CG, Dunn G, Jones AM et al. Novel immunologic classification of aspergillosis in adult cystic fibrosis. *J Allergy Clin Immunol* 2013; **132**: 560–6.

130. Stevens DA, Moss RB, Kurup VP et al. Allergic bronchopulmonary apergillosis in cystic fibrosis – state of the art: Cystic fibrosis Foundation Consensus Conference. *Clin Infect Dis* 2003; **37**: S225–64.

131. Stevens DA, Schwartz HU, Lee JY et al. A randomized trial of itraconazole in allergic bronchopulmonary aspergillosis. *N Engl J Med* 2000; **342**: 756–62.

132. Wark PA, Hensley MJ, Salton N et al. Anti-inflammatory effect of itraconazole in stable allergic bronchopulmonary aspergillosis: A randomised controlled trial. *J Allergy Clin Immunol* 2003; **111**: 952–7.

133. Van der Ent CK, Hoekstra H and Rijkers GT. Successful treatment of Allergic Bronchopulmonary Aspergillosis with recombinant IgE antibody. *Thorax* 2007; **62**: 276–7.

134. Cohen-Cymberknoh M, Blau A Shoseyov D et al. Intravenous monthly pulse methylprednisolone treatment for ABPA in patients with cystic fibrosis. *J Cyst Fibrosis* 2009; **8**: 253–7.

135. Chotirmall SH, O'Donoghue E, Bennett K et al. Sputum *Candida Albicans* presages FEV1 decline and hospital treated exacerbations in Cystic Fibrosis *Chest* 2010; **138**: 1186–95.

17

Pulmonary exacerbations

PATRICK A. FLUME AND DONALD R. VANDEVANTER

INTRODUCTION

The lung disease of cystic fibrosis (CF) is persistent, with chronic signs and symptoms and progressive loss of lung function. The daily symptoms may wax and wane, but there are also intermittent episodes where the symptoms are worse than the seemingly normal variation, these episodes being commonly referred to as pulmonary exacerbations. These events are almost always managed by increased intensity of treatment, including chest physiotherapy, nutrition, and administration of antibiotics. Pulmonary exacerbations appear to be common and frequent events, yet we still have a poor understanding of their etiologies and their optimal management, as the ensuing chapter should make clear.

DEFINING A PULMONARY EXACERBATION

Although a common event, there is no broadly accepted consensus definition of a pulmonary exacerbation.[1] Multiple objective definitions of pulmonary exacerbation have been proposed and employed in CF clinical trials, all of which require the presence of different constellations of clinical presentation.[2-8] These definitions tend to utilize the same key respiratory signs and symptoms (increased cough, increased sputum production, shortness of breath, chest pain, loss of appetite, loss of weight, and lung function decline);[9] however, they differ in sensitivity and are not interchangeable (Table 17.1). Although individual clinicians may be relatively consistent in their approach to exacerbation diagnosis, there can be substantial inconsistency between clinicians with respect to diagnosis.[10]

The different algorithms that have been used to attempt to standardize the diagnosis of exacerbation[2-8] share several common themes. First, some sort of accounting of observed changes in parameters from a patient's stable condition is required in order for an exacerbation to be diagnosed.

Second, changes in four specific parameters (cough, sputum, spirometry, and weight) are found in all of these algorithms. Changes in five other parameters (chest examination, absenteeism, exercise tolerance, chest x-ray, and temperature) are found in a majority of the algorithms, whereas changes in other parameters such as dyspnea, sinus pain, oxygen saturation, and neutrophilia are only occasionally included in definitions. Two of the algorithms also require that treatment, in the form of increased physiotherapy and antibiotics, be administered in order for a definition of exacerbation to be met.[3,4] Interestingly, none of these algorithms include an evaluation of patient-reported status, despite recognition that changes in how a patient feels and functions are highly relevant to the diagnosis and not particularly well captured by objective changes in signs and symptoms.[11,12] A further impediment to reaching a consensus definition of exacerbation results from age-related differences in both clinical presentation and applicability of diagnostic tests, with clinical presentations most associated with an exacerbation diagnosis differing by patient age.[6] Thus, even if a consensus definition were ultimately devised, it would likely require stratification into age groups.

In the absence of an unambiguous method to identify exacerbations based on objective measures collected at presentation, investigators often employ a surrogate indicator of exacerbation: administration of antibiotics in response to acute changes in respiratory signs and symptoms.[9,13-16] This pragmatic approach recognizes that administration of antibiotics is often more comprehensively tracked in patient registries than the many respiratory signs and symptoms that may comprise an exacerbation definition. However, there are several shortcomings to this approach that suggest care should be exercised when interpreting these data. Perhaps most importantly, this approach leaves the diagnosis of exacerbation to the treating clinician, despite recognition of the substantial variability that can exist between clinicians with respect to thresholds for antibiotic intervention.[5,10,17] By this definition, there are no untreated exacerbations in these retrospective analyses, yet it has been shown that

Table 17.1 Published definitions of cystic fibrosis pulmonary exacerbations

	Ramsey (1993)	Fuchs (1994)	CFF (1997)	Rosenfeld (2001)	Rabin (2004)	Blumer (2005)	Kraynack (2009)
Cough	x	x	x	x	x	x	x
Sputum	x	x	x	x	x	x	x
Lung function	x	x	x	x	x	x	x
Weight loss	x	x	x	x	x	x	x
Chest exam		x	x	x	x	x	x
Absenteeism	x		x	x		x	x
Exercise tolerance			x	x		x	x
Chest x-ray		x	x			x	x
Fever	x	x	x				x
Hemoptysis		x			x		x
Dyspnea		x				x	x
Fatigue, malaise		x				x	x
Tachypnea	x		x			x	
Sinus pain	x	x					
SaO$_2$			x				x
Sinus discharge		x					
Neutrophilia	x						
Criteria	2/5 + 1/3	4/12 + antibiotics	3/11	Score	3/4	5/10	Score

Note: Multiple published definitions of the pulmonary exacerbation have been proposed and employed in CF clinical trials. These definitions use similar key respiratory signs and symptoms but they vary in how they are scored.
SaO$_2$, arterial oxygen saturation.

patients with apparently similar respiratory sign and symptom presentations also go untreated in the CF population.[6] Further, there is good evidence that overall clinical thresholds for antibiotic intervention have shifted over time.[14] Thus, a given patient history and clinical presentation may precipitate antibiotic treatment (and thus be considered an exacerbation) in one time and setting but not in another.

Because antibiotic treatments may also be prophylactic in nature[18,19] or administered as part of chronic suppression strategies,[20–24] not all antibiotic usage found in patient registries should be included in algorithms that identify exacerbations by antibiotic treatment. A common approach to reducing or eliminating the inclusion of antibiotic treatments not associated with exacerbation in epidemiologic studies is to limit analyses to treatments involving intravenous (IV) antibiotics.[9,13,25,26] This strategy increases the probability that an event was considered an exacerbation by the treating clinician, particularly in North America, but is less certain to identify diagnosed exacerbations in regions where scheduled IV antibiotic treatments are also employed as part of chronic infection strategies.[22,24] Importantly, this strategy fails to capture a substantial number of exacerbations treated with oral and/or inhaled, but not IV antibiotics.[14,16] Clinicians also tailor exacerbation interventions to an assessment of exacerbation severity based on clinical presentation. Mild exacerbations (with fewer or less pronounced clinical symptoms) are often treated on an outpatient basis with oral or inhaled antibiotics, whereas more severe exacerbations often result in admission to the hospital and administration of IV antibiotics.[14,27] There are other

factors, such as a patient's age and lung disease stage, that likely affect the probability of receiving IV antibiotics for treatment of exacerbation,[15,16] and analyses limited to IV antibiotic treatment of exacerbation underestimate the incidence of exacerbations diagnosed by clinicians in younger patients with less-advanced lung disease.[14,16]

The value of a standardized exacerbation definition is obvious for clinical research such as for the investigation of a chronic therapy meant to prevent an exacerbation. However, there is clearly room to achieve better clinical outcomes through standardization of exacerbation diagnosis and treatment as well.[10] A recent study using clinical vignettes to assess clinicians' determination of an exacerbation found considerable variance between centers and within centers (i.e., multiple clinicians at one center), but there was also inconsistency within individual physicians.[10]

EPIDEMIOLOGY

It should be obvious that our inability to achieve a prospective consensus definition of exacerbation makes the description of the incidence rate of these events and their distribution in the population difficult, if not impossible. Ideally, patient medical records could be retrospectively assessed for specific changes in clinical presentations of signs and symptoms at clinical encounters that would then be scored as meeting a particular definition of exacerbation or not. In practice, epidemiologists have relied heavily on

Current advice is to use the antibiotics that have previously been demonstrated to have been successful in treatment of an exacerbation, and to make changes only when there is an inadequate response. For those patients who are being treated for the first time, or for when a change is considered, sputum or throat-swab cultures are typically used to guide therapy. Antibiotic recommendations for the most common bacteria are offered in Table 17.3. Note that these antibiotics and dosing regimens have not been shown to be optimal, but some antibiotic dosing issues warrant further discussion.

Table 17.3 Antibiotics commonly used for treatment of acute pulmonary exacerbation in cystic fibrosis patients

Antibiotic	Target pathogens	Route	Dose	Frequency	Notes	Toxicity
Tobramycin	PA, BC, AX, AB	IV	10 mg/kg (daily)	Q 8–24 hrs	See dosing parameters in Table 17.4	Ototoxicity Nephrotoxicity Vestibular toxicity
Gentamicin	PA, BC, AX, AB	IV	10 mg/kg (daily)			
Amikacin	PA, BC, AX, AB	IV	30 mg/kg (daily)			
Vancomycin	MSSA, MRSA	IV	15 mg/kg	Q 8 hours	Monitor drug levels	Nephrotoxicity Red man syndrome
Linezolid	MSSA, MRSA	IV PO	600 mg 600 mg	Q 12 hours		Bone marrow suppression Peripheral neuropathy
Ciprofloxacin	PA, BC	IVPO	400 mg 750 mg	Q 8 hours BID or TID		Nausea and vomiting Altered mental status Tendon rupture (rare)
Levofloxacin	PA, BC, SM	IVPO	500 mg 750 mg	Q 24 hours QD or BID		
Sulfamethoxazole-trimethoprim	MSSA, MRSA, BC, SM, HI	IVPO	2.5 mg/kg X mg/kg	Q 6 hours BID or TID	Dose based on trimethoprim	Nephrotoxicity, bone marrow suppression, hyperkalemia, nausea
Chloramphenicol	PA, BC, HI, AX	IV				Bone marrow suppression
Doxycycline	BC, MSSA, MRSA, HI, AX, AB	IVPO	100 mg 100 mg	Q 12 hours BID		
Colistin	PA, AB	IV	2.5–5 mg/kg (daily)	Q 8 hours	maximum of 100 mg/dose	Nephrotoxicity
Amoxicillin (± clavulinate)	MSSA, HI	PO	750–1000 mg	Q 8 hours		Nausea, diarrhea
Cefepime	PA, BC	IV	2 gm	Q 12 hours		Decreased seizure threshold
Ceftazidime	PA, BC	IV	50 mg/kg	Q 8 hours	Maximum dose 3 g	
Piperacillin-tazobactam	PA, BC, HI, AX	IV	90 mg/kg	Q 6 hours	Maximum dose 4.5 g	Decreased seizure threshold Fever and rash Renal failure
Ticarcillin-clavulinate	PA, BC, SM, MSSA, HI	IV	80–100 mg/kg	Q 6 hours	Maximum dose 3.2 g	
Imipenem	PA, BC, MSSA, HI, AX, AB	IV	500 mg	Q 6 hours		Decreased seizure threshold
Meropenem	PA, BC, MSSA, HI, AX, AB	IV	25–40 mg/kg	Q 8 hours	Maximum dose 2 g	

Source: Adapted from Barto TL and Flume PA, *Hosp Pract (1995)*, 2010 Feb;38(1):26–34; Cystic Fibrosis Trust, http://www.cysticfibrosis.org .uk /media/82010/antibiotic-treatment-for-cystic-fibrosis-may-09.pdf, 2009.

Note: Antibiotics often used to treat specific bacteria found in CF sputum cultures. Doses recommended are commonly used, but should be adapted to specific patients' needs and tolerability.

PA, Pseudomonas aeruginosa; BC, Burkholderia cepacia; MSSA, Methicillin-susceptible Staphylococcus aureus; MRSA, Methicillin-resistant Staphylococcus aureus; SM, Stenotrophomonas maltophilia; HI, Hemophilus influenzae; AX, Achromobacter xylosoxidans; AB, Acinetobacter baumannii.

Aminoglycoside antibiotics have concentration-dependent effects on bacteria (i.e., increased killing as concentrations are increased),[123,124] although the optimum maximum concentration for treatment of lung infections in CF has not been established. Dosing of aminoglycosides is limited by potential for nephrotoxicity, ototoxicity, and vestibular toxicity.[49] Traditionally, aminoglycosides had been dosed on a three-times-daily schedule, but more recent data suggest that once-daily dosing would allow for a greater peak concentration that may improve efficacy while reducing the overall exposure to the drug, thus decreasing the risk of toxicity.[125,126] Dosing recommendations are offered in Table 17.3, acknowledging that the optimum pharmacokinetic parameters (e.g., peak and trough concentrations) are not known. An initial dose of aminoglycosides commonly reported in clinical trials are 10 mg/kg/d for tobramycin and gentamicin, and 30 mg/kg/d for amikacin. The expected pharmacokinetic parameters for patients with CF and normal renal function for different dosing intervals are shown in Table 17.4. An increase in the dosing interval (e.g., from every 8 hours to every 24 hours) allows for higher peak concentrations, but at the expense of a potentially longer period where there is an undetectable concentration of drug. This time can be reduced by increasing the dose and raising the peak concentration, but the clinician must decide which dose and dosing interval is best suited for the patient. Since CF patients are likely to experience multiple exacerbations in their lifetime, it is important to consider that toxicity may develop as a result of multiple treatments.[49] In addition, there are some patients who have a genetic susceptibility to aminoglycoside ototoxicity,[127] although the incidence is so low that genetic testing is not recommended. However, the use of aminoglycosides requires periodic monitoring of drug concentration, as dosage adjustment may be necessary. Periodic assessments for nephrotoxicity include weekly measurement of serum creatinine while on active treatment. Audiology may be used to monitor for ototoxicity but it is not clear how best to use this diagnostic testing. That is, although it may seem prudent to monitor weekly, this is not practical in the care of patients, so testing is

recommended for any symptoms of tinnitus, hearing loss, or imbalance.

The CF Pulmonary Guidelines raised the question as to whether to use inhaled and IV aminoglycoside antibiotics simultaneously. An argument for such a strategy is an enhanced killing effect on bacteria by improved drug delivery using two delivery routes. Another may be the reinforcement of a chronic therapy routine, even if there is no measurable acute benefit. An argument against this strategy includes the potential increased risk of toxicity as some of the inhaled drug will be absorbed into the circulation. Recent data have demonstrated that absorption of inhaled tobramycin may cause difficulty in interpreting serum aminoglycoside levels, which are commonly measured to guide IV dosing, especially when the inhaled drug is given in the latter portion of the IV dosing interval.[128]

Beta-lactam antibiotics demonstrate time-dependent pharmacodynamic properties, where maintaining the concentration above the minimum inhibitory concentration for longer portions of the dosing interval is associated with better antibacterial effect, but greater concentrations do not necessarily improve the killing effect.[129] There has been interest in continuous infusion of beta-lactam antibiotics in non-CF infections, but there is no evidence that such a strategy is superior in CF infections, and so this did not get a recommendation in the CF Pulmonary Guidelines.[27]

WHAT IS THE OPTIMAL DURATION OF TREATMENT?

Systematic reviews of the literature have not found any studies that have defined the optimal duration of antibiotic therapy for treatment of a pulmonary exacerbation.[27,130] An assessment of current practice has shown median treatment durations of IV antibiotics of 14.5 days (<18 years of age) to 16.8 days (>18 years); however, there is considerable variability in median treatment durations across CF care centers.[30] Because treatment guidelines[3] suggest that treatment extension may be warranted to achieve response in individual patients (despite a lack of supportive objective evidence), there is also great variability in treatment duration at the individual patient level.[13,131]

Table 17.4 Dosing regimens for aminoglycosides

| Antibiotic | Initial dose (mg/kg/d) | Dosing every 24 hours | | | Dosing every 12 hours | | | Dosing every 8 hours | | |
		Predicted peak (μg/mL)	Predicted trough (μg/mL)	Predicted time below level of detection (hours)	Predicted peak (μg/mL)	Predicted trough (μg/mL)	Predicted time below level of detection (hours)	Predicted peak (μg/mL)	Predicted trough (μg/mL)	Predicted time below level of detection (hours)
Tobramycin	10	25–35	<0.5	9–11	10–16	<0.5	3–4	7–10	<0.5	1–2
Gentamicin	10	25–35	<0.5	9–11	10–16	<0.5	3–4	7–10	<0.5	1–2
Amikacin	30	30–45	<5	9–11	15–20	<5	3–4	10–13	<5	1–2

Source: Flume PA et al., Am J Respir Crit Care Med 2009; 180(9): 802–8. Reprinted with permission.
Note: These values are based on population pharmacokinetics assuming a volume of distribution of 0.25 L/kg and a half-life of 2.5 hours, but individual pharmacokinetic testing is recommended. Standard assays for drug concentrations have a lower level of detection of 0.5 μg/mL.

Unlike the treatment of acute (non-CF) infections, antibiotic treatment of chronic CF airways infection will not result in eradication of the infection. There is a reduction in bacterial density in the sputum, reaching greatest reduction after just 1 week of treatment.[2] Therefore, the treatment goals for a pulmonary exacerbation include resolution of symptoms (e.g., cough, dyspnea) and restoration of lung function (e.g., FEV_1).[3] Patient symptoms and lung function improve with treatment of an exacerbation with symptoms reaching resolution at or before day 10 and FEV_1 response peaking at day 10–13.[13,44] More than 90% of patients will have reached their peak FEV_1 by day 14, but the median time to peak lung function varies by underlying stage of lung disease; those patients with milder lung disease ($FEV_1 > 70\%$ pred) achieve peak earlier than those with more severe disease.[131]

Such results may offer confidence that a treatment duration of 10–14 days will coincide with target goals, but these studies do not yet provide us with the information we need to determine the optimal duration of antibiotic therapy. For example, it may be that clinical parameters would continue to improve even if antibiotics were stopped earlier. Alternatively, it may be that continued antibiotic treatment beyond the point at which a patient reaches his or her baseline might ensure that patient remain stable for a longer period of time. In one retrospective analysis, those patients who were treated for 1 to 2 weeks had the best average outcome.[13] Those patients who were treated for less than 1 week had a poorer average response, raising the question of whether they were undertreated. However, those patients who were treated for more than 2 weeks also had poorer average outcomes; presumably the longer duration of therapy was given because the patients had not improved sufficiently, yet longer therapies did not seem to add benefit.

STEROIDS

The CFF Pulmonary Guidelines on chronic medications to maintain lung health recommended against the routine use of oral or inhaled corticosteroids except for those patient with asthma or allergic bronchopulmonary aspergillosis (ABPA).[27] Although published data had demonstrated a benefit to lung function, there was an increase in adverse events with oral corticosteroids. If this improvement in lung function is because of reduction in inflammation, then a short course of systemic corticosteroids may offer benefit in the treatment of an acute exacerbation without the long-term adverse effects. There have been two studies that have assessed the use of steroids added to standard antibiotic therapy.[132,133] There was improvement in lung function in both studies, but there was no statistically significant difference between the steroid and placebo groups. The CFF Pulmonary Guidelines Committee therefore concluded that there was insufficient evidence to recommend the routine use of corticosteroids in the treatment of an acute exacerbation of pulmonary disease, and recommended that a clinical trial is warranted.[27] Corticosteroids may well be indicated for those patients who also have ABPA, as there could be an allergic aspect to the exacerbation.

AIRWAY CLEARANCE

Airway clearance therapy has long been considered the most important aspect of treatment of CF lung disease[134] and techniques are discussed in detail in Chapter 43. In general, airway clearance therapies should be intensified as part of the treatment of an acute exacerbation. This typically means increased time and frequency of treatment; the ability to accomplish this goal of therapy should play a key role in the decision of where to treat the patient. Interestingly, a small (possibly underpowered) retrospective analysis of adjuvant administration of inhaled hypertonic saline to augment chest physiotherapy during exacerbation treatment in 18 CF adults reported no measurable differences in FEV_1 improvement over that observed with historical controls.[135]

OTHER CHRONIC THERAPIES

The CF Pulmonary Guidelines for treatment of pulmonary exacerbations recommended continuing the chronic medications used by the patient.[27] This was based on the observation that most of the studies reviewed for the guidelines on chronic therapies included patients who were treated for an acute exacerbation, and use of the study agent was not stopped during treatment of the acute exacerbation.[31] There are some chronic therapies that require careful consideration, including inhaled tobramycin discussed earlier, as well as the use of high-dose non-steroidal anti-inflammatory agents, (e.g., ibuprofen) in the setting of IV aminoglycosides, where there is a potential increased risk of nephrotoxicity.[136]

TREATMENT OF OTHER COMORBIDITIES

CF is associated with many other complications, which can be acutely worsened in the setting of a pulmonary exacerbation. CF-related diabetes is present in about 15% of adolescent patients and 32.5% of adult patients[30] and glucose metabolism balance is often upset in the setting of an exacerbation.[39] The nutritional and metabolic derangements were reviewed earlier. Patients will require additional supplemental calories, glucose monitoring, and evaluation by a CF-experienced dietitian. Pain is more common in older patients, although interestingly not necessarily in patients with more advanced lung disease, and has been shown to significantly interfere with airway clearance during pulmonary exacerbation.[137]

Hemoptysis is also a common complication of CF, and its presence is often felt to be a manifestation of an exacerbation.[138] The CFF Pulmonary Guidelines on complications recommended that antibiotics should be a part of the treatment regimen in patients with at least mild hemoptysis.[139] The guidelines also addressed whether to continue with airway clearance therapies and inhaled medications in the setting of hemoptysis as such therapies might impair clot formation and adherence resulting in more bleeding.[140] The consensus was that stopping airway clearance therapies was inappropriate for the patient with scant hemoptysis, but stopping airway clearance therapies was preferred for patients with massive hemoptysis.[139] Similar recommendations were made for inhaled therapies, although there was some greater concern about continuing hypertonic saline because of its propensity to cause cough. It was noted that successful clearance of airway phlegm was critical in the resolution of the exacerbation, so if the hemoptysis was not life-threatening, then the therapies should be continued.

CONCLUSION

Pulmonary exacerbation is a common event in CF, loosely defined as an episode of worsening of the daily respiratory and systemic symptoms and an acute drop in pulmonary function. Although there is not an established definition of an exacerbation, they have become increasingly recognized as an important aspect of CF lung disease, and treatment guidelines have been recommended. These events are almost always managed by increased intensity of treatment, including chest physiotherapy, nutrition, and administration of antibiotics. Pulmonary exacerbations have an adverse impact on CF patients' quality of life and the overall cost of care. Thus, the prevention of pulmonary exacerbations has become a point of emphasis and a common treatment goal for therapies used routinely to maintain lung health.

Practice guidelines have been developed for the treatment of pulmonary exacerbations but perhaps the most revealing aspect of this systematic review is how few objective data exist to inform optimal treatment practices.[27] The development of a standardized definition for a pulmonary exacerbation is of great importance for both research studies as well as providing proper therapies. This would allow for clinical trials comparing interventions, answering the questions offered in the practice guidelines, such as the optimal duration of antibiotic therapy. We may then be able to address the question as to why there is loss of lung function with a pulmonary exacerbations; is it because of a patient-related factor (e.g., inflammation), a disease-related factor (e.g., highly virulent pathogen), or because of a treatment-related factor (e.g., abbreviated antibiotic duration)? Having a standardized definition will help us understand the exacerbation so that we may better attempt to prevent them and/or to treat them.

REFERENCES

1. Ferkol T, Rosenfeld M, Milla CE. Cystic fibrosis pulmonary exacerbations. *J pediatr* 2006; **148**(2): 259–64.
2. Blumer JL, Saiman L, Konstan MW, Melnick D. The efficacy and safety of meropenem and tobramycin vs ceftazidime and tobramycin in the treatment of acute pulmonary exacerbations in patients with cystic fibrosis. *Chest* 2005; **128**(4): 2336–46.
3. Cystic Fibrosis Foundation. Treatment of pulmonary exacerbation of cystic fibrosis. *Clinical Practice Guidelines for Cystic Fibrosis*. Bethesda, MD: Cystic Fibrosis Foundation, 1997.
4. Fuchs HJ, Borowitz DS, Christiansen DH et al. Effect of aerosolized recombinant human DNase on exacerbations of respiratory symptoms and on pulmonary function in patients with cystic fibrosis. The Pulmozyme Study Group. *N Engl J Med* 1994; **331**(10): 637–42.
5. Kraynack NC, McBride JT. Improving care at cystic fibrosis centers through quality improvement. *Semin Respir Crit Care Med* 2009; **30**(5): 547–58.
6. Rabin HR, Butler SM, Wohl ME et al. Pulmonary exacerbations in cystic fibrosis. *Pediatr Pulmonol* 2004; **37**(5): 400–6.
7. Ramsey BW, Dorkin HL, Eisenberg JD et al. Efficacy of aerosolized tobramycin in patients with cystic fibrosis. *New Engl J Med* 1993; **328**(24): 1740–6.
8. Rosenfeld M, Emerson J, Williams-Warren J et al. Defining a pulmonary exacerbation in cystic fibrosis. *J Pediatrics* 2001; **139**(3): 359–65.
9. Goss CH, Burns JL. Exacerbations in cystic fibrosis. 1: Epidemiology and pathogenesis. *Thorax.* 2007; **62**(4): 360–7.
10. Kraynack NC, Gothard MD, Falletta LM, McBride JT. Approach to treating cystic fibrosis pulmonary exacerbations varies widely across US CF care centers. *Pediatr Pulmonol* 2011; **46**(9): 870–81.
11. Abbott J, Holt A, Hart A et al. What defines a pulmonary exacerbation? The perceptions of adults with cystic fibrosis. *J Cyst Fibros* 2009; **8**(5): 356–9.
12. Goss CH, Quittner AL. Patient-reported outcomes in cystic fibrosis. *Proc Am Thorac Soc* 2007; **4**(4): 378–86.
13. Collaco JM, Green DM, Cutting GR, Naughton KM, Mogayzel PJ Jr. Location and duration of treatment of cystic fibrosis respiratory exacerbations do not affect outcomes. *Am J Respir Crit Care Med* 2010; **182**(9): 1137–43.
14. VanDevanter DR, Elkin EP, Pasta DJ, Morgan WJ, Konstan MW. Changing thresholds and incidence of antibiotic treatment of cystic fibrosis pulmonary exacerbations, 1995-2005. *J Cyst Fibros* 2013; **12**(4): 332–7.
15. VanDevanter DR, Yegin A, Morgan WJ, Millar SJ, Pasta DJ, Konstan MW. Design and powering of cystic fibrosis clinical trials using pulmonary exacerbation as an efficacy endpoint. *J Cyst Fibros* 2011; **10**(6): 453–9.
16. Wagener JS, Rasouliyan L, VanDevanter DR et al. Oral, inhaled, and intravenous antibiotic choice for treating pulmonary exacerbations in cystic fibrosis. *Pediatr Pulmonol* 2013; **48**(7): 666–73.
17. Johnson C, Butler SM, Konstan MW, Morgan W, Wohl ME. Factors influencing outcomes in cystic fibrosis: A center-based analysis. *Chest* 2003; **123**(1): 20–7.

18. Smyth A, Walters S. Prophylactic antibiotics for cystic fibrosis. *Cochrane Database Syst Rev* 2003; (3): CD001912.

19. Weaver LT, Green MR, Nicholson K et al. Prognosis in cystic fibrosis treated with continuous flucloxacillin from the neonatal period. *Arch Dis Child* 1994; **70**(2): 84–9.

20. Ballmann M, Smyth A, Geller DE. Therapeutic approaches to chronic cystic fibrosis respiratory infections with available, emerging aerosolized antibiotics. *Respir Med* 2011; **105**(Suppl 2):S2–8.

21. Oermann CM, Retsch-Bogart GZ, Quittner AL et al. An 18-month study of the safety and efficacy of repeated courses of inhaled aztreonam lysine in cystic fibrosis. *Pediatr Pulmonol* 2010; **45**(11): 1121–34.

22. Pedersen SS, Jensen T, Hoiby N, Koch C, Flensborg EW. Management of *Pseudomonas aeruginosa* lung infection in Danish cystic fibrosis patients. *Acta Paediatr Scand* 1987; **76**(6): 955–61.

23. Ramsey BW, Pepe MS, Quan JM et al. Intermittent administration of inhaled tobramycin in patients with cystic fibrosis. Cystic Fibrosis Inhaled Tobramycin Study Group. *New Engl J Med* 1999; **340**(1): 23–30.

24. Szaff M, Hoiby N, Flensborg EW. Frequent antibiotic therapy improves survival of cystic fibrosis patients with chronic Pseudomonas aeruginosa infection. *Acta Paediatr Scand* 1983; **72**(5): 651–7.

25. Konstan MW, Morgan WJ, Butler SM et al. Risk factors for rate of decline in forced expiratory volume in one second in children and adolescents with cystic fibrosis. *J Pediatr* 2007; **151**(2): 134–9, 9 e1.

26. VanDevanter DR, Wagener JS, Pasta DJ et al. Pulmonary outcome prediction (POP) tools for cystic fibrosis patients. *Pediatr Pulmonol* 2010; **45**(12): 1156–66.

27. Flume PA, Mogayzel PJ Jr., Robinson KA et al. Cystic fibrosis pulmonary guidelines: Treatment of pulmonary exacerbations. *Am J Respir Crit Care Med* 2009; **180**(9): 802–8.

28. Schechter MS, McColley SA, Regelmann W et al. Socioeconomic status and the likelihood of antibiotic treatment for signs and symptoms of pulmonary exacerbation in children with cystic fibrosis. *J Pediatr* 2011; **159**(5): 819–24 e1.

29. Rosenfeld M, Ratjen F, Brumback L et al. Inhaled hypertonic saline in infants and children younger than 6 years with cystic fibrosis: The ISIS randomized controlled trial. *JAMA* 2012; **307**(21): 2269–77.

30. Registry CFFP. Annual Data Report to the Center Directors. 2012.

31. Flume PA, O'Sullivan BP, Robinson KA et al. Cystic fibrosis pulmonary guidelines: Chronic medications for maintenance of lung health. *Am J Respir Crit Care Med* 2007; **176**(10): 957–69.

32. Britto MT, Kotagal UR, Hornung RW, Atherton HD, Tsevat J, Wilmott RW. Impact of recent pulmonary exacerbations on quality of life in patients with cystic fibrosis. *Chest* 2002; **121**(1): 64–72.

33. Bradley J, McAlister O, Elborn S. Pulmonary function, inflammation, exercise capacity and quality of life in cystic fibrosis. *Europ Respir J* 2001; **17**(4): 712–5.

34. Orenstein DM, Pattishall EN, Nixon PA, Ross EA, Kaplan RM. Quality of well-being before and after antibiotic treatment of pulmonary exacerbation in patients with cystic fibrosis. *Chest* 1990; **98**(5): 1081–4.

35. Ionescu AA, Nixon LS, Evans WD et al. Bone density, body composition, and inflammatory status in cystic fibrosis. *Am J Respir Crit Care Med* 2000; **162**(3 Pt 1): 789–94.

36. Wieboldt J, Atallah L, Kelly JL et al. Effect of acute exacerbations on skeletal muscle strength and physical activity in cystic fibrosis. *J Cyst Fibros* 2012; **11**(3): 209–15.

37. McColley SA, Stellmach V, Boas SR, Jain M, Crawford SE. Serum vascular endothelial growth factor is elevated in cystic fibrosis and decreases with treatment of acute pulmonary exacerbation. *Am J Respir Crit Care Med* 2000; **161**(6): 1877–80.

38. Roderfeld M, Rath T, Schulz R et al. Serum matrix metalloproteinases in adult CF patients: Relation to pulmonary exacerbation. *J Cyst Fibros* 2009; **8**(5): 338–47.

39. Moran A, Brunzell C, Cohen RC et al. Clinical care guidelines for cystic fibrosis-related diabetes: A position statement of the American Diabetes Association and a clinical practice guideline of the Cystic Fibrosis Foundation, endorsed by the Pediatric Endocrine Society. *Diabetes Care* 2010; **33**(12): 2697–708.

40. Sc NN, Shoseyov D, Kerem E, Zangen DH. Patients with cystic fibrosis and normoglycemia exhibit diabetic glucose tolerance during pulmonary exacerbation. *J Cyst Fibros* 2010; **9**(3): 199–204.

41. Shead EF, Haworth CS, Barker H, Bilton D, Compston JE. Osteoclast function, bone turnover and inflammatory cytokines during infective exacerbations of cystic fibrosis. *J Cyst Fibros* 2010; **9**(2): 93–8.

42. Shead EF, Haworth CS, Gunn E, Bilton D, Scott MA, Compston JE. Osteoclastogenesis during infective exacerbations in patients with cystic fibrosis. *Am J Respir Crit Care Med* 2006; **174**(3): 306–11.

43. Aris RM, Stephens AR, Ontjes DA et al. Adverse alterations in bone metabolism are associated with lung infection in adults with cystic fibrosis. *Am J Respir Crit Care Med* 2000; **162**(5): 1674–8.

44. Regelmann WE, Elliott GR, Warwick WJ, Clawson CC. Reduction of sputum *Pseudomonas aeruginosa* density by antibiotics improves lung function in cystic fibrosis more than do bronchodilators and chest physiotherapy alone. *Am Rev Resp Dis* 1990; **141**(4 Pt 1): 914–21.

45. Sanders DB, Bittner RC, Rosenfeld M, Hoffman LR, Redding GJ, Goss CH. Failure to recover to baseline pulmonary function after cystic fibrosis pulmonary exacerbation. *Am J Respir Crit Care Med* 2010; **182**(5): 627–32.

46. Sanders DB, Bittner RC, Rosenfeld M, Redding GJ, Goss CH. Pulmonary exacerbations are associated with subsequent FEV1 decline in both adults and children with cystic fibrosis. *Pediatr Pulmonol* 2011; **46**(4): 393–400.

47. Bertenshaw C, Watson AR, Lewis S, Smyth A. Survey of acute renal failure in patients with cystic fibrosis in the UK. *Thorax.* 2007; **62**(6): 541–5.

48. Smyth A, Lewis S, Bertenshaw C, Choonara I, McGaw J, Watson A. Case-control study of acute renal failure in patients with cystic fibrosis in the UK. *Thorax* 2008; **63**(6): 532–5.

49. Al-Aloul M, Miller H, Alapati S, Stockton PA, Ledson MJ, Walshaw MJ. Renal impairment in cystic fibrosis patients due to repeated intravenous aminoglycoside use. *Pediatr Pulmonol* 2005; **39**(1): 15–20.

50. Mulheran M, Degg C, Burr S, Morgan DW, Stableforth DE. Occurrence and risk of cochleotoxicity in cystic fibrosis patients receiving repeated high-dose aminoglycoside therapy. *Antimicrob Agents Chemother* 2001; **45**(9): 2502–9.

51. Soulsby N, Bell S, Greville H, Doecke C. Intravenous aminoglycoside usage and monitoring of patients with cystic fibrosis in Australia. What's new? *Int Med J* 2009; **39**(8): 527–31.

52. Ellaffi M, Vinsonneau C, Coste J et al. One-year outcome after severe pulmonary exacerbation in adults with cystic fibrosis. *Am J Respir Crit Care Med* 2005; **171**(2): 158–64.

53. Emerson J, Rosenfeld M, McNamara S, Ramsey B, Gibson RL. *Pseudomonas aeruginosa* and other predictors of mortality and morbidity in young children with cystic fibrosis. *Pediatr Pulmonol* 2002; **34**(2): 91–100.

54. Liou TG, Adler FR, Fitzsimmons SC, Cahill BC, Hibbs JR, Marshall BC. Predictive 5-year survivorship model of cystic fibrosis. *Am J Epidemiol* 2001; **153**(4): 345–52.

55. Mayer-Hamblett N, Rosenfeld M, Emerson J, Goss CH, Aitken ML. Developing cystic fibrosis lung transplant referral criteria using predictors of 2-year mortality. *Am J Respir Crit Care Med.* 2002; **166**(12 Pt 1): 1550–5.

56. Lieu TA, Ray GT, Farmer G, Shay GF. The cost of medical care for patients with cystic fibrosis in a health maintenance organization. *Pediatrics* 1999; **103**(6): e72.

57. Ouyang L, Grosse SD, Amendah DD, Schechter MS. Healthcare expenditures for privately insured people with cystic fibrosis. *Pediatr Pulmonol* 2009; **44**(10): 989–96.

58. Ferkol T. Pathophysiology of a pulmonary exacerbation: An educated guess. *Pediatr Pulmonol* 2009; **44**(Suppl 32): 140–1.

59. Zemanick ET, Wagner BD, Harris JK, Wagener JS, Accurso FJ, Sagel SD. Pulmonary exacerbations in cystic fibrosis with negative bacterial cultures. *Pediatr Pulmonol* 2010; **45**(6): 569–77.

60. Ordonez CL, Henig NR, Mayer-Hamblett N et al. Inflammatory and microbiologic markers in induced sputum after intravenous antibiotics in cystic fibrosis. *Am J Respir Crit Care Med* 2003; **168**(12): 1471–5.

61. Smith AL, Doershuk C, Goldmann D et al. Comparison of a beta-lactam alone versus beta-lactam and an aminoglycoside for pulmonary exacerbation in cystic fibrosis. *J Pediatr* 1999; **134**(4): 413–21.

62. Smith AL, Redding G, Doershuk C et al. Sputum changes associated with therapy for endobronchial exacerbation in cystic fibrosis. *J Pediatr* 1988; **112**(4): 547–54.

63. Stressmann FA, Rogers GB, Marsh P et al. Does bacterial density in cystic fibrosis sputum increase prior to pulmonary exacerbation? *J Cyst Fibros* 2011; **10**(5): 357–65.

64. Tunney MM, Klem ER, Fodor AA et al. Use of culture and molecular analysis to determine the effect of antibiotic treatment on microbial community diversity and abundance during exacerbation in patients with cystic fibrosis. *Thorax* 2011; **66**(7): 579–84.

65. VanDevanter DR, Van Dalfsen JM. How much do Pseudomonas biofilms contribute to symptoms of pulmonary exacerbation in cystic fibrosis? *Pediatr Pulmonol* 2005; **39**(6): 504–6.

66. Nguyen D, Singh PK. Evolving stealth: Genetic adaptation of *Pseudomonas aeruginosa* during cystic fibrosis infections. *Proc Natl Acad Sci USA* 2006; **103**(22): 8305–6.

67. Smith EE, Buckley DG, Wu Z et al. Genetic adaptation by Pseudomonas aeruginosa to the airways of cystic fibrosis patients. *Proc Natl Acad Sci USA* 2006; **103**(22): 8487–92.

68. Carter ME, Fothergill JL, Walshaw MJ, Rajakumar K, Kadioglu A, Winstanley C. A subtype of a *Pseudomonas aeruginosa* cystic fibrosis epidemic strain exhibits enhanced virulence in a murine model of acute respiratory infection. *J Infect Dis* 2010; **202**(6): 935–42.

69. Fothergill JL, Mowat E, Ledson MJ, Walshaw MJ, Winstanley C. Fluctuations in phenotypes and genotypes within populations of *Pseudomonas aeruginosa* in the cystic fibrosis lung during pulmonary exacerbations. *J Med Microbiol* 2010; **59**(Pt 4): 472–81.

70. Aaron SD, Ramotar K, Ferris W et al. Adult cystic fibrosis exacerbations and new strains of Pseudomonas aeruginosa. *Am J Respir Crit Care Med* 2004; **169**(7): 811–5.

71. Lipuma JJ. The changing microbial epidemiology in cystic fibrosis. *Clin Microbiol Rev* 2010; **23**(2): 299–323.

72. Rogers GB, Hoffman LR, Whiteley M, Daniels TW, Carroll MP, Bruce KD. Revealing the dynamics of polymicrobial infections: Implications for antibiotic therapy. *Trends Microbiol* 2010; **18**(8): 357–64.

73. Rogers GB, Carroll MP, Serisier DJ, Hockey PM, Jones G, Bruce KD. Characterization of bacterial community diversity in cystic fibrosis lung infections by use of 16s ribosomal DNA terminal restriction fragment length polymorphism profiling. *J Clin Microbiol* 2004; **42**(11): 5176–83.

74. Zhao J, Schloss PD, Kalikin LM et al. Decade-long bacterial community dynamics in cystic fibrosis airways. *Proc Natl Acad Sci USA* 2012; **109**(15): 5809–14.

75. Sibley CD, Grinwis ME, Field TR et al. Culture enriched molecular profiling of the cystic fibrosis airway microbiome. *PLoS One* 2011; **6**(7): e22702.

76. Tunney MM, Field TR, Moriarty TF et al. Detection of anaerobic bacteria in high numbers in sputum from patients with cystic fibrosis. *Am J Respir Crit Care Med* 2008; **177**(9): 995–1001.

77. Abman SH, Ogle JW, Butler-Simon N, Rumack CM, Accurso FJ. Role of respiratory syncytial virus in early hospitalizations for respiratory distress of young infants with cystic fibrosis. *J Pediatr* 1988; **113**(5): 826–30.

78. Ramsey BW, Gore EJ, Smith AL, Cooney MK, Redding GJ, Foy H. The effect of respiratory viral infections on patients with cystic fibrosis. *Am J Dis Child* 1989; **143**(6): 662–8.

79. van Ewijk BE, van der Zalm MM, Wolfs TF et al. Prevalence and impact of respiratory viral infections in young children with cystic fibrosis: Prospective cohort study. *Pediatrics* 2008; **122**(6): 1171–6.

80. Wang EE, Prober CG, Manson B, Corey M, Levison H. Association of respiratory viral infections with pulmonary deterioration in patients with cystic fibrosis. *New Eng J Med* 1984; **311**(26): 1653–8.

81. Wark PA, Tooze M, Cheese L et al. Viral infections trigger exacerbations of cystic fibrosis in adults and children. *Eur Respir J* 2012; **40**(2): 510–2.

82. Wat D, Gelder C, Hibbitts S et al. The role of respiratory viruses in cystic fibrosis. *J Cyst Fibros* 2008; **7**(4): 320–8.

83. Look DC, Walter MJ, Williamson MR et al. Effects of paramyxoviral infection on airway epithelial cell Foxj1 expression, ciliogenesis, and mucociliary function. *Am J Pathol* 2001; **159**(6): 2055–69.

84. Tarran R, Button B, Picher M et al. Normal and cystic fibrosis airway surface liquid homeostasis. The effects of phasic shear stress and viral infections. *J Biol Chem* 2005; **280**(42): 35751–9.

85. Petersen NT, Hoiby N, Mordhorst CH, Lind K, Flensborg EW, Bruun B. Respiratory infections in cystic fibrosis patients caused by virus, chlamydia and mycoplasma: Possible synergism with *Pseudomonas aeruginosa*. *Acta Paediatr Scand* 1981; **70**(5): 623–8.

86. Hybiske K, Ichikawa JK, Huang V, Lory SJ, Machen TE. Cystic fibrosis airway epithelial cell polarity and bacterial flagellin determine host response to *Pseudomonas aeruginosa*. *Cell Microbiol* 2004; **6**(1): 49–63.

87. Asner S, Waters V, Solomon M et al. Role of respiratory viruses in pulmonary exacerbations in children with cystic fibrosis. *J Cyst Fibros* 2012; **11**(5): 433–9.

88. Colombo C, Costantini D, Rocchi A et al. Cytokine levels in sputum of cystic fibrosis patients before and after antibiotic therapy. *Pediatr Pulmonol* 2005; **40**(1): 15–21.

89. Downey DG, Brockbank S, Martin SL, Ennis M, Elborn JS. The effect of treatment of cystic fibrosis pulmonary exacerbations on airways and systemic inflammation. *Pediatr Pulmonol* 2007; **42**(8): 729–35.

90. Gray RD, Imrie M, Boyd AC, Porteous D, Innes JA, Greening AP. Sputum and serum calprotectin are useful biomarkers during CF exacerbation. *J Cyst Fibros* 2010; **9**(3): 193–8.

91. Harris WT, Muhlebach MS, Oster RA, Knowles MR, Clancy JP, Noah TL. Plasma TGF-beta(1) in pediatric cystic fibrosis: Potential biomarker of lung disease and response to therapy. *Pediatr Pulmonol* 2011;**46**(7): 688–95.

92. Laguna TA, Wagner BD, Luckey HK et al. Sputum desmosine during hospital admission for pulmonary exacerbation in cystic fibrosis. *Chest* 2009; **136**(6): 1561–8.

93. Watts KD, McColley SA. Elevated vascular endothelial growth factor is correlated with elevated erythropoietin in stable, young cystic fibrosis patients. *Pediatr Pulmonol* 2011; **46**(7): 683–7.

94. Reeves EP, Bergin DA, Fitzgerald S et al. A novel neutrophil derived inflammatory biomarker of pulmonary exacerbation in cystic fibrosis. *J Cyst Fibros* 2012; **11**(2): 100–7.

95. Goss CH, Newsom SA, Schildcrout JS, Sheppard L, Kaufman JD. Effect of ambient air pollution on pulmonary exacerbations and lung function in cystic fibrosis. *Am J Respir Crit Care Med* 2004; **169**(7): 816–21.

96. Wolter JM, Bowler SD, Nolan PJ, McCormack JG. Home intravenous therapy in cystic fibrosis: A prospective randomized trial examining clinical, quality of life and cost aspects. *Eur Respir J* 1997; **10**(4): 896–900.

97. Bosworth DG, Nielson DW. Effectiveness of home versus hospital care in the routine treatment of cystic fibrosis. *Pediatr Pulmonol* 1997; **24**(1): 42–7.

98. Bradley JM, Wallace ES, Elborn JS, Howard JL, McCoy MP. An audit of the effect of intravenous antibiotic treatment on spirometric measures of pulmonary function in cystic fibrosis. *Ir J Med Sci* 1999; **168**(1): 25–8.

99. Donati MA, Guenette G, Auerbach H. Prospective controlled study of home and hospital therapy of cystic fibrosis pulmonary disease. *J Pediatri* 1987; **111**(1): 28–33.

100. Esmond G, Butler M, McCormack AM. Comparison of hospital and home intravenous antibiotic therapy in adults with cystic fibrosis. *J Clin Nurs* 2006; **15**(1): 52–60.

101. Gilbert J, Robinson T, Littlewood JM. Home intravenous antibiotic treatment in cystic fibrosis. *Arch Dis Child* 1988; **63**(5): 512–7.

102. Nazer D, Abdulhamid I, Thomas R, Pendleton S. Home versus hospital intravenous antibiotic therapy for acute pulmonary exacerbations in children with cystic fibrosis. *Pediatr Pulmonol* 2006; **41**(8): 744–9.

103. Pond MN, Newport M, Joanes D, Conway SP. Home versus hospital intravenous antibiotic therapy in the treatment of young adults with cystic fibrosis. *Eur Respir J* 1994; **7**(9): 1640–4.

104. Thornton J, Elliott R, Tully MP, Dodd M, Webb AK. Long term clinical outcome of home and hospital intravenous antibiotic treatment in adults with cystic fibrosis. *Thorax* 2004; **59**(3): 242–6.

105. Winter RJ, George RJ, Deacock SJ, Shee CD, Geddes DM. Self-administered home intravenous antibiotic therapy in bronchiectasis and adult cystic fibrosis. *Lancet* 1984; **1**(8390): 1338–9.

106. Yi MS, Tsevat J, Wilmott RW, Kotagal UR, Britto MT. The impact of treatment of pulmonary exacerbations on the health-related quality of life of patients with cystic fibrosis: Does hospitalization make a difference? *J Pediatrics* 2004; **144**(6): 711–8.

107. Gold R, Carpenter S, Heurter H, Corey M, Levison H. Randomized trial of ceftazidime versus placebo in the management of acute respiratory exacerbations in patients with cystic fibrosis. *J Pediatr* 1987; **111**(6 Pt 1): 907–13.

108. Wientzen R, Prestidge CB, Kramer RI, McCracken GH, Nelson JD. Acute pulmonary exacerbations in cystic fibrosis. A double-blind trial of tobramycin and placebo therapy. *Am J Dis Child* 1980; **134**(12): 1134–8.

109. McLaughlin FJ, Matthews WJ Jr., Strieder DJ et al. Clinical and bacteriological responses to three antibiotic regimens for acute exacerbations of cystic fibrosis: Ticarcillin-tobramycin, azlocillin-tobramycin, and azlocillin-placebo. *J Infect Dis* 1983; **147**(3): 559–67.

110. Smith AL, Fiel SB, Mayer-Hamblett N, Ramsey B, Burns JL. Susceptibility testing of *Pseudomonas aeruginosa* isolates and clinical response to parenteral antibiotic administration: Lack of association in cystic fibrosis. *Chest* 2003; **123**(5): 1495–502.

111. Hurley MN, Ariff AH, Bertenshaw C, Bhatt J, Smyth AR. Results of antibiotic susceptibility testing do not influence clinical outcome in children with cystic fibrosis. *J Cyst Fibros* 2012; **11**(4): 288–92.

112. Foweraker JE, Laughton CR, Brown DF, Bilton D. Phenotypic variability of *Pseudomonas aeruginosa* in sputa from patients with acute infective exacerbation of cystic fibrosis and its impact on the validity of antimicrobial susceptibility testing. *J Antimicrob Chemother* 2005; **55**(6): 921–7.

113. Harris JK, De Groote MA, Sagel SD et al. Molecular identification of bacteria in bronchoalveolar lavage fluid from children with cystic fibrosis. *Proc Natl Acad Sci USA* 2007; **104**(51): 20529–33.

114. Parkins MD, Sibley CD, Surette MG, Rabin HR. The Streptococcus milleri group: An unrecognized cause of disease in cystic fibrosis: A case series and literature review. *Pediatr Pulmonol* 2008; **43**(5): 490–7.

115. Conway SP, Pond MN, Watson A, Etherington C, Robey HL, Goldman MH. Intravenous colistin sulphomethate in acute respiratory exacerbations in adult patients with cystic fibrosis. *Thorax* 1997; **52**(11): 987–93.

116. Master V, Roberts GW, Coulthard KP et al. Efficacy of once-daily tobramycin monotherapy for acute pulmonary exacerbations of cystic fibrosis: A preliminary study. *Pediatr Pulmonol* 2001; **31**(5): 367–76.

117. Padoan R, Cambisano W, Costantini D, Crossignani RM, Danza ML, Trezzi G, et al. Ceftazidime monotherapy vs. combined therapy in Pseudomonas pulmonary infections in cystic fibrosis. *Pediatr Infect Dis J* 1987;6(7):648-53.

118. Saiman L, Mehar F, Niu WW et al. Antibiotic susceptibility of multiply resistant *Pseudomonas aeruginosa* isolated from patients with cystic fibrosis, including candidates for transplantation. *Clin Infect Dis* 1996; **23**(3): 532–7.

119. Doring G, Conway SP, Heijerman HG et al. Antibiotic therapy against *Pseudomonas aeruginosa* in cystic fibrosis: A European consensus. *Eur Respir J* 2000; **16**(4): 749–67.

120. Bosso JA, Saxon BA, Matsen JM. Comparative activity of cefepime, alone and in combination, against clinical isolates of *Pseudomonas aeruginosa* and *Pseudomonas cepacia* from cystic fibrosis patients. *Antimicrob Agents Chemother* 1991; **35**(4): 783–4.

121. Tre-Hardy M, Nagant C, El Manssouri N et al. Efficacy of the combination of tobramycin and a macrolide in an in vitro *Pseudomonas aeruginosa* mature biofilm model. *Antimicrob Agents Chemother* 2010; **54**(10): 4409–15.

122. Aaron SD, Vandemheen KL, Ferris W et al. Combination antibiotic susceptibility testing to treat exacerbations of cystic fibrosis associated with

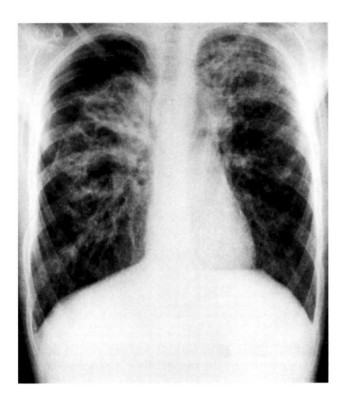

Figure 18.4 Chest radiograph showing widespread pulmonary disease and a right-sided pneumothorax.

"small" and large pneumothoraxes are ≥2 cm.[24] In the case of CF, in adults we suggest that a small air rim <1cm around the lung is mild, moderate up to 2 cm, and large ≥2 cm. Fortunately, pneumothorax is rare in young children with CF, probably because generally they have much less respiratory disease, but the recommendations above may be scaled down for children.

Management is summarized in Figure 18.6 and in the literature.[5,25] Even a small and asymptomatic pneumothorax should be observed in hospital for 24 hours. No treatment may be needed, but the clinician must be satisfied that the pneumothorax is not getting bigger and no associated hemothorax is developing. A moderate or large pneumothorax will require insertion of an intercostal tube. The position is decided after studying the chest radiograph, but the usual position is at the fifth to sixth intercostal space in the midaxillary line. A Seldinger technique should be used, and the tube is directed to the apex of the lung and sufficient length is inserted. An alternative position is the second intercostal space anteriorly. If the pneumothorax does not re-expand quickly, suction should be applied, at a pressure of 5–7 kPa. If it does not re-expand after 4 or 5 days, surgical advice should be obtained. It may take longer for the CF lung to re-expand compared with the healthy lung. If the lung does not re-expand, the clinician faces a dilemma. Extensive pleurectomy, or talc pleurodesis, may make the patient unsuitable for future transplantation. This is because dissection of the pleura would take a long time causing a long ischemic time and there is often extensive bleeding. Despite the high incidence of pneumothoraxes in people with CF, no randomized control trials to compare medical and surgical treatment have been conducted.[25,26] The best treatment at all ages in our view is limited abrasion surgical pleurodesis.[27] In patients not suitable for transplantation, or too ill for surgery, chemical pleurodesis using bleomycin or talc has been used.[25] While the patient has a chest drain, in situ physiotherapy should be continued and intravenous antibiotics given as indicated. SaO_2 should be monitored and oxygen given to help reabsorb the air from the pneumothorax. High dose oxygen, up to 10 L, may be helpful, but $PaCO_2$ must be carefully monitored. High flow oxygen reduces the total pressure of gas in the capillaries, particularly nitrogen, and there is therefore a higher gradient between the pleural capillaries and the pleural cavity, and hence air is reabsorbed. High flow oxygen can increase the rate of reabsorption of air by up to fourfold.[28] Appropriate analgesics should be given. When a pneumothorax is diagnosed, it should be treated quickly with an intercostal tube as re-expansion edema is more common when the lung is reinflated after a period of time.[29] In the case of a tension pneumothorax, the patient should be given oxygen and a 4-cm cannula can be inserted as an emergency procedure into the second intercostal space, midclavicular line above the third rib. Sometimes, Heimlich valves can be used temporarily; but, in our opinion, these are not as effective as an underwater drain seal.

Some patients in chronic respiratory failure are dependent on noninvasive positive pressure ventilation. There is a slightly increased incidence of pneumothorax in these patients, but they can be managed using a ventilator at low pressure.[30] After nonsurgical treatment of a pneumothorax, patients should avoid spirometry for 2 weeks[5] and should be provided with a letter stating they are CF patients who have had a pneumothorax and if they present to any hospital with breathlessness or chest pain a chest radiograph should be performed to exclude recurrence. Patients who have not had surgical procedures should not fly until a chest radiograph has confirmed that the lung is completely up, and for 6 weeks afterward.[31] Most regulatory authorities would prohibit scuba diving in anyone with airflow obstruction, and certainly after a pneumothorax.

Pneumomediastinum and surgical emphysema are usually associated with a pneumothorax, but occasionally they may be present as an isolated finding in an otherwise well CF patient. No treatment is required. Air leaks may rarely be the first presentation of CF[32] and have been described as the presenting feature of ABPA.[33]

LUNG OR LOBAR COLLAPSE

This subject has recently been reviewed.[34] This complication is relatively uncommon if effective antibiotics, airway clearance, and mucoactive agents are prescribed. The commonest cause is mucus plugging, which may be exacerbated by anything that increases sputum viscosity, such as diabetes

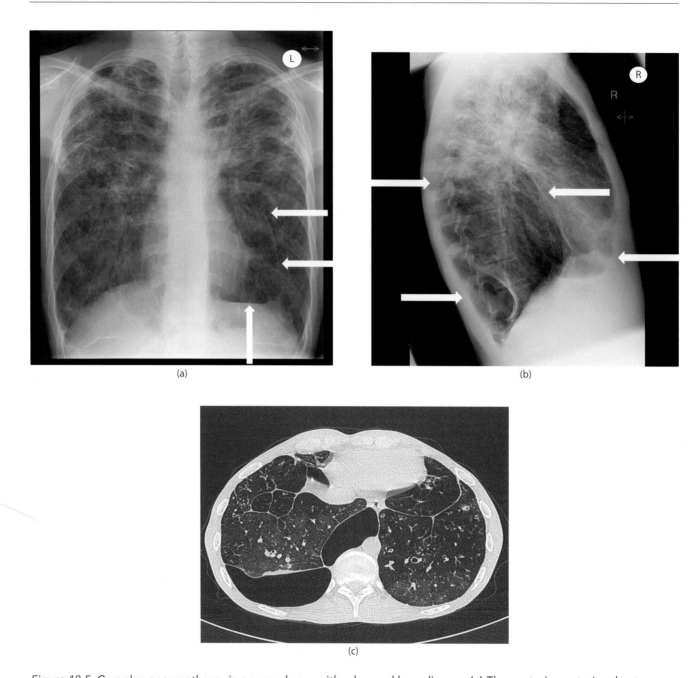

Figure 18.5 Complex pneumothorax in a second case with advanced lung disease. **(a)** The posterior–anterior chest radiograph shows an area of lucency overlying the left lower lobe (white arrows). **(b)** The lateral chest radiograph shows a posterior area of lucency suggestive of a complex pneumothorax (white arrows). **(c)** The computed tomography scan confirms that the posterior area of lucency is a complex pneumothorax with tethering of the visceral and parietal pleura.

or dehydration. Other contributing factors may be poor adherence to treatment, especially airway clearance, and a coincident localized airway malformation. Mucus plugging should also raise the possibility of ABPA[35] (Chapter 16). Other causes include shrinkage, destruction, and fibrosis of a lobe with the central airways patent; airway occlusion by a large blood clot; and, much more rarely, membranous occlusion of an airway.[36] This last cause has been proposed to be related to airway occlusion by an exuberant granulation tissue response (pseudopolyp formation); although usually presenting with localized cavitatory lesions, membranous occlusion enters the differential diagnosis of a complete bronchial obstruction. Anecdotally, a CT scan may help delineate optimal management. If the collapsed lobe is seen to contain a prominent air bronchogram it is likely that there is no proximal mucus plugging, and the changes represent chronic lobar destruction, which is not likely to respond to bronchoscopy and is irreversible. Finally, the possibility of non-CF causes such as foreign body must be remembered.

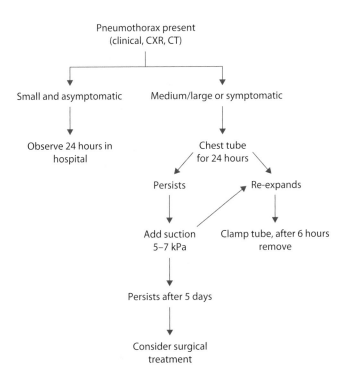

Figure 18.6 Management of pneumothorax in cystic fibrosis.

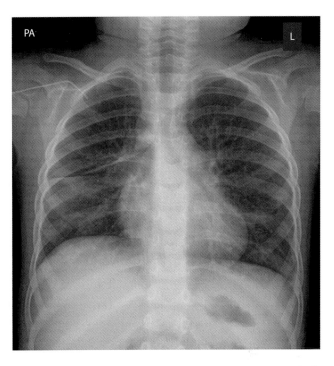

Figure 18.8 Appearances after bronchoscopic removal of large sputum plugs.

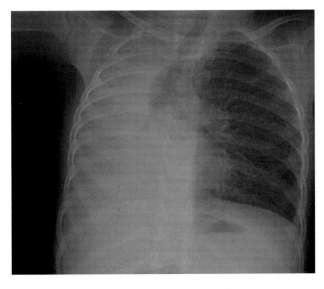

Figure 18.7 Complete collapse of the right lung. Note the left lung herniating across the mediastinum and the abrupt termination of the right upper lobe bronchus and right bronchus intermedius, with no distal air bronchogram.

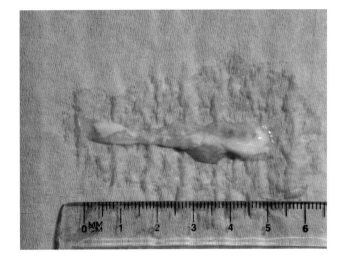

Figure 18.9 A large plug of sputum that totally occluded the left main bronchus in another child. This could only be removed by pulling out the plug together on the end of the flexible bronchoscope.

Treatment is with intensive physiotherapy, possibly augmented by positive airway pressure, either or both rhDNase and HS, and appropriate intravenous and nebulized antibiotics. If this fails, bronchoscopy should be performed, with the largest caliber flexible bronchoscope tolerated by the patient (Figures 18.7 through 18.9). There is evidence from case series that directly instilling rhDNase endobronchially may be beneficial.[37–39] We have also occasionally instilled surfactant endobronchially to facilitate lobar expansion. If there are really tenacious plugs of sputum that cannot be removed using the fiber-optic bronchoscope, rigid bronchoscopy may be considered.

Surgical removal of the collapsed lobe is occasionally contemplated in the patient with well-preserved lung architecture in the other lobes. However, in general a CT scan will reveal that the disease is not truly isolated and there is

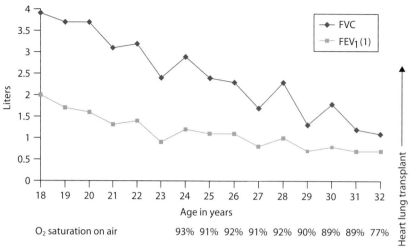

Figure 18.10 Deterioration in pulmonary function over a 14-year period in an adult with cystic fibrosis, despite maximum medical treatment.

widespread bronchiectasis elsewhere. We routinely perform bronchoscopy as part of the workup for lobectomy or pneumonectomy. The presence of infected secretions throughout the bronchial tree would increase our reluctance to advocate surgery. The occasional patient may get short-term benefit from lobectomy,[40,41] but only in the rare case of a destroyed nonfunctional lobe with well-preserved lung elsewhere. Even in such cases, recurrence of CF lung disease is not uncommon.[42]

PULMONARY HYPERTENSION AND SECONDARY CARDIAC COMPLICATIONS

Patients with end-stage CF become severely hypoxic (Figure 18.10), and before that they develop significant desaturation during exercise and sleep.[43] Cor pulmonale is well recognized in patients with hypoxia and pulmonary hypertension. Right heart failure may be present before death in a few patients. The prognosis once heart failure occurs is grave.[44] The mechanism for pulmonary hypertension appears to be pulmonary vasoconstriction and subsequent vascular remodeling.[45] It has been shown that endothelin-1 and nuclear factor-κB may be involved in pulmonary vascular dysfunction.[46] A study of 21 CF patients breathing air and oxygen mixtures showed mean pulmonary artery pressure (PAP) to be abnormally high in 8 of 21, and the PAP correlated with the degree of hypoxia.[47] CF patients who are awaiting transplantation frequently have a mild degree of pulmonary hypertension, and its presence significantly worsens survival.[47] Infection with *B. cepacia* has also been associated with worse pulmonary hypertension.[48] Patients with right heart failure may have electrocardiogram changes (Figure 18.11) such as P-pulmonale, and the chest radiograph may show cardiomegaly (Figure 18.12).

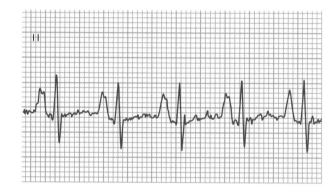

Figure 18.11 Electrocardiogram of a cystic fibrosis patient with right heart failure showing tall P-waves.

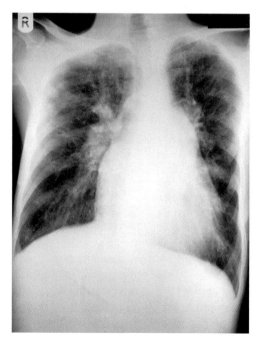

Figure 18.12 Chest radiograph of a cystic fibrosis patient with right heart failure.

Prolonged oxygen therapy has shown no survival advantage[49] but can provide symptomatic relief and should be given to hypoxic patients. Heart failure usually responds well to oxygen and diuretics. Some severely hypoxic patients continue to study or work using an oxygen concentrator at college or in the workplace.

More recently, Doppler echocardiography has been used to study the heart in CF patients. Abnormalities of structure and function of the right ventricle have been shown to be present in early stages of the disease.[50] In some patients, pulmonary hypertension was demonstrated and also significant right ventricular systolic and diastolic dysfunction in patients with severe disease, in the absence of left ventricular abnormalities.[51] In 12 CF patients, circulating atrial natriuretic peptide (ANP) was higher in patients with pulmonary hypertension than in those without.[52] Right ventricular ejection fraction during exercise has been shown to be a strong predictor of outcome among patients awaiting lung transplantation.[53]

Recently, in a number of patients significant alterations in right and left ventricular filling with respiration were demonstrated by Doppler echocardiography. On inspiration, the right heart filling was increased and the left heart filling was reduced. On expiration, the right ventricular filling was reduced; in addition, there was flow reversal into the hepatic veins (Figure 18.13). Reciprocal changes happened in the left heart. Possibly, this picture of disturbed cardiac physiology is somewhat similar to cardiac tamponade caused by a large pericardial effusion or large left pleural effusion. Such a complication may account for some of the unexplained neurological symptoms experienced by some CF patients with severe disease.[54]

Patients with CF may develop arrhythmias, which are usually supraventricular.[55] This is probably caused by ventricular remodeling due to hypoxia, infection, and/or sympathomimetic medication. Disease of the coronary arteries is rare, probably due to the low serum lipid levels found in CF. However, a 48-year-old man with CF, pancreatic insufficiency, and cystic fibrosis-related diabetes (CFRD) was reported as presenting acutely with a symptomatic non-ST elevation myocardial infarction (MSTEMI).[56] It is likely that as the CF population continues to show improved survival more ischemic cardiac disease will present. Some cases of cardiomyopathy have also been seen in CF patients.

RESPIRATORY FAILURE

Patients may develop hypoxic respiratory failure, which leads to pulmonary artery hypertension and cor pulmonale. At the same time, airflow obstruction reduces vital capacity and tidal volume, leading to decreased alveolar ventilation. There may be progressive elevation in carbon dioxide and hypercapnic respiratory failure. It is very common for both hypoxemia and hypercapnia to occur together.

Patients should be given the opportunity to be assessed for pulmonary transplantation if appropriate. Immediate management involves the clearance of pulmonary secretions by physiotherapy techniques including, if necessary, intermittent positive pressure breathing. Appropriate antibiotics should be given intravenously and by aerosol; the presence of antibiotic-resistant or unusual organisms should be sought. Anti-inflammatory drugs, including corticosteroids, dornase alfa, and bronchodilators, should be given. Hypoxia should be treated by controlled oxygen therapy and some patients, especially those with severe nocturnal hypoxia, may benefit from nasal continuous positive airway pressure or positive pressure ventilation (Chapter 19), which allows the patient to eat, talk, and communicate. It is cost-effective as the patient does not need the intensive care unit (ICU). There is no consensus, at least in children,

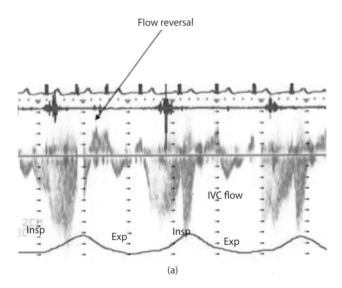

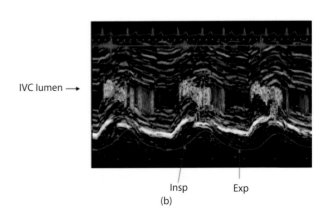

(a) (b)

Figure 18.13 **(a)** Inferior vena cava (IVC) pulsed-wave Doppler velocities in a patient with end-stage cystic fibrosis showing flow reversal during expiration. **(b)** IVC color flow Doppler M-mode in a patient with end-stage cystic fibrosis showing flow reversal (red) during expiration and aliasing velocities (mosaic) during inspiration.

as to when to initiate noninvasive ventilation (NIV), and practice differs widely.[57] In cases of hypercapnia, we find intravenous aminophylline and/or intravenous terbutaline helpful, acting as respiratory stimulants as well as bronchodilators. Finally, if the patient's genotype is unknown it should be determined, in case of eligibility for novel therapies on standard or compassionate grounds. There are nine rare class 3 mutations as well as G551D who are also eligible for Kalydeco.[58] Patients with class 4, class 5, or even class 2 mutations might reasonably be considered for this medication on compassionate grounds.

It is clear that the vast majority of adult CF patients die without being admitted to ICU. Endotracheal intubation is thought to be appropriate in less than 1% of CF patients, and less than 8% of hospital deaths in adults are in ICU.[59] The situation may be different in children—in a recent review of an admittedly small number of deaths, most died in hospital and nearly half were ventilated.[60] It is not possible to determine the appropriateness or otherwise of ICU management in children. There is little place for submitting an adult patient with end-stage respiratory and nutritional failure, who has already had maximal medical treatment including NIV, to intubation and positive pressure ventilation. The patient should be made comfortable and given symptomatic treatment, involving the palliative care team (Chapter 46). However, the rare adult patient may benefit from ICU care and indeed live to leave hospital and subsequently receive a lung transplant. Prediction is difficult—traditional ICU predictive indexes perform poorly in predicting survival in CF patients admitted to ICU.[61]

The role of ICU management in patients with CF has been hotly debated. Two recent surveys have been published[59,61] comprising 94 ICU admissions in 72 CF patients, all with very poor initial lung function. Unsurprisingly, management with NIV is to be preferred and is associated with a better prognosis[61] and indeed is increasingly being used to support CF patients in respiratory failure. Survival rates depend on the reasons for admission. Overall, more than half did not survive to leave hospital.[61] A total of 59% of 22 patients intubated for hemothorax or pneumothorax survived to hospital discharge, whereas only 4 of 12 intubated for infective exacerbation left hospital. However, those who left hospital survived around 15 months post discharge. Poor nutrition in the 2 years prior to intubation and CF-related bone disease were markers of a poor outlook, but not absolute or rate of change of spirometry. By contrast, in another study of ICU admissions, which included the use of NIV without intubation, accelerated FEV_1 decline was a poor prognostic feature.

The appropriateness of a given level of respiratory support should always be considered carefully, whether NIV or intubation in ICU. An important consideration is whether there is a potentially treatable situation, in either an acute episode that will respond to treatment or a realistic hope that an organ for transplantation may become available (it should be noted that the results of transplanting an intubated CF patient are less good than if the patient is breathing

spontaneously) (Chapter 29). Ventilatory support should never be used to prolong the process of dying.

PHARMACOLOGICAL ADJUNCTS TO MUCUS CLEARANCE

These agents can be divided into two classes:

- Altering the abnormal secretions to facilitate sputum clearance
  - rhDNase (well established)
  - N-acetyl cysteine (NAC), popular in some centers, but no convincing evidence (see later)
- Normalizing airway surface liquid volume, attacking what is thought to be the fundamental abnormality in CF
  - 7% HS (well established)
  - Mannitol, an inert naturally occurring sugar alcohol that acts as an osmotic agent (evidence base still being evaluated)
  - Denufosol tetrasodium, which stimulates an alternative chloride channel (recent study led to withdrawal)

These are only adjunctive to mechanical methods of airway clearance, which are reviewed in Chapter 43. The clearest evidence for mucolytic therapy is the use of rhDNase, followed by HS.

rhDNase

rhDNase decreases sputum viscoelasticity in CF patients, and this makes chest physiotherapy easier. Many studies have shown a clinical improvement in patients following treatment.[62,63] A North American study of more than 900 patients showed that patients with moderate lung disease had an improvement of 5.8% in FEV_1 when treated with rhDNase over a 6-month period ($p < .01$).[64] Patients with mild pulmonary disease, i.e., $FEV_1 > 85\%$ predicted, and children aged 5–10 years have also showed a benefit.[65] A 2-year randomized placebo-controlled study showed benefit in young patients.[66] Patients with severe pulmonary disease also benefitted.[67,68] An uncontrolled, open-labeled study followed up patients for 2 years while they were taking rhDNase and showed that the FEV_1 stabilized 6% above baseline.[69] A case-controlled study of rhDNase that evaluated the impact on disease progression over a 4-year period also showed benefit.[70] The European registry reported on patients treated with rhDNase and showed that the treated patients benefited with an improved FEV_1 and reduced pulmonary exacerbations.[71] Registry data showed excellent safety in CF patients of all ages.[72]

rhDNase is equally effective when delivered before or after physiotherapy, but patients chronically infected with P. aeruginosa may derive more improvement in FEV_1 when rhDNase is administered after physiotherapy.[73] Other studies did not show that timing of rhDNase therapy with respect to physiotherapy affects outcome, so timing should be determined by individual preference.[74]

It has been shown that delivery of rhDNase using a smart nebulizer to allow more medication to be delivered to the small airways improves small airways obstruction.[75] rhDNase also improved lung clearance index (LCI) in a short-term study.[76]

The effect of rhDNase on survival is more difficult to prove. Starting treatment was associated with a reduction in mortality in the subsequent year (hazard ratio, 0.85; 97% confidence interval [CI], 0.76–0.95; $p < .005$).[77] CF patients with FEV_1 less than 30% predicted between the years 1990 and 2003 showed that the median survival improved from 1.2 years in the 1990–1991 group to 5.3 years in the 2002–2003 group. This marked improvement in survival began in 1994. Use of rhDNase was associated with a reduced risk of death (hazard ratio, 0.59; 95% CI, 0.44–0.79).[78] The efficacy and safety of rhDNase[72,79] suggest that treatment with dornase alfa should be started in early childhood,[65,66,80] although safety data for the very immature airway are lacking. The possible anti-inflammatory effects of rhDNase are discussed later.

HYPERTONIC SALINE

Sputum induction with HS is a well-established clinical and research procedure. There is a dose–response effect for mucociliary clearance (MCC) up to 6% HS, with no further increase going up to 12%.[81] Addition of amiloride to HS did not improve MCC.[82] It is noted that 7% HS is now commercially available and recommended for use. It should be noted that 10% HS may cause bronchoconstriction but also subsequent bronchodilation, similar to the paradoxical bronchodilatation seen after exercise in some CF patients,[83,84] and a first test dose even of 7% HS should always be performed under medical supervision. Efficacy studies of HS have focused on changes in lung function and changes in the weight of expectorated sputum. Sputum induction and enhanced sputum clearance may not be the same procedure, however. Short-term studies demonstrated increases in pulmonary function with HS similar to those obtained with rhDNase in phase 11 studies.[85,86] There have been two longer term studies. A pediatric trial, in which children were randomly allocated in a crossover design to any of 7% HS, daily rhDNase, or alternate-day rhDNase for 12 weeks, showed that for the group there was no significant change in spirometry over baseline with HS, unlike rhDNase.[87] Looking at individual patients, 35% did have an improvement in FEV_1 of at least 10% on HS, including some children who did not improve with rhDNase. The wide scatter emphasizes that there are important individual differences in response with this as with other treatments in CF. Patients already taking short-acting β-2 agonists were allowed to take them prior to nebulizing HS, and only three were unable to use HS. The study was not powered to show a difference in exacerbation rate. Benefit at 6 weeks was less

than that at 12 weeks, so a 12-week trial was recommended on an individual, n of 1 basis. By contrast, a much smaller short-term study concluded that efficacy for 5.85% HS and rhDNase was similar,[86] but examination of the individual data reveals that there were marked individual differences in response. In the second long-term study, normal saline and hypertonic (7%) given nebulized twice daily were compared over a 1-year period in 164 patients.[88] There was a statistically significant, but clinically trivial (67 mL FEV_1), improvement in the HS group but a dramatic reduction in infective exacerbations (2.74 vs. 1.30 per patient in favor of HS) and improved work attendance. It should be noted that only 18% were using nebulized antibiotics, so it may be that the results are not generally applicable. In an accompanying paper, it was suggested that 7% HS had a prolonged effect on MCC.[89] Curiously, this was abrogated by concurrent amiloride therapy. A recent retrospective study confirmed the benefit of HS in prevention of exacerbations.[90] HS is well tolerated during the exacerbation itself, but a retrospective study showed no benefit in terms of outcomes.[91]

The ISIS study[92] randomized infants aged 4–60 months to either 7% HS ($n = 158$) or 0.9% saline ($n = 163$) nebulized twice daily for 48 weeks. The primary end point was reduction in protocol-defined exacerbations. There was no difference in the primary or any secondary end point. The subgroup that had infant pulmonary function tests performed had a barely significant increase in $FEV_{0.5}$. LCI was, however, improved in the subgroup that had this measured.[93] HS should not be a routine therapy in infants. However, in older children and adults the Cochrane review[94] supports the use of HS in CF, while acknowledging that there are weaknesses in the evidence base. Overall, this cheap treatment may be a useful adjunctive therapy in CF and possibly partially correct the effects of the basic defect by rehydrating the airway surface.

There have been concerns about the effects of HS on airway defenses and its possible proinflammatory potential. Repetitive induction of sputum with HS has been reported to cause increased airway neutrophilia,[95,96] which may be intrinsically undesirable in CF; however, in the large HS study reported earlier[87] HS had no proinflammatory effects and there were no correlations between changes in lung function and changes in inflammatory markers,[97] suggesting that there is no clinically significant proinflammatory effect of HS over at least a 12-week period. Indeed, a recent study suggested that HS might in fact be anti-inflammatory. Glycosaminoglycans (GAGs) bind the neutrophil chemoattractant interleukin (IL)-8, stabilizing it and promoting neutrophil chemotaxis. HS liberates IL-8 from the matrices formed by GAGs, making it vulnerable to proteolytic cleavage and reducing neutrophil chemotaxis.[98] GAGs also bind antimicrobial peptides such as LL-37, such that, although total LL-37 levels are supranormal in CF, free LL-37 is undetectable. As with IL-8, HS liberated IL-37 but in so doing rendered it vulnerable to proteolytic cleavage by neutrophil elastase and cathepsin D.[99] Finally, glutathione is an important antioxidant, and thiocyanate is an important substrate for myeloperoxidase and lactoperoxidase, key enzymes in host defense. Both are transported by cystic fibrosis transmembrane conductance regulator (CFTR), and in a CF mouse model both were reduced at baseline but increased by HS inhalation.[100] Any relevance of these mechanisms in man is unknown.

HS should be considered for use in all CF patients of school age and above; prediction of response is not possible.[101] Its use would be most strongly advocated in patients with multiple exacerbations. HS is recommended as standard therapy by the US Cystic Fibrosis Foundation in CF patients 6 years and older.[102] Traditionally, it is recommended prior to airway clearance; but a recent Cochrane review reported that there is no evidence with respect to alternative timings, and further study is needed.[103] Clearly, treatment burden should be considered; there are already multiple inhaled therapies that may be recommended, and it is important to be realistic in considering what a patient can achieve in terms of treatment time.

Sputum induction, using HS, may also be used diagnostically. This has been routine in the context of HIV and TB, but we have been slower to introduce it in the context of CF. Compared with standard methods of collection of lower respiratory tract secretions, induced sputum was shown to lead to the isolation of more organisms.[104] It may even be that induced sputum is a better "gold standard" than BAL, in which differences in culture results from different lobes in the same patient have been well documented.[105,106] The TB experience is that the technique can be used even in babies.[107] Care must be taken to ensure that sputum induction does not lead to cross infection. There is a need for comparisons between standard methods, such as cough swab and nasopharyngeal aspirates, with sputum induction, the use of cough plates, and BAL.

MANNITOL

Mannitol is a naturally occurring sugar alcohol, used as an indirect airway challenge agent in asthma. Mannitol is given by inhalation of a dry powder, but 10 capsules are needed (capsule dose: 40 mcg/mannitol). Given its role as an airway challenge, it is unsurprising that it causes bronchoconstriction in nearly 25% of CF patients. It was impossible to predict who would fail the challenge, and specifically there was no relationship with atopic status.[108] There have been three large efficacy studies of mannitol in CF. The first was a randomized, three-period crossover study[109] comparing 12 weeks of mannitol, rhDNase, and mannitol and rhDNase combined. It showed that mannitol and rhDNase had equivalent effects on FEV$_1$, but the combination had no effect (this was not seen in other studies). There were marked individual differences in response to the two agents, and mannitol was much less well tolerated than rhDNase. The largest efficacy study in 326 CF patients aged 6 years and over, lasted 26 weeks (double blind phase) followed by a 26-week open label extension.[110] The results showed that there was a 6.5% increase in FEV$_1$ with mannitol, irrespective of whether

the patient also inhaled rhDNase, maintained over the study period and a 35.4% reduction in CF exacerbations. Mannitol was well tolerated, although adverse events were commoner in the mannitol group. The third efficacy study[111] comprised 26 weeks of double-blind therapy with mannitol 400 mg bd ($n = 192$, "treated" group) and with mannitol 50 mg bd ($n = 126$, "control" group) in CF patients aged 6 years and over, with a 26-week open label extension. There was a significant increase in the primary end-point FEV$_1$ in the treated group, but only after a post hoc recalculation of baseline FEV$_1$; so, many would rate this as a negative trial. There was no reduction in exacerbations, but the study was probably underpowered to show this. Adverse events were similar in both groups and, for the most part, mild. Merging the two largest studies,[110,111] there were small improvements in spirometry (FEV$_1$, 73.42 mL; $p < .001$), irrespective of rhDNase use. Interestingly, only adults improved their FEV$_1$. Pulmonary exacerbations were reduced by 29% ($p = .039$) by mannitol.[112] A Cochrane review or meta-analysis on the use of mannitol in CF is awaited.

The mechanism whereby mannitol leads to clinical benefit is unclear. Two weeks of inhaled mannitol led to significant improvements in mucus hydration and surface properties, which correlated with the change in spirometry,[113] but other beneficial effects cannot be excluded. In terms of potential adverse effects, in vitro, mannitol has been shown to stimulate exopolysaccharide production by *Burkholderia cenocepacia*.[114] Mannitol is a growth factor for *S. aureus*, *P. aeruginosa*, and *B. cepacia*. This raises safety concerns, but no clinical study has shown a change in airway infection with inhaled mannitol.

Mannitol is clearly a promising agent in CF treatment. The exact role is currently unclear, but it should certainly be considered in patients who have not responded to rhDNase or HS.

OTHER MUCOLYTICS

NAC: a systematic review identified six randomized controlled trials of NAC in CF, which enrolled 181 patients, and concluded that there was no evidence of benefit for 3 months of therapy.[115] There are no longer term studies. A more recent study reported that NAC administered by metered dose inhaler was well tolerated and improved sputum rheology in vitro.[116] There appears to be an additive beneficial effect on mucus properties when NAC and rhDNase are combined.[117] However, there are no new efficacy studies to report since the systematic review.[115] NAC may have anti-inflammatory properties, reducing neutrophil count, IL-8, and neutrophil elastase in one study.[118] However, this was not confirmed in the phase 2 study.[116] Currently, NAC cannot be recommended as routine therapy in CF.[115]

Denufosol tetrasodium: stimulation of the P2Y$_2$ receptor leads to chloride transport via a non-CFTR channel. A phase 2 study of the P2Y$_2$ agonist denufosol tetrasodium showed it to be safe and well tolerated.[119] A 24-week phase 3 study (TIGER-1; $n = 178$ denufosol, $n = 174$ placebo) showed a statistically significant but clinically trivial improvement in FEV$_1$ (less than 50 mL), and no effect on exacerbations.[120] A further phase 3 study (TIGER-2, 466 patients enrolled in a 48-week study[121]) showed no efficacy at all, so interest in denufosol has waned.

ANTI-INFLAMMATORY THERAPY

There is a widespread assumption that inflammation is a bad thing in CF and must be suppressed.[122] This arose in part from the early prednisolone study[123] (see later) and in part from the study of the impressive catalog of toxic materials released from necrotic neutrophils, which are abundant in the airway. Furthermore, some, but not all, studies (Chapter 7) have suggested that the CF airway is intrinsically proinflammatory, even in the absence of infection. However, it would be wrong to assume that all inflammation is bad. Inflammation is beneficial in many circumstances. Firstly, it is known that congenital immunodeficiencies characterized by absent or reduced lung defenses result in devastating systemic infections, which, other than the feared cepacia syndrome, are unheard of in CF, at least in the untransplanted patient. Thus, the neutrophil must have some protective function in CF. Secondly, early infection with *P. aeruginosa* is frequently overcome and it seems not unlikely that the host immune response is important in this. Thirdly, a recent trial of an anti-inflammatory strategy, LTB$_4$ antagonism,[124] had to be terminated prematurely because of an increase in serious adverse events, in particular infection, in the treated group. Fourthly, even in studies showing that suppression of inflammation is beneficial not all CF patients have benefited equally; for example, prednisolone was only useful in patients chronically infected with *P. aeruginosa*.[125] So the mantra "inflammation bad, anti-inflammation good" should not be applied uncritically. This section reviews the role in CF of currently available anti-inflammatory medications.

ORAL CORTICOSTEROIDS

An initial study stated that prednisolone in a dose of 2 mg/kg on alternate days was beneficial in CF, with no side effects.[123] This finding was tested in a multicenter, double-blind, and randomized controlled trial of prednisolone 2 mg/kg alternate days versus 1 mg/kg alternate days versus placebo.[125] Benefit was shown for both steroid-treated groups but only in patients chronically infected with *P. aeruginosa*. However, predictable side effects led to the high dose limb being halted after 2 years and the lower dose after 4 years. It is unknown whether a much lower dose of prednisolone might be beneficial (say, 5–10 mg/day) nor is that trial likely ever to be done. Currently, prednisolone as an anti-inflammatory agent can only be recommended in patients doing very badly on standard therapy. The high prevalence of CF bone disease, and the potential

role of prednisolone in pathogenesis, mandates extreme caution in the use of this medication unless there is clear likely benefit, for example, in ABPA. The potential immunosuppressive effects of corticosteroids should also not be overlooked. The Cochrane review[126] did not add anything, because there were insufficient studies to perform a meta-analysis. However, it highlighted growth effects, including catch-up growth not starting until 2 years after treatment had ceased and there likely being permanent growth retardation in males.[127,128] The US CFF recommends against the use of oral prednisolone to improve pulmonary function and reduce exacerbation rates in children, but it considered there was insufficient evidence in adults either for or against routine therapy.[102]

There is no place for the routine use of systemic steroids in infective exacerbations of CF. However, intravenous methyl prednisolone has been used with good effect in children with respiratory failure and severe hyperinflation thought to be due to severe inflammation in distal airways that was unresponsive to conventional treatment.[129]

INHALED CORTICOSTEROIDS

Inhaled corticosteroids (ICSs) have been widely prescribed in CF, often without much justification. Prior to the era of newborn screening, infants were sometimes prescribed ICSs because their symptoms were attributed to asthma before the correct diagnosis was made. The word "wheeze" is used very ambiguously, and another reason inhaled steroids are prescribed to known CF patients is the mistaken belief that the noise the patient or family is describing is related to bronchospasm, not airway secretions. Because CF is not known to be protective against asthma, one would expect by chance that 5%–10% of the CF clinic will have coincident asthma and benefit from ICS, but the diagnosis is very difficult to establish. Pointers in favor would be the presence of a personal or family history of atopy, acute reversibility to bronchodilator, (when available) a raised rather than the more characteristically lower than normal exhaled nitric oxide, and sputum eosinophilia. A recent large multicenter study of withdrawal of ICSs showed no evidence of harm, in terms of time to next exacerbation.[130] However, there was patient selection in the CF-WISE study; for ethical reasons, patients most likely to benefit from ICSs were excluded from the study.

The role of ICSs has been further explored in two database studies.[131,132] The first showed that initiation of ICSs was associated with a slowing of the rate of decline of spirometry, but reduced linear growth and increased use of insulin and oral hypoglycemic agents.[131] The patient age range was 6–17 years, and there were nearly 3000 patients in the study. A smaller study ($n = 852$ patients) showed benefit in terms of a lower rate of decline in FEV$_1$ only for children aged 6–12 years.[132] For all ages combined, baseline FEV$_1$ was lower in the ICS users, suggesting they had been selected as a subgroup not doing well, in whom treatment may also have been intensified in other ways.

Considering these apparently conflicting results, what are the indications for ICSs in CF? An unequivocal indication for using them in CF is if coincident asthma has been diagnosed, and in that context ICSs should be used exactly as if the patient has asthma.[133] This means that every effort should be made to document one or more features of asthma (earlier); if age is appropriate, the response should be assessed using a period of home peak flow monitoring; and at each clinic visit, an active decision should be taken as to whether the dose can be reduced. More controversial is their use in the generality of CF patients. The CF-WISE study shows clearly that ICSs have been overprescribed in CF patients in the United Kingdom, but it does not show that they should never be prescribed. The database studies may be confounded by reverse causation (patients doing badly started on ICSs and other treatments also intensified) but do at least suggest that ICSs should be considered in CF patients who are not doing well, in particular in school age. The Cochrane review[134] was unable to give definite recommendations; the US CFF has recommended against the general use of ICSs.[102]

However, high-dose ICSs may cause serious side effects such as hypoglycemia[135] and permanent growth retardation,[136] so caution with their use is mandatory. Fears have been expressed that inhaled steroids may actually increase the likelihood of infection with *P. aeruginosa*, leading to premature termination of a trial[137]; however, the result did not reach statistical significance and has not been replicated.[138] Nonetheless, ICSs have been shown in other contexts to increase the risk of pneumonia, tuberculosis, and atypical mycobacterial infection.[139–141]

MACROLIDES

There is considerable interest in the immunomodulatory and other properties of macrolides, which have been reviewed in detail elsewhere in the literature.[142] Diffuse panbronchiolitis is a neutrophilic disease that is similar to CF, which afflicts almost exclusively middle-aged people in the Far East.[143] Presentation is with cough, chronic sputum production, and breathlessness, with coarse crackles heard on auscultation. There is a mixed obstructive and restrictive pattern physiologically. High-resolution CT scanning reveals bronchiectasis. Sputum cultures are positive for *Haemophilus influenzae*; *S. aureus*; and, most strikingly, mucoid *P. aeruginosa*. Serendipitously, it became clear that long-term, low-dose erythromycin dramatically improved prognosis, changing 10-year survival from less than 20% to more than 90%.[144] A series of elegant studies established that diffuse panbronchiolitis is characterized by a neutrophilic bronchoalveolar lavage and that macrolide treatment therapy reduced lavage neutrophil chemoattractant activity and neutrophil counts.[145] Importantly, the response did not depend on the patient being chronically infected with mucoid *P. aeruginosa*.[146] Treatment with erythromycin or, if this fails, clarithromycin is essentially curative of a once fatal condition. This extraordinary result led to interest in the use of macrolides in CF, first in a series of case reports and a case study and then in randomized controlled trials. These have all been performed in school-aged children and adults; there is an ongoing study in newborn screened infants in Australasia, the results of which are keenly anticipated.

Since the first case reports and case series, randomized controlled trials have established the beneficial effects of azithromycin in CF, summarized in the Cochrane review.[147] Interestingly, clarithromycin appears to be ineffective.[148] It is noted that 10 of 31 studies summarized, amounting to nearly 1000 patients, showed that azithromycin therapy led to a mean increase in FEV_1 of just under 4% after 6 months of treatment. There was also a significant reduction in pulmonary exacerbations and antibiotic usage, with adverse events being infrequent. Any benefit is lost within 28 days of discontinuing therapy.[149] A number of important points arise from the various studies, some of which may help to elucidate mechanisms of benefit of macrolides, which are as yet unknown. CF patients who are not infected with *Pseudomonas* still derive benefit from treatment.[150] Even CF patients with essentially normal spirometry have a clinically and statistically significant reduction in pulmonary exacerbations.[151] There is marked individual variation in response to treatment.[152,153] There is little in the way of more long-term data, although in an open-label extension study benefit appeared to be maintained out to a year.[154] Emerging macrolide resistance is a concern, and there has been a suggestion based on in vitro data that azithromycin might select for atypical mycobacterial infection,[155] although a clinical effect has not been seen, and recent studies are reassuring in this respect.[156]

It is not clear which of the numerous actions of azithromycin are important in the benefit seen with macrolides in CF. It is clearly not correction of the electrophysiological defect.[157,158] Antipseudomonal effects seem unlikely to be important, given infection with this organism is not a prerequisite for benefit, although this is not to say that some such actions may not be therapeutically useful, such as reducing the minimal inhibitory concentration of antipseudomonal antibiotics in biofilms.[159] One study showed small reductions in systemic inflammatory markers with azithromycin, but the results were neither dramatic nor consistent within the study.[160] In patients with diffuse panbronchiolitis, benefit would appear to be related to reduction of airway neutrophilia. However, there is no reason to suppose the mechanism is necessarily the same in CF, and in fact no group has been able to identify the actual mechanism. There is a real practical need to find the mechanism; there are many hundreds of naturally occurring macrolides with differing properties, and a designer macrolide, targeting a specific mechanism, could be highly beneficial. Finally, it should be remembered that beneficial though azithromycin is in CF the extent of benefit falls well short of what is seen in diffuse panbronchiolitis. The results of the azithromycin studies should stimulate a search for a better macrolide.

The Cochrane review notes evidence of benefit from 6 months of therapy[147]; the US CFF recommends chronic macrolide therapy for all patients of 6 years and over to improve lung function and reduce exacerbations but surprisingly restricting therapy to those chronically infected with *P. aeruginosa*.[102] We recommend a trial of therapy for 6 months in those patients old enough to perform spirometry who have either impaired lung function or multiple pulmonary exacerbations, discontinuing if no benefit is seen. The optimum dosing regime is not known; most would use 250 mg in those < 40 kg of body weight and 500 mg in those ≥ 40 kg, either 3 days a week or daily.

NONSTEROIDAL ANTI-INFLAMMATORY AGENTS

A logical anti-inflammatory approach, given that oral steroids are too toxic and inhaled steroids are relatively ineffective, would be a nonsteroidal anti-inflammatory medication such as ibuprofen. The Cochrane review[161] was largely dominated by two randomized controlled studies[162,163] and suggested that ibuprofen slowed the rate of decline of lung function, particularly in young children (in a post hoc analysis). Major adverse events were not reported, but the power of the review was not sufficiently great to be confident of safety. However, in the first major ibuprofen trial[162] the dose was carefully titrated and it was impossible to predict blood levels, so these had to be measured. There is animal data that high-dose ibuprofen is anti-inflammatory, but low-dose ibuprofen may be proinflammatory[164]; so, at least in theory, regular monitoring is necessary.

Confirmatory data for a beneficial role of ibuprofen came from an analysis of the US registry data.[165] The authors compared 1365 CF patients treated with ibuprofen with 8690 untreated controls with a similar baseline level of disease severity and showed there was a slower rate of decline in spirometry in the ibuprofen group. There was a small increased risk of acute gastrointestinal hemorrhage with ibuprofen, which was not thought to outweigh the benefits of active treatment. By contrast, a pragmatic, single center study showed no benefit with ibuprofen therapy[166]; furthermore, nearly half the patients discontinued therapy because of side effects. In addition to gastrointestinal bleeding, ibuprofen may contribute to acute renal failure, especially with concurrent aminoglycoside treatment.[167–169]

Overall, the role of ibuprofen in CF is unclear, and more data are needed. Complications are probably rare but devastating when they occur. The need to monitor blood levels, and the theoretical risk of doing harm if the dose is wrong, also indicates the need for caution. At the moment, we cannot recommend ibuprofen as a routine CF therapy. But the US CFF in fact does, although acknowledging the evidence is not conclusive[102]; there may be scope for related but safer agents to be used in the future. The ibuprofen studies do, however, provide further proof of concept that anti-inflammatory strategies may be useful in CF.

OTHERS

The US CFF concluded there was insufficient evidence to recommend leukotriene receptor antagonists and cromolyns as routine therapies.[102]

RHDNASE AS AN ANTI-INFLAMMATORY AGENT

The strong physiological evidence for benefit of rhDNase therapy has been reviewed earlier. There have been suggestions in the literature of both pro- and anti-inflammatory effects. An initial in vitro study suggested that addition of bovine rhDNase to CF sputum led to the release of IL-8, which had been bound to DNA by electrostatic forces.[170] However, a 3-month trial of rhDNase also looked at the change in sputum IL-8 and neutrophil elastase levels and showed no change.[171] A recent study has suggested that there may be an additional, anti-inflammatory benefit of rhDNase.[172] There was no effect on inflammation in those who had no neutrophilia in the initial lavage. In those with an initial neutrophilia who were randomized to rhDNase, there was no increase in lavage neutrophils; the placebo group showed increasing neutrophilia. It could be that the known effect of rhDNase in reducing exacerbations could have led to fewer neutrophils in the airway; unfortunately, exacerbations were not reported. More recently, it was shown that dornase alfa therapy reduces markers of inflammation and neutrophil-associated metalloproteins in CF, suggesting a potential benefit from using this therapy early in the disease.[65,66,80,173,174]

BRONCHODILATORS

Hypersensitivity of the airways in CF has long been recognized,[175] and many patients with CF wheeze. This may be due to bronchospasm, mucosal edema, or retained secretions in the airways. In such cases, ABPA and gastroesophageal reflux should be excluded or treated and reversible airflow obstruction sought.

β-Adrenergic agonists enhance ciliary beat frequency and may affect mucus secretion.[176] Terbutaline has been shown to stimulate chloride ion secretion in the lumen and may increase hydration of the airway.[177] All patients with CF should be tested to see if their spirometry improves after the use of a bronchodilator.[178–182] Patients should have the bronchodilator stopped if no benefit is demonstrated. More than half the patients in the European and US databases are taking regular bronchodilators.[183,184] During acute exacerbations patients may benefit from a bronchodilator, and there is evidence, in some cases, that intravenous administration may be more beneficial.[185]

Long-acting β-agonists have also been shown to be beneficial in some patients,[186–189] but long-term studies are required. The Cochrane review concluded that short-term and long-acting β-2 agonists can be beneficial in both the short term and the long term in individuals with demonstrable bronchodilator response.[190] Theophylline increases MCC, diaphragmatic contractivity, and central nervous system drive[191] and may also be anti-inflammatory, at least in the context of asthma in the non-CF patient in low dose.[192] It is of interest that theophyllines reduce neutrophil chemotaxis and thus airway inflammation in a more relevant model, namely, chronic obstructive pulmonary disease,[193] possibly also by inducing neutrophil apoptosis,[194] and they may restore steroid sensitivity,[195] all of which could be highly relevant in CF. However, there are no in vivo CF data to match these intriguing results. If theophylline is to be used in CF, careful monitoring is required to avoid toxicity, especially nausea and vomiting. Some studies have shown theophylline to be beneficial.[196–198] Intravenous aminophylline can be helpful in acute exacerbations associated with carbon dioxide retention.

NOVEL THERAPIES

Here, we discuss briefly the anecdotal use of non-CF-specific treatments that have been used more extensively in other contexts and that may bring unexpected benefit to the occasional patient.

POTENTIAL CURRENT OPTIONS

Intravenous immunoglobulin infusions

Intravenous immunoglobulin (IVIG) has been used in asthma with questionable benefit. A case series has shown that IVIG in selected patients may allow reduction of steroid dosage, with no deterioration in lung function.[199] Our current practice in CF children is to use a 6-month trial in those with particularly distal airway disease, with minor or no sputum production and not much proximal bronchiectasis. Response is unpredictable but occasionally dramatic.

Cytotoxic agents

CF patients who have undergone orthotopic liver transplantation may show stabilization or even improvement in lung function. One of several possible explanations is the posttransplant use of immunosuppressive agents. There are a few anecdotal reports of the use of immunosuppression with methotrexate[200] and cyclosporin A[201] in the pretransplant stage. Intravenous cyclosporin A has been used in combination with intravenous antibiotics and oral prednisolone to treat cepacia syndrome.[202] Clearly, they all have side effects, and the risks of a therapeutic trial must be balanced against benefit. In particular, cyclosporin is nephrotoxic and may therefore worsen aminoglycoside and diabetes-associated renal impairment. The recently developed nebulized preparations of cyclosporin may offer a useful therapy for the future.[203] The potential for opportunistic infections, including invasive aspergillosis, must not be forgotten if immunosuppression is intensified.[204]

MANAGEMENT OF THE CYSTIC FIBROSIS PATIENT NEEDING SURGERY

Surgery may be needed as a result of CF-related complications (e.g., nasal polyps and insertion of gastrostomy) or for an unrelated condition. In all cases, the anesthetic and surgical team should liaise closely with the CF center. Such close liaison may even preclude the need for surgery, for example, medical management of distal intestinal obstruction syndrome (DIOS) may obviate the need for a laparotomy.

The ideal is for procedures to be performed close to the CF unit, by surgeons and anesthetists who are familiar with CF and the treatment protocols. If this is not possible, the members of the whole CF multidisciplinary team need to liaise with their counterparts in the surgical service, to ensure airway clearance and nutritional and gastrointestinal issues are not neglected just because the patient is undergoing an orthopedic procedure for a fracture. As with much of CF care, recommendations are not evidence based. It is also important that at all stages routine care and detection of complications is not neglected because the team is preoccupied with CF-related issues.

PREOPERATIVE PLANNING

If a CF patient is to have a general anesthetic, it is worth briefly considering whether other procedures should be performed opportunistically, particularly obtaining lower airway secretions from a patient who is unable to expectorate. This may be by either blind suction below the vocal cords performed by the anesthetist or fiber-optic bronchoscopy. If surgery is performed away from the CF center, it is essential that the sample is cultured in a CF-accredited microbiology. We have also used the opportunity of a general anesthetic to perform research bronchoscopy, with appropriate ethical approval, informed consent from the carers, and age-appropriate assent from the child.

PREOPERATIVE ASSESSMENT OF THE PATIENT

General

Ideally, the anesthetist and the CF physician should jointly see the patient. If this is not possible, at least a discussion of the current CF issues should take place. However, these should not distract from the routine preoperative checks normally carried out by the anesthetist. In addition, there are a number of special CF-related issues that should be considered.

RESPIRATORY ISSUES

Preoperative oxygen saturation in all CF patients, and spirometry in all those over age 5, should be recorded unless pain or another severe illness precludes this. All results should be compared with the patient's usual values at the CF center. For elective procedures, the patient's respiratory status should be optimized with intensive physiotherapy and antibiotics in particular. It is wise to obtain a sputum or cough swab culture prior to surgery, where this is practical. For all but minor procedures in well patients, a course of intravenous antibiotics should be considered, starting at least 48 hours prior to the procedure and continuing until the patient is pain free and has made a complete recovery. The anesthetist should enquire about current or past oral or high-dose ICS therapy; the need for per- and postoperative steroid treatment should be judged on standard criteria. If there is any doubt about the patient's respiratory status, a preoperative chest x-ray should be obtained to exclude a pneumothorax, or localized collapse, which might be treated with preoperative bronchoscopy. The possibility of bronchospasm should be considered, although this is rare.

OTHER ISSUES

Nutritional status should be assessed and postponement of all but emergency surgery considered if there is scope for optimizing this. Sodium and potassium depletion, with metabolic alkalosis, is not uncommon in hot weather,[204,205] and urea and electrolytes may need to be measured and any imbalance corrected. Any constipation or DIOS should be treated vigorously, to avoid postoperative bowel obstruction. Gastroesophageal reflux is common in CF, and it should be noted whether this is present. CF patients on insulin should be managed using standard insulin-dependent diabetes protocols, but the anesthetist should be aware that the stress of surgery may precipitate hyperglycemia in the CF patient with borderline endocrine pancreatic function. Diabetic ketoacidosis is not a usual feature of CF-related diabetes. Finally, the potential for drug interaction should be noted. The patient is usually already taking several other medications; there may be liver disease (which may also cause clotting factor deficiency, and thrombocytopenia if there is also hypersplenism) and renal insufficiency, particularly if multiple previous courses of aminoglycosides have been prescribed[206] or the patient has CF-related diabetes.[207]

PEROPERATIVE MANAGEMENT

Although gastroesophageal reflux is common, aspiration during anesthesia is rare and there is no need to routinely use a rapid-sequence induction. Suxamethonium should probably be avoided because this agent may cause postoperative pain, which will impede physiotherapy. Standard peroperative monitoring is performed. The patient should be ventilated in such a way as to prevent as far as possible postoperative

atelectasis. The anesthetist should be aware of the possibility of the buildup of secretions causing V:Q mismatch, or even blocking the endotracheal tube. In general, peroperative chest physiotherapy while the patient is anesthetized has not been shown to be useful.[208] Pre- and postoperatively, oxygen and other inhaled gases should be humidified. Drugs that might cause postoperative suppression of cough, or constipation, should be avoided. Consideration should be given to inserting a regional blockade with, for example, marcaine, while the patient is still anesthetized.

POSTOPERATIVE CARE

Adequate pain relief without cough suppression, to ensure efficient airway clearance, is essential. The continued close involvement of expert physiotherapists for airway clearance and mobilization of the patient is crucial. Opiates and dehydration may predispose to constipation, which should be treated aggressively to avoid progression to subacute bowel obstruction. If the postoperative phase is prolonged and nutrition is difficult, a nasogastric tube can be used for feeding using a predigested feed. If a prolonged period of ileus or other cause of failure of enteral nutrition is anticipated, then total parenteral nutrition should be instituted early. It is better for the patient to have adequate calories than to worry about the theoretical effects of intravenous intralipid on pulmonary gas exchange.

TRAVELING AND THE CYSTIC FIBROSIS PATIENT

Increasing numbers of adolescents and adults with CF wish to travel, often for long distances. This should be encouraged if their health permits. They should be advised to take travel insurance, making sure CF is covered. They should take with them a letter documenting regular medications, lung function, and sputum microbiology in case they need to see a doctor abroad. It is sensible to take contact details of the nearest CF center. Medication should be carried in hand baggage in case the flight is delayed. Certainly all medications required in flight must be in the hand baggage. Patients should take with them the medications they are expected to need while away from home, together with a reserve supply of appropriate antibiotics. A letter should list any medications and air compressors, needles, and or syringes that they may be carrying. Usually, patients should have all appropriate immunizations advised for healthy travelers. However, immunosuppressed transplant patients should avoid live vaccines. Patients visiting hot countries should take salt supplements. Patients with CF are advised to visit countries with good health-care services should they become ill. *Burkholderia pseudomallei*, which is found in Thailand, Malaysia, Vietnam, and Northern Australia, can cause severe pneumonia and patients are advised to avoid these areas.[209]

Commercial aircraft cruise between 10,000 and 50,000 ft above sea level. The cabin pressure is approximately 5,000–6,000 ft above sea level, and the partial pressure of oxygen is reduced to 80% of the sea-level values, e.g., a patient who already has a PaO_2 of 9.6 kPa will drop to 6.3 kPa or less at an altitude to 8,000 ft after breathing air for 45 minutes.[210] The drop will be greater if the patient falls asleep,[211] and in noncommercial flights the airplane cabin may not be pressurized and an even lower FiO_2 may be encountered. Both the American Thoracic Society[212] and the British Thoracic Society[213] guidelines recommend that a PaO_2 > 6.6 kPa (50 mmHg) be maintained during flight. Patients with a sea-level PaO_2 < 9.30 kPa or SaO_2 of 92% should be advised to have oxygen in flight. However, it has been pointed out that chronically hypoxic CF patients are often asymptomatic at these levels.[214] It has been recommended that CF patients with a baseline FEV_1 < 60% and PaO_2 < 10.5kPA are most likely to need in-flight oxygen.[215] It is recommended that a hypoxic inhalation test is carried out on this group of patients using 15% oxygen and 85% nitrogen breathed for 15minutes. If the saturation drops below 85%, the CF patient should have oxygen in flight. It should be acknowledged that the risk of short periods of hypoxia in a CF patient is unknown and that obtaining oxygen for flights on commercial airlines may be expensive; however, the cost of diverting a commercial jet because someone has become unwell may be more than £20,000 and cause inconvenience to other passengers, so flight assessments should not be undertaken lightly. The British Thoracic Society has recently updated its guidelines on fitness to fly.[31]

It has been reported that patients who went on skiing holidays at high altitude without consulting their clinicians developed right ventricular failure.[204] When discussing holiday arrangements with patients, clinicians should take into account the altitude they wish to visit. Patients with any pneumothorax should not fly—it will expand as the aircraft altitude rises, unless effectively drained. Patients attending a CF unit should be encouraged to discuss their holiday arrangements with their physician so that all the aforementioned issues can be fully discussed.

VIDEO

- *Video 18.1 (http://goo.gl/Oa0t9E)*: Bronchial arterial embolization in a patient with life theatening hemoptsis.

REFERENCES

1. Schidlow DV, Taussig LM, Knowles MR. Cystic Fibrosis Foundation consensus conference report on pulmonary complications of cystic fibrosis. *Pediatr Pulmonol* 1993; **15**: 187–198.
2. Flume PA, Yankaskas JR, Ebeling M, Hulsey T, Clark LL. Massive hemoptysis in cystic fibrosis. *Chest* 2005; **128**: 729–38.
3. Youssef AI, Escalante-Glorsky S, Bonnet RB, Chen YK. Hemoptysis secondary to bronchial varices associated with alcoholic liver cirrhosis and portal hypertension. *Am J Gastroenterol* 1994; **89**: 1562–3.
4. Sosa Lozano LA, Shahir K, Akbar M, Goodman LR. A case of tracheal varices: An unusual but important cause of mural nodules in the trachea. *Br J Radiol* 2011; **84**: 262–4.
5. Flume PA, Mogayzel PJ, Jr., Robinson KA, Rosenblatt RL, Quittell L, Marshall BC; Clinical Practice Guidelines for Pulmonary Therapies Committee; Cystic Fibrosis Foundation Pulmonary Therapies Committee. Cystic fibrosis pulmonary guidelines: Pulmonary complications: Hemoptysis and pneumothorax. *Am J Respir Crit Care Med* 2010; **182**: 298–306.
6. Magee G, Williams MH, Jr. Treatment of massive hemoptysis with intravenous pitressin. *Lung* 1982; **160**: 165–9.
7. Bilton D, Webb AK, Foster H et al. Life threatening haemoptysis in cystic fibrosis: An alternative therapeutic approach. *Thorax* 1990; **45**: 975–6.
8. Graff GR. Treatment of recurrent severe hemoptysis in cystic fibrosis with tranexamic acid. *Respiration* 2001; **68**: 91–4.
9. Hurley M, Bhatt J, Smyth A. Treatment massive haemoptysis in cystic fibrosis with tranexamic acid. *J R Soc Med* 2011; **104**(Suppl 1): S49–52.
10. Moua J, Nussbaum E, Liao E, Randhawa IS. Beta-blocker management of refractory hemoptysis in cystic fibrosis: A novel treatment approach. *Ther Adv Respir Dis* 2013; **7**: 217–23. PMID: 23539159.
11. Fairfax AJ, Ball J, Batten JC et al. A pathological study following bronchial artery embolization for haemoptysis in cystic fibrosis. *Br J Dis Chest* 1980; **74**: 345–52.
12. Sweezey NB, Fellows KE. Bronchial artery embolization for severe hemoptysis in cystic fibrosis. *Chest* 1990; **97**: 1322–6.
13. Stern RC, Wood RE, Boat TF et al. Treatment and prognosis of massive hemoptysis in cystic fibrosis. *Am Rev Respir Dis* 1978; **117**: 825–8.
14. Cohen AM. Haemoptysis—role of angiography and embolisation. *Pediatr Pulmonol* 1992; **S8**: 85–6.
15. Daliri A, Probst NH, Jobst B, Lepper PM, Kickuth R, Szucs-Farkas Z et al. Bronchial artery embolization in patients with hemoptysis including follow-up. *Acta Radiol* 2011; **52**: 143–7.
16. Barben J, Robertson D, Olinsky A et al. Bronchial artery embolization for hemoptysis in young patients with cystic fibrosis. *Radiology* 2002; **224**: 124–30.
17. Pestana Knight EM, Novelli PM, Joshi SM. Cerebral and systemic infarcts after bronchial artery embolization. *Pediatr Neurol* 2011; **45**: 324–7.
18. Hurt K, Bilton D. Haemoptysis: Diagnosis and treatment. *Acute Med* 2012; **11**: 39–45.

19. Schramel FM, Postmus PE, Vanderschueren RG. Current aspects of spontaneous pneumothorax. *Eur Respir J* 1997; **10**: 372–9.

20. Penketh AR, Knight RK, Hodson ME et al. Management of pneumothorax in adults with cystic fibrosis. *Thorax* 1982; **37**: 850–3.

21. Spector ML, Stern RC. Pneumothorax in cystic fibrosis: A 26-year experience. *Ann Thorac Surg* 1989; **47**: 204–7.

22. Flume PA, Strange C, Ye X et al. Pneumothorax in cystic fibrosis. *Chest* 2005; **128**: 720–8.

23. Flume PA. Pneumothorax in cystic fibrosis. *Curr Opin Pulm Med* 2011 Jul; **17**(4): 220–5. doi: 10.1097/MCP.0b013e328345e1f8.

24. MacDuff A, Arnold A, Harvey J; BTS Pleural Disease Guideline Group. Management of spontaneous pneumothorax: British Thoracic Society Pleural Disease Guideline 2010. *Thorax* 2010; **65**(Suppl 2): ii18–31.

25. Amin R, Noone PG, Ratjen F. Chemical pleurodesis versus surgical intervention for persistent and recurrent pneumothoraces in cystic fibrosis. *Cochrane Database Syst Rev* 2012 Dec 12; **12**: CD007481.

26. Rolla M, D'Andrilli A, Rendina EA, Diso D, Venuta F. Cystic fibrosis and the thoracic surgeon. *Eur J Cardiothorac Surg* 2011; **39**: 716–25.

27. O'Lone E, Elphick HE, Robinson PJ. Spontaneous pneumothorax in children: When is invasive treatment indicated? *Pediatr Pulmonol* 2008; **43**: 41–6.

28. Northfield TC. Oxygen therapy for spontaneous pneumothorax. *Br Med J* 1971; **4**(779): 86–8.

29. Miller WC, Toon R, Palat H et al. Experimental pulmonary edema following re-expansion of pneumothorax. *Am Rev Respir Dis* 1973; **108**: 654–6.

30. Haworth CS, Dodd ME, Atkins M et al. Pneumothorax in adults with cystic fibrosis dependent on nasal intermittent positive pressure ventilation (NIPPV): A management dilemma. *Thorax* 2000; **55**: 620–2.

31. Shrikrishna D, Coker RK; Air Travel Working Party of the British Thoracic Society Standards of Care Committee. Managing passengers with stable respiratory disease planning air travel: British Thoracic Society recommendations. *Thorax* 2011; **66**: 831–3.

32. Davies J, Chaudry R, Larovere J, Hansell D, Dawson M, Abrahamson E. Cystic fibrosis presenting as acute upper airway obstruction. *Thorax* 2006; **61**: 92.

33. Sutrave H, Ward A, Smyth AR, Bhatt J. Pneumomediastinum as a presenting feature of allergic bronchopulmonary aspergillosis in a child with cystic fibrosis. *J R Soc Med* 2012; **105**(Suppl 2): S36–9.

34. Flight WG, Hildage J, Webb AK. Progressive unilateral lung collapse in cystic fibrosis—a diagnostic challenge. *J R Soc Med* 2012; **105**: S44–9.

35. Cakir E, Uyan ZS, Ersu RH, Karadag F, Dagli E. Mucoid impaction: An unusual form of allergic bronchopulmonary aspergillosis in a patient with cystic fibrosis. *Pediatr Pulmonol* 2006; **41**: 1103–7.

36. Colin A, Tsiligiannis T, Nose V, Waltz DA. Membranous obliterative bronchitis: A proposed unifying model. *Pediatr Pulmonol* 2006; **41**: 126–32.

37. Shah PL, Scott S, Hodson ME. Lobar atelectasis in cystic fibrosis and treatment with recombinant human Dnase 1. *Respir Med* 1994; **88**: 313–5.

38. Slattery DM, Waltz DA, Denham B, O'Mahoney M, Greally P. Bronchoscopically administered human Dnase for lobar atelectasis in cystic fibrosis. *Pediatr Pulmonol* 2001; **31**: 383–8.

39. McLaughlin AM, McGrath E, Barry R, Egan JJ, Gallagher CG. Treatment of lobar atelectasis with bronchoscopically administered recombinant human deoxyribonuclease in cystic fibrosis? *Clin Respir J* 2008; **2**: 123–6.

40. Lucas J, Connett GJ, Lea R, Rolles CJ, Warner JO. Lung resection in cystic fibrosis patients with localised pulmonary disease. *Arch Dis Child* 1996; **74**: 449–51.

41. Camargos P, Le Bourgeois M, Revillon Y et al. Lung resection in cystic fibrosis: A survival analysis. *Pediatr Pulmonol* 2008; **43**: 72–6.

42. Lucas J, Connett G, Fairhurst J. Long term results of lung resection in cystic fibrosis patients with localised lung disease. *Arch Dis Child* 2002; **86**; 66.

43. Coffey MJ, FitzGerald MX, McNicholas WT. Comparison of oxygen desaturation during sleep and exercise in patients with cystic fibrosis. *Chest* 1991; **100**: 659–62.

44. Stern RC, Borkat G, Hirschfeld SS et al. Heart failure in cystic fibrosis. Treatment and prognosis of cor pulmonale with failure of the right side of the heart. *Am J Dis Child* 1980; **134**: 267–72.

45. Bright-Thomas RJ, Webb AK. The heart in cystic fibrosis. *J R Soc Med* 2002; **95**(Suppl 41): 2–10.

46. Henno P, Maurey C, Danel C, Bonnette P, Souilamas R, Stern M et al. Pulmonary vascular dysfunction in end-stage cystic fibrosis: Role of NF-kappa B and endothelin-1. *Eur Respir J* 2009; **34**: 1329–37.

47. Venuta F, Tonelli AR, Anile M, Diso D, De Giacomo T, Ruberto F et al. Pulmonary hypertension is associated with higher mortality in cystic fibrosis patients awaiting lung transplantation. *J Cardiovasc Surg (Torino)* 2012; **53**: 817–20.

48. Fauroux B, Hart N, Belfar S, Boulé M, Tillous-Borde I, Bonnet D et al. *Burkholderia cepacia* is associated with pulmonary hypertension and increased mortality among cystic fibrosis patients. *J Clin Microbiol* 2004; **42**: 5537–41.

49. Zinman R, Corey M, Coates AL et al. Nocturnal home oxygen in the treatment of hypoxemic cystic fibrosis patients. *J Pediatr* 1989; **114**: 368–77.

50. Baño-Rodrigo A, Salcedo-Posadas A, Villa-Asensi JR, Tamariz-Martel A, Lopez-Neyra A, Blanco-Iglesias E. Right ventricular dysfunction in adolescents with mild cystic fibrosis. *J Cyst Fibros* 2012; **11**: 274–80.

51. Florea VG, Florea ND, Sharma R et al. Right ventricular dysfunction in adult severe cystic fibrosis. *Chest* 2000; **118**: 1063–8.

52. Burghuber OC, Hartter E, Weissel M et al. Raised circulating plasma levels of atrial natriuretic peptide in adolescent and adult patients with cystic fibrosis and pulmonary artery hypertension. *Lung* 1991; **169**: 291–300.

53. Selimovic N, Andersson B, Bech-Hanssen O, Lomsky M, Riise GC, Rundqvist B. Right ventricular ejection fraction during exercise as a predictor of mortality in patients awaiting lung transplantation: A cohort study. *Br Med J Open* 2013 Apr 8; **3**(4): e002108.

54. Ketchell RL, Gyi KM, Badawi R et al. Cardiac compromise in end-stage cystic fibrosis. *Pediatric Pulmonol* 2004; **38**(S27): 312.

55. Sullivan MM, Moss RB, Hindi RD et al. Supraventricular tachycardia in patients with cystic fibrosis. *Chest* 1986; **90**: 239–42.

56. Perrin FM, Serino W. Ischaemic heart disease—a new issue in cystic fibrosis? *J R Soc Med* 2010 Jul; **103**(Suppl 1): S44–8.

57. Collins N, Gupta A, Wright S, Gauld L, Urquhart D, Bush A. Survey of the use of non-invasive positive pressure ventilation in UK and Australasian children with cystic fibrosis. *Thorax* 2011; **66**: 538–9.

58. Yu H, Burton B, Huang CJ et al. Ivacaftor potentiation of multiple CFTR channels with gating mutations. *J Cyst Fibros* 2012; **11**: 237–45.

59. Jones A, Bilton D, Evans TW, Finney SJ. Predictors of outcome in patients with cystic fibrosis requiring endotracheal intubation. *Respirology* 2013; **18**: 630–6.

60. Urquhart DS, Thia LP, Francis J et al. Deaths in childhood from cystic fibrosis: 10-Year analysis from two London specialist centres. *Arch Dis Child* 2013; **98**: 123–7.

61. Texereau J, Jamal D, Choukroun G et al. Determinants of mortality for adults with cystic fibrosis admitted in Intensive Care Unit: A multicentre study. *Respir Res* 2006; **7**: 14.

62. Ranasinha C, Assoufi B, Shak S et al. Efficacy and safety of short-term administration of aerosolised recombinant human DNase I in adults with stable stage cystic fibrosis. *Lancet* 1993; **342**: 199–202.

63. Ramsey BW, Astley SJ, Aitken ML et al. Efficacy and safety of short-term administration of aerosolized recombinant human deoxyribonuclease in patients with cystic fibrosis. *Am Rev Respir Dis* 1993; **148**: 145–51.

64. Fuchs HJ, Borowitz DS, Christiansen DH et al. Effect of aerosolized recombinant human DNase on exacerbations of respiratory symptoms and on pulmonary function in patients with cystic fibrosis. The Pulmozyme Study Group. *N Engl J Med* 1994; **331**: 637–42.

65. Accurso FJ. Aerosolised dornase alfa in cystic fibrosis patients with clinically mild lung disease. *Dornase Alfa Clinical Series* 2006; **2**: 1–6.

66. Quan JM, Tiddens HA, Sy JP et al. A two-year randomized, placebo-controlled trial of dornase alfa in young patients with cystic fibrosis with mild lung function abnormalities. *J Pediatr* 2001; **139**: 813–20.

67. Shah PI, Bush A, Canny GJ et al. Recombinant human DNase I in cystic fibrosis patients with severe pulmonary disease: A short-term, double-blind study followed by six months open-label treatment. *Eur Respir J* 1995; **8**: 954–8.

68. McCoy K, Hamilton S, Johnson C. Effects of 12-week administration of dornase alfa in patients with advanced cystic fibrosis lung disease. Pulmozyme Study Group. *Chest* 1996; **110**: 889–95.

69. Shah PL, Scott SF, Geddes DM et al. Two years experience with recombinant human DNase I in the treatment of pulmonary disease in cystic fibrosis. *Respir Med* 1995; **89**: 499–502.

70. Shah PL, Conway S, Scott SF et al. A case-controlled study with dornase alfa to evaluate impact on disease progression over a 4-year period. *Respiration* 2001; **68**: 160–4.

71. Hodson ME, McKenzie S, Harms HK et al. Dornase alfa in the treatment of cystic fibrosis in Europe: A report from the Epidemiologic Registry of Cystic Fibrosis. *Pediatr Pulmonol* 2003; **36**: 427–32.

72. McKenzie SG, Chowdhury S, Strandvik B, Hodson ME; Investigators of the Epidemiologic Registry of Cystic Fibrosis. Dornase alfa is well tolerated: Data from the epidemiologic registry of cystic fibrosis. *Pediatr Pulmonol* 2007; **42**: 928–37.

73. Fitzgerald DA, Hilton J, Jepson B et al. A crossover, randomized, controlled trial of dornase alfa before versus after physiotherapy in cystic fibrosis. *Pediatrics* 2005; **116**: e549–54.

74. Dentice R, Elkins M. Timing of dornase alfa inhalation for cystic fibrosis. *Cochrane Database Syst Rev* 2011; (5): CD007923.

75. Bakker EM, Volpi S, Salonini E, van der Wiel-Kooij EC, Sintnicolaas CJ, Hop WC et al. Improved treatment response to dornase alfa in cystic fibrosis patients using controlled inhalation. *Eur Respir J* 2011; **38**: 1328–35.

76. Amin R, Subbarao P, Lou W, Jabar A, Balkovec S, Jensen R et al. The effect of dornase alfa on ventilation inhomogeneity in patients with cystic fibrosis. *Eur Respir J* 2011; **37**: 806–12.

186. Bargon J, Viel K, Dauletbaev N et al. Short-term effects of regular salmeterol treatment on adult cystic fibrosis patients. *Eur Respir J* 1997; **10**: 2307–11.

187. Hordvik NL, Sammut PH, Judy CG et al. Effects of standard and high doses of salmeterol on lung function of hospitalized patients with cystic fibrosis. *Pediatr Pulmonol* 1999; **27**: 43–53.

188. Salvatore D, D'Andria M. Effects of salmeterol on arterial oxyhemoglobin saturations in patients with cystic fibrosis. *Pediatr Pulmonol* 2002; **34**: 11–5.

189. Hordvik NL, Sammut PH, Judy CG, Colombo JL. Effectiveness and tolerability of high-dose salmeterol in cystic fibrosis. *Pediatr Pulmonol* 2002; **34**: 287–96.

190. Halfhide C, Evans HJ, Couriel J. Inhaled bronchodilators for cystic fibrosis. *Cochrane Database Syst Rev* 2005 Oct 19; (4): CD003428.

191. Vaz Fragoso CA, Miller MA. Review of the clinical efficacy of theophylline in the treatment of chronic obstructive pulmonary disease. *Am Rev Respir Dis* 1993; **147**: S40–7.

192. Lim S, Tomita K, Caramori G, Jatakanon A, Oliver B, Keller A et al. Low-dose theophylline reduces eosinophilic inflammation but not exhaled nitric oxide in mild asthma. *Am J Respir Crit Care Med* 2001; **164**: 273–6.

193. Culpitt SV, de Matos C, Russell RE, Donnelly LE, Rogers DF, Barnes PJ. Effect of theophylline on induced sputum inflammatory indices and neutrophil chemotaxis in chronic obstructive pulmonary disease. *Am J Respir Crit Care Med* 2002; **165**: 1371–6.

194. Yasui K, Agematsu K, Shinozaki K, Hokibara S, Nagumo H, Nakazawa T et al. Theophylline induces neutrophil apoptosis through adenosine A2A receptor antagonism. *J Leukoc Biol* 2000; **67**: 529–35.

195. To Y, Ito K, Kizawa Y, Failla M, Ito M, Kusama T et al. Targeting phosphoinositide-3-kinase-delta with theophylline reverses corticosteroid insensitivity in chronic obstructive pulmonary disease. *Am J Respir Crit Care Med* 2010; **182**: 897–904.

196. Larsen GL, Barron RJ, Landay RA, Cotton EK, Gonzalez MA, Brooks JG. Intravenous aminophylline in patients with cystic fibrosis. Pharmacokinetics and effect on pulmonary function. *Am J Dis Child* 1980; **134**: 1143–8.

197. Pan SH, Canafax DM, Le CT et al. Bronchodilation from intravenous theophylline in patients with cystic fibrosis: Results of a blinded placebo-controlled crossover clinical trial. *Pediatr Pulmonol* 1989; **6**: 172–9.

198. Yankaskas JR, Marshall BC, Sufian B et al. Cystic fibrosis adult care: Consensus conference report. *Chest* 2004; **125**(Suppl 1): 1S–39S.

199. Balfour-Lynn I, Mohan U, Bush A, Rosenthal M. Intravenous immunoglobulin for cystic fibrosis lung disease: A case series of 16 children. *Arch Dis Child* 2004; **89**: 315–9.

200. Bhal GK, Maguire SA, Bowler IM. Use of cyclosporin A as a steroid sparing agent in cystic fibrosis. *Arch Dis Child* 2001; **84**: 89.

201. Gilchrist FJ, Webb AK, Bright-Thomas RJ, Jones AM. Successful treatment of cepacia syndrome with a combination of intravenous cyclosporine, antibiotics and oral corticosteroids. *J Cyst Fibros* 2012; **11**: 458–60.

202. Iacono AT, Johnson BA, Grgurich WF et al. A randomised trial of inhaled cyclosporine in lung-transplant recipients. *N Engl J Med* 2006; **354**: 141–50.

203. Brown K, Rosenthal M, Bush A. Fatal invasive aspergillosis in an adolescent with cystic fibrosis. *Pediatr Pulmonol* 1999; **27**: 130–3.

204. Speechly-Dick ME, Rimmer SJ, Hodson ME. Exacerbations of cystic fibrosis after holidays at high altitude—a cautionary tale. *Respir Med* 1992; **86**: 55–6.

205. Kennedy JD, Dinwiddie R, Daman-Willems C, Dillon MJ, Matthew DJ. Pseudo-Bartter's syndrome in cystic fibrosis. *Arch Dis Child* 1990; **65**: 786–7.

206. Al-Aloul M, Miller H, Alapati S, Stockton PA, Ledson MJ, Walshaw M. Renal impairment in cystic fibrosis patients due to repeated intravenous aminoglycoside use. *Pediatr Pulmonol* 2005; **39**: 15–30.

207. Quon BS, Mayer-Hamblett N, Aitken ML, Smyth AR, Goss CH. Risk factors for chronic kidney disease in adults with cystic fibrosis. *Am J Respir Crit Care Med* 2011; **184**: 1147–52.

208. Tannenbaum E, Prasad SA, Main E, Stocks J. The effect of chest physiotherapy on cystic fibrosis patients undergoing general anaesthesia for an elective surgical procedure. *Pediatr Pulmonol* 2001; (Suppl 22) **32**: 315.

209. Hirche TO, Bradley J, d'Alquen D, De Boeck K, Dembski B, Elborn JS et al.; European Centres of Reference Network for Cystic Fibrosis (ECORN-CF) Study Group. Travelling with cystic fibrosis: Recommendations for patients and care team members. *J Cyst Fibros* 2010; **9**: 385–99.

210. Dillard TA, Berg BW, Rajagopal KR et al. Hypoxemia during air travel in patients with chronic obstructive pulmonary disease. *Ann Intern Med* 1989; **111**: 362–7.

211. BuchdahlRM, Babiker A, Bush A, Cramer D. Predicting hypoxaemia during flights in children with cystic fibrosis. *Thorax* 2001; **56**: 877–9.

212. Standards for the diagnosis and care of patients with chronic obstructive pulmonary disease (COPD) and asthma. This official statement of the American

Thoracic Society was adopted by the ATS Board of Directors, November 1986. *Am Rev Respir Dis* 1987; **136**: 225–44.

213. British Thoracic Society Standards of Care Committee. Managing passengers with respiratory disease planning air travel: British Thoracic Society recommendations. *Thorax* 2002; **57**: 289–304.

214. Fischer R, Lang SM, Bruckner K et al. Lung function in adults with cystic fibrosis at altitude: Impact on air travel. *Eur Respir J* 2005; **25**: 718–24.

215. Peckham D, Watson A, Pollard K et al. Predictors of desaturation during formal hypoxic challenge in adult patients with cystic fibrosis. *J Cyst Fibros* 2002; **1**: 281–6.

20

Delivering therapy to the cystic fibrosis lung

BRUCE K. RUBIN AND RONALD W. WILLIAMS

INTRODUCTION

There are many advantages in delivering medication directly to the airway by aerosol, broadly encompassing issues of efficacy, safety, efficiency, and adherence. For a drug to be helpful, it first must reach the site of action in sufficient quantity to give relief, but not so much as to cause harm. The airway is attractive either as the intended target for therapy or the gateway for systemic delivery. Inhaled medicines need not be designed to be stable to exposure to gastrointestinal fluids, first-pass hepatic metabolism,[1] and interaction with ingested foods, but they must be stable to aerosolization forces and remain active at the airway surface. Changes in gastrointestinal absorption, whether physiologic or related to illness, do not affect aerosol delivery.[2] Palatability, an issue important for drug delivery to children, is much less of a consideration and may improve adherence.

When the lung is the target of therapy, aerosols may reduce side effects by decreasing systemic delivery,[3] and lower dosing may be possible by avoiding gastrointestinal exposure.[2] This also allows for use of higher local drug concentrations with less risk for systemic toxicity.[4] Finally, by avoiding the delays associated with gastrointestinal absorption, effects of the drug often occur more rapidly.

TARGETING AEROSOLS TO SPECIFIC REGIONS OF THE LUNG

In the healthy lung, aerosol deposition is targeted by using aerosol and device characteristics, and with controlled breathing techniques.[3] Particle size (mass median aerodynamic diameter [MMAD]) and size distribution (geometric standard deviation [GSD]), strongly influence the site of airway deposition. Particles with diameter between 1 and 5 μm are more likely to deposit in the conducting airways[5] with central deposition favored at the high end of this range.[6] A valved holding chamber (VHC) is commonly used to improve coordination of inhalation and the dynamic characteristics of the aerosol jet. An aerosol leaving the VHC has an MMAD about 25% smaller than when it first exits the pressurized metered dose inhaler (pMDI) because of propellant evaporation and sedimentation of larger particles.[7,8] Newer aerosol generators have been designed to produce particle sizes to achieve better therapeutic deposition of medications.

Inspiratory flow also significantly affects deposition of aerosol particles, with higher velocity flow depositing particles more proximally. Oral deposition can be minimized by limiting the aerosol velocity, limiting flow generated by patients, or training the patient in slow inhalation technique. VHCs again serve as a good example. Activation of a pMDI releases an aerosol with high velocity. If delivered directly into the mouth, there is greater likelihood that particles will deposit in the oropharynx secondary to inertia. Discharge into a VHC reduces aerosol velocity and increases delivery to the lung.[8]

Aerosol deposition changes in the diseased CF lung, especially during exacerbations, when secretions are abundant and breathing patterns are altered.[9] Obstructed air flow is turbulent when the Reynolds number increases, and this favors deposition centrally and at sites of obstruction.[2,5,10] Delivery of aerosols in CF patients may become more difficult as lung disease worsens.[11] This is not necessarily a detriment, and may in fact enhance deposition of mucoactive agents at the sites of mucus plugging.

INHALATION DELIVERY SYSTEMS

JET NEBULIZERS

Arguably the most recognizable devices for delivering aerosols to the lung, jet nebulizers use pressurized air to force a liquid through a small orifice and an arrangement of baffles to produce droplets.[5] These are entrained into the air stream created when the patient inhales. A fraction of the droplets created have MMAD in the range of 2–5 μm, making them suitable for use with drugs targeted to the conducting airways.

These devices can be used to aerosolize drug solutions or suspensions. In general liquids with higher vapor pressure, lower viscosity and surface tension similar to water more readily promote droplet formation, and this imposes some limitations on use. Surfactants tend to foam when nebulized because of very low surface tension, and oils are too viscous and have vapor pressures too low to nebulize effectively.[12] Drugs in suspension are nebulized less efficiently than those in solution.

The simplest devices produce a continuous aerosol. This is inefficient, as the drug released during patient exhalation is lost.[13] In combination with the large nonrespirable fraction of droplets, the mean delivery of drug is 10% of the original amount at best.[7] Efficiency of nebulizers can be improved with the use of aerosol reservoirs, which is the most commonly employed solution, or by matching aerosol generation to patient inhalation. Breath-enhanced devices create an aerosol continuously but this is released only when the patient inhales. Commercially available products of this type include: the PARI LC® Plus (PARI, Midlothian, Virginia), the NebuTech® (Salter Labs, Arvin, California), the Sidestream® Plus (Respironics, Cedar Grove, New Jersey), and Ventstream® Pro (Philips Respironics, Murrysville, Pennsylvania).[14] With the PARI LC Plus in particular, the volume of tobramycin delivered to the lung is doubled in comparison to a standard jet nebulizer, though overall delivery time is increased.[15]

Breath-activated nebulizers (BANs) generate aerosol only during inhalation, so there is no need for an aerosol reservoir or recycling chamber to conserve medication. Commercial products of this type are the AeroEclipse® BAN and AeroEclipse II BAN (Monaghan Medical Corporation, Plattsburgh, New York).[14] When using the same loading volume as traditional jet nebulizers, the AeroEclipse BAN will have much longer delivery times. These devices are generally most appropriate in patients older than 4 years,[13] as younger patients may have difficulty triggering the valve. To date, this device has not been studied for use in CF therapy.

Effective delivery of an aerosol requires a "closed circuit" with the airway. This is achieved when the patient maintains a seal on the nebulizer mouthpiece, or when an attached mask is kept fully in contact with the patient's face.[16] It is not uncommon for the constant output devices to be used with a "blow-by" technique, especially in infants and children. This practice is ineffective,[17] as even small leaks around a facemask can decrease aerosol delivery by half, and this rapidly declines with increasing distance from the face,[18] an effect attributed to aerosol dilution from air entrained around the mask.[19]

ULTRASONIC NEBULIZERS

Ultrasonic nebulizers operate by vibrating a piezoelectric crystal submerged in a liquid, or with liquid deposited onto the crystal. Ultrasound waves are transmitted to the liquid creating ripple disturbances at the surface. With lower intensity ultrasonic waves, the surface will cavitate and form bubbles, and these will rupture to form droplets. Higher intensity waves create micro-geysers that erupt droplets. In either case, air flowing across the surface during patient inhalation entrains the droplets and carries them to the patient lung.[12] These devices require tuning of sound waves based on viscosity, surface tension, and vapor pressure of the intended liquid, but ultimately produce droplets with MMAD in the range of 3.0–3.6 μm.[15]

There are some drawbacks to this technology. Energy used to produce droplets also heats the liquid, and the higher intensity vibrations often needed for medical solutions can fragment drug molecules.[12] Heat also enhances evaporation. The remaining solids can deposit on the piezoelectric crystal and reduce efficiency. Ultrasonic devices are expensive, require maintenance, and must be cleaned after each use.[15] Still, in one study of 10 CF subjects, an ultrasonic nebulizer (Multisonic compact® 2.4 MHz, Schill, Probstzella, Germany) produced greater peripheral lung deposition compared to the PARI LC Plus Turbo (PARI, Starnberg, Germany).[4] This technology does not lend itself to all aerosol therapies.

PRESSURIZED METERED-DOSE INHALERS

pMDIs were developed in the 1950s. Though they can only deliver a small volume of medicine with each actuation, they are convenient, reliable, and inexpensive. There are both manual and breath-activated pMDIs, but each is powered by a propellant in a liquid state when under pressure and forms a solution or suspension with the drug. When triggered, a fixed volume of propellant and drug is released into an expansion chamber. There is a rapid phase change in the propellant, with a shift toward a gaseous state, as the lower pressure allows the propellant to boil. The pressurized gas–drug mixture is forced through a small orifice, the actuator nozzle, creating an aerosol of droplets.[12] In chlorofluorocarbon (CFC) inhalers, the orifice diameter is one of the key determinants of droplet size, with smaller diameters generally yielding smaller MMADs and greater fine particle fractions (FPF).[8] A smaller actuator orifice also increases fine particle mass with hydrofluoroalkane (HFA) propellants when some drugs enter solution (rather than suspension) without significantly changing droplet size.[8]

Accessory devices: Spacers and valved holding chambers

Spacer and VHC devices can improve aerosol size and velocity, simplify inhalation technique (only the VHC), and decrease side effects by decreasing systemic exposure to the drug. A spacer decreases aerosol velocity by allowing the propellant to evaporate and larger droplets to deposit inside the spacer.[8] The net result is that the aerosol has a smaller MMAD and GSD that favors deposition in the lungs. A corollary is that only a single dose should be administered for each inhalation, as drug will be lost with multiple actuations from increased deposition on spacer walls.[5]

VHC have the added benefit of simplifying coordination of device actuation and patient inhalation, which can be especially important for children.[7] The VHC has an added benefit over a simple spacer, in that the valve protects the aerosol cloud from being lost by inadvertent exhalation once the mouthpiece or mask is in place. Since more medicine bypasses the oropharynx, there are fewer side effects related to swallowing the medication. With inhaled corticosteroids, there is also decreased incidence of oral candidiasis and dysphonia caused by oral and pharyngeal deposition.[8]

The CFC propellant previously used with pMDIs cools as it expands, which is why this was used in refrigerators. When delivered directly into the mouth, the high-velocity aerosol cloud could reach the throat and startle the patient sufficiently to stop inhalation. This "cold Freon" effect[7] was eliminated with the addition of an accessory device.

With polycarbonate accessory devices, electrostatic polarity of the aerosol can lead to static charge rain out, with as much as 80% loss of inhaled mass within the device. Using an electrically shielded chamber made of metal or nonconducting polymers, or a VHC with a detergent coating, reduces this loss.[16] Devices with detergent coatings should be cleaned regularly with a low concentration dishwashing detergent and allowed to air dry, as this will maintain a detergent layer.[5] As with nebulizers, a facemask can be attached to a VHC to allow it to be used in small children, although this reduces delivery to the lungs by at least half.[20]

DRY POWDER INHALERS

In the dry powder inhaler (DPI), an aerosol is created when a patient-generated airflow passes through a loose powder of drug and carrier particles. The trade-off for not needing propellant is the need for higher inspiratory flow, and this generally makes it more difficult for children younger than 6 years to use a DPI.[8] In contrast to the long and slow inhalation needed with pMDIs, a brisk and more forceful inhalation is needed with most DPIs to generate the necessary turbulence to separate the drug and powder aggregates.[5,7,21] This is especially true with DPIs that have higher flow resistance, such as the Pulmicort Flexhaler®. Low-resistance devices, such as the Diskus®, require less patient effort, but in general do not deliver as much drug to the lungs.[7]

NEWER TECHNOLOGY FOR DRUG DELIVERY IN CYSTIC FIBROSIS

Each available device offers advantages in different areas (Tables 20.1 and 20.2), and ultimately this may translate to better pairing of devices with patients.

SMALL-VOLUME LIQUID INHALERS

AERx (Aradigm Corporation, Hayward, California) has developed two devices. One is microprocessor controlled and designed to deliver drug to the alveoli for systemic delivery, e.g., delivering insulin for diabetes management or opioids for pain control.[13] The other is, AERx Essence®, a mechanical airway delivery device, making it less costly and simpler than the first system, but with precise control of aerosol generation maintained by the perforated AERx Strip® that is inserted into the delivery device.[22] The handheld component synchronizes aerosol generation with inhalation and limits flow, with greater than 50% loading dose reliably delivered to the lung. This device has effectively delivered proteins, including dornase alfa[22] and small molecules. Neither device is currently approved for use with CF medications.

VIBRATING MESH NEBULIZERS

The technology for these devices varies somewhat by manufacturer, but all produce aerosols via a microporous plate or mesh that is in contact with a liquid drug. A piezoelectric crystal or horn vibrates either the plate or the liquid, and droplets are produced as the liquid passes through the pores. The size of the pores is matched to the drug used and the target within the lung.[23] In active systems, the vibrations serve to pull liquid through the pores,[5] creating micropumps that generate the aerosol.[13] In a passive device, the plate is attached to an ultrasonic horn, and the energy of the piezoelectric crystal pushes liquid through the mesh to create the aerosol.[5]

These technologies offer advantages in portability, convenience, delivery time, and efficiency over traditional jet nebulizers, but they are more expensive, and require frequent cleaning and maintenance. Although they may allow nebulization of more fragile molecules because of lower sheer stress,[13] the mesh is prone to clogging, which decreases output. It follows that these devices are not suitable for viscous or high osmolarity solutions. Because the mesh pores are matched to specific drugs, it is possible that using a medication not tested for a specific device will damage or clog the mesh, and may significantly change the effectiveness of medication delivery. It is not clear at this time whether a patient will need a different device for each medication, or whether parts of a device may ultimately be customizable for different medications.

The PARI eFlow® is an active vibrating mesh nebulizer (VMN). It is capable of operating at very low residual volume, ideal for more potent or expensive drugs, or at volumes comparable to traditional jet nebulizers. It is currently approved for use with nebulized aztreonam (Cayston®, Gilead Sciences, Foster City, California) in the United States, and is being studied with other drugs. Early results suggest that it is more efficient than the PARI LC Star jet nebulizer for nebulizing dornase alfa,[24] and that it can deliver tobramycin to the lungs in amounts comparable to the PARI LC Plus, but with half the loading dose, and in about one-quarter of the time.[25]

The I-neb AAD (adaptive aerosol delivery) system (Philips Respironics, Chichester, United Kingdom) is a passive VMN combined with a microprocessor that analyzes the patient's breathing pattern and adapts aerosol release for enhanced lung deposition.[26] The characteristics of the generated aerosol are comparable to other VMNs, so it is the integrated software that separates this into the category of "intelligent" nebulizers. More than just limiting aerosol

Table 20.1 Novel aerosol devices

Device	Advantages	Disadvantages
Breath-activated, nebulizers AeroEclipse	Delivers medication only during inhalation Less medication wasted	Needs sufficient flow to trigger Takes longer to deliver medication More expensive
Breath-enhanced nebulizers Adaptive aerosol delivery (iNeb)AJQTA patient-individualized therapy	Targeted delivery Less wasted medication Delivery adapts to patient's breathing Can monitor patient adherence	Very expensive devices Not ventilator enabled Can be "confused" by incorrect use
Vibrating-mesh nebulizers Aeroneb Go, Pro Omron MicroAir PARI eFlow ODEM Touch Spray	Fast, quiet, portable Self-contained power source Can optimize particle size for specific drugs	More expensive Not compatible with viscous liquids or those that crystallize on drying Cleaning can be difficult Medication dosage must be adjusted if transition from a jet nebulizer
Aerosol Hood (Child Hood)	Easy to apply May be used for small infants in mild respiratory distress	Not well validated Facial deposition and environmental contamination by aerosol Unpredictable aerosol deposition
Metered-dose liquid inhalers Respimat Soft Mist inhaler	Easier to use than a pressurized metered-dose inhaler Gives feedback Very effective aerosol delivery	More expensive Small dosing chamber Not suitable for use with a mechanical ventilator
Engineered particles Technospheres PulmoSpheres	Can use a very simple and inexpensive dry-powder inhaler device Breath-activated	More difficult to manufacture particles Not for use with all medications May require larger number of inhalations then usual dry powder inhaler
High-flow nasal cannula delivery	Able to deliver drug to patient in respiratory distress No need to stop oxygen to deliver medication	No clinical data yet to support use or provide dosing guidelines May not be useful for some drugs Higher upper-airway deposition

Source: Rubin, BK, Respir Care, 56, 9, 1411–23, 2011. With permission.

Table 20.2 Approved devices and medications

Device	Medication
PARI eFlow®	Aztreonam (Cayston®)
PARI LC® Plus	Tobramycin (TOBI®, Bramitob®) Colistimethate
PARI LC® Star	Dornase alfa Hypertonic saline Colistimethate
Prodose AAD System®	Colistimethate (Promixin®)
I-neb AAD®	Colistimethate
TOBI® Podhaler®	Tobramycin dry powder
Turbospin®	Colistimethate dry powder
Colobreathe®	Colistimethate dry powder
Hudson T Up-draft® II	Dornase alfa
Marquest Acorn® II	Dornase alfa
PARI LC® Jet	Dornase alfa
PARI Baby®	Dornase alfa
Durable Sidestream®	Dornase alfa
Bronchitol inhaler device	Mannitol dry powder (Bronchitol®)

release to the patient's inhalation phase, the goal is to target release to the period of inhalation likely to increase deposition at the intended lung site. This device has been used with CF patients in Europe for delivery of colistimethate.[27]

The first implementation of this technology was the HaloLite AAD system (Profile Therapeutics, Bognor Regis, United Kingdom), released in 1997,[27] which analyzed three patient breaths and then controlled aerosol release to the first half of the inhalation phase.[7] The second implementation was the Prodose AAD System (Bayer Schering Pharma AG, Berlin, Germany), released in 2002, and in Europe was approved for use in CF to deliver Promixin (colistimethate). This device provided continuous breathing analysis and adjusted aerosol delivery dynamically.[28] It was also able to adjust the total dose delivered based on breathing characteristics, rather than using preset doses. These devices were based on jet nebulizer technology. Though nebulization times are longer with AAD systems using the same loading doses required for continuous flow jet nebulizers, the higher efficiency of these devices allows reductions in drug volume, and therefore administration time, while achieving the same clinical effect.[29]

The I-neb AAD system is the third-generation AAD technology, and offers two modes of operation. The first is tidal breathing mode, and is similar to the operation of the Prodose system. The second is targeted inhalation mode, and this uses a flow-restricting mouthpiece and tactile patient cues to control breathing dynamics.[13] This was studied in a group of 42 subjects with CF, who used it to administer colistimethate sodium, salbutamol, dornase alfa, tobramycin, and hypertonic saline. The authors were able to demonstrate 40%–50% reductions in time to complete therapies, and increased adherence, but the study did not investigate clinical response.[30]

Activaero pairs AAD technology with the PARI LC Plus in the AKITA® JET, and with the PARI eFlow in the AKITA² APIXNEB™. In addition to synchronizing aerosol generation with patient breathing, this system uses positive pressure to deliver each dose.[5] Though its use in treating CF is limited at this time, one study with the APIXNEB that included seven subjects with CF having mild-to-moderate lung disease (mean $FEV_1\%$ 62 ± 15) demonstrated that it was well tolerated, and that central and peripheral lung deposition was comparable to that of healthy controls.[31]

NEWER DRY POWDER INHALERS

Devices now available for treating CF showcase advancements in both device and particle engineering that allow delivery of much larger doses. A dry powder formulation of tobramycin is now approved for chronic antipseudomonal therapy, and is delivered via the TOBI® Podhaler® (Novartis AG, Basel, Switzerland).[32] The Turbospin® (PH&T, Milan, Italy) is a breath-activated, handheld, reusable inhaler that is available in Europe to administer a dry powder formulation of colistimethate, and has shown efficacy and tolerability in treating pulmonary infection by *Pseudomonas aeruginosa* in CF patients 6 years and older.[33] Finally, a dry powder formulation of mannitol, Bronchitol® (Pharmaxis, New South Wales, Australia), is available as an adjunct to airway clearance therapy in Australia and Europe.

ENGINEERED PARTICLES

Another approach to enhancing the effectiveness of aerosol therapy is to improve the drug particles. A particle must be large enough to contain the drug while maintaining an MMAD in the 1–5 μm range for lung deposition. A secondary goal is that the particle be physically larger than 5 μm to delay phagocytosis by macrophages, thus increasing the time for drug activity between doses.[34]

An example of this is the PulmoSphere® (Novartis AG, Basel, Switzerland). With a stabilized surfactant molecule as its base, a porous, spherical shell forms around the drug yielding a spherical particle with a large physical diameter but low density (low MMAD).[35] Because of their shape, there is minimal contact surface with other particles, thus these particles have high dispersibility.[36] PulmoSphere technology has been successfully combined with tobramycin, designed

for delivery via the TOBI Podhaler. This is approved for use in Europe, Chile, Canada,[32] and in the United States. There are also active clinical trials of PulmoSphere formulations of ciprofloxacin and amphotericin B.[35]

The use of liposomes as engineered carrier particles has also been evaluated. The phospholipid bilayer of liposomes is biocompatible, but this can possibly alter the pharmacokinetics and pharmacodynamics of the encapsulated drug.[37] Though drug leakage can potentially lead to toxicity,[38] lipids can be manipulated to favor fusion with cell membranes, retention of carrier particles in the airway, and drug release rate.[7] This has been demonstrated in an animal model, showing that liposomal salbutamol delivered by aerosol is retained in the lungs up to three times longer than the conventional salbutamol formulation.[39] An inhaled liposomal formulation of amikacin has been studied in subjects with CF,[40] liposomal cyclosporine has been investigated in lung transplant patients,[41] and investigations are proceeding with formulations of ciprofloxacin, tobramycin,[7] colistin,[42] dornase, and amphotericin.[43]

With the variety of devices available to facilitate delivery of aerosol medications for the treatment of lung disease, it is important to consider the abilities, needs, and desires of each patient to match them with the most appropriate device. When clinical focus shifts from "population" to "the CF patient in front of me" the most effective device is often one the patient is willing to use every day, as not using it clearly delivers no medicine. Also important is the patient's or caregiver's ability to prepare the medicine for use, and using proper inhalation technique for the device.[44] For each intended dose, failure to use, prepare, or correctly inhale a medicine, are considered critical errors. An observational study by Molimard et al., involving approximately 3800 subjects using various nebulizers, pMDIs, and DPIs to deliver asthma and chronic obstructive pulmonary disease (COPD) medications, found at least one critical error in 49%–76% patients, varying with device.[45]

ADHERENCE TO THERAPY

For therapy to be most effective, adherence is critically important. Poor adherence is not necessarily related to a patient's age. Adherence with inhaled dornase therapy was retrospectively assessed in 90 adult patients with CF. Only 24% filled prescriptions for at least 8 of 12 months, whereas the self-reported measure of good compliance was 80%.[46] Another study looked at adherence to inhaled dornase and oral ADEK vitamins in adolescents with CF, and found about 27% adherence with dornase and about 65% adherence with ADEK. The results were weakly correlated with parental impressions of disease severity and perceived medication benefit.[47] In adult CF patients, Sawicki et al. found there was a higher perceived burden correlated with the number of nebulized therapies needed in a day.[48]

Factors contributing to adherence are the patient's impression of physician empathy, clear explanations and education provided by the physician, and specific, rather than general, recommendations for improving health.[49] For example, rather than just asking a patient to add dornase alfa treatments to their airway clearance therapy, there should be specific recommendations about the proper choice of nebulizer, care and cleaning of equipment, and how to incorporate this medicine into their existing regimen.

Often overlooked as affecting adherence is the extent to which physicians follow published care guidelines.[50,51] The CF Foundation Annual Report 2008 reported prescribing adherence of only 67% for aerosol tobramycin and 76% for dornase.

THERAPY AND ADHERENCE

Poor patient adherence is often attributed to increasing complexity of therapy.[52,53] Though difficult to define in this context,[54] complexity seems to encompass many factors, including number of medications, the frequency and time needed for individual treatments, the expected duration of therapy, and the need for medical devices or assistance to complete therapy.[55] By any measure, the long-term treatment of CF is complex.[54,56]

Aerosol therapy in CF is primarily used for health maintenance and prevention of complications. As such the consequences of nonadherence tend to develop over time and the connection between cause and effect tends to blur.[57] In a retrospective longitudinal study of 95 CF patients, there was an association between poor adherence and the need for IV antibiotics to treat a respiratory exacerbation with lower baseline lung function, though poor adherence did not predict decline in lung function.[58] Contemporary research on inhaled tobramycin, azithromycin, and other preventive therapies, indirectly suggests an association between nonadherence and increased morbidity. Briesacher's study, for example, showed the risk for hospitalization decreased by 60% in patients who adhered to preventive therapy with inhaled tobramycin.[59]

PATIENT AND ADHERENCE

The patient causes of therapy non-adherence have been classified as those related to misunderstandings, competing demands or disorganization, and active decision making.[60] Problems with understanding, which has been called unwitting non-adherence, often originate in the health-care setting. Inadequate patient education about disease and therapy, misunderstanding by the patient, or poor recall can lead to non-adherence.[52] Improved adherence may be gained with physician attention to education to improve the patient's understanding of medications and benefits.[61] A variant of this is when patients are given incorrect information by the care provider, increasing confusion, frustration,

and non-adherence. Specifically considering aerosol therapy, estimates are that 28%–68% patients cannot correctly use their prescribed pMDI or DPI and that 39%–67% health-care providers cannot correctly describe or demonstrate these devices.[62]

When a patient tries to maintain adherence but fails at times because of competing demands on time, either actual or resulting from disorganization, then adherence is erratic. Adherence is often better when medication effects are easily and quickly observed.[49] Thus in persons with CF, adherence to taking pancreatic enzymes with meals is uniformly reported to be far greater than adherence to taking aerosol medication or using airway clearance.

The last category is willful non-adherence or contrivance. This is a personal choice by the patient, made after receiving appropriate education and with understanding of the consequences. There is evidence to suggest that a patient's perception of their disease severity differs significantly from the physician's and that they may feel certain treatments are not needed or not appropriate for them.[63] Reported predictors for non-adherence in this respect are concerns for medication effectiveness and side effects.[64]

IMPROVING ADHERENCE

A first step in improving adherence is identifying and addressing deficiencies on the health-care side of the physician–patient relationship (Table 20.3). The CF Center at Cincinnati Children's Hospital Medical Center assessed its own compliance with published care guidelines, and having found deficiencies undertook efforts to address them. In only 3 months, the measured compliance for all therapies improved from 62% to 87%.[50]

From the patient side, improving adherence can only begin after identifying the patients needing intervention. Increasing attention has been given to the need to review medications and adherence at all clinical encounters, and it is essential to have a strong physician–patient relationship as the foundation to improve chances of success.[65] Still, efforts are typically limited to reports from the patient and to the physician's judgment based on subjective and objective assessments of the patient's health. Unfortunately, both have been shown inaccurate for assessing adherence,[58,66] as they are complicated by recall bias and fabrication, and most likely overestimate adherence.[56,62] One study illustrating this involved 63 adults with CF, where the median values for self-reporting and physician estimates were about 80% and 60%, respectively, compared to about 36% indicated by electronic monitoring.[49,56]

In general, adherence with nebulized medications used for CF care is low.[63] Though not widely available at this time, electronic monitoring with the device has been shown more accurate in assessing adherence compared to patient self-reporting, physician assessment, and prescribing history.[64,67] It is well suited for adaptation to aerosol devices, and when augmented by frequent feedback to the patient, has contributed to improvements in adherence.[50,68] The more

Table 20.3 Therapy adherence

Barriers	Interventions
Health-care system	Foster strong doctor–patient relationships
	Follow established guidelines
	Ask the patient about adherence
Socioeconomic factors	Follow-up on missed appointments and refills
Disease-related factors	Stress that parents have primary responsibility for medication administration
	Frequent education and review
Complexity of therapy	Simplify therapy when possible
Patient misunderstanding	Frequent education and review
	Provide written care plans with clear expectations
	Demonstrate and review techniques for inhalation therapy
Competing demands	Offer suggestions for optimizing delivery of multiple therapies
Contrivance	Discuss the patient's views influencing their decision

sophisticated devices record each use, the duration of each session when applicable, and the amount of dose delivered.[65,69]

INHALATION TECHNIQUE AND DEVICE SELECTION

Age is often the first consideration in aerosol device selection. Children under the age of 3 years generally cannot perform controlled breathing techniques, so compressed air nebulizers with the aerosol delivered through a facemask, or a pMDI with VHC and mask are typically used.[5,58] Since crying and faster breathing decreases aerosol delivery to the lungs, quiet breathing is desired for the duration of treatment.[23,66] Nebulization hoods, though less common in an outpatient setting, have been shown to be as effective as nebulizers in a study of 14 wheezing infants aged 1–19 months and no history of prematurity,[70] and 10 infants with bronchopulmonary dysplasia.[71]

In a study of 12 infants given nebulization treatments when asleep, the median percentage dose delivered to the lung in older controls was 6% by oral inhalation and 2.7% by nasal inhalation. In infants, the median percentage delivered was 1.3%, but the percent deposition by body weight (a reasonable surrogate for airway surface) was the same.[72] To improve delivery, it is suggested that infants be supine and that the facemask be fitted correctly.

Beyond age of 3 years most children are able to perform the slow, deep breathing needed for effective use of the pMDI with VHC or the steady quiet breathing needed with a nebulizer. Breathing assessments in 96 patients with CF suggests that by age 6 years most will also be able to use DPIs effectively.[21]

The force, frequency, and depth of breathing during aerosol inhalation all influence the efficiency of medication delivery. Using slow, deep (i.e., larger tidal volume) inhalation will enhance delivery to the peripheral lung,[5,7,9] and breath holding at the end of inhalation helps to maximize deposition.[7,9] In CF patients with mildly impaired lung function, using this technique yields deposition efficiency approaching that of persons with normal lung function.[6] For pMDIs and DPIs in particular, meta-analyses suggest that with appropriate inhalation technique the various available devices can produce equivalent therapeutic results,[73] but often patients are not provided education or they choose not to follow recommendations.[5]

Aerosol delivery devices are now designed to assist patients in using proper breathing techniques. One of the better recognized, and simplest, solutions is the addition of a VHC to pMDIs. In addition to simplifying the coordination between device activation and patient inhalation, some of these attachments produce a whistle when inspiratory effort is too vigorous. Some newer devices use high-resistance mouthpieces to promote slower inhalation.[26]

AEROSOL MEDICATIONS

For a formulation to be effective, it should not cause airway inflammation. Extremes of pH, osmolarity, or tonicity have been shown to cause coughing, bronchoconstriction, or mucosal irritation.[7,9,15] Early investigations with inhaled aztreonam used the IV formulation that contained an arginine salt. This was poorly tolerated, and there were concerns that long-term use would worsen airway inflammation by augmenting nitric oxide production. This led to substitution by a lysine salt.[74–76]

Except for therapies meant to promote effective cough (e.g., hyperosmolar saline) another consideration may be to delay clearance of a drug via cough, the mucociliary escalator, and macrophage uptake. Longer residence times may permit lower dosing and may allow less frequent administration, both of which have been shown to improve patient adherence.[7]

BRONCHODILATORS

Short-acting beta-agonists are widely used for the management of CF lung disease. It is reported that use exceeds 80% of patients,[77] and the CF Foundation recommends that salbutamol be used, although there are few data showing clinical benefit.[78] Historically reported uses include dilating airways to improve lung function, enhancing the effectiveness of the mucociliary clearance apparatus, improving antibiotic deposition, and preventing bronchospasm triggered by other inhaled therapies, but there are few data demonstrating effectiveness in CF.[79,80]

Bronchodilation and improved lung function

Though there are reports of an increased risk of atopy in CF patients,[81] bronchodilator reversibility is not inherently demonstrated as it is in asthma. After more than two decades of investigation, the conclusions are inconsistent, especially with respect to age and disease severity.[82] A small case–control study in patients younger than age 18 months, testing responses to metaproterenol, asserts that infants with CF have greater basal airway tone that can be relieved with beta-agonists.[83] A cross-sectional study of 25 older children and teens demonstrated greater bronchodilator reversibility in CF subjects with FEV_1 above 70% predicted than those with more severe disease. In sicker patients, there was evidence to suggest that smooth muscle relaxation increased collapse of the damaged airways, which worsened lung function measurements.[84] A similar conclusion had previously been reported after finding that bronchodilator use was associated with a less effective cough in patients with more severe disease.[85] Other reports show short-term improvements in lung function, but no long-lasting benefits.[78] Bronchodilator use has also been found to impair lung function in some patients more significantly during exercise,[86] even in patients known to demonstrate significant bronchodilator reversibility at baseline.[87]

Enhancing mucociliary clearance

Physiologic mucociliary clearance results from coordination between production of airway surface fluid and mucus, and function of the ciliated cells that propel mucus. This involves fluid, ion, and mucus transport into the airway lumen to regulate periciliary fluid volume. There was increased chloride and water secretion in dog trachea following treatment with terbutaline.[88] In vitro studies with human, canine, rat, and cat airway cells have shown that beta-agonists increase cilia beat frequency and improve whole lung mucociliary clearance, but the effects are attenuated in patients with lung disease.[89] Chloride secretion seems to decline with beta-agonist dosing,[90] leading to lower airway surface fluid volumes and impaired cilia function. Mucin secretion from human airway cells does not seem to be effected by beta-agonist stimulation.[89,90]

Bronchospasm and particle deposition

It has been recommended that beta-agonist administration precede inhalation of antibiotics and mucolytics in CF treatment to reduce the risk of bronchoconstriction or to improve medication delivery.[91,92] The US CF Foundation recommends chronic use to improve lung function, but does not discuss medication-induced bronchospasm.[78]

Bronchoconstriction has been reported following inhalation of tobramycin,[93,94] colistimethate,[95] and aztreonam,[96] but generally this was using the parenteral formulations. Using a radiolabeled inhalation formulation of tobramycin, antibiotic deposition was measured in 24 subjects with CF. Pulmonary scintigraphy studies showed significantly decreased deposition of drug in almost all lung regions when preceded by salbutamol and airway clearance therapy. Deposition decreased with increasing severity of lung disease.[97]

Beta-agonist use before mucolytic therapy, especially hypertonic saline, is also recommended, but evidence is conflicting. An early case–control study assessing tolerance of hypertonic saline to induce sputum expectoration in asthma patients showed greater drops in FEV_1 and increased reports of discomfort following pretreatment with placebo compared to salbutamol.[98] It has also been investigated for use in bronchoprovocation studies with asthmatics.[99] In CF patients, hypertonic saline has been found to be safe and well tolerated when preceded by beta-agonist therapy,[100] but it is difficult to find studies that did not include pretreatment as part of the protocol for all subjects.[101] One study of 45 patients assessing tolerability did not specifically control beta-agonist use, but it was administered only to subjects already using salbutamol as chronic therapy (78%). A clinically significant decline in FEV_1 was noted in only three patients, all of whom had used salbutamol. Twenty-six others showed declines in FEV_1 that were not clinically significant, with a correlation between increasing age and greater decline, perhaps more due to dynamic collapse of the airway with coughing than to bronchospasm.[102]

Anticholinergics

Currently there are no long-term data on regular use of anticholinergic bronchodilators in CF. Short-term studies have shown bronchodilation in some CF patients, usually those with previously recognized bronchodilator reversibility to beta-agonists, but results are variable over time.[82] Similar findings have been reported for anticholinergic and short-acting beta-agonist combination therapy, without significant additive effects.[103] A Cochrane review and a CF Foundation Guideline are in agreement that evidence is insufficient to recommend for or against routine use of anticholinergic bronchodilators in CF.[78,104]

INHALED ANTIBIOTICS

The role of inhaled antibiotic therapy for treating CF has evolved from early off-label use of parenteral formulations to evidence-based use of specially developed inhalation formulations. There are many advantages to using inhaled antibiotics, including ease of use, convenience, and decreased systemic exposure, the latter offering improved safety and lower side-effect profiles. As *P. aeruginosa* has traditionally been the organism most closely linked to respiratory morbidity,[105] it is also the primary target in the development of antibiotic inhalation therapies. Currently available inhalation

6. Brand P, Meyer T, Häussermann S et al. Optimum peripheral drug deposition in patients with cystic fibrosis. *J Aerosol Med* 2005; **18**(1): 45–54.

7. Labiris NR, Dolovich MB. Pulmonary drug delivery. Part II: The role of inhalant delivery devices and drug formulations in therapeutic effectiveness of aerosolized medications. *Br J Clin Pharmacol* 2003; **56**(6): 600–12.

8. Smyth HD. Propellant-driven metered-dose inhalers for pulmonary drug delivery. *Expert Opin Drug Deliv* 2005; **2**(1): 53–74.

9. Monteiro APAF, Sexauer WP, Stremler N, Fiel SB. Aerosolized antibiotics in cystic fibrosis. *Semin Respir Crit Care Med* 2003; **42**(1): 33–8.

10. Geller DE. Aerosol antibiotics in cystic fibrosis: Yesterday, today and tomorrow. *Respir Drug Deliv* 2008; **1**: 37–46.

11. Ilowite JS, Gorvoy JD, Smaldone GC. Quantitative deposition of aerosolized gentamicin in cystic fibrosis. *Am Rev Respir Dis* 1987; **136**(6): 1445–9.

12. Leong KH. Theoretical principles and devices used to generate aerosols for research. In: Hickey AJ (Ed). *Pharmaceutical Inhalation Aerosol Technology.* Informa Healthcare; 2003. pp. 253–78.

13. Geller DE. The science of aerosol delivery in cystic fibrosis. *Pediatr Pulmonol* 2008; **43**(Suppl 9): S5–S17.

14. Ari A, Hess DR, Myers T, Rau J. Small-volume nebulizers. In: *A Guide to Aerosol Delivery Devices for Respiratory Therapists.* Irving, TX: American Association for Respiratory Care; 2009. pp. 10–20.

15. Le J, Ashley ED, Neuhauser MM et al. Consensus summary of aerosolized antimicrobial agents: Application of guideline criteria. *Pharmacotherapy* 2010; **30**(6): 562–84.

16. Smaldone GC, Berg E, Nikander K. Variation in pediatric aerosol delivery: Importance of facemask. *J Aerosol Med* 2005; **18**(3): 354–63.

17. National Institute of Health. Managing asthma long term in children 0–4 years of age and 5–11 years of age. In: *Expert Panel Report 3: Guidelines for the Diagnosis and Management of Asthma.* Bethesda, MD: NIH; 2007. pp. 281–319.

18. Ari A, Hess DR, Myers T, Rau J. Neonatal and pediatric aerosol drug delivery. In: *A Guide to Aerosol Delivery Devices for Respiratory Therapists.* Irving, TX: American Association for Respiratory Care; 2009. pp. 45–6.

19. Janssens HM, Devadason SG, Hop WC et al. Variability of aerosol delivery via spacer devices in young asthmatic children in daily life. *Eur Respir J* 1999; **13**(4): 787–91.

20. National Institute of Health. Control of environmental factors and comorbid conditions that affect asthma. In: *Expert panel report 3: Guidelines for the Diagnosis and Management of Asthma.* Bethesda, MD: NIH; 2007. pp. 165–90.

21. Tiddens HA, Geller DE, Challoner P et al. Effect of dry powder inhaler resistance on the inspiratory flow rates and volumes of cystic fibrosis patients of six years and older. *J Aerosol Med* 2006; **19**(4): 456–65.

22. Geller D, Thipphawong J, Otulana B et al. Bolus inhalation of rhDNase with the AERx system in subjects with cystic fibrosis. *J Aerosol Med* 2003; **16**(2): 175–82.

23. Rubin BK. Pediatric aerosol therapy: New devices and new drugs. *Respir Care* 2011; **56**(9): 1411–23.

24. Burchell J, Ng EN, Annese T et al. Validation of methods to determine optimal delivery of cystic fibrosis medications from vibrating membrane (mesh) nebulizers. *Respir Drug Deliv* 2010; **3**: 887–90.

25. Coates AL, Denk O, Leung K et al. Higher tobramycin concentration and vibrating mesh technology can shorten antibiotic treatment time in cystic fibrosis. *Pediatr Pulmonol* 2011; **46**(4): 401–8.

26. McCormack P, McNamara PS, Southern KW. A randomised controlled trial of breathing modes for adaptive aerosol delivery in children with cystic fibrosis. *J Cyst Fibros* 2011; **10**(5): 343–9.

27. Denyer J, Nikander K. The I-neb adaptive aerosol delivery (AAD) system. *MedicaMundi* 2010; **54**: 54–8.

28. Denyer J, Nikander K, Smith NJ. Adaptive aerosol delivery (AAD®) technology. *Expert Opin Drug Deliv* 2004; **1**(1): 165–76.

29. Dhand R. Intelligent nebulizers in the age of the internet: The I-neb adaptive aerosol delivery (AAD) system. *J Aerosol Med Pulm Drug Deliv* 2010; **23**(Suppl 1): iii–v.

30. Denyer J, Black A, Nikander K et al. Domiciliary experience of the target inhalation mode (TIM) breathing maneuver in patients with cystic fibrosis. *J Aerosol Med Pulm Drug Deliv* 2010; **23**(Suppl 1): S45–54.

31. Brand P, Schulte M, Wencker M et al. Lung deposition of inhaled alpha1-proteinase inhibitor in cystic fibrosis and alpha1-antitrypsin deficiency. *Eur Respir J* 2009; **34**(2): 354–60.

32. Vandevanter DR, Geller DE. Tobramycin administered by the TOBI® Podhaler® for persons with cystic fibrosis: A review. *Medical Devices: Evidence and Research* 2011; **4**: 179–88.

33. Schuster A, Haliburn C, Doring G et al. Safety, efficacy and convenience of colistimethate sodium dry powder for inhalation (Colobreathe DPI) in patients with cystic fibrosis: A randomised study. *Thorax* 2013; **68**(4): 344–50.

34. Yang Y, Bajaj N, Xu P et al. Development of highly porous large PLGA microparticles for pulmonary drug delivery. *Biomaterials* 2009; **30**(10): 1947–53.

35. Geller DE, Weers J, Heuerding S. Development of an inhaled dry-powder formulation of tobramycin using PulmoSphere™ technology. *J Aerosol Med Pulm Drug Deliv* 2011; **24**(4): 175–82.

36. Edwards DA, Hanes J, Caponetti G et al. Large porous particles for pulmonary drug delivery. *Science* 1997; **276**(5320): 1868–71.

37. Misra A, Jinturkar K, Patel D et al. Recent advances in liposomal dry powder formulations: Preparation and evaluation. *Expert Opin Drug Deliv* 2009; **6**(1): 71–89.

38. Meenach SA, Kim YJ, Kauffman KJ et al. Synthesis, optimization, and characterization of camptothecin-loaded acetalated dextran porous microparticles for pulmonary delivery. *Mol Pharm* 2012; **9**(2): 290–8.

39. Chen X, Huang W, Wong BC et al. Liposomes prolong the therapeutic effect of anti-asthmatic medication via pulmonary delivery. *Int J Nanomedicine* 2012; **7**: 1139–48.

40. Okusanya OO, Bhavnani SM, Hammel J et al. Pharmacokinetic and pharmacodynamic evaluation of liposomal amikacin for inhalation in cystic fibrosis patients with chronic pseudomonal infection. *Antimicrob Agents Chemother* 2009; **53**(9): 3847–54.

41. Behr J, Zimmermann G, Baumgartner R et al. Lung deposition of a liposomal cyclosporine A inhalation solution in patients after lung transplantation. *J Aerosol Med Pulm Drug Deliv* 2009; **22**(2): 121–30.

42. Wallace SJ, Li J, Nation RL et al. Interaction of colistin and colistin methanesulfonate with liposomes: Colloidal aspects and implications for formulation. *J Pharm Sci* 2012; **101**(9): 3347–59.

43. Fauvel M, Farrugia C, Tsapis N et al. Aerosolized liposomal amphotericin B: Prediction of lung deposition, in vitro uptake and cytotoxicity. *Int J Pharmaceutics* 2012; **436**(1–2): 106–10.

44. Weers J, Ung K, Glusker M. Minimizing human factors effects through improved inhaler design. *Respir Drug Deliv* 2012; **1**: 217–26.

45. Molimard M, Raherison C, Lignot S et al. Assessment of handling of inhaler devices in real life: An observational study in 3811 patients in primary care. *J Aerosol Med* 2003; **16**(3): 249–54.

46. Burrows JA, Bunting JP, Masel PJ, Bell SC. Nebulised dornase alpha: Adherence in adults with cystic fibrosis. *J Cyst Fibros* 2002; **1**(4): 255–9.

47. Zindani GN, Streetman DD, Streetman DS, Nasr SZ. Adherence to treatment in children and adolescent patients with cystic fibrosis. *J Adolesc Health* 2006; **38**(1): 13–7.

48. Sawicki GS, Sellers DE, Robinson WM. High treatment burden in adults with cystic fibrosis: Challenges to disease self-management. *J Cyst Fibros* 2009; **8**(2): 91–6.

49. Bernard RS, Cohen LL. Increasing adherence to cystic fibrosis treatment: A systematic review of behavioral techniques. *Pediatr Pulmonol* 2004; **37**(1): 8–16.

50. McPhail GL, Weiland J, Acton JD et al. Improving evidence-based care in cystic fibrosis through quality improvement. *Arch Pediatr Adolesc Med* 2010; **164**(10): 957–60.

51. Pham JC, Kelen GD, Pronovost PJ. National study on the quality of emergency department care in the treatment of acute myocardial infarction and pneumonia. *Acad Emerg Med* 2007; **14**(10): 856–63.

52. Vermeire E, Hearnshaw H, Van Royen P, Denekens J. Patient adherence to treatment: Three decades of research. A comprehensive review. *J Clin Pharm Ther* 2001; **26**(5): 331–42.

53. Stange D, Kriston L, Wolff von A et al. Medication complexity, prescription behaviour and patient adherence at the interface between ambulatory and stationary medical care. *Eur J Clin Pharmacol* 2013; **69**(3): 573–80.

54. Kettler LJ, Sawyer SM, Winefield HR, Greville HW. Determinants of adherence in adults with cystic fibrosis. *Thorax* 2002; **57**(5): 459–64.

55. Sawicki GS, Tiddens H. Managing treatment complexity in cystic fibrosis: Challenges and opportunities. *Pediatr Pulmonol* 2012; **47**(6): 523–33.

56. Daniels T, Goodacre L, Sutton C et al. Accurate assessment of adherence: Self-report and clinician report vs electronic monitoring of nebulizers. *Chest* 2011; **140**(2): 425–32.

57. Zemanick ET, Harris JK, Conway S et al. Measuring and improving respiratory outcomes in cystic fibrosis lung disease: Opportunities and challenges to therapy. *J Cyst Fibros* 2010; **9**(1): 1–16.

58. Eakin MN, Bilderback A, Boyle MP et al. Longitudinal association between medication adherence and lung health in people with cystic fibrosis. *J Cyst Fibros* 2011; **10**(4): 258–64.

59. Briesacher BA, Quittner AL, Saiman L et al. Adherence with tobramycin inhaled solution and health care utilization. *BMC Pulm Med* 2011; **11**(5): 1–6.

60. Rand CS. "I took the medicine like you told me, doctor": Self-report of adherence with medical regimens. In: Stone A, Turkkan JS, Bachrach CA et al. (Eds). *The Science of Self-Report: Implications For Research and Practice*. Mahwah, NJ: Lawrence Erlbaum Associates; 2000. pp. 257–76.

61. Efficace F, Baccarani M, Rosti G et al. Investigating factors associated with adherence behaviour in patients with chronic myeloid leukemia: An observational patient-centered outcome study. *Br J Cancer* 2012; **107**(6): 904–9.

62. Fink JB, Rubin BK. Problems with inhaler use: A call for improved clinician and patient education. *Respir Care* 2005; **50**(10): 1360–74.

63. Geller DE, Madge S. Technological and behavioral strategies to reduce treatment burden and improve adherence to inhaled antibiotics in cystic fibrosis. *Respir Med* 2011; **105**(S2): S24–31.

64. Collaco JM, Kole AJ, Riekert KA et al. Respiratory medication adherence in chronic lung disease of prematurity. *Pediatr Pulmonol* 2012; **47**(3): 283–91.

65. Santus P, Picciolo S, Proietto A et al. Doctor-patient relationship: A resource to improve respiratory diseases management. *Eur J Intern Med* 2012; **23**(5): 442–6.

66. Finney JW, Hook RJ, Friman PC et al. The overestimation of adherence to pediatric medical regimens. *Child Health Care* 1993; **22**(4): 297–304.

67. Denyer J. Adherence monitoring in drug delivery. *Expert Opin Drug Deliv* 2010; **7**(10): 1127–31.

68. Nikander K, Pearce L, Smith N, Pritchard J. The impact of electronic monitors on patients' adherence to inhaled medications. *Respir Drug Deliv* 2012; **1**: 673–8.

69. McNamara PS, McCormack P, McDonald AJ et al. Open adherence monitoring using routine data download from an adaptive aerosol delivery nebuliser in children with cystic fibrosis. *J Cyst Fibros* 2009; **8**(4): 258–63.

70. Amirav I, Balanov I, Gorenberg M et al. Nebuliser hood compared to mask in wheezy infants: Aerosol therapy without tears! *Arch Dis Child* 2003; **88**(8): 719–23.

71. Kugelman A, Amirav I, Mor F et al. Hood versus mask nebulization in infants with evolving bronchopulmonary dysplasia in the neonatal intensive care unit. *J Perinatol* 2006; **26**(1): 31–6.

72. Chua HL, Collis GG, Newbury AM et al. The influence of age on aerosol deposition in children with cystic fibrosis. *Eur Respir J* 1994; **7**(12): 2185–91.

73. Dolovich MB, Ahrens RC, Hess DR et al. Device selection and outcomes of aerosol therapy: Evidence-based guidelines. *Chest* 2005; **127**(1): 335–71.

74. Gibson RL, Retsch-Bogart GZ, Oermann C et al. Microbiology, safety, and pharmacokinetics of aztreonam lysinate for inhalation in patients with cystic fibrosis. *Pediatr Pulmonol* 2006; **41**(7): 656–65.

75. McCoy KS, Quittner AL, Oermann CM et al. Inhaled aztreonam lysine for chronic airway *Pseudomonas aeruginosa* in cystic fibrosis. *Am J Respir Crit Care Med* 2008; **178**(9): 921–8.

76. Retsch-Bogart GZ, Quittner AL, Gibson RL et al. Efficacy and safety of inhaled aztreonam lysine for airway pseudomonas in cystic fibrosis. *Chest* 2009; **135**(5): 1223–32.

77. Traylor BR, Wheatley CM, Skrentny TT et al. Influence of genetic variation of the β2-adrenergic receptor on lung diffusion in patients with cystic fibrosis. *Pulm Pharmacol Ther* 2011; **24**(5): 610–6.

78. Flume PA, O'Sullivan BP, Robinson KA et al. Cystic fibrosis pulmonary guidelines. *Am J Respir Crit Care Med* 2007; **176**(10): 957–69.

79. Robay A, Toumaniantz G, Leblais V, Gauthier C. Transfected beta3- but not beta2-adrenergic receptors regulate cystic fibrosis transmembrane conductance regulator activity via a new pathway involving the mitogen-activated protein kinases extracellular signal-regulated kinases. *Mol Pharmacol* 2005; **67**(3): 648–54.

80. Bossard F, Silantieff E, Lavazais-Blancou E et al. β1, β2, and β3 adrenoceptors and Na+/H+ exchanger regulatory factor 1 expression in human bronchi and their modifications in cystic fibrosis. *Am J Respir Cell Mol Biol* 2011; **44**(1): 91–8.

81. Ormerod LP, Thomson RA, Anderson CM, Stableforth DE. Reversible airway obstruction in cystic fibrosis. *Thorax* 1980; **35**(10): 768–72.

82. Cropp GJ. Effectiveness of bronchodilators in cystic fibrosis. *Am J Med* 1996; **100**(1A): 19S–29S.

83. Hiatt P, Eigen H, Yu P, Tepper RS. Bronchodilator responsiveness in infants and young children with cystic fibrosis. *Am J Respir Crit Care Med* 1988; **137**(1): 119–22.

84. Macfarlane PI, Heaf D. Changes in airflow obstruction and oxygen saturation in response to exercise and bronchodilators in cystic fibrosis. *Pediatr Pulmonol* 1990; **8**(1): 4–11.

85. Zach MS, Oberwaldner B, Forche G, Polgar G. Bronchodilators increase airway instability in cystic fibrosis. *Am Rev Respir Dis* 1985; **131**(4): 537–43.

86. Kusenbach G, Friedrichs F, Skopnik H, Heimann G. Increased physiological dead space during exercise after bronchodilation in cystic fibrosis. *Pediatr Pulmonol* 1993; **15**(5): 273–8.

87. Serisier DJ, Coates AD, Bowler SD. Effect of albuterol on maximal exercise capacity in cystic fibrosis. *Chest* 2007; **131**(4): 1181–7.

88. Davis B, Marin MG, Yee JW, Nadel JA. Effect of terbutaline on movement of Cl- and Na+ across the trachea of the dog in vitro. *Am Rev Respir Dis* 1979; **120**(3): 547–52.

89. Bennett WD. Effect of beta-adrenergic agonists on mucociliary clearance. *J Allergy Clin Immunol* 2002; **110**(6): S291–7.

90. Finkbeiner WE, Zlock LT, Morikawa M et al. Cystic fibrosis and the relationship between mucin and chloride secretion by cultures of human airway gland mucous cells. *AJP Lung Cell Mol Physiol* 2011; **301**: L402–14.

91. Cystic Fibrosis Trust. Nebulised antibiotics. In: *Antibiotic Treatment for Cystic Fibrosis*. Bromley, United Kingdom: Cystic Fibrosis Trust; 2002. pp. 25–33.

92. Doring G, Conway SP, Heijerman HG et al. Antibiotic therapy against *Pseudomonas aeruginosa* in cystic fibrosis: A European consensus. *Eur Respir J* 2000; **16**(4): 749–67.

93. Ramagopal M, Lands LC. Inhaled tobramycin and bronchial hyperactivity in cystic fibrosis. *Pediatr Pulmonol* 2000; **29**(5): 366–70.

94. Alothman GA, Alsaadi MM, Ho BL et al. Evaluation of bronchial constriction in children with cystic fibrosis after inhaling two different preparations of tobramycin. *Chest* 2002; **122**(3): 930–4.

95. Alothman GA, Ho B, Alsaadi MM et al. Bronchial constriction and inhaled colistin in cystic fibrosis. *Chest* 2005; **127**(2): 522–9.

96. Plosker GL. Aztreonam lysine for inhalation solution in cystic fibrosis. *Drugs* 2010; **70**(14): 1843–55.

97. Grotta MB, Etchebere EC de SC, Ribeiro AF et al. Pulmonary deposition of inhaled tobramycin prior to and after respiratory therapy and use of inhaled albuterol in cystic fibrosis patients colonized with *Pseudomonas aeruginosa*. *J Bras Pneumol* 2009; **35**(1): 35–43.

98. Popov TA, Pizzichini MM, Pizzichini E et al. Some technical factors influencing the induction of sputum for cell analysis. *Eur Respir J* 1995; **8**(4): 559–65.

99. Araki H, SLY P. Inhalation of hypertonic saline as a bronchial challenge in children with mild asthma and normal children. *J Allergy Clin Immunol* 1989; **84**(1): 99–107.

100. Dellon EP, Donaldson SH, Johnson R, Davis SD. Safety and tolerability of inhaled hypertonic saline in young children with cystic fibrosis. *Pediatr Pulmonol* 2008; **43**(11): 1100–6.

101. Rosenfeld M, Davis S, Brumback L et al. Inhaled hypertonic saline in infants and toddlers with cystic fibrosis: Short-term tolerability, adherence, and safety. *Pediatr Pulmonol* 2011; **46**(7): 666–71.

102. Suri R, Marshall LJ, Wallis C et al. Safety and use of sputum induction in children with cystic fibrosis. *Pediatr Pulmonol* 2003; **35**(4): 309–13.

103. Ziebach R, Pietsch-Breitfeld B, Bichler M et al. Bronchodilatory effects of salbutamol, ipratropium bromide, and their combination: Double-blind, placebo-controlled crossover study in cystic fibrosis. *Pediatr Pulmonol* 2001; **31**(6): 431–5.

104. Halfhide C, Evans HJ, Couriel J. Inhaled bronchodilators for cystic fibrosis. *Cochrane Database Syst Rev (Online)* 2005; (4): CD003428.

105. Newhouse M, Labiris NR, Freitag A. Inhaled antibiotics: Why TOBI® and other aminoglycosides have such clinical importance. *Respir Drug Deliv* 2009; **1**: 35–48.

106. Littlewood KJ, Higashi K, Jansen JP et al. A network meta-analysis of the efficacy of inhaled antibiotics for chronic *Pseudomonas* infections in cystic fibrosis. *J Cyst Fibros* 2012; **11**(5): 419–26.

107. Chuchalin A, Amelina E, Bianco F. Tobramycin for inhalation in cystic fibrosis: Beyond respiratory improvements. *Pulm Pharmacol Ther* 2009; **22**(6): 526–32.

108. Geller DE, Pitlick WH, Nardella PA et al. Pharmacokinetics and bioavailability of aerosolized tobramycin in cystic fibrosis. *Chest* 2002; **122**(1): 219–26.

109. Wallace SJ, Li J, Rayner CR et al. Stability of colistin methanesulfonate in pharmaceutical products and solutions for administration to patients. *Antimicrob Agents Chemother* 2008; **52**(9): 3047–51.

110. Westerman EM, Le Brun PPH, Touw DJ et al. Effect of nebulized colistin sulphate and colistin sulphomethate on lung function in patients with cystic fibrosis: A pilot study. *J Cyst Fibros* 2004; **3**(1): 23–8.

111. Li J, Milne RW, Nation RL et al. Stability of colistin and colistin methanesulfonate in aqueous media and plasma as determined by high-performance liquid chromatography. *Antimicrob Agents Chemother* 2003; **47**(4): 1364–70.

112. Hodson M, Gallagher C, Govan J. A randomised clinical trial of nebulised tobramycin or colistin in cystic fibrosis. *Eur Respir J* 2002; **20**(3): 658–64.

113. Taccetti G, Campana S, Festini F et al. Early eradication therapy against *Pseudomonas aeruginosa* in cystic fibrosis patients. *Eur Respir J* 2005; **26**(3): 458–61.

114. Valerius NH, Koch C, Hoiby N. Prevention of chronic *Pseudomonas aeruginosa* colonisation in cystic fibrosis by early treatment. *Lancet* 1991; **338**(8769): 725–6.

115. Hansen CR, Pressler T, Hoiby N. Early aggressive eradication therapy for intermittent *Pseudomonas aeruginosa* airway colonization in cystic fibrosis patients: 15 years experience. *J Cyst Fibros* 2008; **7**(6): 523–30.

116. McCoy KS. Compounded colistimethate as possible cause of fatal acute respiratory distress syndrome. *N Engl J Med* 2007; **357**(22): 2310–1.

117. Mccoy KS. Personal communication with the physician of record. 2012.

118. Assael BM. Aztreonam inhalation solution for suppressive treatment of chronic *Pseudomonas aeruginosa* lung infection in cystic fibrosis. *Expert Rev Anti Infect Ther* 2011; **9**(11): 967–73.

119. Geller DE. Aerosol antibiotics in cystic fibrosis. *Respir Care* 2009; **54**(5): 658–70.

120. Pesaturo KA, Horton ER, Belliveau P. Inhaled aztreonam lysine for cystic fibrosis pulmonary disease-related outcomes. *Ann Pharmacother* 2012; **46**(7-8): 1076–85.

121. Oermann CM, Retsch-Bogart GZ, Quittner AL et al. An 18-month study of the safety and efficacy of repeated courses of inhaled aztreonam lysine in cystic fibrosis. *Pediatr Pulmonol* 2010; **45**(11): 1121–34.

122. Oermann CM, McCoy KS, Retsch-Bogart GZ et al. *Pseudomonas aeruginosa* antibiotic susceptibility during long-term use of aztreonam for inhalation solution (AZLI). *J Antimicrob Chemother* 2011; **66**(10): 2398–404.

123. Retsch-Bogart GZ, Burns JL, Otto KL et al. A phase 2 study of aztreonam lysine for inhalation to treat patients with cystic fibrosis and *Pseudomonas aeruginosa* infection. *Pediatr Pulmonol* 2008; **43**(1): 47–58.

124. Assael BM, Pressler T, Bilton D et al. Inhaled aztreonam lysine vs. inhaled tobramycin in cystic fibrosis: A comparative efficacy trial. *J Cyst Fibros* 2013; **12**(2): 130–40. Available at http://dx.doi.org/10.1016/j.jcf.2012.07.006

125. Proesmans M, Vermeulen F, Vreys M, De Boeck K. Use of nebulized amphotericin B in the treatment of allergic bronchopulmonary aspergillosis in cystic fibrosis. *Int J Pediatr* 2010; **2010**: 1–9.

126. Hayes D, Murphy BS, Lynch JE, Feola DJ. Aerosolized amphotericin for the treatment of allergic bronchopulmonary aspergillosis. *Pediatr Pulmonol* 2010; **45**(11): 1145–8.

127. Slobbe L, Boersma E, Rijnders BJA. Tolerability of prophylactic aerosolized liposomal amphotericin-B and impact on pulmonary function: Data from a randomized placebo-controlled trial. *Pulm Pharmacol Ther* 2008; **21**(6): 855–9.

128. Kuiper L, Ruijgrok EJ. A review on the clinical use of inhaled amphotericin B. *J Aerosol Med Pulm Drug Deliv* 2009; **22**(3): 213–27.

129. Tolman JA, Nelson NA, Son YJ et al. Characterization and pharmacokinetic analysis of aerosolized aqueous voriconazole solution. *Eur J Pharm Biopharm* 2009; **72**(1): 199–205.

130. Cystic Fibrosis Foundation. Drug Development Pipeline. Available at http://www.cff.org/research/DrugDevelopmentPipeline/; accessed on October 1, 2012.

131. ARIKACE® (Inhaled liposomal amikacin). INSMED 2010. Available at http: //www.insmed.com/arikace.php; accessed on September 30, 2012.

132. Rubin BK. Mucolytics, expectorants, and mucokinetic medications. *Respir Care* 2007; **52**(7): 859–65.

133. Balsamo R, Lanata L, Egan CG. Mucoactive drugs. *Eur Respir Rev* 2010; **19**(116): 127–33.

134. Phillips GJ, James SL, Lethem MI. Rheological properties and hydration of airway mucus. In: Rogers DF, Lethem MI (Eds). *Airway Mucus: Basic Mechanisms and Clinical Perspectives*. Basel, Switzerland: Birkhäuser Basel; 1997. pp. 117–48.

135. Fuchs HJ, Borowitz DS, Christiansen DH et al. Effect of aerosolized recombinant human DNase on exacerbations of respiratory symptoms and on pulmonary function in patients with cystic fibrosis. The Pulmozyme Study Group. *N Engl J Med* 1994; **331**(10): 637–42.

136. Wilmott RW, Amin RS, Colin AA et al. Aerosolized recombinant human DNase in hospitalized cystic fibrosis patients with acute pulmonary exacerbations. *Am J Respir Crit Care Med* 1996; **153**(6 Pt 1): 1914–7.

137. Frederiksen B, Pressler T, Hansen A et al. Effect of aerosolized rhDNase (Pulmozyme) on pulmonary colonization in patients with cystic fibrosis. *Acta Paediatr* 2006; **95**(9): 1070–4.

138. Giessen LVD. Does the timing of inhaled dornase alfa matter? *J Cyst Fibros* 2009; **8**(S1): S6–S9.

139. Donaldson SH, Bennett WD, Zeman KL et al. Mucus clearance and lung function in cystic fibrosis with hypertonic saline. *N Engl J Med* 2006; **354**(3): 241–50.

140. Bye PTP, Elkins MR. Other mucoactive agents for cystic fibrosis. *Paediatr Respir Rev* 2007; **8**(1): 30–9.

141. Wills PJ, Hall RL, Chan W, Cole PJ. Sodium chloride increases the ciliary transportability of cystic fibrosis and bronchiectasis sputum on the mucus-depleted bovine trachea. *J. Clin. Invest.* 1997; **99**(1): 9–13.

142. Kishioka C, Okamoto K, Kim J-S, Rubin BK. Hyperosmolar solutions stimulate mucus secretion in the ferret trachea. *Chest* 2003; **124**(1): 306–13.

143. Greiff L, Andersson M, Wollmer P, Persson CGA. Hypertonic saline increases secretory and exudative responsiveness of human nasal airway in vivo. *Eur Respir J* 2003; **21**(2): 308–12.

144. Kim C-H, Hyun Song M, Eun Ahn Y et al. Effect of hypo-, iso- and hypertonic saline irrigation on secretory mucins and morphology of cultured human nasal epithelial cells. *Acta Otolaryngol* 2005; **125**(12): 1296–300.

145. Henke MO, Renner A, Huber RM et al. MUC5AC and MUC5B mucins are decreased in cystic fibrosis airway secretions. *Am J Respir Cell Mol Biol* 2004; **31**(1): 86–91.

146. Henke MO, John G, Germann M et al. MUC5AC and MUC5B mucins increase in cystic fibrosis airway secretions during pulmonary exacerbation. *Am J Respir Crit Care Med* 2007; **175**(8): 816–21.

147. Rogers DF. Mucoactive agents for airway mucus hypersecretory diseases. *Respir Care* 2007; **52**(9): 1176–93.

148. Elkins MR, Robinson M, Rose BR et al. A controlled trial of long-term inhaled hypertonic saline in patients with cystic fibrosis. *N Engl J Med* 2006; **354**(3): 229–40.

149. Ropper AH. Hyperosmolar therapy for raised intracranial pressure. *N Engl J Med* 2012; **367**(8): 746–52.

150. Bragadottir G, Redfors B, Ricksten S-E. Mannitol increases renal blood flow and maintains filtration fraction and oxygenation in postoperative acute kidney injury: A prospective interventional study. *Crit Care* 2012; **16**(4): R159.

151. Robinson M, Daviskas E, Eberl S et al. The effect of inhaled mannitol on bronchial mucus clearance in cystic fibrosis patients: A pilot study. *Eur Respir J* 1999; **14**(3): 678–85.

152. Jaques A, Daviskas E, Turton JA et al. Inhaled mannitol improves lung function in cystic fibrosis. *Chest* 2008; **133**(6): 1388–96.

153. Minasian C, Wallis C, Metcalfe C, Bush A. Comparison of inhaled mannitol, daily rhDNase and a combination of both in children with cystic fibrosis: A randomised trial. *Thorax* 2010; **65**(1): 51–6.

154. Teper A, Jaques A, Charlton B. Inhaled mannitol in patients with cystic fibrosis: A randomised open-label dose response trial. *J Cyst Fibros* 2011; **10**(1): 1–8.

155. Aitken ML, Bellon G, De Boeck K et al. Long-term inhaled dry powder mannitol in cystic fibrosis: An international randomized study. *Am J Respir Crit Care Med* 2012; **185**(6): 645–52.

156. Yaghi A, Zaman A, Dolovich MB. The direct effect of hyperosmolar agents on ciliary beating of human bronchial epithelial cells. *J Aerosol Med Pulm Drug Deliv* 2012; **25**(2): 88–95.

157. King M, Rubin BK. Pharmacological approaches to discovery and development of new mucolytic agents. *Adv Drug Deliv Rev.* 2002; **54**(11): 1475–90.

158. Bilton D, Bellon G, Charlton B et al. Pooled analysis of two large randomised phase III inhaled mannitol studies in cystic fibrosis. *J Cyst Fibros* 2013; **12**(4): 367–76.

159. Trapnell BC. Inhaled dry powder mannitol: A solution for cystic fibrosis. *Am J Respir Crit Care Med* 2012; **185**(6): 596–8.

160. Chan J, Chan HK, Kwok P et al. Rapid delivery of solubilized mannitol for treatment of cystic fibrosis. *Respir Drug Deliv* 2011; **1**: 515–8.

161. Chan JGY, Kwok PCL, Young PM et al. Mannitol delivery by vibrating mesh nebulisation for enhancing mucociliary clearance. *J Pharm Sci* 2011; **100**(7): 2693–702.

162. Dueholm M, Nielsen C, Thorshauge H et al. N-acetylcysteine by metered dose inhaler in the treatment of chronic bronchitis: A multi-centre study. *Respir Med* 1992; **86**(2): 89–92.

163. Decramer M, Rutten-van Mölken M, Dekhuijzen PNR et al. Effects of N-acetylcysteine on outcomes in chronic obstructive pulmonary disease (Bronchitis Randomized on NAC Cost-Utility Study, BRONCUS): A randomised placebo-controlled trial. *Lancet* 2005; **365**(9470): 1552–60.

164. Duijvestijn YC, Brand PL. Systematic review of N-acetylcysteine in cystic fibrosis. *Acta Paediatr* 1999; **88**(1): 38–41.

165. Nash EF, Stephenson A, Ratjen F, Tullis E. Nebulized and oral thiol derivatives for pulmonary disease in cystic fibrosis. *Cochrane Database Syst Rev (Online)* 2009; (1): CD007168.

166. Knowles M, Gatzy J, Boucher R. Increased bioelectric potential difference across respiratory epithelia in cystic fibrosis. *N Engl J Med* 1981; **305**(25): 1489–95.

167. Kohler D, App E, Schmitz-Schumann M et al. Inhalation of amiloride improves the mucociliary and the cough clearance in patients with cystic fibroses. *Eur J Respir Dis Suppl* 1986; **146**: 319–26.

168. Konig J. The cystic fibrosis transmembrane conductance regulator (CFTR) inhibits ENaC through an increase in the intracellular Cl- concentration. *EMBO Rep* 2001; **2**(11): 1047–51.

169. Cuthbert AW. New horizons in the treatment of cystic fibrosis. *Br J Pharmacol* 2011; **163**(1): 173–83.

170. Qadri YJ, Rooj AK, Fuller CM. ENaCs and ASICs as therapeutic targets. *AJP Cell Physiol* 2012; **302**(7): C943–65.

171. Conese M, Romano M, Furnari ML et al. New genetic and pharmacological treatments for cystic fibrosis. *Curr Pediatr Rev* 2009; **5**(1): 8–27.

172. Hirsh AJ, Sabater JR, Zamurs A et al. Evaluation of second generation amiloride analogs as therapy for cystic fibrosis lung disease. *J Pharmacol Exp Ther* 2004; **311**(3): 929–38.

173. Voynow JA, Rubin BK. Mucins, mucus, and sputum. *Chest* 2009; **135**(2): 505–12.

174. Chmiel J, Konstan M. Inflammation and anti-inflammatory therapies for cystic fibrosis. *Clin Chest Med* 2007; **28**(2): 331–46.

175. Dezateux C, Walters S, Balfour-Lynn I. Inhaled corticosteroids for cystic fibrosis. *Cochrane Database Syst Rev (Online)* 2000; (2): CD001915.

176. Pressler T. Targeting airway inflammation in cystic fibrosis in children: Past, present, and future. *Paediatr Drugs* 2011; **13**(3): 141–7.

177. Grimbert D, Vecellio L, Delépine P et al. Characteristics of EPI-hNE4 aerosol: A new elastase inhibitor for treatment of cystic fibrosis. *J Aerosol Med* 2003; **16**(2): 121–9.

178. Cantin AM, Berthiaume Y, Cloutier D, Martel M. Prolastin aerosol therapy and sputum taurine in cystic fibrosis. *Clin Invest Med* 2006; **29**(4): 201–7.

179. Griese M, Latzin P, Kappler M et al. Alpha1-antitrypsin inhalation reduces airway inflammation in cystic fibrosis patients. *Eur Respir J* 2007; **29**(2): 240–50.

180. Rhoads J. Warning letter. 2005; available online at: http://www.fda.gov/iceci/enforcementactions/warningletters/2005/.

181. Ruf K, Hebestreit H. Exercise-induced hypoxemia and cardiac arrhythmia in cystic fibrosis. *J Cyst Fibros* 2009; **8**(2): 83–90.

182. Fauroux B. Why, when and how to propose noninvasive ventilation in cystic fibrosis? *Minerva Anestesiol* 2011; **77**(11): 1108–14.

183. Gozal D. Nocturnal ventilatory support in patients with cystic fibrosis: Comparison with supplemental oxygen. *Eur Respir J* 1997; **10**(9): 1999–2003.

184. Young AC, Wilson JW, Kotsimbos TC, Naughton MT. The impact of nocturnal oxygen desaturation on quality of life in cystic fibrosis. *J Cyst Fibros* 2011; **10**(2): 100–6.

185. Suratwala D, Chan JSH, Kelly A et al. Nocturnal saturation and glucose tolerance in children with cystic fibrosis. *Thorax* 2011; **66**(7): 574–8.

186. Bass JL, Corwin M, Gozal D et al. The effect of chronic or intermittent hypoxia on cognition in childhood: A review of the evidence. *Pediatrics* 2004; **114**(3): 805–16.

187. Balfour-Lynn IM, Field DJ, Gringras P et al. BTS guidelines for home oxygen in children. *Thorax* 2009; **64**(S2): ii1–ii26.

188. Elphick HE, Mallory G. Oxygen therapy for cystic fibrosis. *Cochrane Database Syst Rev (Online)* 2009; (1): CD003884.

189. Nixon PA, Orenstein DM, Curtis SE, Ross EA. Oxygen supplementation during exercise in cystic fibrosis. *Am Rev Respir Dis* 1990; **142**(4): 807–11.

190. Dodd ME, Haworth CS, Webb AK. A practical approach to oxygen therapy in cystic fibrosis. *J R Soc Med* 1998; **91**(S34): 30–9.

21

Upper airway disease

ROMANA KUCHAI AND WILLIAM E. GRANT

INTRODUCTION

Cystic fibrosis (CF) is an autosomal recessive disease with multisystem involvement, and with particularly devastating respiratory impact. The respiratory tract can be considered to extend from the lips and nostrils to the alveoli, being divided into an upper airway and a lower airway at the level of the larynx, and is lined throughout with respiratory pseudostratified ciliated epithelium. Although the dominant features relate to lower respiratory tract infections and pancreatic insufficiency, the upper airway sites most significantly affected by the disease are the nose and paranasal sinuses.

Thickened viscid secretions overwhelm mucociliary clearance mechanisms and lead to mucus stasis and infection in the paranasal sinuses and lower segmental airways alike. Chronic inflammation in the nasal airways may lead to nasal polyposis, a condition rarely seen in childhood outside CF. Significant sinonasal symptoms arise in some 30%–45% of sufferers, and these may be debilitating. Chronic catarrhal and cough symptoms with nasal obstruction, anosmia, and headache are typical presenting features. The sinuses may become chronically infected by organisms such as *Pseudomonas aeruginosa*.[1] Interestingly, the incidence of primary otological disease, or of dysfunction secondary to Eustachian tube failure due to chronic sinonasal disease, appears to be no higher than that in the general population.[2,3]

Physicians focusing on the life-threatening lower respiratory symptoms suffered by these patients may undertreat and underappreciate the extent, impact, and significance of sinonasal disease in this condition. The inflammatory burden of upper airway disease may contribute, by mechanisms that are as yet not fully understood but involving sinobronchial reflex pathways, eosinophilia, and humoral mechanisms, to the worsening of already profound lower respiratory tract dysfunction.

Improved medical management and surgical management of sinonasal disease, both of which have seen dramatic developments in recent years, contribute to secondary improvement in control of pulmonary inflammatory and infective disease in non-CF patients.[4–8] As might be expected given the underlying pathophysiology of CF, studies in this population show varied, but less dramatic, response of the lower airway to improved upper airway disease management.

As CF patients are recognized to underreport upper airway symptoms, optimal treatment of upper airway disease will ideally involve input from rhinologically specialized ear, nose, throat (ENT) practitioners in a multidisciplinary setting. Improved management may thus not only result in benefits for the primary nasal symptoms but also improve lower respiratory manifestations of the disease.

PATHOPHYSIOLOGY

Mucus stasis inevitably leads to secondary infection and, in the nose, sinus ostial obstruction with failure in ventilation and drainage, which are the major predisposing factors in the development of sinus disease in normal subjects.[9] Infective organisms isolated from the sinuses tend to be *P. aeruginosa*, *Staphylococcus aureus*, *Haemophilus influenzae*, and anaerobes.[1]

Rhinosinusitis is considered an inflammatory process of multifactorial etiology. The predisposing pathologies are a combination of infection, allergy, mucosal edema, and rarely physical obstruction. Either one or more of pathologies may result in mucociliary impairment. Disease manifestations are likely to result from a combination of inflammation secondary to the failure to clear thickened secretions, sinus ostial obstruction, and superadded infection, rather than simply being primarily infective.

MUCOCILIARY FUNCTION

CF patients are traditionally thought to have reduced mucociliary clearance.[10,11] More recently, a study aimed at differentiating primary (cystic fibrosis transmembrane conductance regulator [CFTR] ion transport related) from secondary (inflammatory) causes of delayed mucociliary clearance challenged the idea that CFTR dysfunction on its own caused delayed clearance from the nose.[12] Fifty children with CF, primary ciliary dyskinesia, and no respiratory disease were studied. Normal and CF children had normal mucociliary clearance times and proinflammatory cytokine levels. The finding that CF children actually had normal mucociliary function suggests that adults with CF had impaired ciliary clearance secondary to inflammatory airway changes. There is no doubt that chronic inflammation results in secondary changes including goblet cell hyperplasia, as well as squamous metaplasia and loss of ciliated cells. Bacterial toxins, such as the pyocyanin and 1-hydroxyphenazine produced by *Pseudomonas* spp.,[13,14] as well as inflammatory by-products such as neutrophil elastase can further impair ciliary motility.[15] Progressive respiratory disease seems to be secondary to chronic infection and the onset of neutrophil-dominated inflammation.[16] The neutrophil necrosis releasing proteolytic enzymes and their effect are thought to result in the damage to underlying epithelium. This, coupled with the greatly increased mucus viscosity, results in severely disturbed mucociliary clearance.

Within paranasal sinuses, alteration in the viscoelastic properties of the mucus in CF contributes to a mechanical obstruction of the sinus ostia. The secondary mucostasis, infection, and inflammation that develops results in intrasinus hypoxia, hypercarbia, and reduction in pH, leading to further mucosal inflammation, edema, and yet further mucociliary impairment and the opportunity for bacterial infection and colonization.

NASAL POLYPOSIS

Nasal polyposis in children is exceptionally rare outside the CF population, and once identified the diagnosis of CF must be pursued.

The incidence of nasal polyposis in CF was probably underestimated in earlier studies before the advent of endoscopic techniques, and more recent figures quoting a range of 32%–45% are probably more accurate.[2,17] Hadfield et al. report an incidence of 37% in 211 adults with CF from the Royal Brompton Hospital.[18] Slieker reports half the children in a series of 140 children with CF had polyps, but that only 59% of these were symptomatic.[19]

However, the pathophysiology of the development of nasal polyposis in CF is unclear, as indeed it is in non-CF polyposis. There appears to be a higher incidence of colonization of *Pseudomonas* in CF patients with sinonasal polyps than those

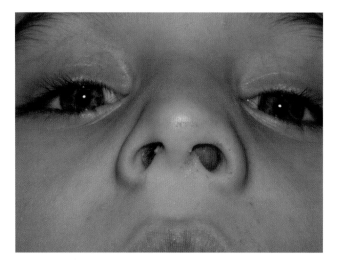

Figure 21.1 Photograph demonstrating nasal polyposis with complete occlusion of left nasal airway and broadening of nasal dorsum secondary to extensive anterior ethmoid polyposis.

without. Why some patients develop symptomatic sinusitis; some remain relatively asymptomatic; and some, but by no means all, go on to develop nasal polyposis is not understood. Tos has hypothesized that polyps result from nasal mucosal inflammation where epithelial damage allows prolapse of the lamina propria and suggested a similar pathogenesis in inflammatory and non-CF polyps, based on histological appearance.[20] However, subsequent studies (later) have shown that the histological features of CF polyps demonstrate specific differences to the polyps in chronic rhinosinusitis.

The presence of expansive polypoid disease in the ethmoids may result in the widening of the nasal bridge and the appearance of hypertelorism[2] (see Figure 21.1). The relatively elastic bones of younger children with massive polyposis in the ethmoid labyrinth may be responsible for the broad nasal dorsum sometimes seen in pediatric cystic polyposis—a pseudohypertelorism or Woakes syndrome. In CF, the anterior ethmoid grows faster than the posterior compartment, which may also relate to the broadening of the nasal dorsum seen with massive polyps. There is a higher frequency of chronic lower airway infection with *P. aeruginosa* in CF patients with nasal polyps compared with patients with no polyps.[21]

MICROBIOLOGY

Whereas in the non-CF population haemophilus and streptococcal organisms are predominantly responsible for chronic infective rhinosinusitis, in CF *P. aeruginosa* and *Staphylococcus aureus* are more frequently cultured. The majority of the bacterial isolates recovered from the sinuses are also present in sputum cultures, as demonstrated by genotyping of the bacteria.[22] Other potential pathogens that

Table 21.1 Bent and Kuhn classification for AFS

Major
1. Type 1 hypersensitivity confirmed by history
2. Nasal polyposis
3. Characteristic CT scan signs
4. Positive fungal smear

Minor
1. Asthma
2. Unilateral predominance
3. Serum eosinophilia
4. Radiographic bone erosion
5. Fungal culture
6. Charcot–Leyden crystals

are isolated with increasing frequency include atypical myco-bacteria, *Stenotrophomonas maltophilia*, and *Achromobacter xylosoxidans*. Mainz et al. in 2009 published data analyzing the microbial colonization of upper and lower airways. Their work identified the role of the upper airway as a reservoir of infection for *P. aeruginosa* and *Staphylococcus* aureus in CF patients. In practice, however, it remains a fact that lower respiratory tract culture specimens are often considered easier to obtain than upper respiratory tract culture specimens.

There has been little in the literature regarding fungal disease in CF in spite of debate in recent years regarding the role of fungi in chronic rhinosinusitis and nasal polyposis in the general population. One group found that fungal cultures were positive in 33.3% of cases.[23] Within the CF population, *Candida albicans* was the commonest, with one each of *Aspergillus fumigatus*, *Penicillium* spp., *Exserohilum*, and *Bipolaris*. There appeared to be no correlation between presence of fungal isolates and requirement for revision surgery. Two patients were diagnosed as having allergic fungal sinusitis (AFS), according to the criteria of Bent and Kuhn.[24] This is described in Table 21.1.

The role of these fungi in the pathogenesis of sinonasal disease in CF is unclear at this time, and while they may be incidental isolates in some patients, in particular those with *Aspergillus* spp., chronic low-grade presence may provoke IgE-mediated hypersensitivity and AFS in a manner similar to allergic bronchopulmonary mycosis. Stressman et al., in their study in 2011, confirmed microbial diversity of common and novel species of bacteria within the upper respiratory tract.

SINONASAL SYMPTOMS

There is a low self-reporting of symptoms by CF patients and poor correlation between symptoms and disease severity.[25–27] Patients may accept upper airway symptoms as normal because they may have been present from an early age.[26] Common symptoms include nasal obstruction, purulent rhinorrhea, headache, anosmia, facial pain, snoring, and voice change.[28,29] Headache and periorbital pain are the commonest reported symptoms in those with chronic rhinosinusitis, and anosmia is the commonest symptom in those with polyps.[30] Headache is difficult to quantify but tends to be reported more in adolescent and adult patients. Mucoceles are rare in children and can be associated with a variance of symptoms including epiphora and chronic rhinosinusitis. Such symptoms alongside endoscopic findings may raise a high suspicion of CF if not previously suspected.

Imaging in the form of computed tomography (CT) scanning is the investigation of choice to establish the extent of sinonasal disease. Mucoceles are managed with surgical drainage, which are now successfully amenable to endoscopic surgical drainage.

CLINICAL AND ENDOSCOPIC FINDINGS

Much can be gleaned from simple inspection of the child or adult in the clinic. Observation of mouth breathing tendencies may point to severity of nasal obstructive disease. Typical "adenoid"-type facies, due to nasal obstruction, may be evident. Broadening of the nasal bridge along with pseudohypertelorism is a further common clinical finding[30] (Figure 21.1). Physical findings may, however, be absent. Intranasal examination can be performed with a bright headlight or perhaps with an otoscope following the application of a topical decongestant. Rhinitic inferior turbinates are frequently misinterpreted as polyps, and referral for examination by a collaborative rhinologist with an interest in this condition is ideal. Although gross polyps are easily seen; up to 25% of polyps can be missed by just direct visualization alone.[30] Inspection is ideally carried out with either a rigid 2.7-mm Hopkins rod endoscope in adults and older children or a flexible endoscope in younger children (see Figures 21.2 and 21.3). This commonly reveals degrees of nasal polyposis, purulent secretions emanating from one or more of the recognized drainage pathways, or medial bulging of the lateral nasal wall. Appraisal of the postnasal space for obstructive

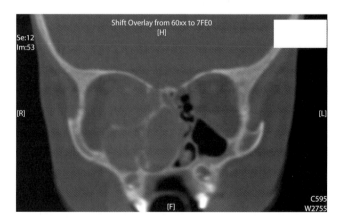

Figure 21.2 Coronal of computed tomography (CT) scans revealing the extent of an ethmoidal mucocele in a child.

adenoid enlargement may allow for a simple intervention that might improve the nasal airway and function. A workup for coexisting allergy should be undertaken. A complete ENT examination should be considered on a regular basis in the interest of overall well-being of the CF patient.[31]

ALLERGY

Most studies demonstrate increased atopy based on skin prick tests in patients with CF, and specifically increased hypersensitivity to *Aspergillus* spp. It has been noted that consequently an increase in AFS is considered more likely.

Atopy does not appear to influence the development of nasal polyps,[18,32] but *Aspergillus* allergy is commoner in CF patients with polyps than those without.[33] A genetic link between CF and allergic bronchopulmonary aspergillosis (ABPA) is suggested by the finding of a high frequency of homozygous and heterozygous *CFTR* gene mutations in patients with ABPA and normal sweat tests and without CF.[34,35] The term sinobronchial allergic mycosis has been proposed for coexisting ABPA and AFS.[36] At the moment, there is no direct association of allergy contributing to the development of nasal polyposis, asthma, or progressive lung disease; however, as 20% of patients with CF also suffers from allergy, it is important to consider the optimization of its treatment.

POSTTRANSPLANT LYMPHOPROLIFERATIVE DISORDER

Posttransplant lymphoproliferative disorder (PTLD) may be defined as uncontrolled lymphoproliferation in a setting of pharmacological immunosuppression. Sinonasal PTLD is rare,[37] and early detection is prognostically critical. Chronic rhinosinusitis is extremely common in CF and can cause numerous problems, placing the patients at risk of life-threatening illness. Clinician awareness that post-transplant immunosuppressed patients may not simply be suffering with a further recurrence of CF nasal polyposis is therefore of great importance.

IMAGING

Plain sinus radiographs have little if any role[38] as they may appear abnormal in most cases of CF. The imaging modality of choice in the evaluation of paranasal sinus disease is the CT scan. These scans play an important role in determining the extent and nature of disease and are indispensable in guiding surgical intervention where this is required. Rapid acquisition spiral CT techniques are satisfactorily tolerated, and radiation exposure is relatively low. CT findings in CF patients almost invariably show extensive pan-sinus opacification, with demineralization of the uncinate and medial

displacement of the lateral nasal wall; findings specific to this population are not seen in chronic sinusitis in non-CF patients.

CT may not always clearly distinguish between polyp and fluid, whether pus or retained secretions. Varying signal return may indicate the presence of pus of varying degrees of inspissation, fluid, and polyp. Normal CT scans are exceptionally rare in CF, most series reporting almost universal opacification.[8,28,30]

Features representative of CF may be the following:
1. Extensive paranasal sinus opacification (see Figures 21.2 and 21.3).
2. Sinus agenesis or hypoplasia (see Figure 21.4).
3. Bulging of the lateral nasal wall with thinning or loss of bony landmarks (see Figure 21.5).

These are the hall marks of CF sinus disease.

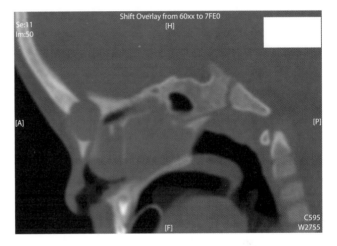

Figure 21.3 A sagittal view of CT scans revealing the extent of an ethmoidal mucocele in a child.

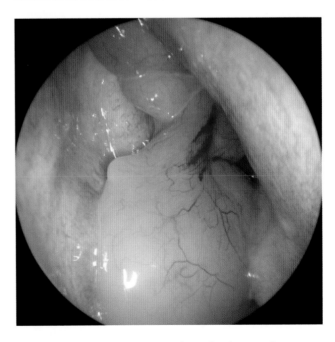

Figure 21.4 Endoscopic view of nasal polyposis, hypoplastic sinus with nasal polyposis.

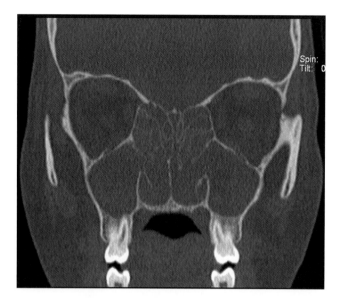

Figure 21.5 CT scan showing extensive pan-sinus opacification with no airway patency and middle meatal expansion.

The common finding of medialization of the lateral nasal wall is particularly interesting and the pathogenesis is incompletely understood. This medial bulging of the lateral nasal wall has been defined as a soft tissue mass extending medially from the maxillary sinus in the area of the middle meatus to at least half the distance from the lamina papyracea (medial orbital bony plate) to the nasal septum[40] (see Figure 21.5). However, the condition appears to be distinct from simple mucocele formation, as multiloculated collections of pus and thickened infected secretions are surrounded by gross thickening of the maxillary lining, which is frequently polypoid; therefore, the terms mucopyosinusitis and pseudomucocele have been proposed. Thinning of the bone of the medial wall and expansion of the natural maxillary sinus ostium from a few millimeters in healthy individuals to many times this is a common finding (see Figure 21.5). The destruction of the bony walls of the antrum may be attributable to osteitis,[42] pressure necrosis, demineralization,[43] or osteolysis. Pseudomucocele of the antrum may be age related, being present in all CF children under 5 years and more than 85% in the age group 5–8 but in only 60% of CF adolescents.[2] When present, it is usually bilateral.

The frontal sinuses classically remain hypoplastic as do the sphenoid sinuses. This is thought to reflect failure to develop due to inadequate ventilation, which reduces pneumatization in a fashion analogous to the sclerotic mastoid bone system with reduced air cell development seen in chronic suppurative ear disease.[44] Primary ciliary dyskinesia is the only other disease with a clear association with frontal sinus hypoplasia. However, agenesis of one or both frontal sinuses can be seen in the absence of any sinonasal disease in 10% of healthy individuals (see Figure 21.6).[45]

In summary, CT imaging of the paranasal sinuses is recommended in symptomatic sinusitis and polyposis and where significant medial bulging of the lateral nasal wall is perceived. There is, nevertheless, at times a poor correlation between severity of symptoms and CT findings.

Magnetic resonance imaging (MRI) tends to be very sensitive to inflammatory change and can be used to monitor treatment; but it does not reveal bony detail, so it is less used in sinus imaging. In a comparative study of CT with MRI in CF patients, by Eggesbo et al.,[46] MRI was able to differentiate opacification secondary to thickened mucosa as opposed to mucopurulent discharge. The gadolinium enhancemen of T1 weighted images allows distinction between mucosal edema and fluid/secretions. Patients who have undergone functional endoscopic sinus surgery (FESS) may be monitored postoperatively with MRI imaging (STIR and T1) to detect pus-filled loculations that can be eradicated with further surgery, avoiding both unnecessary further irradiation and unnecessary surgery for misdiagnosed simple mucosal disease.[47]

A new field of molecular imaging that includes radionucleotide-based methods such as planar γ-scintigraphy and single photon emission CT can be applied in combination with positron emission tomography scans within a standardized protocol to ensure uniformity. This can ensure that both clinicians and patients are able to assess and evaluate the condition and the therapeutic outcome in a more sophisticated multidisciplinary approach.[48]

HISTOPATHOLOGY

Nasal polyps in non-CF patients are benign mucosal swellings histologically characterized by edema, goblet cell hyperplasia of the epithelium, thickening of the basement membrane, and presence of numerous leukocytes, predominantly eosinophils.[49] Many histological similarities exist between polyps in CF and non-CF patients.[50] All nasal polyps show focal edema, hyperplasia, atrophy, or squamous metaplasia of the epithelium. The lamina propria is moderately populated with small blood vessels and mucus glands and shows focal accumulation of inflammatory cells.

Ultrastructurally, CF polyps differ significantly from non-CF polyps. Histological features specific to nasal polyposis in CF are a thin delicate basement membrane of surface epithelium, lack of extensive infiltration with eosinophils, and a preponderance of acid mucin in glands and cysts of the polyps (characteristically neutral in "allergic polyps") (Figure 21.7).[51–53]

The CF nasal polyps show specific characteristics of (1) minimal damage to surface epithelium, (2) presence of a mucus blanket lining the apical epithelium, (3) occasional intracytoplasmic lumina, (4) continuous and fenestrated type capillaries, (5) numerous degranulated mast cells, (6) many plasma cells often morphologically atypical and with intracisternal Russell bodies, and (7) a smaller number of eosinophils in comparison with non-CF polyps.[51]

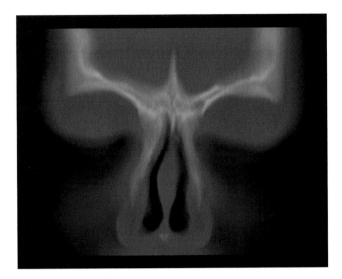

Figure 21.6 CT scan showing typical frontal sinus agenesis.

Further evidence in support of a different etiology for CF and non-CF nasal polyposis is becoming available from biochemical and molecular genetic studies. Nasal polyps from CF patients have different glycohistochemical properties from non-CF polyps, showing higher levels of lectin reactive galactoside residues.[52] Studies of innate markers like human β-defensins and toll-like receptors and inflammatory mediators such as myeloperoxidase, IgE, and interleukins (ILs) have shown significant differences between CF and non-CF nasal polyps.[53] IL-8 and myeloperoxidase have been shown to be significantly elevated in CF nasal polyposis in comparison with control or non-CF polyposis.

Inflammatory cell and cytokine pathways have been well documented in the lower respiratory tract and in chronic rhinosinusitis, but relatively little has been reported regarding these mechanisms in chronic rhinosinusitis in patients with CF. Sinus mucosal specimens were found to have higher numbers of neutrophils, macrophages, and cells expressing messenger RNA for interferon-γ and IL-8 in patients with CF than in patients with chronic rhinosinusitis or controls. Conversely, the number of eosinophils and cells expressing RNA for IL-4, IL-5, and IL-10 was higher in patients with chronic sinusitis in non-CF patients. These differing inflammatory mechanisms may in part explain differences in response to treatments in the CF group.[54]

NITRIC OXIDE

Nitric oxide is synthesized in the nasal sinuses and may be low in the presence of normal synthetic activity if the sinus ostia are blocked, e.g., in nasal polyposis.[55] Children with CF have been shown to have lowered nasal levels of nitric oxide but exhaled NO levels in the normal range.[56,57] Lowered nasal airway concentration of nitric oxide results from reduced nitric oxide synthase expression in the upper respiratory tract and may be in part responsible for the reduction in elimination of bacteria such as *Pseudomonas*.[58]

MEDICAL MANAGEMENT

Medical management involves the use of anti-inflammatory and antimicrobial therapy coupled with attempts at promoting clearance of static secretions with irrigation techniques. Most medical treatment strategies derive from those used in non-CF polyposis and rhinosinusitis and have a limited evidence base for their use in either condition and must be considered empiric. Combinations of oral and topical treatments are used depending on clinical symptom severity. The recognition that sinonasal disease in CF is incurable leads to efforts to control the disease medically, reserving surgery for those with more severe symptoms. Topical decongestants aim to open sinus ostia occluded by mucosal edema and promote sinus ventilation and drainage in acute infective exacerbation only; in the chronic situation, there is little role for topical decongestant therapy. There is increasing enthusiasm for nasal saline irrigations, either isotonic or hypertonic, to aid in clearing thick secretions, and trials in non-CF patients have shown benefit in chronic rhinosinusitis in symptom reduction, endoscopic appearance, and quality of life outcome measures.[59] Hypertonic solutions provide an osmotic gradient favoring fluid transport into the nose, resulting in an "osmotic decongestion" of sinus mucosa and may be more effective than isotonic solutions. Although medical management with nasal irrigation, appropriate antibiotics, and nasal steroid agents may provide both symptomatic relief and prolong the intervals between surgical procedures. It is important to consider the relevance of surgical procedures on failure of medical therapy.

CORTICOSTEROIDS

There is good evidence for the use of systemic steroids to bring about reduction in polyps and symptoms in studies in non-CF patients with persistent rhinosinusitis with nasal polyposis. There also exists good evidence to support a role for the use of postoperative steroids in reducing polyp recurrence postoperatively.[60] β-Methasone drops may significantly reduce polyp size compared to placebo.[61] Concerns regarding systemic adrenal suppression with long-term nasal steroid drop therapy lead to the recommendation that this form of treatment might alternate or rotate with periods of simple nasal steroid sprays in which systemic bioavailability is much lower.

ANTIBIOTICS

Infection secondary to thickened secretions and impaired ciliary function have led to the use of protracted courses of oral antibiotic treatment. The choice of antibiotic therapy is governed by likely infective organisms. The nasal sinuses, like the lungs, may become chronically infected by *Pseudomonas* and *Staphylococcus*, as well as nontypeable *H. influenzae*.[1,22] Empirical oral antibiotic treatment for sinusitis is recommended for a duration of 3–6 weeks for subjective increases in postnasal drainage, congestion, and cough symptoms.[62,63]

Complete eradication of *Pseudomonas* is unlikely.[64] Macrolides may be beneficial in chronic rhinosinusitis in non-CF children,[65,66] but there are no studies of macrolide therapy in CF sinonasal disease.

Some authors have recommended regular nasal and postsinus surgical sinus cavity irrigation with tobramycin, particularly in lung transplant patients, to reduce the risk of *Pseudomonas* pulmonary seeding and infection from infected sinuses.[67,68] Aminoglycosides such as tobramycin are known to cause ototoxicity resulting in labyrinthine damage and sensorineural hearing loss with prolonged use and, therefore, their application must be carefully considered.

Although nebulized formulations may be beneficial for lung infections, it has yet to be confirmed a standard in the treatment of sinonasal disease.

DEOXYRIBONUCLEASE

Recombinant human deoxyribonuclease 1 (dornase alfa) lyses extracellular DNA released by leucocytes involved in airway infection and inflammation, thereby reducing mucus viscosity. There is some evidence for benefit from nasal applications in patients undergoing sinus surgery.[64,69]

SURGICAL MANAGEMENT

Approximately 20%–25% of patients eventually necessitate surgical treatment for refractory sinonasal disease. Surgical options range from simple nasal polypectomy, where the polyps are simply amputated or avulsed, to meticulous clearance of all diseased mucosa with removal of the ethmoid labyrinth, usually with preservation of the turbinate structures and wide opening of the maxillary, and if present sphenoid and frontal sinuses (see Figure 21.6). The time to recurrence to some extent appears to depend on the extent of surgical disease clearance. Simple polypectomy surgery was associated with a tendency to earlier recurrence[70] than polypectomy with efforts to clear disease more thoroughly at intranasal ethmoidectomy.[3,71]

The basic tenet of endoscopic sinus surgery in sinusitis is that restoration of ventilation and drainage of a sinus cavity allows restoration of normal function with return of chronically inflamed mucosa to normal. Endoscopic sinus surgical techniques have been hugely successful in the general population in restoring nasal function.

There was early enthusiasm that improved lung function might be brought about by sinus surgery in CF patients. As the lower respiratory tract suffers from the identical

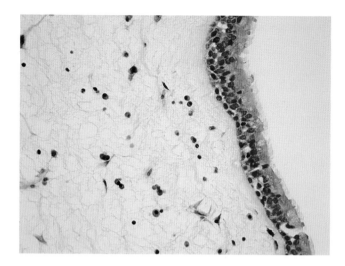

Figure 21.7 Area of polypoid mucosa showing subsurface edema with chronic inflammatory cells (few eosinophils). H&E stain and X200 magnification.

difficulties of greatly thickened mucus and secondary mucociliary failure, it is not surprising that problems persist in spite of adequate and maximal surgical and medical sinus treatment.

Although nasal polyposis is frequently the obvious disease on inspection of the nasal cavities, the presence of trapped and infected pockets of mucopus within the obstructed ethmoid chambers and within the antrum is the usual finding at surgery (see Figures 21.8 and 21.9). It is often an oversimplification to consider polyposis and chronic rhinosinusitis as separate entities, and polyps may be best considered as "the extreme outcome of unchecked mucosal inflammation in the ethmoid sinuses."[72] The degree of polyp formation, however, varies from extensive to little at all, for reasons that remain obscure but may be related to manifestations of different *CFTR* mutations. In turn, such differing disease may indicate the likelihood of different response to surgery.[73]

While accepting the incurability of sinonasal disease, this is not to say that considerable benefit may not be conferred by surgery. The aim of surgery is the relief of symptoms, clearance of disease and its inflammatory burden, elimination of reservoirs of infected mucus (especially in the severely affected population undergoing heart–lung transplant surgery), and minimization of likelihood of recurrence of disease. The excision of the ethmoid labyrinth of many small bony compartments, creating an open cavity, along with the creation of large drainage and ventilation antrostomies into the maxillary antra that might allow gravitational drainage, helped by irrigation with saline sprays and douches, would seem likely to help reduce mucus stasis and infection and allow ingress of medication and therefore decrease infection and inflammation.

In spite of almost universal disease presence on CT imaging, surgery has in the main been offered to patients with more severely diseased noses as they have been the ones associated with more severe symptoms. Some authors have recommended conservative surgery on the basis that the disease is highly likely to recur and that prolonged procedures and anesthetics should be avoided in this population with respiratory and occasional coagulation compromise.[74] Others advocate that if a procedure is to be undertaken as definitive a disease clearance as possible should be achieved with optimization of anatomy for future management. This would include the addition of adenoidectomy in children and, for example, septoplasty where indicated. A recent study demonstrated

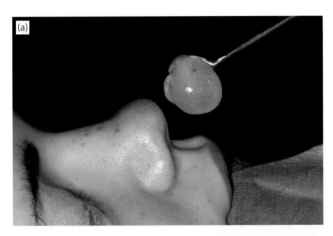

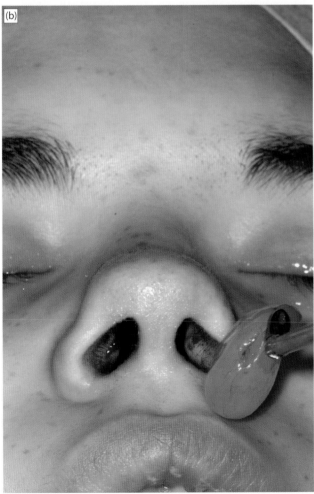

Figure 21.8 **(a)** Nasal polyp. **(b)** Nasal polyp on delivery.

the recurrence of frontal sinus restenosis being higher in CF patients following definitive frontal sinus surgery, endorsing the view that the pathway for long-term management must consider this group of patients carefully.

Balloon catheter sinuplasty is currently used in the treatment of chronic rhinosinusitis. It enables a mucus-sparing technique that has been proved to be safe; however, its use is limited in polypoid disease and therefore its application in CF patients is limited. Surgery can be considered a contraindication and even inappropriate in those with severe pulmonary disease where general anesthesia poses an unacceptable risk to the patient; however, a limited procedure may be performed under local anesthesia.

SYMPTOM BENEFIT

Improvement following nonendoscopic[75,76] and subsequently endoscopic sinus surgery[2,70,71,77–79] of symptoms relating to nasal polyposis and chronic rhinosinusitis is universally reported. Recurrence of sinonasal disease is ultimately the rule, and persistence of radiological abnormality on CT imaging is inevitable.[81–83] The correlation, however, between radiological findings and clinical symptoms in CF patients remains unclear.

Most studies are retrospective case series, and the duration of follow-up frequently varies. In one prospective study of patients undergoing endoscopic sinus surgery with a mean follow-up of 34 months, improvements in nasal obstructive symptoms, olfactory acuity, and reduction in purulent nasal discharge[29] were reported. A mucopyocele-like disease process affecting the ethmoid and maxillary sinuses was frequent, but in spite of addressing this surgically the nasal cavities remained abnormal (Figure 21.9).

In another study, patients became asymptomatic or improved in most cases.[74] They found on endoscopic appraisal of the nasal cavities that there was a 50% chance of returning to preoperative state by 18–24 months. They

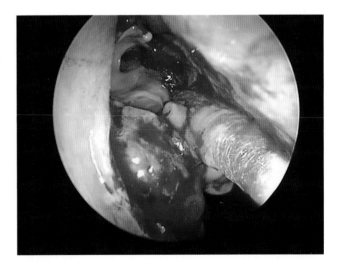

Figure 21.9 Endoscopic photograph showing both polyp and release of pocket of *Pseudomonas* pus from infected ethmoid air cell.

suggest that surgery was more effective at relieving infective processes than preventing recurrence of aggressive polyposis. Half of a subset who had had prior surgery in childhood had an average symptom-free period of 11.3 years before recurrence in adulthood. Postoperative antibiotic sinus lavage has been considered to reduce revision surgery; however, Rickert et al. have shown a less than 30% rate of revision surgery in CF patients without the use of antibiotic lavage.

There remains a need for further studies of the impact of surgery in CF patients where outcome measures should assess the quality of life and frequency of admissions with acute upon chronic upper and lower respiratory tract infections.

IMPACT ON PULMONARY FUNCTION

Although small studies have reported an improvement in lung function after sinus surgery, most have shown no change.[64,81–83] It must be borne in mind that this population is prone to a wide variation in pulmonary function depending on infective exacerbations and intercurrent treatment, and this may render flawed small studies looking at pulmonary function at a given postoperative time point. The most recent study by Osborn et al., looking at a retrospective review of young pre-lung transplant CF patients, showed no improvement of pulmonary function tests and no change in microbial pathogens within the respiratory tract following endoscopic sinus surgery.[86]

BENEFIT TO LUNG TRANSPLANT PATIENTS

Patients with advanced lung damage who are candidates for heart–lung transplantation have been recommended to undergo sinus surgery to reduce the likelihood of sinuses acting as reservoirs for *Pseudomonas* infection. One pretransplant protocol consists of FESS and wide antrostomy with postoperative saline and tobramycin irrigation to avoid pseudomonal and related pulmonary infection, with reports of only rare recurrent polyposis and success in preventing pseudomonal pulmonary infection, although the time frame is not described.[74]

Another group reported a significant decrease in the need for revision surgery with the use of postsinus surgical tobramycin irrigation in nontransplant CF patients.[75] *Pseudomonas* strain typing suggested that the sinuses were likely to be acting as a reservoir for bacterial spread, indicating that disease eradication or reduction in the sinuses might result in less secondary pulmonary infection.[84]

COMPLICATIONS

CF patients with significant respiratory compromise are not ideal candidates for protracted surgical procedures under general anesthesia.[74] The potential for disturbed clotting pathways secondary to vitamin K deficiency, malabsorption,

and thrombocytopenia secondary to hypersplenism is further cited as a risk factor for this surgery. Despite this, a retrospective review of surgical experience over a 42-year period found no complications from general anesthesia and no excessive bleeding or hypoxia postoperatively.[81] Complications are reported to be similar in frequency and type to the non-CF population.[85]

CONCLUSION

CF is a complex multiorgan disease. The same pathophysiological processes affect the upper and lower airways alike. Chronic rhinosinusitis, with or without nasal polyposis, is manifest in a high proportion of sufferers. Developments in endoscopic and imaging techniques and improved understanding of disease mechanisms have led to improvements in diagnosis and treatment. Adequate management of sinonasal disease results in improved overall well-being and reduction in upper airway symptoms and may have further impact in secondary benefit to lower respiratory function.

There is reasonable evidence to support the role of surgery to address symptomatic sinonasal disease in terms of improvement in symptom scores. The impact on lower respiratory function is less clear; but patients, in particular transplant patients, may benefit from the removal of reservoirs of infection in obstructed sinuses. However, the disease must be considered an incurable sinopathy and recurrence is inevitable. The time to recurrence appears to be related to the extent of disease clearance achieved at surgery. The extent of surgery undertaken should at least restore the airway and allow the disease to be controlled medically for prolonged periods. The factors that contribute to increased revision sinus surgery are currently being studied, and this may further our understanding of the methods by which we are further able to optimize our management of sinonasal disease in this patient group for the future.

REFERENCES

1. Shapiro ED, Milmoe GJ, Wald ER, Rodnan JB, Bowen AD. Bacteriology of the maxillary sinuses in patients with cystic fibrosis. *J Infect Dis* 1982 Nov; **146**(5): 589–93.
2. Brihaye P, Jorissen M, Clement PA. Chronic rhinosinusitis in cystic fibrosis (mucoviscidosis). *Acta Otorhinolaryngol Belg* 1997; **51**(4): 323–37.
3. Cepero R, Smith RJ, Catlin FI, Bressler KL, Furuta GT, Shandera KC. Cystic fibrosis—an otolaryngologic perspective. *Otolaryngol Head Neck Surg* 1987 Oct; **97**(4): 356–60.
4. Adinoff AD, Cumming NP. Sinusitis and its relationship to asthma. *Pediat Ann* 1989; **18**: 785.
5. Rachelefsky GS, Katz RM, Siegel SC. Chronic sinus disease with associated reactive airway disease in children. *Pediatrics* 1984 Apr; **73**(4): 526–9.

6. McFadden EA, Kany RJ, Fink JN, Toohill RJ. Surgery for sinusitis and aspirin triad. *Laryngoscope* 1990 Oct; **100**(10 Pt 1): 1043–6.

7. Nishioka GJ, Cook PR, Davis WE et al. Functional endoscopic sinus surgery in patients with chronic sinusitis and asthma. *Otolaryngol Head Neck Surg* 1994; **110**: 494.

8. Parsons DS, Phillips SE. Functional endoscopic surgery in children: A retrospective analysis of results. *Laryngoscope* 1993 Aug; **103**(8): 899–903.

9. Stammberger H, Posawetz W. Functional endoscopic sinus surgery. Concept, indications and results of the Messerklinger technique. *Eur Arch Otorhinolaryngol* 1990; **247**(2): 63–76; Review.

10. Rutland J, Cole PJ. Nasal mucociliary clearance and ciliary beat frequency in cystic fibrosis compared with sinusitis and bronchiectasis. *Thorax* 1981 Sep; **36**(9): 654–8.

11. Armengot M, Escribano A, Carda C, Sanchez C, Romero C, Basterra J. Nasal mucociliary transport and ciliary ultrastructure in cystic fibrosis. A comparative study with healthy volunteers. *Int J Pediatr Otorhinolaryngol* 1997 May 4; **40**(1): 27–34.

12. McShane D, Davies JC, Wodehouse T, Bush A, Geddes D, Alton EW. Normal nasal mucociliary clearance in CF children: Evidence against a CFTR-related defect. *Eur Respir J* 2004 Jul; **24**(1): 95–100.

13. Wilson R, Pitt T, Taylor G, Watson D, MacDermot J, Sykes D et al. Pyocyanin and 1-hydroxyphenazine produced by *Pseudomonas aeruginosa* inhibit the beating of human respiratory cilia in vitro. *J Clin Invest* 1987 Jan; **79**(1): 221–9.

14. Munro NC, Barker A, Rutman A, Taylor G, Watson D, McDonald-Gibson WJ et al. Effect of pyocyanin and 1-hydroxyphenazine on in vivo tracheal mucus velocity. *J Appl Physiol* 1989 Jul; **67**(1): 316–23.

15. Amitani R, Wilson R, Rutman A, Read R, Ward C, Burnett D et al. Effects of human neutrophil elastase and *Pseudomonas aeruginosa* proteinases on human respiratory epithelium. *Am J Respir Cell Mol Biol* 1991 Jan; **4**(1): 26–32.

16. Osborn AJ, Leung R, Ratjen F, James AL. Effect of endoscopic sinus surgery on pulmonary function and microbial pathogens in a pediatric population with cystic fibrosis. *Arch Otolaryngol Head Neck Surg* 2011 Jun; **137**(6): 542–7.

17. Coste A, Gilain L, Roger G, Sebbagh G, Lenoir G, Manach Y et al. Endoscopic and CT-scan evaluation of rhinosinusitis in cystic fibrosis. *Rhinology* 1995 Sep; **33**(3): 152–6.

18. Hadfield PJ, Rowe-Jones JM, Mackay IS. The prevalence of nasal polyps in adults with cystic fibrosis. *Clin Otolaryngol Allied Sci* 2000 Feb; **25**(1): 19–22.

19. Slieker MG, Schilder AG, Uiterwaal CS, van der Ent CK. Children with cystic fibrosis: Who should visit the otorhinolaryngologist? *Arch Otolaryngol Head Neck Surg* 2002 Nov; **128**(11): 1245–8.

20. Tos M, Mogensen C, Thomsen J. Nasal polyps in cystic fibrosis. *J Laryngol Otol* 1977 Oct; **91**(10): 827–35.

21. Henriksson G, Westrin KM, Karpati F, Wikstrom AC, Stierna P, Hjelte L. Nasal polyps in cystic fibrosis: Clinical endoscopic study with nasal lavage fluid analysis. *Chest* 2002 Jan; **121**(1): 40–7.

22. Taylor RF, Morgan DW, Nicholson PS, Mackay IS, Hodson ME, Pitt TL. Extrapulmonary sites of *Pseudomonas aeruginosa* in adults with cystic fibrosis. *Thorax* 1992 Jun; **47**(6): 426–8.

23. Wise SK, Kingdom TT, McKean L, DelGaudio JM, Venkatraman G. Presence of fungus in sinus cultures of cystic fibrosis patients. *Am J Rhinol* 2005 Jan–Feb; **19**(1): 47–51.

24. Bent JP 3rd, Kuhn FA. Diagnosis of allergic fungal sinusitis. *Otolaryngol Head Neck Surg* 1994 Nov; **111**(5): 580–8.

25. King VV. Upper respiratory disease, sinusitis, and polyposis. *Clin Rev Allergy* 1991 Spring–Summer; **9**(1–2): 143–57.

26. Kerrebijn JD, Poublon RM, Overbeek SE. Nasal and paranasal disease in adult cystic fibrosis patients. *Eur Respir J* 1992 Nov; **5**(10): 1239–42.

27. Cuyler JP, Monaghan AJ. Cystic fibrosis and sinusitis. *J Otolaryngol* 1989 Jun; **18**(4): 173–5.

28. Nishioka GJ, Barbero GJ, Konig P, Parsons DS, Cook PR, Davis WE. Symptom outcome after functional endoscopic sinus surgery in patients with cystic fibrosis: A prospective study. *Otolaryngol Head Neck Surg* 1995 Oct; **113**(4): 440–5.

29. Brihaye P, Clement PA, Dab I, Desprechin B. Pathological changes of the lateral nasal wall in patients with cystic fibrosis (mucoviscidosis). *Int J Pediatr Otorhinolaryngol* 1994 Jan; **28**(2–3): 141–7.

30. Gentile VG, Isaacson G. Patterns of sinusitis in cystic fibrosis. *Laryngoscope* 1996 Aug; **106**(8): 1005–9.

31. Nishioka GJ, Cook PR. Paranasal sinus disease in patients with cystic fibrosis. *Otolaryngol Clin North Am* 1996 Feb; **29**(1): 193–205.

32. Raj P, Stableforth DE, Morgan DW. A prospective study of nasal disease in adult cystic fibrosis. *J Laryngol Otol* 2000 Apr; **114**(4): 260–3.

33. Cimmino M, Cavaliere M, Nardone M, Plantulli A, Orefice A, Esposito V et al. Clinical characteristics and genotype analysis of patients with cystic fibrosis and nasal polyposis. *Clin Otolaryngol Allied Sci* 2003 Apr; **28**(2): 125–32.

34. Miller PW, Hamosh A, Macek M, Jr., Greenberger PA, MacLean J, Walden SM et al. Cystic fibrosis transmembrane conductance regulator (*CFTR*) gene mutations in allergic bronchopulmonary aspergillosis. *Am J Hum Genet* 1996 Jul; **59**(1): 45–51.

35. Marchand E, Verellen-Dumoulin C, Mairesse M, Delaunois L, Brancaleone P, Rahier JF et al. Frequency of cystic fibrosis transmembrane

conductance regulator gene mutations and 5T allele in patients with allergic bronchopulmonary aspergillosis. *Chest* 2001 Mar; **119**(3): 762–7.

36. Venarske DL, deShazo RD. Sinobronchial allergic mycosis: The SAM syndrome. *Chest* 2002 May; **121**(5): 1670–6.

37. Pickhardt PJ, Siegel MJ, Hayashi RJ, Kelly M. Posttransplantation lymphoproliferative disorder in children: Clinical, histopathologic, and imaging features. *Radiology* 2000 Oct; **217**(1): 16–25.

38. McAlister WH, Lusk R, Muntz HR. Comparison of plain radiographs and coronal CT scans in infants and children with recurrent sinusitis. *Am J Roentgenol* 1989 Dec; **153**(6): 1259–64.

39. Nishioka GJ, Cook PR, McKinsey JP, Rodriguez FJ. Paranasal sinus computed tomography scan findings in patients with cystic fibrosis. *Otolaryngol Head Neck Surg* 1996 Mar; **114**(3): 394–9.

40. Kim HJ, Friedman EM, Sulek M, Duncan NO, McCluggage C. Paranasal sinus development in chronic sinusitis, cystic fibrosis, and normal comparison population: A computerized tomography correlation study. *Am J Rhinol* 1997 Jul–Aug; **11**(4): 275–81.

41. Krzeski A, Kapiszewska-Dzedzej D, Jakubczyk I, Jedrusik A, Held Ziolkowska M. Extent of pathological changes in the paranasal sinuses of patients with cystic fibrosis: CT analysis. *Am J Rhinol* 2001 May–Jun; **15**(3): 207–10.

42. Mackay IS, Djazaeri B. Chronic sinusitis in cystic fibrosis. *J R Soc Med* 1994; **87**(Suppl 21): 17–9.

43. Kim HJ, Friedman EM, Sulek M, Duncan NO, McCluggage C. Paranasal sinus development in chronic sinusitis, cystic fibrosis, and normal comparison population: A computerized tomography correlation study. *Am J Rhinol* 1997 Jul–Aug; **11**(4): 275–81.

44. Davidson TM, Murphy C, Mitchell M, Smith C, Light M. Management of chronic sinusitis in cystic fibrosis. *Laryngoscope* 1995 Apr; **105**(4 Pt 1): 354–8.

45. Bolger WE, Woodruff WW, Jr., Morehead J, Parsons DS. Maxillary sinus hypoplasia: Classification and description of associated uncinate process hypoplasia. *Otolaryngol Head Neck Surg* 1990 Nov; **103**(5(Pt 1)): 759–65.

46. Mainz JG, Naehrlich L, Schien M, Käding M, Schiller I, Mayr S et al. Concordant genotype of upper and lower airways *P. aeruginosa* and *S. aureus* isolates in cystic fibrosis. *Thorax* 2009 Jun; **64**(6): 535–40. doi: 10.1136/thx.2008.104711. [Epub 2009 Mar 11].

47. Eggesbo HB, Dolvik S, Stiris M, Sovik S, Storrosten OT, Kolmannskog F. Complementary role of MR imaging of ethmomaxillary sinus disease depicted at CT in cystic fibrosis. *Acta Radiol* 2001 Mar; **42**(2): 144–50.

48. Stressmann FA, Rogers GB, Chan SW, Howarth PH, Harries PG, Bruce KD et al. Characterization of bacterial community diversity in chronic rhinosinusitis

infections using novel culture-independent techniques. *Am J Rhinol Allergy* 2011 Jul–Aug; **25**(4): e133–40. doi: 10.2500/ajra.2011.25.3628.

49. Hellquist HB. Nasal polyps update. Histopathology. *Allergy Asthma Proc* 1996 Sep–Oct; **17**(5): 237–42.

50. Tos M, Mogensen C, Thomsen J. Nasal polyps in cystic fibrosis. *J Laryngol Otol* 1977 Oct; **91**(10): 827–35.

51. Beju D, Meek WD, Kramer JC. The ultrastructure of the nasal polyps in patients with and without cystic fibrosis. *J Submicrosc Cytol Pathol* 2004 Apr; **36**(2): 155–65.

52. Hassid S, Choufani G, Decaestecker C, Delbrouck C, Dawance S, Pelc P et al. Glycohistochemical characteristics of nasal polyps from patients with and without cystic fibrosis. *Arch Otolaryngol Head Neck Surg* 2000 Jun; **126**(6): 769–76.

53. Claeys S, Van Hoecke H, Holtappels G, Gevaert P, De Belder T, Verhasselt B et al. Nasal polyps in patients with and without cystic fibrosis: A differentiation by innate markers and inflammatory mediators. *Clin Exp Allergy* 2005 Apr; **35**(4): 467–72.

54. Sobol SE, Christodoulopoulos P, Manoukian JJ, Hauber HP, Frenkiel S, Desrosiers M et al. Cytokine profile of chronic sinusitis in patients with cystic fibrosis. *Arch Otolaryngol Head Neck Surg* 2002 Nov; **128**(11): 1295–8.

55. Colantonio D, Brouillette L, Parikh A, Scadding GK. Paradoxical low nasal nitric oxide in nasal polyposis. *Clin Exp Allergy* 2002 May; **32**(5): 698–701.

56. Balfour-Lynn IM, Laverty A, Dinwiddie R. Reduced upper airway nitric oxide in cystic fibrosis. *Arch Dis Child* 1996 Oct; **75**(4): 319–22.

57. Lundberg JO, Nordvall SL, Weitzberg E, Kollberg H, Alving K. Exhaled nitric oxide in paediatric asthma and cystic fibrosis. *Arch Dis Child* 1996 Oct; **75**(4): 323–6.

58. Dotsch J, Puls J, Klimek T, Rascher W. Reduction of neuronal and inducible nitric oxide synthase gene expression in patients with cystic fibrosis. *Eur Arch Otorhinolaryngol* 2002 Apr; **259**(4): 222–6.

59. Rabago D, Pasic T, Zgierska A, Mundt M, Barrett B, Maberry R. The efficacy of hypertonic saline nasal irrigation for chronic sinonasal symptoms. *Otolaryngol Head Neck Surg* 2005 Jul; **133**(1): 3–8.

60. Fokkens W, Lund V, Bachert C, Clement P, Helllings P, Holmstrom M et al.; EAACI. EAACI position paper on rhinosinusitis and nasal polyps executive summary. *Allergy* 2005 May; **60**(5): 583–601.

61. Hadfield PJ, Rowe-Jones JM, Mackay IS. A prospective treatment trial of nasal polyps in adults with cystic fibrosis. *Rhinology* 2000 Jun; **38**(2): 63–5.

62. Ramsey B, Richardson MA. Impact of sinusitis in cystic fibrosis. *J Allergy Clin Immunol* 1992 Sep; **90**(3 Pt 2): 547–52.

63. Halvorson DJ, Dupree JR, Porubsky ES. Management of chronic sinusitis in the adult cystic fibrosis patient. *Ann Otol Rhinol Laryngol* 1998 Nov; **107**(11 Pt 1): 946–52.

64. Raynor EM, Butler A, Guill M, Bent JP 3rd. Nasally inhaled dornase alfa in the postoperative management of chronic sinusitis due to cystic fibrosis. *Arch Otolaryngol Head Neck Surg* 2000 May; **126**(5): 581–3.

65. Iino Y, Sasaki Y, Miyazawa T, Kodera K. Nasopharyngeal flora and drug susceptibility in children with macrolide therapy. *Laryngoscope* 2003 Oct; **113**(10): 1780–5.

66. Hashiba M, Baba S. Efficacy of long-term administration of clarithromycin in the treatment of intractable chronic sinusitis. *Acta Otolaryngol Suppl* 1996; **525**: 73–8.

67. Davidson TM, Murphy C, Mitchell M, Smith C, Light M. Management of chronic sinusitis in cystic fibrosis. *Laryngoscope* 1995 Apr; **105**(4 Pt 1): 354–8.

68. Lewiston N, King V, Umetsu D, Starnes V, Marshall S, Kramer M et al. Cystic fibrosis patients who have undergone heart-lung transplantation benefit from maxillary sinus antrostomy and repeated sinus lavage. *Transplant Proc* 1991 Feb; **23**(1 Pt 2): 1207–8.

69. Cimmino M, Nardone M, Cavaliere M, Plantulli A, Sepe A, Esposito V et al. Dornase alfa as postoperative therapy in cystic fibrosis sinonasal disease. *Arch Otolaryngol Head Neck Surg* 2005 Dec; **131**(12): 1097–101.

70. Rowe-Jones JM, Mackay IS. Endoscopic sinus surgery in the treatment of cystic fibrosis with nasal polyposis. *Laryngoscope* 1996 Dec; **106**(12 Pt 1): 1540–4.

71. Yung MW, Gould J, Upton GJ. Nasal polyposis in children with cystic fibrosis: A long-term follow-up study. *Ann Otol Rhinol Laryngol* 2002 Dec; **111**(12 Pt 1): 1081–6.

72. Moss RB, King VV. Management of sinusitis in cystic fibrosis by endoscopic surgery and serial antimicrobial lavage. Reduction in recurrence requiring surgery. *Arch Otolaryngol Head Neck Surg* 1995 May; **121**(5): 566–72.

73. Jarrett WA, Militsakh O, Anstad M, Manaligod J. Endoscopic sinus surgery in cystic fibrosis: Effects on pulmonary function and ideal body weight. *Ear Nose Throat J* 2004 Feb; **83**(2): 118–21.

74. Davidson TM, Murphy C, Mitchell M, Smith C, Light M. Management of chronic sinusitis in cystic fibrosis. *Laryngoscope* 1995 Apr; **105**(4 Pt 1): 354–8.

75. Drake-Lee AB, Morgan DW. Nasal polyps and sinusitis in children with cystic fibrosis. *J Laryngol Otol* 1989 Aug; **103**(8): 753–5.

76. Crockett DM, McGill TJ, Healy GB, Friedman EM, Salkeld LJ. Nasal and paranasal sinus surgery in children with cystic fibrosis. *Ann Otol Rhinol Laryngol* 1987 Jul–Aug; **96**(4): 367–72.

77. Duplechain JK, White JA, Miller RH. Pediatric sinusitis. The role of endoscopic sinus surgery in cystic fibrosis and other forms of sinonasal disease. *Arch Otolaryngol Head Neck Surg* 1991 Apr; **117**(4): 422–6.

78. Cuyler JP. Follow-up of endoscopic sinus surgery on children with cystic fibrosis. *Arch Otolaryngol Head Neck Surg* 1992 May; **118**(5): 505–6.

79. Jones JW, Parsons DS, Cuyler JP. The results of functional endoscopic sinus (FES) surgery on the symptoms of patients with cystic fibrosis. *Int J Pediatr Otorhinolaryngol* 1993 Dec; **28**(1): 25–32.

80. Madonna D, Isaacson G, Rosenfeld RM, Panitch H. Effect of sinus surgery on pulmonary function in patients with cystic fibrosis. *Laryngoscope* 1997 Mar; **107**(3): 328–31.

81. Umetsu DT, Moss RB, King VV, Lewiston NJ. Sinus disease in patients with severe cystic fibrosis: Relation to pulmonary exacerbation. *Lancet* 1990 May 5; **335**(8697): 1077–8.

82. Rosbe KW, Jones DT, Rahbar R, Lahiri T, Auerbach AD. Endoscopic sinus surgery in cystic fibrosis: Do patients benefit from surgery? *Int J Pediatr Otorhinolaryngol* 2001 Nov 1; **61**(2): 113–9.

83. Schulte DL, Kasperbauer JL. Safety of paranasal sinus surgery in patients with cystic fibrosis. *Laryngoscope* 1998 Dec; **108**(12): 1813–5.

84. Holzmann D, Speich R, Kaufmann T, Laube I, Russi EW, Simmen D et al. Effects of sinus surgery in patients with cystic fibrosis after lung transplantation: A 10-year experience. *Transplantation* 2004 Jan 15; **77**(1): 134–6.

85. Albritton FD, Kingdom TT. Endoscopic sinus surgery in patients with cystic fibrosis: An analysis of complications. *Am J Rhinol* 2000 Nov–Dec; **14**(6): 379–85.

86. Osborn AJ, Leung R, Ratjen F, James AL. Effect of endoscopic sinus surgery on pulmonary function and microbial pathogens in a pediatric population with cystic fibrosis. *Arch Otolaryngol Head Neck Surg* 2011 Jun; **137**(6): 542–7.

22

Gastrointestinal disease in cystic fibrosis

ALAN STEEL AND DAVID WESTABY

INTRODUCTION

The gastrointestinal (GI) tract in cystic fibrosis (CF) patients is a source of significant morbidity and mortality. Its importance has been noted since the early descriptions of the disease.[1] Abnormalities of GI function can be detected in utero[2] and can progress throughout adulthood, with functional bowel disease, with no structural pathological changes identified,[3] pancreatic exocrine failure, or GI cancer particularly relevant to the aging CF population.

Although there are CF-specific GI conditions (meconium ileus [MI], distal intestinal obstruction syndrome [DIOS], fibrosing colonopathy), some GI conditions have particular features related to CF (malabsorption, gastroesophageal reflux disease [GERD]), but most manifestations of CF GI disease share similarities in presentation and treatment with the non-CF population. The burden of GI disease in CF patients is substantial, but true prevalence data are often lacking (Table 22.1).

MOLECULAR BIOLOGY/ PATHOPHYSIOLOGY

Before the seminal description of the genetic defect responsible for CF in 1989,[25–27] the GI complications of CF suggested electrolyte and water movements across the intestinal mucosa were impaired. The cystic fibrosis transmembrane conductance regulator (*CFTR*) gene encodes an adensoine triphosphate– and cyclic adenosine monophosphate–dependent chloride channel that is found in the apical border of epithelial cells lining exocrine glands such as the pancreas but can also be demonstrated throughout the GI tract. The primary function of the CFTR protein is as a chloride channel. The regulation of this chloride channel is complex and dependent on multiple kinases, sequential phosphorylation, and dephosphorylation that allow

flux of Cl^- anions through the transmembrane domain of the CFTR protein.[28] The consequence of the Cl^- flux is a negative potential on the luminal surface, which pulls Na^+ across epithelial tight junctions into the lumen with water following by osmosis. There is increasing evidence that the CFTR mutation results in changes of Na^+ channel function with reduced inhibition of Na^+ absorption in CF as well as impairment of other chloride channels. These functional alterations of ion transport across epithelial surfaces result in reduced flow of water into the intestinal lumen, with consequent dehydrated inspissated secretions.

There are now more than 1900 *CFTR* genetic mutations described, and these can be classified according to level of functional CFTR[29] (Table 22.2). The most common mutation, ΔF508, has been consistently associated with more severe phenotype.[30,31] Classification of the functional deficit allows demonstration of milder phenotype with heterozygotes or those with class IV or V mutations. The extraintestinal manifestations of this genotype : phenotype relationship has been covered more extensively in earlier sections, but has specific relevance to pancreatic function, where mild phenotypic disease has a genetically determined predictable risk of pancreatitis.[32]

ABNORMAL FINDINGS IN CF

It has long been possible to demonstrate abnormal pathological and physiological findings in CF. Since normal GI tract physiology and homeostasis is incompletely understood and often difficult to study, it should not be surprising that we do not fully understand the mechanisms by which CF abnormalities translate into distinct GI pathological presentations.

Whether the abnormal findings are a primary defect of CF or arise secondary to reduced fluid volume and pH in the GI tract, with mucus accumulation, altered gut microbiome and consequent modified host immunological

Table 22.1 Prevalence of gastrointestinal conditions in cystic fibrosis

Pancreatic insufficiency	85%	Ref. [4]
Small bowel bacterial overgrowth	30%–55%	Refs. [5] and [6]
Gastroesophageal reflux disease	20%–80%	Refs. [7] and [8]
Constipation	26%–47%	Refs. [9] and [10]
Distal intestinal obstruction syndrome	16%	Refs. [11] and [12]
Meconium ileus	6%–20%	Ref. [13]
Clostridium difficile carriage	22%–32%	Ref. [14]
Clostridium difficile toxin symptomatic	Case reports/post-transplant	Ref. [15]
Helicobacter pylori	10%–60%	Ref. [16]
Rectal prolapse	10%–20%	Ref. [17]
Intussusception	1%	Ref. [18]
Appendicitis	1%–2%	Ref. [19]
Celiac disease	0.4%–1.2%	Ref. [20]
Crohn's disease	0.22%	Ref. [21]
Volvulus	Case reports	Ref. [9]
Peptic ulcer	Rare	Ref. [22]
Fibrosing colonopathy	Historical	Ref. [23]
Eosinophillic esophagitis	Case reports	Ref. [24]

Table 22.2 Classification of CFTR mutations and their functional effect

Class	Functional effect of mutation
I	Defective protein production
II	Defective protein processing
III	Defective protein regulation
IV	Defective protein conductance
V	Quantitative deficiency of protein on epithelial surface

responses are difficult to ascertain, but may become clearer with the increased use of animal and further clinical investigation.

There is no naturally occurring animal model of CF, but following the specific genetic description animal models have been developed.[33–35] The early animal models of CF developed in mice, targeting the CFTR gene, produced intestinal pathology in keeping with current perceptions of pathophysiology leading to intestinal obstruction and perforation, but did not produce characteristic lung, pancreatic, or liver pathology. Development of more complex models and using long-lived variants has now produced consistent progressive multiorgan pathology similar to the human descriptions.[36] The discordant outcomes in these early animal models provided evidence that defects in CFTR function could be overcome by alternate Cl⁻ channels.[37]

HISTOPATHOLOGY

Early descriptions of inspissated mucus and dilated glands in the upper GI tract have been supplemented with multiple abnormalities in cellular ultrastructure.[38–40] Cellular transport and metabolic mechanisms can be examined with electron microscopy and immunohistochemistry. Whether these abnormalities are primary such as impaired Golgi apparatus function or secondary: as a response to viscid pathological mucus, abnormal bacterial colonization of the GI tract, or intestinal inflammation is largely open to conjecture and future investigation. Reports of pathognomonic changes in GI tissue are not generally useful.[41]

RADIOLOGY

As radiological modalities have waxed and waned in availability and popularity descriptions of radiological abnormalities in CF have arrived in the medical literature.[19] Essentially, there is thickening of mucosal folds and the intestinal wall. These findings have been demonstrated by oral contrast radiography, ultrasound, computed tomography (CT), and subsequently magnetic resonance imaging (MRI). Radiological findings of pneumatosis intestinalis are reported and appear to share the benign prognosis of other chronic respiratory conditions.

pH STUDIES

Intestinal bicarbonate is reduced in CF due to failure of pancreatic and upper GI tract (duodenal) bicarbonate secretion. This results in lowered luminal pH within the proximal small bowel although pH may be normal in distal small bowel.[42] The role of impaired acid buffering in the duodenum will be explored below, but lowered duodenal pH is not entirely ameliorated by the use of acid-secreting suppressive medications such as proton pump inhibitors (PPIs) or H₂ antagonists.

MOTILITY

Delayed transit of intestinal contents can be demonstrated in CF. Upper GI tract motility is relatively easy to study, but there is limited evidence of impairment associated with CF, exemplified by a small study of 12 adult and pediatric patients who shows large variation in measured parameters without definitive impact on outcome.[43] Small intestinal motility is demonstrably delayed and may be secondary to thickened mucosal folds, abnormally viscous secretions, or abnormal bacterial colonization of the intestine. Therapies to improve lumen hydration can improve intestinal motility, bacterial overgrowth, and intestinal transit.

INFLAMMATION

There is evidence of intestinal inflammation in the CF population. Gut lavage demonstrates nonspecific measures of inflammation with fecal markers such as calprotectin or proinflammatory cytokines.[44,45] These markers do not specify type or location of inflammation. The precise etiology and consequence of this inflammation are unknown, but it may be that intestinal inflammation, mucosal histological/radiological abnormalities, and intestinal permeability are linked. Proinflammatory signals in the GI tract can be detected by measuring nuclear transcripts in cell isolates, cell phenotype, and function or by measuring systemic markers of intestinal damage and translocation of bacterial cell products. These changes are not specific to CF and more work will need to be done to assess the importance of GI inflammation in CF.

CLINICAL SYNDROMES WITH CF ASSOCIATIONS

The adoption of widespread pediatric genetic screening for CF has revolutionized the presentation of pediatric CF in the United Kingdom, which means that GI disease usually presents within the context of known CF. Cases will continue to present with CF-specific GI conditions due to immigrant populations, incomplete uptake of screening, and rare disease-causing mutations. Furthermore, despite a clear diagnosis the clinical syndromes described below continue to develop and present persistent problems of clinical management.

MALABSORPTION

The consequences of long-term malabsorption can be devastating with permanent stunting of growth, cognitive dysfunction, and more rapid decline in respiratory function.[2,46] Presentation of CF-related malabsorption is most often in infancy, but the management and consequences will persist throughout life.

Pancreatic exocrine failure

The predominant cause of intestinal malabsorption in the CF population is pancreatic exocrine insufficiency due to acinar gland destruction as a result of deceased volume and increased viscosity of pancreatic secretions. This results in poor flow of enzymes and bicarbonate out of the pancreatic ductal system and activation of these enzymes within the gland causing autodigestion and glandular destruction. More than 80% of the UK CF population are pancreatic insufficient, with prevalence increasing with age, and characteristic radiological appearances of fatty replacement of pancreatic tissue noted on cross-sectional imaging (Figure 22.1).

Pancreatic insufficiency (PI) in infancy can be suspected when other CF manifestations have arisen or can be the presenting feature. Human breast milk contains low levels of amylase and lipase, which can delay presentation until after weaning. PI can be masked by increased calorie intake; however, during intercurrent illness, the calorie intake falls and weight loss becomes evident.[47] These presentations should become rare in the United Kingdom as newborn genetic screening for common CF mutations is now performed.[48] Progressive loss of pancreatic function with age, rare disease-causing CF mutations, and immigration will continue to provide new PI CF cases. Adult CF patients developing PI demonstrate features shared with the non-CF PI population with the classic features of abdominal distension and discomfort, steatorrhea, floating stools, flatus, and weight loss. Pancreatic exocrine failure results in the inability to breakdown complex carbohydrate, protein, and fat due to amylase, protease, and lipase deficiencies, respectively. Fat malabsorption is prominent as lipase action is further impaired by reduced pancreatic bicarbonate secretion, favoring acid denaturation of these enzymes.

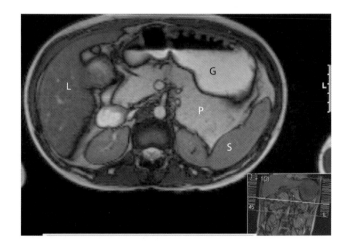

Figure 22.1 Magnetic resonance imaging (MRI) of cystic fibrosis (CF) patient demonstrating complete replacement of pancreatic gland with high signal material characteristic of fat. L, liver; S, spleen; G, gastric contents; P, pancreatic position.

The genotype and class of functional CFTR defect determines the risk and severity of PI. Class IV and V mutations are associated with pancreatic sufficiency (PS) even if there is one severe functional mutation.[31]

Despite optimization of dietary intake and pancreatic enzyme therapies, it is clear that many CF patients continue to demonstrate intestinal malabsorption, evidenced by fat malabsorption. Failure to reproduce physiological pancreatic enzyme concentrations with appropriate timing with regard to food intake results in suboptimal fat absorption, despite the best endeavors to optimize the dosing of replacement enzymes.[49] Further reasons for therapeutic failure of pancreatic enzyme replacement therapy (PERT) are independent causes of malabsorption and these are explored below.

In the past, pancreatic exocrine sufficiency testing required invasive pancreatic stimulation with CCK–secretin or by the obviously unpopular three-day fecal fat collection. The introduction of a highly sensitive (98%–100%) and specific (93%–100%) enzyme-linked immunosorbent assay to detect human fecal pancreatic elastase has largely replaced other testing, including chymotrypsin. The test can be performed on a single stool sample and requires no medication omissions.[50–52] Objective monitoring of response to therapy still requires stool analysis for fat,[50,53] most commonly by microscopy.

Once the need for PERT has been established, therapy is based on oral replacement of pancreatic enzymes. Numerous preparations are available, but all UK products are of porcine origin. Modern formulations with enteric coating of microspheres, microtablets, or granules have greatly improved delivery of active enzymes to the small bowel. Timing of PERT around meals and dosage adjustment should be undertaken with expectation that dose adjustment from day to day is normal as intake varies, and dietetic input is essential. In the pediatric setting, PERT requirements will vary with age and developmental stage.

In 2004, the Food and Drug Administration (FDA) ruled that pancreatic enzyme supplements should undergo efficacy and safety studies. This led to a series of studies fulfilling FDA requirements but failing to address dose–response effects.[54–59]

Dosing of PERT is thus determined by the Committee on Safety of Medicines whose recommendations were based in the aftermath of fibrosing colonopathy cases described in CF children in the United Kingdom[60]: case reports of fibrosing colonopathy were described in children using high doses of PERT. Subsequent case–control studies suggested that high enzyme dose and methacrylic acid copolymer used as an acid-resistant coating were responsible.[23] Withdrawal of the polymer and limitation of enzyme dosing to below 10,000 U/kg/day of lipase has been associated with a lack of new cases of fibrosing colonopathy developing.

Dose recommendations are the following: 2,500 U of lipase/kg per meal or 10,000 U lipase/kg per day, or alternative dose by grams of fat ingested at 4,000 U of lipase/g of fat per day. If dosing is by lipase per kilogram, half doses

should be given with snacks. PERT use with nocturnal feeding requires pragmatic dosing doses taken before, during, and after tube feeding, or the use of an elemental feed.

Failure of intestinal and pancreatic bicarbonate secretion

Duodenal and pancreatic bicarbonate secretion is diminished in CF,[61,62] with consequent reduced intestinal pH that impairs fat digestion and absorption, possibly because of impaired mucus production and impaired lipid translocation to the intestinal cells.[63] Reduced intestinal pH is associated with increased fat malabsorption in CF patients treated with enzyme replacement therapy.[64]

Intestinal bicarbonate deficiency compounds pancreatic exocrine failure since residual pancreatic enzymes and bile acids are inactivated by gastric acid.

Despite this strong association, and the underlying pathology apparently clear, the clinical trial evidence for using acid-suppressing therapy routinely in CF patients receiving PERT is not clear[65]; however, persistent fat malabsorption that responds to PPI therapy can be demonstrated in many patients, and failure to respond may merely be indicative of the presence of other causes of fat malabsorption.

Small bowel bacterial overgrowth (SBBO)

The intestinal lumen in CF has reduced water content with contents being abnormally thick and acidic. This causes accumulation of mucus in the intestine,[66] promoting abnormal bacterial colonization of the intestinal tract. Symptoms of SBBO are nonspecific and can include bloating and pain as well as diarrhea and malabsorption, which does not distinguish this from many other CF presentations. Testing for bacterial overgrowth with breath tests for hydrogen or methane can be difficult to perform reliably in any population, as validity is compromised by antibiotic use. Endoscopic sampling of intestinal contents is not well standardized, although commonly used. Novel wireless technologies, i.e., pill-sized cameras/monitors that are ingested and transmit diagnostic data to recording devices during passage through the GI tract, offer minimally invasive testing but are not risk free with intestinal obstruction, requiring surgical intervention occurring in up to 5% cases,[67–69] although identifying high-risk cases with suspected strictures or adhesions should mandate the prior use of dummy capsules that establish intestinal patency, but dissolve if unable to pass.

Management of SBBO is primarily with further antibiotics such as ciprofloxacin, tetracycline, metronidazole, or rifaximin, which can be used according to local protocols and with regard to the presence of any relevant drug-resistant organisms found in the chest of these patients. Improvements in fat absorption in selected CF patients have been reported after antibiotic use.[70]

Bile salt fecal loss and bile acid homeostasis

Bile salt physiology is abnormal in CF. There is increased loss of bile acids in stool. The normal enterohepatic circulation of bile acids is impaired by diminished ileal reabsorption of bile acids, which can occur due to viscid mucous secretions or SBBO. Bile acid loss can be compensated with increased bile acid synthesis, but not all bile acids are synthesized equally in this event, leading to altered ratios of taurine and glycine.[71]

The alterations of bile acid composition lead to impairment of fat absorption in the context of abnormal duodenal pH due to differences in bile acid solubility in glycine and taurine conjugated bile acids. The relative reduction of taurine-conjugated bile acids could, therefore, be used as a therapeutic target. There is conflicting evidence of taurine supplementation[72,73] in CF, but given some positive data it is not unreasonable to try supplemental taurine for CF patients with persistent fat malabsorption despite correction of other parameters.

Meconium ileus

The earliest GI manifestation of CF is MI: a neonatal bowel obstruction associated with the most severe CFTR mutations. Despite the association with this genotype, genome-wide association studies demonstrate that <20% of phenotypic variability of MI presentation can be explained by CFTR status.[74] Fatal complications of MI were widely reported, but, with modern management, long-term survival of MI patients reflects that of other CF patients.[13]

MI can be detected in the antenatal period by ultrasound examination; however, this is poorly sensitive even when parental genetic analysis has been shown that the fetus is at risk of CF,[75,76] nevertheless suggestive antenatal ultrasound findings should be acted on.[77] MI presents as neonatal bowel obstruction and requires intervention to relieve the blockage. There is an association with more severe CFTR mutations, especially those associated PI but MI is not unique to CF and can also be found in congenital PI and also in pancreatic sufficient CF and also rarely in otherwise normal babies; thus, the diagnosis of CF should always be confirmed. The prevalence in the neonatal CF population is reported as 6%–20%[13] with alternate diagnoses outlined in Table 22.3.

Table 22.3 Differential diagnosis of fetal hyperechogenic bowel

No pathology
Cystic fibrosis
Congenital infection
Intrauterine growth retardation
Gastrointestinal malformation
Chromosomal abnormality
Major congenital gastrointestinal malformations

MI is caused by an accumulation of abnormally viscid meconium, which becomes inspissated and obstructive. MI presents within 48 hours of birth with intestinal obstruction. Passage of meconium per rectum does not exclude the diagnosis. The first sign of MI may be of peritonitis associated with perforation, but delayed or progressive presentation scan show bile stained vomit, abdominal distension, dilated bowel, palpable bowel loops or masses. Investigation with abdominal radiography reveals calcification in 25% of cases,[78] right lower quadrant ground-glass in up to 50%, but these signs are not specific to CF. Up to 40% of MI cases are complicated by intestinal atresia, volvulus, or antenatal perforation with peritonitis. Although these complications are not unique to CF, they are associated with significant morbidity.

Therapy of uncomplicated MI is aimed at increasing the fluid content of the intestine and relieving the obstruction with enemas of Gastrografin®.[79] Warmed saline and N-acetyl-cysteine can augment this or be used when enemas fail and surgical intervention is required. Irrigation of the obstructed segment can be undertaken at surgery via the dilated small bowel or appendiceal stump.

If the meconium obstruction is found within the colon, a similar but distinct clinical entity can be seen. The meconium plug syndrome presents with abdominal distension and failure to pass meconium; however, apart from a tight anal canal there are no other features suggestive of MI. Twenty-five percent of meconium plug syndrome patients will have CF suggesting a shared pathophysiology.[80,81]

GERD

GERD is simply reflux of gastric contents across the lower esophageal sphincter (LES) in a retrograde fashion. The contents of the stomach therefore define the characteristics of the refluxate. This has been recognized in expert gastroenterological opinion definitions describing acid reflux, superimposed acid reflux, weakly acid reflux, and weakly alkaline reflux.[82] GERD has significant effects in CF, adversely impacting on quality of life, nutritional status, and respiratory function.

GERD is common in CF with prevalence above 20%[83] and up to 80% in CF populations. These symptom-reporting studies are supported by uncontrolled data demonstrating objectively measured acid reflux in 55%–80%.[7,84]

The pathogenesis of GERD is multifactorial and can result from a number of pathological conditions. The LOS is a poorly defined 3–4 cm segment of the lower esophagus that, under the influence of a vagal reflex, relaxes in response to gastric distension. Relaxation of this sphincter allows venting of gaseous distention—belching. In addition to such desirable physiological processes, the function of the LOS is normally augmented by close apposition of the diaphragm. In the setting of a hiatus hernia, the diaphragmatic crus sits below the lower esophageal sphincter, promoting reflux when the intra-abdominal pressure is raised, as happens during coughing. A persistently hypotensive

CONSTIPATION

Constipation is often reported in the CF population, but as in the non-CF population should always be clearly defined as lay definitions can often be different from those of the clinician. Constipation can be defined as reduced stool frequency or increased consistency of the passed stool.[12] Constipation symptoms are often more concerning when in association with secondary symptoms of abdominal bloating and pain. The pathophysiology of constipation in CF is defective CFTR function in the GI tract[120] resulting in altered composition of the intestinal fluid, which is compounded by the often low fiber diets followed. This mainstay of therapy is with laxatives to increase the fluid composition of the intestinal contents. Assessment of constipation is primarily by history and clinical assessment with plain abdominal radiography used to differentiate from DIOS, although serial abdominal radiographs should not be used to monitor or screen for constipation, principally due to poor sensitivity.[10]

INTUSSUSCEPTION

Intussusception is an important complication found in CF populations. The etiology of intussusception, where one segment of bowel invaginates into an adjoining segment of bowel is poorly understood but is thought to require a lead point around which the peristalsing bowel can work to invaginate a proximal bowel segment. In CF, the thickened bowel contents are thought to provide this starting point. Asymptomatic intussusception is reported in CF,[121] with ileocolic and cecocolic most common.[18] Radiographic demonstration of the intussuscepted segment is possible with standard modalities. Symptomatic cases require intervention, which can be surgical resection as ischemic necrosis can ensue.

APPENDICITIS

Historical descriptions of CF appendix pathology are established[122]; however, the incidence of acute appendicitis requiring emergency medical/surgical intervention does not appear to be elevated. Appendicitis can present with obvious clear-cut signs and symptoms; however, CF patients often report abdominal pain, have blood tests compatible with acute appendicitis (elevated white cell count, C-reactive protein, and erythrocyte sedimentation rate), and have alternate intra-abdominal pathology. Mucus accumulation in appendix goblet cells is suggestive of CF, which should be actively excluded with these histological findings. The role of the appendix is poorly defined in healthy populations, non-CF colitides, and CF.

VOLVULUS

Volvulus, whereby the intestine twists on its mesentery, so obstructing arterial supply and venous drainage of the affected bowel can occur not only as a consequence of MI but can also occur spontaneously as in the non-CF population.

Early recognition is key to avoiding surgical resection of ischemic or infarcted intestine.

RECTAL PROLAPSE

Rectal prolapse occurs in as many as 20% of undiagnosed pediatric CF patients and should be actively excluded in pediatric patients presenting with rectal prolapsed as CF is present in 11% of such cases.[17,123] The differential diagnosis of rectal prolapsed in pediatric patients is shown in Table 22.4. Once CF is recognized and therapy with nutritional support and PERT instigated, the tendency to prolapse is relieved.

ENTERIC INFECTION

Helicobacter pylori

H. pylori infection is associated with significant disease burden with upper GI ulceration of the stomach and duodenum. CF patients have defective bicarbonate secretion, which may predispose to peptic ulceration as suggested by autopsy series.[22] Diagnosis of *H. pylori* infection can be undertaken by urease breath testing, stool antigen testing, endoscopic near patient testing for enzymatic activity, histological examination, and when treatment has previously failed *H. pylori* culture and sensitivity from endoscopic biopsy. Prevalence varies with geographical location.

Clostridium difficile

Clostridium difficile carriage is high in the CF population with reported incidence up to 43%,[14] although reported symptomatic infection with clostridium difficile toxin (CDT) is rarely reported.[124] Risk factors identified for clostridium difficile carriage and infection include exposure to antibiotics, impaired immunity, and reduced gastric acidity.[125] Nosocomial disease outbreaks further add to the risk of clostridium difficile in the CF population. Clinical presentation of clostridium difficile disease can be masked by multiple GI symptoms in the CF population. Diagnosis is made by stool analysis: current testing algorithms include use of polymerase chain reaction tests for clostridium genomic markers and enzyme immunoassay testing for the toxin characteristic of pathological infection. Flexible sigmoidoscopy demonstrates pseudomembranous

Table 22.4 Differential diagnosis of pediatric rectal prolapse

Constipation
Diarrhea
Connective tissue disease
Imperforate anus
Malnutrition
Pertussis
Rectal polyps/tumors
Hemorrhoids

colitis. Current therapeutic strategies include withdrawal of PPI and quinolone antibiotics where possible. Active treatment with oral metronidazole 400 mg tds for 7–14 days or oral vancomycin 125 mg four times daily for 10 days, although more recently fidaxomicin[126] has been licensed and fecal transplantation, where clostridium difficile negative donor feces is instilled via oral or anal routes, is gaining increasing acknowledgment of efficacy despite unsurprising reservations[127] and limited understanding of therapeutic mechanisms.

Post-transplant CDT positivity has been reported to have a particularly poor prognosis,[15] but this is not reflected in the non-CF literature and should merely serve as a reminder to consider CDT disease in the CF population, rather than as a tool to select patients unsuitable for transplantation.

EOSINOPHILLIC ESOPHAGITIS

Eosinophillic esophagitis is a chronic immune-mediated inflammatory condition associated with symptomatic esophageal dysfunction with dysphagia and recurrent bolus obstruction. There are thought to be no shared pathophysiological processes, but again there is significant overlap with features of CF GI disease, particularly with GERD.[24] Investigation is done by endoscopic biopsy of esophagus at esophago–gastro–duodenoscopy with therapy directed at acid suppression and topical steroid therapy.

ENDOSCOPIC PROCEDURES IN CF

To diagnose, monitor, and treat many of the GI conditions described above, invasive endoscopic procedures have to be undertaken. All invasive endoscopic procedures carry risk. Specific risk data for CF patients are unsurprisingly not reported. Local practice and expertise will determine the optimum investigation strategy for CF patients that may require endoscopic investigation/therapy. GI endoscopic investigation is often routine, safe, and diagnostic. Careful case selection is important. GI cancer screening may be warranted if further increases in life expectancy in CF cohorts are reported and the original CF cancer registry data are replicated, but for now, only those cases with clear suggestive history/examination/investigations should be offered endoscopic investigation. The post-transplant cancer data and associated immunosuppression will likely lead to increased cancer screening in the post-transplant cohort, although there are little hard data to support this.

CONCLUSION

CF is a multiorgan disease with the GI tract presenting many diagnostic and management problems. These problems can be identified in the antenatal period, and with increased life expectancy in the CF population, there will be increased recognition of the clinical problems identified

above. Prospective clinical trials in CF patients with GI tract pathology will be difficult to conduct, as has been recognized in Cochrane reviews of gastrostomy feeding in CF patients. Increased appreciation of the role of the gut microbiome in systemic disease and targeted animal model research will lead to further progress in the treatment of GI disease in CF.

REFERENCES

1. Andersen DH. Cystic fibrosis of the pancreas and its relation to celiac disease: A clinical and pathological study. *Am J Dis Child* 1938; **56**(2): 344–399.
2. Farrell PM, Kosorok MR, Rock MJ, Laxova A, Zeng L, Lai HC, et al. Early diagnosis of cystic fibrosis through neonatal screening prevents severe malnutrition and improves long-term growth. Wisconsin Cystic Fibrosis Neonatal Screening Study Group. *Pediatrics* 2001; **107**(1): 1–13.
3. Thompson WG, Longstreth GF, Drossman DA, Heaton KW, Irvine EJ, Muller-Lissner SA. Functional bowel disorders and functional abdominal pain. *Gut* 1999; **45** (Suppl 2): II43–7.
4. Walkowiak J, Lisowska A, Blaszczynski M. The changing face of the exocrine pancreas in cystic fibrosis: Pancreatic sufficiency, pancreatitis and genotype. *Eur J Gastroenterol Hepatol* 2008; **20**(3): 157–60.
5. Lewindon PJ, Robb TA, Moore DJ, Davidson GP, Martin AJ. Bowel dysfunction in cystic fibrosis: Importance of breath testing. *J Pediatr Child Health* 1998; **34**(1): 79–82.
6. Fridge JL, Conrad C, Gerson L, Castillo RO, Cox K. Risk factors for small bowel bacterial overgrowth in cystic fibrosis. *J Pediatr Gastroenterol Nutr* 2007; **44**(2): 212–8.
7. Gustafsson PM, Fransson SG, Kjellman NI, Tibbling L. Gastro-oesophageal reflux and severity of pulmonary disease in cystic fibrosis. *Scand J Gastroenterol* 1991; **26**(5): 449–56.
8. Ledson MJ, Tran J, Walshaw MJ. Prevalence and mechanisms of gastro-oesophageal reflux in adult cystic fibrosis patients. *J R Soc Med* 1998; **91**(1): 7–9.
9. Rubinstein S, Moss R, Lewiston N. Constipation and meconium ileus equivalent in patients with cystic fibrosis. *Pediatrics* 1986; **78**(3): 473–9.
10. van der Doef HP, Kokke FT, Beek FJ, Woestenenk JW, Froeling SP, Houwen RH. Constipation in pediatric cystic fibrosis patients: An underestimated medical condition. *J Cyst Fibros* 2010; **9**(1): 59–63.
11. Cleghorn GJ, Stringer DA, Forstner GG, Durie PR. Treatment of distal intestinal obstruction syndrome in cystic fibrosis with a balanced intestinal lavage solution. *Lancet* 1986; **1**(8471): 8–11.
12. Houwen RH, van der Doef HP, Sermet I, Munck A, Hauser B, Walkowiak J, et al. Defining DIOS and constipation in cystic fibrosis with a multicentre study on the incidence, characteristics, and treatment of DIOS. *J Pediatr Gastroenterol Nutr* 2010; **50**(1): 38–42.

13. Coutts JA, Docherty JG, Carachi R, Evans TJ. Clinical course of patients with cystic fibrosis presenting with meconium ileus. *Br J Surg* 1997; **84**(4): 555.

14. Peach SL, Borriello SP, Gaya H, Barclay FE, Welch AR. Asymptomatic carriage of Clostridium difficile in patients with cystic fibrosis. *J Clin Pathol* 1986; **39**(9): 1013–8.

15. Yates B, Murphy DM, Fisher AJ, Gould FK, Lordan JL, Dark JH, et al. Pseudomembranous colitis in four patients with cystic fibrosis following lung transplantation. *Thorax* 2007; **62**(6): 554–6.

16. Ramos AF, de Fuccio MB, Moretzsohn LD, Barbosa AJ, Passos MD, Carvalho RS, et al. Cystic fibrosis, gastroduodenal inflammation, duodenal ulcer, and H. pylori infection: The "cystic fibrosis paradox" revisited. *J Cyst Fibros* 2013; **12**(4): 377–83.

17. Stern RC, Izant RJ Jr, Boat TF, Wood RE, Matthews LW, Doershuk CF. Treatment and prognosis of rectal prolapse in cystic fibrosis. *Gastroenterology* 1982; **82**(4): 707–10.

18. Holsclaw DS, Rocmans C, Shwachman H. Intussusception in patients with cystic fibrosis. *Pediatrics* 1971; **48**(1): 51–8.

19. Robertson MB, Choe KA, Joseph PM. Review of the abdominal manifestations of cystic fibrosis in the adult patient. *Radiographics* 2006; **26**(3): 679–90.

20. Fluge G, Olesen HV, Gilljam M, Meyer P, Pressler T, Storrosten OT, et al. Co-morbidity of cystic fibrosis and celiac disease in Scandinavian cystic fibrosis patients. *J Cyst Fibros* 2009; **8**(3): 198–202.

21. Lloyd-Still JD. Crohn's disease and cystic fibrosis. *Dig Dis Sci* 1994; **39**(4): 880–5.

22. Vawter GF, Shwachman H. Cystic fibrosis in adults: An autopsy study. *Pathol Ann* 1979; **14** (Pt 2): 357–82.

23. Prescott P, Bakowski MT. Pathogenesis of fibrosing colonopathy: The role of methacrylic acid copolymer. *Pharmacoepidemiol Drug Saf* 1999; **8**(6): 377–84.

24. Goralski JL, Lercher DM, Davis SD, Dellon ES. Eosinophilic esophagitis in cystic fibrosis: A case series and review of the literature. *J Cyst Fibros* 2013: **12**(1); 9–14.

25. Kerem B, Rommens JM, Buchanan JA, Markiewicz D, Cox TK, Chakravarti A, et al. Identification of the cystic fibrosis gene: Genetic analysis. *Science* 1989; **245**(4922): 1073–80.

26. Kerem BS, Buchanan JA, Durie P, Corey ML, Levison H, Rommens JM, et al. DNA marker haplotype association with pancreatic sufficiency in cystic fibrosis. *Am J Hum Genet* 1989; **44**(6): 827–34.

27. Riordan JR, Rommens JM, Kerem B, Alon N, Rozmahel R, Grzelczak Z, et al. Identification of the cystic fibrosis gene: Cloning and characterization of complementary DNA. *Science* 1989; **245**(4922) 1066–73.

28. Vankeerberghen A, Cuppens H, Cassiman JJ. The cystic fibrosis transmembrane conductance regulator: An intriguing protein with pleiotropic functions. *J Cyst Fibros* 2002; **1**(1): 13–29.

29. Kristidis P, Bozon D, Corey M, Markiewicz D, Rommens J, Tsui LC, et al. Genetic determination of exocrine pancreatic function in cystic fibrosis. *Am J Human Genet* 1992; **50**(6): 1178–84.

30. Kerem E, Corey M, Kerem BS, Rommens J, Markiewicz D, Levison H, et al. The relation between genotype and phenotype in cystic fibrosis—Analysis of the most common mutation (delta F508). *N Engl J Med* 1990; **323**(22): 1517–22.

31. Santis G, Osborne L, Knight RA, Hodson ME. Independent genetic determinants of pancreatic and pulmonary status in cystic fibrosis. *Lancet* 1990; **336**(8723): 1081–4.

32. Ooi CY, Dorfman R, Cipolli M, Gonska T, Castellani C, Keenan K, et al. Type of CFTR mutation determines risk of pancreatitis in patients with cystic fibrosis. *Gastroenterology* 2011; **140**(1): 153–61.

33. Snouwaert JN, Brigman KK, Latour AM, Malouf NN, Boucher RC, Smithies O, et al. An animal model for cystic fibrosis made by gene targeting. *Science* 1992; **257**(5073): 1083–8.

34. Dorin JR, Dickinson P, Alton EW, Smith SN, Geddes DM, Stevenson BJ, et al. Cystic fibrosis in the mouse by targeted insertional mutagenesis. *Nature* 1992; **359**(6392): 211–5.

35. Kent G, Iles R, Bear CE, Huan LJ, Griesenbach U, McKerlie C, et al. Lung disease in mice with cystic fibrosis. *J Clin Invest* 1997; **100**(12): 3060–9.

36. Durie PR, Kent G, Phillips MJ, Ackerley CA. Characteristic multiorgan pathology of cystic fibrosis in a long-living cystic fibrosis transmembrane regulator knockout murine model. *Am J Pathol* 2004; **164**(4): 1481–93.

37. Rozmahel R, Wilschanski M, Matin A, Plyte S, Oliver M, Auerbach W, et al. Modulation of disease severity in cystic fibrosis transmembrane conductance regulator deficient mice by a secondary genetic factor. *Nat Genet* 1996; **12**(3): 280–7.

38. Freye HB, Kurtz SM, Spock A, Capp MP. Light and electron microscopic examination of the small bowel of children with cystic fibrosis. *J Pediatr* 1964; **64**: 575–9.

39. Zhang L, Aleksandrov LA, Riordan JR, Ford RC. Domain location within the cystic fibrosis transmembrane conductance regulator protein investigated by electron microscopy and gold labelling. *Biochim Biophys Acta* 2011; **1808**(1): 399–404.

40. Wu X, Amorn MM, Aujla PK, Rice S, Mimms R, Watson AM, et al. Histologic characteristics and mucin immunohistochemistry of cystic fibrosis sinus mucosa. *Arch Otolaryngol Head Neck Surg* 2011; **137**(4): 383–9.

41. Rosenstein BJ. What is a cystic fibrosis diagnosis? *Clin Chest Med* 1998; **19**(3): 423–41, v.

42. Gregory PC. Gastrointestinal pH, motility/transit and permeability in cystic fibrosis. *J Pediatr Gastroenterol Nutr* 1996; **23**(5): 513–23.

43. Taylor CJ, Hillel PG, Ghosal S, Frier M, Senior S, Tindale WB, et al. Gastric emptying and intestinal transit of pancreatic enzyme supplements in cystic fibrosis. *Arch Dis Child* 1999; **80**(2): 149–52.

44. Bruzzese E, Raia V, Gaudiello G, Polito G, Buccigrossi V, Formicola V, et al. Intestinal inflammation is a frequent feature of cystic fibrosis and is reduced by probiotic administration. *Aliment Pharm Therap* 2004; **20**(7): 813–9.

45. Smyth RL, Croft NM, O'Hea U, Marshall TG, Ferguson A. Intestinal inflammation in cystic fibrosis. *Arch Dis Child* 2000; **82**(5): 394–9.

46. Konstan MW, Butler SM, Wohl ME, Stoddard M, Matousek R, Wagener JS, et al. Growth and nutritional indexes in early life predict pulmonary function in cystic fibrosis. *J Pediatr* 2003; **142**(6): 624–30.

47. Imrie CW, Connett G, Hall RI, Charnley RM. Review article: Enzyme supplementation in cystic fibrosis, chronic pancreatitis, pancreatic and periampullary cancer. *Aliment Pharmacol Therap*; **32** (Suppl 1): 1–25.

48. O'Sullivan BP, Baker D, Leung KG, Reed G, Baker SS, Borowitz D. Evolution of pancreatic function during the first year in infants with cystic fibrosis. *J Pediatr* 2013; **162**(4): 808–12.e1.

49. Taylor JR, Gardner TB, Waljee AK, Dimagno MJ, Schoenfeld PS. Systematic review: Efficacy and safety of pancreatic enzyme supplements for exocrine pancreatic insufficiency. *Aliment Pharmacol Therap* 2010; **31**(1): 57–72.

50. Walkowiak J, Nousia-Arvanitakis S, Cade A, Kashirskaya N, Piotrowski R, Strzykala K, et al. Fecal elastase-1 cut-off levels in the assessment of exocrine pancreatic function in cystic fibrosis. *J Cyst Fibros* 2002; **1**(4): 260–4.

51. Walkowiak J, Herzig KH, Witt M, Pogorzelski A, Piotrowski R, Barra E, et al. Analysis of exocrine pancreatic function in cystic fibrosis: One mild CFTR mutation does not exclude pancreatic insufficiency. *Eur J Clin Invest* 2001; **31**(9): 796–801.

52. Walkowiak J, Herzig KH, Strzykala K, Przyslawski J, Krawczynski M. Fecal elastase-1 is superior to fecal chymotrypsin in the assessment of pancreatic involvement in cystic fibrosis. *Pediatrics* 2002; **110** (1 Pt 1): e7.

53. Daftary A, Acton J, Heubi J, Amin R. Fecal elastase-1: Utility in pancreatic function in cystic fibrosis. *J Cyst Fibros* 2006; **5**(2): 71–6.

54. Trapnell BC, Strausbaugh SD, Woo MS, Tong SY, Silber SA, Mulberg AE, et al. Efficacy and safety of PANCREAZE® for treatment of exocrine pancreatic insufficiency due to cystic fibrosis. *J Cyst Fibros* 2011; **10**(5): 350–6.

55. Borowitz D, Stevens C, Brettman LR, Campion M, Chatfield B, Cipolli M. International phase III trial of liprotamase efficacy and safety in pancreatic-insufficient cystic fibrosis patients. *J Cyst Fibros* 2011; **10**(6): 443–52.

56. Patchell CJ, Desai M, Weller PH, Macdonald A, Smyth RL, Bush A, et al. Creon 10,000 minimicro-spheres vs. Creon 8,000 microspheres—An open randomised crossover preference study. *J Cyst Fibros* 2002; **1**(4): 287–91.

57. Munck A, Duhamel JF, Lamireau T, Le Luyer B, Le Tallec C, Bellon G, et al. Pancreatic enzyme replacement therapy for young cystic fibrosis patients. *J Cyst Fibros* 2009; **8**(1): 14–8.

58. Wooldridge JL, Heubi JE, Amaro-Galvez R, Boas SR, lake KV, Nasr SZ, et al. EUR-1008 pancreatic enzyme replacement is safe and effective in patients with cystic fibrosis and pancreatic insufficiency. *J Cyst Fibros* 2009; **8**(6): 405–17.

59. Trapnell BC, Maguiness K, Graff GR, Boyd D, Beckmann K, Caras S. Efficacy and safety of Creon 24,000 in subjects with exocrine pancreatic insufficiency due to cystic fibrosis. *J Cyst Fibros* 2009; **8**(6): 370–7.

60. Powell CJ. Colonic toxicity from pancreatins: A contemporary safety issue. *Lancet* 1999; **353**(9156): 911–5.

61. Tang L, Fatehi M, Linsdell P. Mechanism of direct bicarbonate transport by the CFTR anion channel. *J Cyst Fibros* 2009; **8**(2): 115–21.

62. Hallberg K, Abrahamsson H, Dalenback J, Fandriks L, Strandvik B. Gastric secretion in cystic fibrosis in relation to the migrating motor complex. *Scand J Gastroenterol* 2001; **36**(2): 121–7.

63. Wouthuyzen-Bakker M, Bodewes FA, Verkade HJ. Persistent fat malabsorption in cystic fibrosis: Lessons from patients and mice. *J Cyst Fibros* 2011; **10**(3): 150–8.

64. Robinson PJ, Smith AL, Sly PD. Duodenal pH in cystic fibrosis and its relationship to fat malabsorption. *Digest Dis Sci* 1990; **35**(10): 1299–304.

65. Ng SM, Francini AJ. Drug therapies for reducing gastric acidity in people with cystic fibrosis. *Cochrane Database Syst Rev* 2012; (4): CD003424.

66. Borowitz D, Durie PR, Clarke LL, Werlin SL, Taylor CJ, Semler J, et al. Gastrointestinal outcomes and confounders in cystic fibrosis. *J Pediatr Gastroenterol Nutr* 2005; **41**(3): 273–85.

67. Cave D, Legnani P, de Franchis R, Lewis BS, ICCE. ICCE consensus for capsule retention. *Endoscopy* 2005; **37**(10): 1065–7.

68. Gelfond D, Ma C, Semler J, Borowitz D. Intestinal pH and Gastrointestinal Transit Profiles in Cystic Fibrosis Patients Measured by Wireless Motility Capsule. *Digest Dis Sci* 2013; **58**(8): 2275–81.

69. Lisowska A, Wojtowicz J, Walkowiak J. Small intestine bacterial overgrowth is frequent in cystic fibrosis: Combined hydrogen and methane measurements are required for its detection. *Acta Biochim Pol* 2009; **56**(4): 631–4.

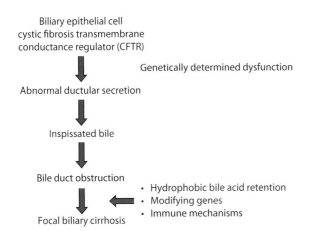

Biliary epithelial cell
cystic fibrosis transmembrane
conductance regulator (CFTR)

⬇ Genetically determined dysfunction

Abnormal ductular secretion

⬇

Inspissated bile

⬇

Bile duct obstruction

⬇ ⬅ • Hydrophobic bile acid retention
• Modifying genes
• Immune mechanisms

Focal biliary cirrhosis

Figure 23.1 Pathogenesis of chronic liver disease in cystic fibrosis (CF).

cholelithiasis (5%–25%).[8] Fatty liver (steatosis) is thought to be present in 25%–75% of CF patients, but this is likely to be related to poor nutrition and/or insulin resistance rather than a direct genetic defect.[9]

The characteristic hepatic lesion in CF is a nonuniform, focal biliary cirrhosis consistent with that seen in partial biliary obstruction due to damage to intrahepatic bile ducts leading to portal abnormalities and eventual fibrosis (Figures 23.2 and 23.3).

BILE DUCT PLUGGING

The plugging of intrahepatic bile ducts due to the enhanced viscosity of bile has been compared to that seen in the pancreatic ducts of CF patients,[10] i.e., it is a direct expression of the basic underlying gene defect.[11] The CFTR has been

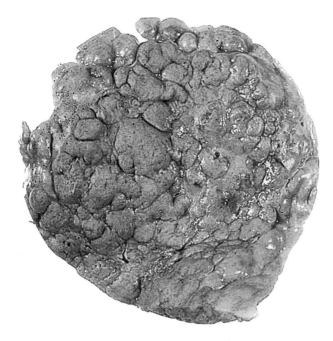

Figure 23.2 Postmortem specimen showing the typical multifocal nodularity of CF-related cirrhosis.

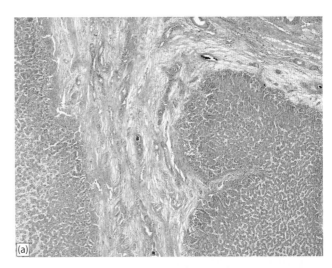

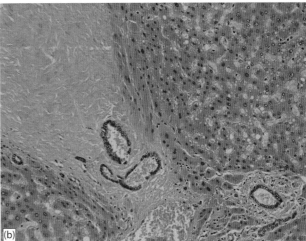

Figure 23.3 (a) Biliary type bridging fibrosis with bile casts occluding bile ducts (H&E, 20× magnification). (b) Bile ducts containing eosinophilic secretions in a sclerosed large portal tract and a steatotic background (H&E, 400× magnification).

localized to the apical membrane of the intrahepatic bile ducts.[12] Enhanced bile viscosity is likely to be due to the abnormalities of chloride transport inhibiting the hydration and alkalinization of the canalicular-produced bile as well as the excessive production by intrahepatic biliary epithelial cells of mucus composed of proteoglycans.[13] Patchy plugging of the intrahepatic ducts with this high-viscosity bile results in an initial focal distribution of cirrhotic changes. Obstruction of biliary ductules with thick eosinophilic material results in periductal inflammation, bile duct proliferation, and periportal fibrosis. The activation of hepatic stellate cells results in the production of collagen and profibrogenic cytokines like interleukin-4.[8] With increasing ductular involvement over a variable time span, the process gradually becomes much more diffuse in a small percentage of CF children, producing a fully established biliary cirrhosis with extensive liver involvement and consequent portal hypertension. This process may take years to decades.

BILE ACID–RELATED TOXICITY

Whether biliary duct obstruction alone is sufficient to account for this process remains controversial. A light and electron microscopic study of CF liver disease demonstrated features more in keeping with a destructive bile duct lesion than a purely obstructive phenomenon.[14] Similar findings have been reported from a murine model of CF.[15] A bile-related toxin has been suggested as the most likely explanation for these findings. Initial analyses showed no significant difference in the serum bile acid profile between those with and without evidence of liver disease. However, given the significantly lower volume and thus higher concentration of bile produced in the presence of the *CFTR* gene defect,[16,17] it could be speculated that bile reflux and retention caused by the partial or complete obstruction of ducts seen in CFALD dramatically increases the exposure of hepatocytes to potentially hepatotoxic lipophilic bile acids. A recent study has revisited the relationship between the bile acid profile and the presence of CFALD in children.[18] These authors identified an inverse correlation between the level of endogenous serum ursodeoxycholic acid (UDCA) and CFALD and suggested that this might represent a protective factor against liver injury. Why higher levels of endogenous UDCA levels are found in some patients has not been explained.

RISK FACTORS

Although the above provides a possible etiological basis for chronic CFALD, it does not account for the absence of liver involvement in such a large proportion of patients and the wide spectrum of severity in those in whom liver disease does occur, independent of the CFTR mutations carried. A number of possible contributing or associated factors have been proposed.

Genetic influences

Attempts to match a specific CF genotype with expression of liver disease have failed to show any significant correlation.[19] However, there is evidence that the presence of a severe genotype (class I, II, and III mutations), associated with complete or virtually complete loss of CFTR function, has an independent association with the development of CFALD.[7,20,21] A relationship between human leukocyte antigen (HLA) status has been reported with a significant increased prevalence of DQ6 in those with CFALD.[22] There is now accumulating evidence that other genetic factors may be extremely important in the pathogenesis of liver disease. Modifier genes are inherited independently of the CFTR mutation but may attenuate or exacerbate the CF phenotype by their influence on such factors as host defense and the inflammatory response. Several candidate genes have been studies but so far only the SERPINA1 Z allele (formerly alpha-1 antitrypsin) has been found to be strongly associated with CFALD and portal hypertension.[23] SERPINA1 protein is a serine protease inhibitor mainly expressed in hepatocytes. The protein encoded by the Z allele is misfolded and accumulates in the endoplasmic reticulum, triggering hepatocyte death, inflammation, and fibrosis.[2] The SERPINA1 polymorphism is relatively uncommon in CF—only 2% of patients are carriers—however, the odds ratio (OR) for association with CFALD is relatively high at 5.04. It does not appear to be a modifier of lung disease.

It is also noteworthy that the relatively common UGT1A1 promoter mutation associated with Gilbert's syndrome is a risk factor for gallstone formation in CF (OR 7.3).[24]

Meconium ileus (MI)

A history of MI has been identified as a risk factor for CFALD in a number of reports.[5,7] A study reporting autopsy findings suggested that viscous mucus might accumulate simultaneously in the intestine, gallbladder, and biliary tree leading to chronic damage.[25] Other studies have failed to confirm an association with MI,[20,26] and as only a small proportion of patients who develop CFALD have a history of MI this should only be considered a possible contributory factor at most.

Male gender

A male preponderance among CFALD patients has been reported in several studies.[6,7] There is further evidence that in female patients liver disease occurred only before puberty, wheras male patients presented up to the age of 18 years.[7] This male predominance may in part reflect the possible survival benefit of males in CF.[27] However, a role for estrogens and their receptors in modulating the development of CFALD should be considered.

Common bile duct obstruction

Distal common bile duct compression by pancreatic fibrosis is a well-recognized cause of obstructive biliary injury in patients with chronic pancreatitis and has been postulated as a factor in the development of liver disease in CF.[28] However, imaging of the extrahepatic biliary tree in CFALD has shown this to be an unusual phenomenon and at best only a contributory factor in a small proportion of cases.[29]

Additional contributing factors

The presence of a subpopulation of lymphocytes, cytotoxic to hepatocytes and directed toward the liver-specific lipoprotein, suggests that immune mechanisms might also be involved in the pathogenesis of CF liver disease.[30] Factors that may exacerbate existing liver injury include poor nutritional status (total parenteral nutrition may accelerate disease progression), drug toxicity, sepsis, medical treatment or compliance, and recent abdominal surgery.[4,11]

CLINICAL FEATURES OF LIVER DISEASE

Deep cholestasis secondary to common bile duct obstruction with inspissated bile may be the earliest manifestation of CF.[31,32] This condition rarely results in clinically significant liver disease, typically resolving spontaneously during the first months of life.

Most patients with CFALD remain asymptomatic even when multilobular cirrhosis develops.[33] The diagnosis of CFALD is usually clinically evident by the end of the first decade. Portal hypertension, and its sequelae, is more often a feature than hepatocellular failure. The commonest clinical presentation is the finding of hepatomegaly on routine examination[33]; however, this may also arise from fatty liver without CFALD.

Fatty infiltration (steatosis) of the liver may sometimes produce massive hepatomegaly and abdominal distension, complicated by hypoglycemia.[34,35] It is the most frequent hepatic lesion associated with CF but does not seem to be caused directly by the CF secretory defect, being rather a consequence of the disease process outside the liver (e.g., conditions associated with insulin resistance[36]) and the effect of circulating cytokines resulting from chronic infection by respiratory pathogens.[37] Malnutrition has also been implicated in its pathogenesis; deficiencies in carnitine, fatty acids, trace elements, and minerals may be associated.[35] A risk of progression to cirrhosis has not been specifically identified in CF but is recognized in children with other etiological causes of fatty liver.[38] Steatosis alone has previously been considered a relatively benign condition in CF, separate from the development of the CFALD phenotype. However, increasing knowledge of the development of nonalcoholic steatohepatitis into cirrhosis in adults may lead to a reexamination of this issue.[33]

Evidence of underlying cirrhosis may occur at any time, but new diagnoses are most frequently made during the first two decades of life and usually as part of routine follow-up in patients with an established diagnosis of CF. Abnormal liver function tests (LFTs) are common in CF but may be of little significance. Many large centers have established routine surveillance including sequential ultrasound scanning (USS) (see later). This approach has identified a small proportion of patients with no other clinical or laboratory evidence of liver disease. Many CF patients with cirrhosis will develop signs of portal hypertension and present with related complications, particularly variceal bleeding, during their second and third decades. Variceal bleeding may be the presenting feature of established portal hypertension and may occur in the absence of any other signs of decompensation. As in other types of biliary cirrhosis, portal hypertension may occur in a precirrhotic phase because of the presinusoidal component to portal vascular resistance. In such cases, the degree of portal hypertension can be quite out of keeping with the amount of liver fibrosis. Decompensated biliary cirrhosis including jaundice, ascites, or encephalopathy are very unusual presenting features. Similarly, the classical peripheral signs of chronic liver disease such as spider naevi, palmar erythema, clubbing, jaundice, fluid retention, caput medusae are late and uncommon signs.

Overall, the clinical picture is one of a slowly progressive liver disease, the natural history of which is usually interrupted by premature mortality related to pulmonary disease. The long natural history of cirrhosis in CF is not dissimilar to that seen in other biliary cirrhotic disease such as primary biliary cirrhosis or primary sclerosing cholangitis.[39,40]

Controversy remains as to whether the adverse effect of liver disease in CF is restricted to the 3% of patients who have overt liver decompensation and a further 2% who experience variceal bleeding. There is some evidence that liver disease may have an adverse effect on the prognosis in CF independent of specific complications. A large time-dependent multiple regression analysis of survival risk factors in CF reported liver disease as an independent predictor of premature mortality, in addition to pulmonary function and nutrition.[41] As is typical in liver diseases characterized by initial involvement of bile ducts and later impairment of hepatocyte function, the systemic and pulmonary hemodynamic abnormalities of cirrhosis are often earlier and more prominent manifestations than features of liver failure per se.[42,43] Low peripheral vascular resistance, high cardiac output, and increased pulmonary shunting might be expected to adversely affect patients with advanced pulmonary disease. However, recent studies provide evidence that impact on clinical course (with regard to pulmonary and nutritional complications) is not significant until the most advanced stages of liver disease are reached.[7,44]

OUTCOME OF CFALD

A recent study by Rowland et al.[45] followed up 42 children with CFLD and their age- and sex-matched controls with CF only, over a 7-year period. The investigators found that even in the short to medium term, having liver disease in the setting of CF has a substantial negative clinical impact. Apart from having reduced life expectancy overall, about 10% of CFLD patients are at risk of dying from liver complications or needing a liver transplant, and 30% will develop varices. CFALD patients are also at risk of a more severe disease phenotype, with worse nutritional parameters, and a higher risk of CF-related diabetes. Another recent study found that in addition to diabetes, gender, and respiratory function, CFALD was also associated with an increased risk of mortality in CF (Cox hazard ratio 1.3, 95% confidence interval 1.0–1.7).[46]

Interestingly, in the study by Rowland et al. eight children (22%) with evidence of CFALD at baseline had no clinical evidence of liver disease as adults. There are currently no biomarkers to indicate which patients will develop progressive liver disease or which children might benefit from therapeutic or nutritional interventions (see the later section "Management of Liver Disease").

DIAGNOSIS OF CFALD

Diagnostic criteria are not well-defined and universal. Early diagnosis is particularly challenging, and there is no "gold standard" confirmatory investigation for early disease, before portal hypertension is established. Hepatomegaly is found in a third of CF patients and can be due to CFALD or secondary to cor pulmonale with liver congestion. The recent European Association for the Study of the Liver guidelines suggest serum liver tests be performed annually and if abnormal, an ultrasound examination of the abdomen.[47] The diagnosis of CFALD would also depend on excluding other causes of liver disease and abnormal serum liver tests, such as drugs, toxins, viral hepatitis, sepsis, biliary atresia, gall stones, autoimmune hepatitis, primary sclerosing cholangitis, alpha-1 antitrypsin deficiency, celiac disease, Wilson's disease, etc.

More rigid diagnostic criteria for liver disease in CF according to one group are as follows[48]:

1. Positive liver histology (focal biliary cirrhosis, multilobular cirrhosis)
2. At least two of the following or at least two consecutive examinations over a 1-year period:
   a. Hepatomegaly confirmed by USS
   b. Two abnormal serum LFT levels
   c. USS abnormalities other than hepatomegaly (e.g., nodularity, irregular margin, splenomegaly)

LIVER FUNCTION TESTS

Standard laboratory liver-related tests have reasonable sensitivity but poor specificity as predictive factors for CF liver disease. This is not surprising as many potential factors might influence these tests (especially serum aminotransferase), including infection, hypoxemia, and medications. Markers of a biliary component such as the alkaline phosphatase and gamma glutamine transpeptidase may be more helpful particularly when levels are elevated by a factor of 3, and this is sustained over a period of months.[49] A small proportion of patients with established cirrhosis will have entirely normal LFTs.[6,49] The most important role for these standard LFTs is to initiate a search for possible underlying liver disease through imaging.

IMAGING

Transabdominal ultrasound

The availability of high-quality transabdominal USS has provided a cheap and widely available means of detecting underlying chronic liver disease. In experienced hands ultrasound imaging provides diagnostic information with respect to a diffuse cirrhotic process as well as detecting earlier focal abnormalities.[50] Splenomegaly, a dilated portal vein, and the presence of collateral vessels are all important markers of portal hypertension.[50]

Parenchymal irregularity, periportal fibrosis, and irregularity of the liver edge (Figure 23.4) are the factors incorporated in an ultrasound scoring system deemed effective in documenting established cirrhosis in adults (Table 23.1).[43] Ultrasound can be highly predictive for the development of portal hypertension in CFALD.[51]

The use of Doppler studies allows the detection of portal or splenic vein thrombosis, which has an increased prevalence in CF, usually as a consequence of associated chronic pancreatitis. Transabdominal ultrasound has been widely adopted for the routine screening of CF populations.[49]

However, USS cannot diagnose early liver disease and only has a positive predictive value of around 30% and sensitivity of less than 60%.[51] Ultrasound is highly sensitive for detecting fatty liver/steatosis, but this is nonspecific and not necessarily predictive of genuine CFALD.

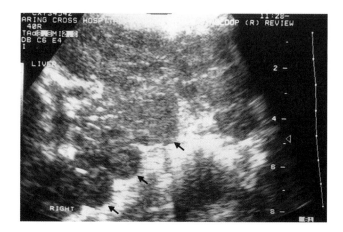

Figure 23.4 Hepatic ultrasound scan showing the surface nodularity of established cirrhosis (arrowed).

Table 23.1 The ultrasound scoring system

	Score		
	1	2	3
Hepatic parenchyma	Normal	Coarse	Irregular
Liver edge	Smooth	–	Nodular
Periportal fibrosis	None	Moderate	Severe

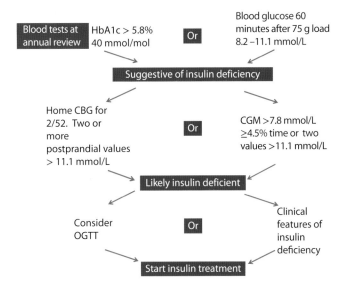

Figure 24.3 Possible scheme for a pragmatic screening sequence to look for impaired glucose metabolism. This is derived from a synthesis of observations in CF and has not been validated for sensitivity or specificity.

However, for reasons of practical organization, patient preference, and uncertainty about the timing of intervention in relation to an abnormal glucose tolerance test, currently many centers do not routinely perform OGTTs. Most centers make an assessment of glucose metabolism at least annually (often on each admission) and this may be by postprandial capillary blood glucose monitoring (CBGM), continuous glucose monitoring system (CGMS), or blood glucose levels with confirmation by OGTT if necessary. A suggested pathway of screening tests and interventions is shown in Figure 24.3.

DIAGNOSTIC THRESHOLDS FOR DIABETES

The WHO defines diabetes mellitus as "a metabolic disorder of multiple etiology characterized by chronic hyperglycemia with disturbances of carbohydrate, fat, and protein

metabolism resulting from defects in insulin secretion, insulin action, or both." Plasma glucose levels form part of a continuum and the precise point at which the level of glycemia does harm varies according to various factors (not all of which have yet been identified) including the level, duration, and variability of hyperglycemia and the target organ or tissue that is being affected. Current diagnostic thresholds for diabetes are based on retinopathy and the influence of glycemia on fetal growth (Table 24.2). In CF pulmonary damage, pulmonopathy may have a different threshold.

Improvements in the standardization of the measurement of HbA1c over the last 20 years have made the test much more accurate and reproducible so that it is now recommended for use in the diagnosis of type 2 diabetes.[49] Despite years of study, there is still much controversy over the best screening tests and thresholds for diagnosis particularly in gestational diabetes where factors other than the glycemic level may contribute to fetal growth and macrosomia. This experience closely parallels the current challenge of establishing appropriate screening tests and diagnostic threshold for CFRD.

The current thresholds for the diagnosis of CFRD are based on the cutoff points for retinopathy in non-CF-population-based studies around the world.[46] However, the threshold for impact on nutritional status and lung damage may be closer to the glycemic threshold for impact on fetal growth than retinopathy. It has been suggested that the criteria for the diagnosis of diabetes in CF should be set at the level where the risk of other complications, particularly lung disease (pulmonopathy) arises.[34] However, it is not yet clear which test best predicts these complications. What is clear is that the tests used for the diagnosis of diabetes perform differently in the CF population.

ORAL GLUCOSE TOLERANCE TEST AND VENOUS PLASMA GLUCOSE

The OGTT is a standardized test that is used for the diagnosis of diabetes in the non-CF population where the fasting glucose level is reproducible and predictive of retinopathy.

Table 24.2 Current diagnostic criteria for diabetes and prediabetes: WHO and ADA criteria

	HbA1c mmol/mmol (%)	Fasting plasma glucose mmol/L	2-Hour 75-g OGTT glucose mmol/L	Others
Diabetes (WHO and ADA)[46,47]	≥48 (6.5)[a]	≥7.0[a]	≥11.1[a]	RPG ≥ 11.1 mmol/L with symptoms
Prediabetes (WHO)[46]	42–47 (6.0–6.4)	6.0–6.9 IFG	7.8–11.0 IGT	
Prediabetes (ADA)[48]	38–47(5.7–6.4)	5.6–6.9 IFG	7.8–11.0 IGT	
Gestational DM (WHO)[46]		≥7.0	≥7.8	
Gestational DM (ADA)[48]		≥5.1	≥8.5	1-Hour 75-g OGTT glucose ≥ 10.0 mmol/L

[a] Any one of these tests can indicate a diagnosis of diabetes; two positive tests are required to make the diagnosis in asymptomatic individuals.

The 2-hour glucose level is less reproducible even in the non-CF population. Each of 685 subjects in the National Health and Nutrition Examination Survey (NHANES) study had 2 OGTTs carried out in a 2-week period. Two-hour glucose levels were more variable than either fasting glucose or HbA1c (within person coefficient of variation of 16.7% for 2-hour vs. 5.7% for fasting and 3.6% for HbA1c).[50] Glucose level varies from minute to minute according to intake of food and dispersal and uptake of glucose into the tissues. Its level varies with the site from which blood is drawn (so that capillary glucose measurements are different from whole blood or venous plasma measurements) and the way the sample is handled so that a 25–40 minute delay in the processing of a plasma glucose sample reduces the measured glucose by 10 mg/dL or 0.5 mmol/L.[51]

The test has further limitations when transposed to the CF population. The 2-hour OGTT is only a snapshot of glucose handling with two venous plasma glucose measurements taken before and 2 hours after a 75 g oral glucose load (effectively a provocation test). In CF, not only is the first phase insulin response reduced but there is a delay in the insulin peak in response to glucose, so the peak glucose level usually occurs 30–60 minutes after a glucose load and the OGTT will tend to underestimate abnormal glucose handling in CF unless additional sampling is undertaken.[49,52] A recent study in CF showed the maximum glucose level correlates with reduction in FEV_1 irrespective of whether the criteria for diabetes are met.[53] The OGTT only identifies individuals who meet the diagnostic criteria when presented with a pure glucose load and may fail to identify those with postprandial glucose levels in the diabetes range on their usual diet. The test may fail to identify individuals who could benefit from early intervention such as patients with IGT with prolonged periods of elevated airway glucose concentrations.[54]

As a standardized test, the OGTT is carried out, while the patient is in a stable clinical state, not taking any medications that can affect the test, with the patient on a "normal diet" for 3 days before the test, fasting before the test, and resting during the test—if these conditions are not met, the test is invalid. This means that the test cannot be used to diagnose diabetes in many patients with CF who have prolonged or regular periods of clinical instability, variable diets or who are taking medications that may affect the test such as oral steroids or azoles. In these situations, random glucose measurements may be used to make the diagnosis. The use of a non-fasting OGTT in CF has not been studied but would be preferable for many patients.

The 2-hour glucose level, which is the level most likely to achieve a diagnosis of diabetes in CF, is recognized to have a high variability both in CF and non-CF populations. As two abnormal tests are required to make the diagnosis of diabetes in asymptomatic individuals, some patients who reach the diagnostic criterion for diabetes on a first test may not achieve a diagnostic level of glucose on a repeated test. Many patients fall into a grey area, having had a test that meets the diagnostic criteria for diabetes but where repeat testing is

normal. The recent US guidelines address this issue by setting the date of diagnosis of diabetes as "the date a person with CF first meets the diagnostic criteria even if hyperglycemia subsequently abates."[4] In many centers, the regular use of the OGTT has been abandoned as a "gold standard" as other diagnostic techniques such as postprandial CBGM, continuous glucose monitoring (CGM), or blood glucose profiles give an earlier indication of insulin deficiency and the onset of diabetes.

HbA1c

HbA1c reflects the average plasma glucose over the previous 8 to 12 weeks. It can be performed at any time of the day and does not require any special preparation such as fasting. HbA1c has now been recommended for use as a diagnostic test for diabetes.[55] An HbA1c of 6.5% (48 mmol/mol) is recommended as the point for diagnosing diabetes, however a lower value does not exclude diabetes. In the general population, the performance of HbA1c is similar to fasting or 2-hour plasma glucose in detecting those at risk of diabetes retinopathy.[56]

In CF, early reports supported the use of HbA1c in detecting CFRD[57] and suggested that it had a high sensitivity (83%) when used to detect CFRD[58]; however, subsequent studies showed poor correlation between HbA1c and 2-hour glucose level in OGTT.[59,60] The relationship between HbA1c and mean plasma glucose (as assessed by 7-point glucose profiles) is not constant,[61] but there is a strong correlation between HbA1c and mean plasma glucose as assessed by area under curve in CGMS[54,62] suggesting that HbA1c may pick up some of the effects of the characteristic early glucose excursions in CF missed by both the OGTT and 7-point glucose profiles. Interestingly, in two large studies, HbA1c did not correlate with plasma glucose levels in OGTT but did show a significant negative correlation with FEV_1.[62,63]

Several factors may affect the performance of HbA1c in CF including reduced red blood cell turnover time and liver disease. Raised levels of HbA1c indicate risk of microvascular complications. CFRD patients with retinopathy and/or microalbuminuria had higher average levels of HbA1c (8.0%, 64 mmol/mol) over 10 years than those who had no eye or kidney disease (HbA1c 5.8%, 40 mmol/mol) and 83% of those with microvascular complications had an HbA1c $\leq$ 7.0%, 53 mmol/mol.[64] A raised HbA1c is associated with increased mortality in CF.[65]

BLOOD GLUCOSE MONITORING AND CONTINUOUS GLUCOSE MONITORING

CBGM is widely used in the assessment of diabetes control to enable titration of treatments to target and to detect hypo- or hyperglycemia. It is quick, simple to use, widely available, and measurements can be taken by the patient. It is not routinely used for the diagnosis of diabetes because of the high coefficient of variation of results, but can be helpful in building a picture of glycemic control in response to changes in diet and treatment. As with the OGTT, CBGM can miss or underestimate glucose excursions. A typical 7-point glucose profile taken with readings before and 2 hours after the three main meals and before bed would miss the peak of glucose excursions in CF, which typically occur 30–60 minutes after a meal (Figure 24.4).

CGM has been used widely in CF to identify individuals with clinically significant glucose excursions. CGM gives a picture of glucose handling over time with estimates of interstitial glucose carried out every 5 minutes over the duration of the test (usually 3–7 days). The test can be carried out at home in conditions that reflect the "real life" of the patient. Patients usually complete a food and activity diary during the test so there is an opportunity to check calorie intake and dietary content. The test can be used to identify individuals who spend a disproportionate amount of time with glucose levels above the pulmonary and renal thresholds for glucose and who may be at increased risk for pulmonary complications or metabolic effects of such raised glucose levels. The area under the curve on CGM correlates with HbA1c unlike CBGM.[54,61] It can be used to identify a subgroup of patients with glucose levels in the diabetic range who could have been diagnosed with diabetes if a random venous plasma glucose had been taken at an appropriate time.[66] These patients are at higher risk of achieving a diagnosis of diabetes over time, have worse lung function, and have the potential to benefit from early intervention. The CGMS has been shown to be reproducible with low intrasubject variability on repeat testing in CF.[67]

A recent study has identified that patients with a CGM time spent above 7.8 mmol/L ≥4.5% had a fall of ≥3% in FVC% over the preceding 12 months.[68] This pulmonary decline was also associated with a blood glucose level at any time during the OGTT ≥8.2 mmol/L. These interesting findings suggest that it may be possible to use CGM to define new thresholds of blood glucose, which are correlated with pulmonary decline, the major cause of morbidity and mortality in CF.

PREDIABETES

The WHO recognizes an intermediate group of individuals who do not have CF and whose glucose levels, although not meeting criteria for diabetes, are nevertheless too high to be considered normal. These persons are defined as having impaired fasting glucose (IFG) (fasting plasma glucose [FPG] levels 6.1–6.9 mmol/L, or IGT 2-hour values in the OGTT of 7.8–11.0 mmol/L).[46] It should be noted that the American Diabetic Association (ADA) defines the cut off for IFG at 5.6 mmol/L.[10] Individuals with IFG and/or IGT have been referred to as having prediabetes, indicating relatively high risk for the future development of diabetes. Several prospective studies in the general population have used HbA1c to predict the progression to diabetes.

The ADA considers an HbA1c in the range of 5.7%–6.4% as prediabetes.[47] Prediabetes in CF is associated with a deterioration in health status for 2–6 years before the diagnosis of CFRD.[18,32,35] Various strategies have been used to identify individuals within this phase who will progress to diabetes over time and in whom intervention to prevent or reverse clinical deterioration may be justified. Patients with IGT appear to be at an increased risk of progression over the next few years whereas those with a hypoglycemic OGTT[69] or FH[70] may have a lower risk of progression at least in the short term.

Studies of interventions in prediabetes in CF have shown improvements in lung function and nutritional status when patients with impaired glucose handling are treated with insulin. Dobson et al.[37] showed a reversal of the decline in pulmonary function tests (PFTs) in 4 patients with normal glucose tolerance but who had postprandial CGM readings >11.1 mmol/L. Modest improvements in BMI z-score and lung function were seen in six patients with IGT treated

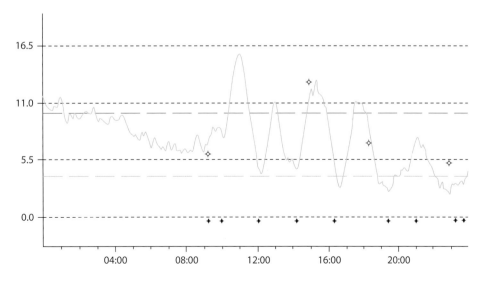

Figure 24.4 CGMS trace in a CF patient with normal glucose tolerance on OGTT and symptoms of hypoglycemia. Open diamonds represent patient's capillary glucose readings taken fasting and 1–2 hours after main meals.

with insulin over a median of 1.4 years.[71] Mozzillo et al.[72] used low-dose insulin glargine to treat 22 patients who had glucose levels >7.8 mmol/L on an OGTT or CGMS at any time, and showed improvements in lung function (mean FEV_1 increased from 68.2% to 77.1%) over a 12-month period. However 9 of the 22 patients met the criteria for the diagnosis of CFRD. A 3-year prospective study of children with CF, IGT, and reduced first phase insulin release treated with low-dose insulin showed improvements in nutritional status and stabilization of FEV_1 when compared to a parallel group of CF children with normal glucose tolerance (NGT) who remained without insulin treatment.[73] However, a recent randomized control trial of long-acting insulin in IGT in CF failed to show any benefit.[74]

SUMMARY

The OGTT is the current recommended screening test for CFRD but it has significant limitations in CF. The OGTT is unpopular with patients and it may fail to identify individuals with clinically significant glycemic excursions who have early insulin deficiency and may benefit from early intervention. Studies of insulin treatment in prediabetes have had variable outcomes mainly reflecting a lack of consistency in the selection criteria for these studies. A pragmatic scheme for screening for insulin deficiency is shown in Figure 24.3.

MANAGEMENT OF CYSTIC FIBROSIS-RELATED DIABETES

MULTIDISCIPLINARY CARE

The management of CFRD should be undertaken in the context of a multidisciplinary team with expertise in CF and diabetes.[4,45] Good communication between the team members and patient with CFRD is essential to avoid conflicting information and to allow the management of CFRD to take an appropriate place in medical management and the holistic care of the patient.[75] Patient education and involvement in the day-to-day management of diabetes and the setting and achievement of treatment goals is an essential component of care.

INSULIN TREATMENT

Patients with CFRD are relatively insulin deficient, and thus insulin is the logical treatment. CF patients on insulin therapy who achieve glycemic control demonstrate improvement in weight, protein anabolism, pulmonary function, and survival (Table 24.3). These studies reported improved outcomes associated with the use of insulin in patients with CFRD, including those without FH. Reported outcomes

Table 24.3 Published studies addressing insulin therapy as an intervention in CFRD

Study reference	Intervention	Number treated	Patient group	Study type	Study duration	Outcomes
Lanng et al.[38]	Insulin	18	CFRD	Case control before and after	2 years	↑ BMI, FEV_1, FVC
Nousia-Arvantakis et al.[39]	Biphasic insulin	6	CFRD	Case control	6 months	↑ BMI, FEV_1
Rolon et al.[40]	Insulin	21	CFRD	Case control	1–5 years	↑ BMI, ↓FEV_1 decline and HbA1c
Franzese et al.[76]	Glargine	8	CFRD	Case control before and after	6 months	↓Lung infections, no effect on HbA1c or BMI
Rafii et al.[77]	Insulin	3	CFRD	Before and after	6 months	↑ Protein synthesis, fat mass and % body fat
Mohan et al.[78]	Bolus only Basal only Basal bolus	31 2 9	CFRD	Before and after	3 years	↑ BMI, FEV_1, FVC, delayed decline in FEV_1
Hardin et al.[79]	Insulin pump	9	CFRD	Before and after	6 months	↑ Weight, lean body mass, ↓HbA1c and protein catabolism
Moran et al.[80]	Aspart (Novorapid)	23 7	CFRD IGT	RCT	12 months	Insulin-reversed weight loss. No difference in FEV_1, HbA1c, or acute illness

included improved lung function, improved nutritional status, improved blood glucose/HbA1c control, decreased pulmonary exacerbation rates (one study), and decreased mortality (one study).

Although the studies of insulin treatment in CFRD have used several different insulin regimens, there is little evidence to show which insulin regimens work best in CFRD. Clinical judgment should be used to choose the best regimen for each patient, which can then be tailored to their individual requirements. In patients with postprandial excursions, rapid-acting insulin can be used with carbohydrate counting to match insulin requirements.

CFRD with FH requires the use of intermediate or long-acting insulin to supplement basal insulin supply. Patients with more complex requirements, including those with nocturnal hypoglycemia or those who require very frequent administration of insulin to cover high-calorie snacks may benefit from rapid-acting insulin by continuous subcutaneous infusion (insulin pump).[62,79–81] Insulin requirements may rise rapidly during acute illness or systemic glucocorticoid treatment.[82,83] At the same time, patient's eating habits may change either through reduced appetite or through the need to increase dietary intake and nutritional supplements. Once illness resolves, it may take several weeks for insulin

requirements to return gradually to baseline. The patient's insulin regimen needs to be adjusted to reflect these changing requirements. Careful monitoring for hypoglycemia is required during this period.

ORAL HYPOGLYCAEMIC AGENTS

Oral hypoglycemic agents have been used in CF, however their side effect profile and theoretical risks in CF mean that they have had a limited place in the treatment of CFRD. Four studies have compared oral agents to insulin in CFRD including one randomized control trial,[80] one randomized crossover trial,[84] and two cohort studies[85,86] (Table 24.4). The observational studies found no difference in lung function, nutritional status, or HbA1c between patients receiving oral hypoglycemic agents and between those receiving insulin treatments. However, the two randomized studies suggested that oral hypoglycemic agents were not as effective as insulin in improving nutritional status, blood glucose HbA1c control, and insulin deficiency as measured by insulin area under the curve. Insulin is the cornerstone of treatment of CFRD, although oral agents may be used in selected patients as a bridge to insulin treatment.

Table 24.4 Studies of oral hypoglycemic agents in CFRD and IGT

Study reference	Intervention	Number treated	Patient group	Study type	Study duration	Outcomes
Culler et al.[87]	Glipizide	6	IGT	Before and after	6 months	↓Urine glucose and HbA1c ↑FPIR
Bertele-Harms et al.[88]	Glibenclamide	20	CFRD	Before and after	0–15 years	↓Urine glucose ↓HbA1c
Kentrup et al.[89]	Acarbose	12	IGT	RCT	14 days	↓Mean and peak glucose
Moran et al.[84]	Repaglinide/ insulin	7	CFRD FH	Case–control crossover	Single dose	Insulin ↓peak glucose and glucose AUCRepaglinide ↓5-hour glucose
Rosenecker et al.[86]	Glibenclamide/ insulin	11 34	CFRD	Before and after	3–7 years	No difference in most recent FEV$_1$, FVC, or BMI
Ballman et al. 2003[90]	Glibenclamide (6 transferred to insulin after 14–24 months)	19	CFRD	Before and after	2 years	No change in PFTs on Glibenclamide if HbA1c was stable
Onady et al. 2006[85]	Sulfonylurea/ metformin/ thiazolidinedione/ insulin	5 4 3 8	CFRD	Before and after	10 years	No difference in HbA1c, weight or FEV$_1$ between treatments
Moran et al. 2009[80]	Repaglinide/ insulin/placebo	26 30 25	CFRD FH/IGT	RCT	12 months	Insulin-reversed weight loss. No difference in FEV$_1$, HbA1c, or acute illness

NUTRITION IN CYSTIC FIBROSIS-RELATED DIABETES

The overarching goal for nutrition in CFRD is to achieve and maintain good nutritional status while optimizing glycemia. People with CF require a high-calorie, high-fat diet, which is usually 120%–150% of the daily recommended intake for age. The increased requirements in CF are due to an increased resting energy expenditure and increased loss of calories through malabsorption. A diet providing 35%–40% of calories as fat, 20% as protein, and 40%–45% as carbohydrates is recommended but this is often difficult to achieve. Prescriptive caloric restriction to maintain euglycemia should be avoided and may not be appropriate in normal or underweight patients with CFRD, depending on careful dietary assessment. The timing of carbohydrate intake and covering insulin treatment need to be matched to avoid glucose excursions and/or hypoglycemia.[91] Carbohydrate counting may be used as a guide to insulin therapy. Dietetic advice from a dietician experienced in CF and diabetes is essential.

Glucose levels should be checked in those patients with CF commenced on enteral tube feeding. CBGM testing is required pre feed, 2 hours into the feed, and immediately post feed to ascertain whether additional insulin is required. The type and dose of insulin prescribed depends on the profile of glucose levels observed during the feed and should be monitored if there is a change in feed type, volume, or duration. There is a risk of hypoglycemia if the feed is interrupted after insulin has been given to cover it or if the feed is not completed or regurgitated. Overnight percutaneous endoscopic gastrostomy (PEG) feeding pumps should have an appropriate alarm that sounds if the feed stops so that patients do not become hypoglycemic.

MANAGEMENT GOALS IN CYSTIC FIBROSIS-RELATED DIABETES

The management goals in diabetes are predominately based on the need to reduce the risk of acute and chronic complications of diabetes (see the section on "Complications of Cystic Fibrosis-Related Diabetes"). The target range for HbA1c has not been established in CF, but HbA1c correlates with microvascular complications in CFRD. The fact that the glycemic threshold for pulmonary disease, renal disease, and mortality appears to be lower in CFRD than in non-CF diabetes suggests that glycemic targets in CFRD should be tighter than those in diabetes in non-CF patients. To date there are no long-term interventional studies that show a reduction in the risk of these complications if lower targets are set in CFRD.

COMPLICATIONS OF CYSTIC FIBROSIS-RELATED DIABETES

As in other forms of diabetes, the clinical phenotype of CFRD is diverse with some individuals who appear to have a lower risk of progressive insulin loss and a lower risk of complications of diabetes. Individuals who meet the criteria for diabetes but in whom islet function is relatively preserved, so that they still maintain normal fasting glucose levels 10 years after the diagnosis, have a lower risk of diabetes complications. One study found that patients who maintained a fasting glucose level of <7 mmol/L had no retinopathy or microalbuminuria compared with 16% and 14%, respectively, patients with CFRD who had raised fasting glucose levels.

ACUTE COMPLICATIONS OF CYSTIC FIBROSIS-RELATED DIABETES

The reported acute complications of CFRD are predominantly metabolic and include diabetic ketoacidosis and hypoglycemia. Diabetic ketoacidosis is rare as absolute insulin deficiency is rare in CFRD.[30] Type 1 diabetes and CFRD can coexist, but this does not appear to happen any more frequently than would be expected by chance—the expected prevalence of type 1 diabetes would be 0.4% in adult patients with CF—so patients are not routinely taught to test for ketones.

Hypoglycemia is common in CF even in patients who do not have CFRD. It can be seen on routine OGTT in 13% patients and represents a mismatch between the prompt absorption of an oral glucose solution and delayed first phase insulin secretion in CF.[92] Patients with a hypo OGTT may revert to NGT or progress to diabetes but do not appear to be at an additional risk of progression to diabetes.[69] Patients with reactive hypoglycemia may be symptomatic and need advice on avoidance of hypoglycemia by dietary modification. Fasting hypoglycemia in CF patients without CFRD is less common and may reflect malnutrition, liver disease, or adrenal suppression—particularly related to oral or inhaled steroid use, or the use of azoles.[93]

Hypoglycemia related to treatment with insulin or oral hypoglycemic agents can occur in CFRD as in any patient receiving these therapies. Although CF patients do not have a good glucagon response to hypoglycemia, the catecholamine response is usually retained. Education on prevention and treatment of hypoglycemia is important and regular CBGM to check the matching of insulin supply to demand is necessary. The effect of hypoglycemia on driving and the importance of monitoring glucose before driving should be explained.

Severe hypoglycemia appears to be less common in CFRD than in type 1 diabetes where complete insulin replacement is required from an early stage. Risk factors for severe hypoglycemia (hypoglycemia requiring the assistance of a third party) and hypoglycemia unawareness are duration of diabetes, repeated episodes of asymptomatic hypoglycemia, and the presence of nocturnal hypoglycemia. Patients should be asked about their symptoms of hypoglycemia. Severe hypoglycemia or the loss of awareness of hypoglycemia are diabetic emergencies, can be associated with significant morbidity and mortality, and the report of either should prompt an urgent review of diabetes treatment.

56. Tapp RJ, Tikellis G, Wong TY et al. Longitudinal association of glucose metabolism with retinopathy: Results from the Australian Diabetes Obesity and Lifestyle (AusDiab) study. *Diabetes Care* 2008; **31**(7): 1349–54.

57. Stutchfield PR, O'Halloran S, Teale JD, Isherwood D, Smith CS, Heaf D. Glycosylated haemoglobin and glucose intolerance in cystic fibrosis. *Arch Dis Child* 1987; **62**(8): 805–10.

58. Yung B, Kemp M, Hooper J, Hodson ME. Diagnosis of cystic fibrosis related diabetes: A selective approach in performing the oral glucose tolerance test based on a combination of clinical and biochemical criteria. *Thorax* 1999; **54**(1): 40–3.

59. Elder DA, Wooldridge JL, Dolan LM, D'Alessio DA. Glucose tolerance, insulin secretion, and insulin sensitivity in children and adolescents with cystic fibrosis and no prior history of diabetes. *J Pediatr* 2007; **151**(6): 653–8.

60. Holl RW, Buck C, Babka C, Wolf A, Thon A. HbA(1c) is not recommended as a screening test for diabetes in cystic fibrosis. *Diabetes Care* 2000; **23**(1): 126.

61. Godbout A, Hammana I, Potvin S et al. No relationship between mean plasma glucose and glycated haemoglobin in patients with cystic fibrosis-related diabetes. *Diabetes Metab* 2008; **34**(6): 568–73.

62. Franzese A, Valerio G, Buono P et al. Continuous glucose monitoring system in the screening of early glucose derangements in children and adolescents with cystic fibrosis. *J Pediatr Endocrinol Metab* 2008; **21**(2): 109–16.

63. Solomon MP, Wilson DC, Corey M et al. Glucose intolerance in children with cystic fibrosis. *J Pediatr* 2003; **142**(2): 128–32.

64. Schwarzenberg SJ, Walk D, Thomas W et al. Microvascular complications in cystic fibrosis-related diabetes. *Diabetes Care* 2007; **30**(5): 1056–61.

65. Adler AI, Shine B, Haworth C, Leelarathna L, Bilton D. Hyperglycemia and death in cystic fibrosis-related diabetes. *Diabetes Care* 2011; **34**(7): 1577–8.

66. Schiaffini R, Brufani C, Russo B et al. Abnormal glucose tolerance in children with cystic fibrosis: The predictive role of continuous glucose monitoring system. *Eur J Endocrinol* 2010; **162**(4): 705–10.

67. O'Riordan SM, Hindmarsh P, Hill NR et al. Validation of continuous glucose monitoring in children and adolescents with cystic fibrosis: A prospective cohort study. *Diabetes Care* 2009; **32**(6): 1020–2.

68. Hameed S, Morton JR, Jaffe A et al. Early glucose abnormalities in cystic fibrosis are preceded by poor weight gain. *Diabetes Care* 2010; **33**(2): 221–6.

69. Radike K, Molz K, Holl RW, Poeter B, Hebestreit H, Ballmann M. Prognostic relevance of hypoglycemia following an oral glucose challenge for cystic fibrosis-related diabetes. *Diabetes Care* 2011; **34**(4):e43.

70. Frohnert BI, Ode KL, Moran A et al. Impaired fasting glucose in cystic fibrosis. *Diabetes Care* 2010; **33**(12): 2660–4.

71. Bizzarri C, Lucidi V, Ciampalini P, Bella S, Russo B, Cappa M. Clinical effects of early treatment with insulin glargine in patients with cystic fibrosis and impaired glucose tolerance. *J Endocrinol Invest* 2006; **29**(3): RC1–4.

72. Mozzillo E, Franzese A, Valerio G et al. One-year glargine treatment can improve the course of lung disease in children and adolescents with cystic fibrosis and early glucose derangements. *Pediatric Diabetes* 2009; **10**(3): 162–7.

73. Kolouskova S, Zemkova D, Bartosova J et al. Low-dose insulin therapy in patients with cystic fibrosis and early-stage insulinopenia prevents deterioration of lung function: A 3-year prospective study. *J Pediatr Endocrinol Metab* 2011; **24**(7–8): 449–54.

74. Minicucci L, Haupt M, Casciaro R et al. Slow-release insulin in cystic fibrosis patients with glucose intolerance: A randomized clinical trial. *Pediatr Diabetes* 2012; **13**(2): 197–202.

75. Collins S, Reynolds F. How do adults with cystic fibrosis cope following a diagnosis of diabetes? *J Adv Nurs* 2008; **64**(5): 478–87.

76. Franzese A, Spagnuolo MI, Sepe A, Valerio G, Mozzillo E, Raia V. Can glargine reduce the number of lung infections in patients with cystic fibrosis-related diabetes? *Diabetes Care* 2005; **28**(9): 2333.

77. Rafii M, Chapman K, Stewart C et al. Changes in response to insulin and the effects of varying glucose tolerance on whole-body protein metabolism in patients with cystic fibrosis. *Am J Clin Nutr* 2005; **81**(2): 421–6.

78. Mohan K, Israel KL, Miller H, Grainger R, Ledson MJ, Walshaw MJ. Long-term effect of insulin treatment in cystic fibrosis-related diabetes. *Respiration* 2008; **76**(2): 181–6.

79. Hardin DS, Rice J, Rice M, Rosenblatt R. Use of the insulin pump in treating cystic fibrosis related diabetes. *J Cyst Fibros* 2009; **8**(3): 174–8.

80. Moran A, Pekow P, Grover P et al. Insulin therapy to improve BMI in cystic fibrosis related diabetes without fasting hyperglycemia: Results of the CFRDT trial. *Diabetes Care* 2009; **32**(10): 1783–8.

81. Grover P, Thomas W, Moran A. Glargine versus NPH insulin in cystic fibrosis related diabetes. *J Cyst Fibros* 2008; **7**(2): 134–6.

82. Hardin DS, Leblanc A, Lukenbaugh S, Seilheimer DK. Insulin resistance is associated with decreased clinical status in cystic fibrosis. *J Pediatr* 1997; **130**(6): 948–56.

83. Hardin DS, Rice J, Hale K. Use of the insulin pump to treat CF related diabetes. *Pediatr Pulmonol* 2001; **32**(S22): A483.

84. Moran A, Phillips J, Milla C. Insulin and glucose excursion following premeal insulin lispro or repaglinide in cystic fibrosis-related diabetes. *Diabetes Care* 2001; **24**(10): 1706–10.

85. Onady GM, Langdon LJ. Insulin versus oral agents in the management of cystic fibrosis related diabetes: A case based study. *BMC Endoc Disord* 2006; **6**: 4.

86. Rosenecker J, Eichler I, Barmeier H, der Hardt H. Diabetes mellitus and cystic fibrosis: Comparison of clinical parameters in patients treated with insulin versus oral glucose-lowering agents. *Pediatr Pulmonol* 2001; **32**(5): 351–5.

87. Culler FL, Mckean LP, Buchanan CN, Caplan DB, Meacham LR. Glipizide treatment of patients with cystic-fibrosis and impaired glucose-tolerance. *J Pediatr Gastroenterol Nutr* 1994; **18**(3): 375–8.

88. Bertele-Harms RM, Harms HK. Sulfonylurea (SU) in the treatment of CF related diabetes mellitus (CFDM). A 15 years experience. *Pediatr Pulmonol* 1996; **22**(Suppl 13): 380A.

89. Kentrup H, Bongers H, Spengler M, Kusenbach G, Skopnik H. Efficacy and safety of acarbose in patients with cystic fibrosis and impaired glucose tolerance. *Eur J Pediatr* 1999; **158**(6): 455–9.

90. Ballmann M, Mueller-Brandes C. Longitudinal follow-up of clinical and laboratory data in pediatric patients with cystic fibrosis related diabetes (CFRD) after initial treatment with an oral antidiabetic drug (Glibenclamide). *J Cyst Fibros* 2003; **2**(Suppl 1): S79.

91. de Valk HW, van der Graaf EA. Cystic fibrosis-related diabetes in adults: Where can we go from here? *Rev Diabet Stud* 2007; **4**(1): 6–12.

92. Battezzati A, Battezzati PM, Costantini D et al. Spontaneous hypoglycemia in patients with cystic fibrosis. *Eur J Endocrinol* 2007; **156**(3): 369–76.

93. Gilchrist FJ, Cox KJ, Rowe R et al. Itraconazole and inhaled fluticasone causing hypothalamic-pituitary-adrenal axis suppression in adults with cystic fibrosis. *J Cyst Fibros* 2013; **12**(4): 399–402.

94. van den Berg JM, Morton AM, Kok SW, Pijl H, Conway SP, Heijerman HG. Microvascular complications in patients with cystic fibrosis-related diabetes (CFRD). *J Cyst Fibros* 2008; **7**(6): 515–9.

95. Andersen HU, Lanng S, Pressler T, Laugesen CS, Mathiesen ER. Cystic fibrosis-related diabetes—The presence of microvascular diabetes complications. *Diabetes Care* 2006; **29**(12): 2660–3.

96. Yung B, Landers A, Mathalone B, Gyi KM, Hodson ME. Diabetic retinopathy in adult patients with cystic fibrosis-related diabetes. *Respir Med* 1998; **92**(6): 871–2.

97. Sullivan MM, Denning CR. Diabetic microangiopathy in patients with cystic-fibrosis. *Pediatrics* 1989; **84**(4): 642–7.

98. Dobson L, Stride A, Bingham C, Elworthy S, Sheldon CD, Hattersley AT. Microalbuminuria as a screening tool in cystic fibrosis-related diabetes. *Pediatr Pulmonol* 2005; **39**(2): 103–7.

99. Lind-Ayres M, Thomas W, Holme B, Mauer M, Caramori ML, Moran A. Microalbuminuria in patients with cystic fibrosis. *Diabetes Care* 2011; **34**(7): 1526–8.

100. Yahiaoui Y, Jablonski M, Hubert D et al. Renal involvement in cystic fibrosis: Diseases spectrum and clinical relevance. *Clin J Am Soc Nephrol* 2009; **4**(5): 921–8.

101. Westall GP, Binder J, Kotsimbos T et al. Nodular glomerulosclerosis in cystic fibrosis mimics diabetic nephropathy. *Nephron Clin Pract* 2004; **96**(3): c70–5.

102. Quon BS, Mayer-Hamblett N, Aitken ML, Smyth AR, Goss CH. Risk factors for chronic kidney disease in adults with cystic fibrosis. *Am J Respir Crit Care Med* 2011; **184**(10): 1147–52.

103. Rhodes B, Nash EF, Tullis E et al. Prevalence of dyslipidemia in adults with cystic fibrosis. *J Cyst Fibros* 2010; **9**(1): 24–8.

104. Murphy HR, Roland JM, Skinner TC et al. Effectiveness of a regional prepregnancy care program in women with type 1 and type 2 diabetes: Benefits beyond glycemic control. *Diabetes Care* 2010; **33**(12): 2514–20.

105. Burden C, Ion R, Chung Y, Henry A, Downey DG, Trinder J. Current pregnancy outcomes in women with cystic fibrosis. *Eur J Obstet Gynecol Reprod Biol* 2012; **164**(2): 142–5.

106. McMullen AH, Pasta DJ, Frederick PD et al. Impact of pregnancy on women with cystic fibrosis. *Chest* 2006; **129**(3): 706–11.

107. Odegaard I, Stray-Pedersen B, Hallberg K, Haanaes OC, Storrosten OT, Johannesson M. Maternal and fetal morbidity in pregnancies of Norwegian and Swedish women with cystic fibrosis. *Acta Obstet Gynecol Scand* 2002; **81**(8): 698–705.

108. Hofer M, Schmid C, Benden C et al. Diabetes mellitus and survival in cystic fibrosis patients after lung transplantation. *J Cyst Fibros* 2012; **11**(2): 131–6.

109. Bradbury RA, Shirkhedkar D, Glanville AR, Campbell LV. Prior diabetes mellitus is associated with increased morbidity in cystic fibrosis patients undergoing bilateral lung transplantation: An 'orphan' area? A retrospective case-control study. *Intern Med J* 2009; **39**(6): 384–8. Epub 2009/02/18.

110. Hadjiliadis D, Madill J, Chaparro C et al. Incidence and prevalence of diabetes mellitus in patients with cystic fibrosis undergoing lung transplantation before and after lung transplantation. *Clin Transplant* 2005; **19**(6): 773–8.

111. Fridell JA, Wozniak TC, Reynolds JM et al. Bilateral sequential lung and simultaneous pancreas transplant: A new approach for the recipient with cystic fibrosis. *J Cyst Fibros* 2008; **7**(4): 280–4.

112. Mekeel KL, Langham MR Jr., Gonzalez-Peralta R, Reed A, Hemming AW. Combined en bloc liver pancreas transplantation for children with CF. *Liver Transplant* 2007; **13**(3): 406–9.

25

Growth and puberty

NICOLA BRIDGES

INTRODUCTION

For individuals with cystic fibrosis (CF) or any other life-long chronic disease, normal growth in childhood, pubertal development at a similar age to peers, and achieving an acceptable adult height are important to psychological well-being, integration into society, and employment chances. Because nutrition is a vital part of the management of CF, height and normal growth are also markers of clinical status. The improvements in management of individuals with CF over the decades have resulted in adult height expectations much nearer to the rest of the population. There are multiple factors contributing to the poor growth seen in CF. Length is reduced at birth compared to the rest of the population. Poor nutrition results in impaired growth in infancy, and later on in childhood, inflammation and infection (or the use of steroids) can impair growth hormone (GH) secretion and action. The same factors can result in delayed pubertal development and reduced pubertal growth. The relationship between sex steroids and bone density means that impaired pubertal development can have an effect on bone density. The most obvious treatment for the growth and pubertal issues in CF is to reduce infection and improve nutrition, and better and earlier management has improved height outcome. There is an increasing understanding of the role of insulin deficiency in reducing nutritional status in CF, and insulin replacement has a growth-promoting action. A number of other growth-promoting drugs such as GH have been tried in CF both as a way of improving height, but also for potential benefits to lung function and other clinical markers.

CHANGING HEIGHT OUTCOMES IN CF

For unknown reasons, babies with CF are shorter than average at birth. Several studies have demonstrated reduced birth length in CF; in a group of 139 children with CF,

mean birth length standard deviation score (SDS) was −0.5 (±0.13) in girls and −0.3 (±0.14) in boys, and birth weight SDS was −0.83 (±0.13) in girls and −0.44 (±0.13) in boys.[1] A study in Italy also found that the parents of children with CF were short for the population and target heights for their CF-affected children were shorter than average,[2] although this finding was not reproduced in a study in a US population.[3]

Without newborn screening, most individuals with CF are diagnosed in infancy because of poor linear growth and weight gain, will be shorter and lighter than average at the time of diagnosis, and then are likely to have catch-up growth at the start of treatment.[4] Children with CF have a deficit in height compared with their peers throughout growth, but the difference between children with CF and the normal population has decreased over the years as treatments have improved. In a group of children studied in the 1960s, Sproul et al. report average height between the 3rd and the 10th centile.[5] In a study published in 1993, height and weight for children with CF followed the 25th centile.[1] In a study using the US CF registry for 1993, the mean height and weight percentiles for children with CF were 30th and 20th, respectively; for 15- to 18-year-olds, 19% of boys and 29% of girls had height below the 5th centile.[6] The UK CF registry report for 2010 showed the mean height percentile for children with CF was 41.0 at 2 years of age, falling to 32.2 at 15 years of age, with weight percentile 54.8 at 2 years and 32.5 at 15 years.[7] Haeusler's study in 1994 reports mean adult height in CF on the 25th centile.[1] Reports of more recent cohorts have demonstrated improved adult height but still reduced compared with the unaffected population.[8] The shorter stature of children with CF does not appear to be associated with significant bone age delay; bone age in prepubertal children with CF is no different to the normal population although there is significant bone age delay in adolescents with CF, probably explained by delay of puberty.[9,10]

The introduction of newborn screening has resulted in improved adult height outcomes. Without newborn screening there is a decline in height and weight during the time between birth and diagnosis—in a group diagnosed at mean age of 0.59 years, height SDS at diagnosis was −1.08 (±1.13) and weight SDS −1.60 (±1.35).[11] In a study in New South Wales looking at the height at age 19 years of individuals who were diagnosed by newborn screening, compared with those diagnosed in the 3 years before screening started in 1981, screened individuals were 6.4(±2.05) cm taller and 6.9(±2.2) kg heavier than the unscreened group.[12] The screened group was still shorter and lighter than the unaffected population. A smaller US cohort, diagnosed by newborn screening after 1983 had height and weight centiles that were the same as the unaffected population at age 15 years, compared with unscreened individuals who were on the 20th and 18th centiles for height and weight, respectively.[13] A study using the UK CF registry[4] compared children aged 1–10 years who were diagnosed by neonatal screening (N=162), with clinically diagnosed (404 in an early diagnosed group diagnosed within 2 months of birth, and 542 in a late-diagnosed group, after 2 months of birth). Height SDS scores were −0.41, −0.49 and −0.70 for the newborn screening, early, and late clinical diagnosis groups, respectively, with 25%, 24%, and 40% of individuals with height below the 10th centile. This suggests that earlier diagnosis (and shorter periods of poor nutrition) results in a better height outcome.

FACTORS AFFECTING GROWTH IN CF

Reasons for reduced growth outcomes in CF include poor nutrition, infection and inflammatory factors, and drugs such as steroids. These factors have complex effects on growth, including changes in GH secretion and action. Growth and lung function are interrelated, with poor lung function predicting poor growth. Low weight and height at 3 years of age did not correlate with poor lung function at that age but predicted poor lung function at 6 years of age.[14]

In CF, and in other disorders characterized by long-term inflammation (such as inflammatory bowel disease), a relationship has been demonstrated between inflammatory markers and growth factors and growth rate. Studies have demonstrated reduced insulin-like growth factor 1 (IGF-1) levels in CF.[15,16] A study looking at a pig model of CF demonstrated reduced IGF-1 levels at birth, suggesting that inflammation may not be the only explanation for reduced IGF-1 concentrations.[17] In a study looking at inflammatory markers in CF patients, growth rate correlated positively with IGF-1 levels,[16] and the inflammatory markers tumor necrosis factor or(TNF-α) and interleukin-6 (IL-6) correlated with factors in the IGF-1/IGF-binding protein (IGFBP) system. Studies in children with inflammatory bowel disease have supported a relationship between inflammation and the IGF-1/IGFBP system. There were low IGF-1 levels at diagnosis, and remission after treatment resulted in an increase in IGF-1 levels, increases in IGFBP3

(which is positively correlated with GH), and decreases in IGFBP2 (which is negatively correlated with GH).[18] In inflammatory bowel disease, TNF-α and IL-6 appear to act to reduce IGF-1 production in the liver and it is likely similar effects occur in CF.[19,20]

Reduced insulin secretion is likely to also be a factor in poor growth in children and adolescents with CF. Studies looking at this in CF are limited, but insulin secretion is known to be closely linked to growth in other circumstances. There is increased insulin secretion and insulin resistance during pubertal growth, and low insulin levels or severe insulin resistance can cause stunting in a range of clinical situations (including Mauriac syndrome and insulin receptor defects). Cheung et al. demonstrated reduced height velocity in adolescents in the years before a diagnosis of CF-related diabetes (CFRD), although there was not a significant improvement with treatment with insulin.[21] In a study looking at oral glucose tolerance tests in adolescents with CF, there was a positive correlation between insulin secretion (measured as insulin area under the curve), height velocity, and IGFBP3 levels.[22]

The adverse effect of steroid treatment on growth velocity and on adult height is well documented, although studies looking specifically at CF are limited. Long-term steroid use in a number of clinical settings has been shown to impact on height—the typical pattern of growth is that at the start of treatment there is a significant slowing of growth velocity, then children grow at a normal velocity but do not make up the initial loss. A study of long-term prednisolone treatment in CF demonstrated catch-up growth after treatment stopped, with catch-up growth better in girls than in boys.[23] The effect of steroid treatment may be difficult to separate from the impact of underlying pathology and clinically it may be difficult to determine how much steroids are to blame for growth effects. In inflammatory bowel disease in children and adolescents, studies have shown that height outcome is influenced by disease severity, but not all have shown a clear adverse impact of steroids, with reports of normal growth and final height after long-term steroid treatment at lower doses.[24]

Steroids have effects on the GH/IGF-1 axis at various levels and also a direct effect on the growth plate. Steroid treatment can reduce GH secretion and also result in relative GH resistance with lowering of circulating IGF-1 levels.[25] Steroid treatment causes apoptosis of the proliferative chondrocytes within the growth plate, which then becomes thinner and grows slower as a result.[26] Inhaled as well as systemic steroids have been demonstrated to affect height; in a study comparing continuous inhaled fluticasone with a placebo in children with CF over 2 years, there was a significant fall in height SDS in those receiving fluticasone (change in height SDS of −0.38 (0.09) in the fluticasone group versus −0.01 (0.07) in the placebo group).[27] In a large group of children with asthma given 2 years treatment with budesonide with nedocromil or placebo, the adult height of the steroid-treated children was 1.2 cm lower than the placebo group, and children who received higher steroid doses

46. Alemzadeh R. Anabolic effects of growth hormone treatment in young children with cystic fibrosis. *J Am Coll Nutr* 1998; **17**(5): 419.

47. Hardin DS, Stratton R,Kramer JC, Reyes de la Rocha S, Govaerts K, Wilson DP. Growth hormone improves weight velocity and height velocity in prepubertal children with cystic fibrosis. *Horm Metab Res* 1998; **30**(10): 636–41.

48. Hardin DS, Ellis KJ, Dyson M, Rice J, McConnell R, Seilheimer DK. Growth hormone decreases protein catabolism in children with cystic fibrosis. *J Clin Endocrinol Metab* 2001; **86**(9): 4424–8.

49. Hutler M, Schnabel D, Staab D et al. Effect of growth hormone on exercise tolerance in children with cystic fibrosis. *Med Sci Sports Exerc* 2002; **34**(4): 567.

50. Schibler A, von der Heiden R, Birrer P, Mullis PE. Prospective randomised treatment with recombinant human growth hormone in cystic fibrosis. *Arch Dis Child* 2003; **88**(12): 1078–81.

51. Darmaun D, Hayes V, Schaeffer D, Welch S, Mauras N. Effects of glutamine and recombinant human growth hormone on protein metabolism in prepubertal children with cystic fibrosis. *J Clin Endocrinol Metab* 2004; **89**(3): 1146–52.

52. Hardin DS, Ferkol T, Ahn C et al. A retrospective study of growth hormone use in adolescents with cystic fibrosis. *Clin Endocrinol* 2005; **62**(5): 560.

53. Hardin DS, Ahn C, Prestidge C, Seilheimer DK, Ellis KJ. Growth hormone improves bone mineral content in children with cystic fibrosis. *J Pediatr Endocrinol Metab* 2005; **18**(6): 589.

54. Hardin DS, Adams-Huet B, Brown D et al. Growth hormone treatment improves growth and clinical status in prepubertal children with cystic fibrosis: Results of a multicenter randomized controlled trial. *J Clin Endocrinol Metab* 2006; **91**(12): 4925–9.

55. Schnabel D, Grasemann C, Staab D, Wollmann H, Ratjen F. A multicenter, randomized, double-blind, placebo-controlled trial to evaluate the metabolic and respiratory effects of growth hormone in children with cystic fibrosis. *Pediatrics* 2007; **119**(6): e1230–e8.

56. Schwab J, Kulin HE, Susman EJ et al. The role of sex hormone replacement therapy on self-perceived competence in adolescents with delayed puberty. *Child Develop* 2001; **72**(5): 1439–50.

57. Houchin LD, Rogol AD. Androgen replacement in children with constitutional delay of puberty: The case for aggressive therapy. *Bailliere's Clin Endocrinol Metab* 1998; **12**(3): 427–40.

58. Coste J, Pouchot J, Carel J-C. Height and health-related quality of life: A nationwide population study. *J Clin Endocrinol Metab* 2012; **97**(9): 3231–9.

59. Christensen TL, Djurhuus CB, Clayton P, Christiansen JS. An evaluation of the relationship between adult height and health-related quality of life in the general UK population. *Clin Endocrinol* 2007; **67**(3): 407–12.

60. Sandberg DE, Colsman M. Growth hormone treatment of short stature: Status of the quality of life rationale. *Hormone Res* 2005; **63**(6): 275–83.

26

Bone disease

JENNIFER L. GORALSKI AND ROBERT M. ARIS

INTRODUCTION

Therapeutic advances in cystic fibrosis (CF) have led to substantially improved survival rates, and today a child born with CF can have a reasonable expectation to live into the sixth decade. An ever-increasing survival rate in CF means that formerly underappreciated comorbid conditions, such as osteoporosis, are increasingly recognized, and can cause significant complications. Early attention to bone health can prevent pain, fractures, and increased health-care costs. Reduced bone mineral density (BMD) in CF is common, with some estimates reporting up to 70% adults with osteopenia.[1] A recent pooled meta-analysis of 1055 young adults with cystic fibrosis[2] revealed prevalence rates of 23.5% for osteoporosis and 38% for osteopenia with vertebral fractures present in 14% and nonvertebral fractures present in 20%. According to the Cystic Fibrosis Foundation (CFF) registry, the prevalence of bone disease in CF is approximately 10% in adolescents and 20%–25% in adults, even in the modern day setting of high-fat diets, pancreatic enzyme replacement, and vitamin D supplementation. More severe bone disease correlates with progressive lung disease, and rates of osteoporosis are particularly high in patients undergoing lung transplantation. Osteopenic bone is more likely to fracture; this fracture risk may limit access to organ transplantation, because glucocorticoids not only are a mainstay of posttransplant immunosuppression, but are also strongly correlated with diminished BMD.

The rate of declining BMD in children is much less well defined; however, it has been noted that otherwise well children with CF gain only about half of the BMD compared to healthy peers, measured longitudinally over 1- to 2-year intervals. For example, one longitudinal study of 85 patients with CF aged 5 to 18 years demonstrated a significantly lower gain in total body and lumbar spine BMD over 2 years when compared to controls, even after adjustment for age, sex, and height Z-scores.[3] In addition to a failure to accrue bone mass at the normal rate,[4] adolescents and

adults also lose bone mass at an increased rate as evidenced by year-long studies that showed young adults with CF lost bone mass at a rate approximating that of postmenopausal women.[4]

The etiology of increased risk for decreased BMD in CF is multifactorial and includes nutritional causes, adverse effects of medications, chronic inflammation, low physical activity, and possibly the underlying cystic fibrosis transmembrane conductance regulator (CFTR) mutation, among others (Figure 26.1). Both prophylactic and treatment regimens can reduce the complications of low BMD in CF. Most experts believe that bone disease in CF begins in childhood, and hence attention to this important parameter is best observed by pediatricians.

NORMAL BONE PHYSIOLOGY AND ABNORMAL PHYSIOLOGY IN CYSTIC FIBROSIS

Bone is composed of a highly specialized cell matrix that is made up primarily of osteoblasts, cells responsible for laying down new bone and increasing mineralization, and osteoclasts, which resorb mineralized bone. The bony matrix, or osteoid, is composed of type 1 collagen and noncollagenous proteins, primarily osteocalcin. Calcium and phosphate salts complex to increase the hardness of the bone; the serum levels of these essential minerals are regulated by vitamin D and parathyroid hormone (PTH).[5] Bone mineralization begins before birth and continues throughout childhood and adolescence. Peak acquisition of bone mirrors the adolescent growth spurt, and bone formation exceeds resorption until the time of peak bone mass stage, which occurs sometime between 25 and 30 years old. In general, if vitamin D levels are deficient during rapid skeletal growth as occurs in childhood, the clinical manifestation is of rickets, with cupping and widening of metaphyseal lines; however, this complication rarely occurs in CF even

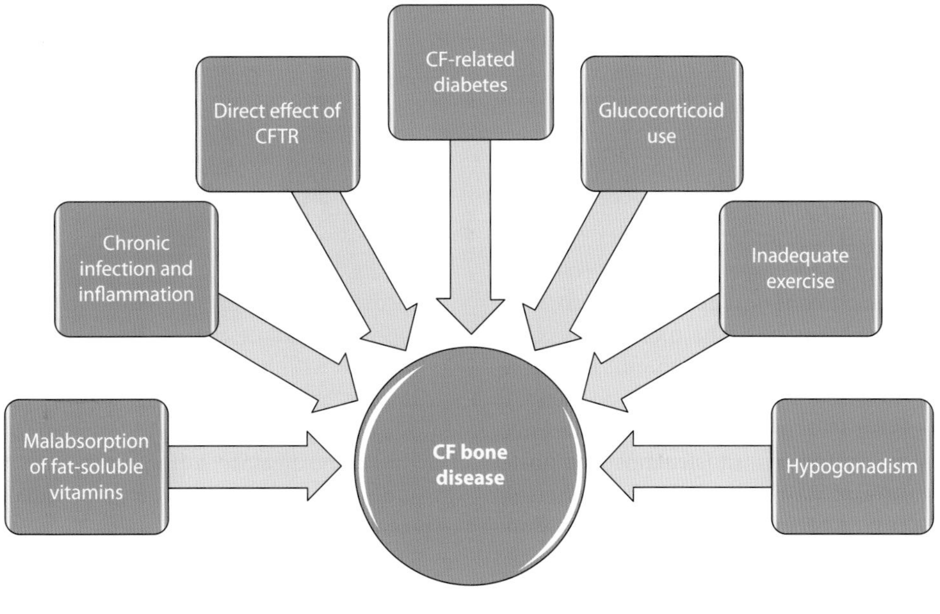

Figure 26.1 CF-specific factors that contribute to early onset of osteopenia in CF adolescents and young adults.

in the presence of vitamin D deficiency. If vitamin D deficiency occurs following the completion of growth or after closure of growth plates, osteopenia and osteomalacia are the norm, as demineralized osteoid replaces mineralized bone during remodeling.[5] Age-related bone loss occurs in both sexes as part of the aging process, where bone resorption exceeds formation.

In CF, studies of bone histology have shown a decrease in both cortical and trabecular bone volume, decrease in osteoblast numbers and function, and increase in osteoclast numbers and activity.[6,7] This confirms that the low BMD found via screening examinations does in fact have a pathologic counterpart. Despite the frequency of vitamin D deficiency in CF, however, osteomalacia has not been shown to be a factor in CF bone disease.[6]

PATHOGENESIS/RISK FACTORS

The underlying pathophysiology of CF bone disease has not been clearly delineated, although many risk factors contribute to disease, as shown in Figure 26.1. There is an apparent increase in bone reabsorption and decrease in mineralized bone deposition.[8] Risk factors are discussed individually below.

MALNUTRITION AND PANCREATIC INSUFFICIENCY

Poor nutrition is common in CF, attributed to pancreatic exocrine insufficiency as well as frequent infections and chronic inflammation leading to a generalized catabolic state. Several studies have documented an association between low BMD and low body mass index (BMI)

in patients with CF.[9–12] This may be particularly important during the time of increased adolescent growth velocity, which is also a time when weight gain may be particularly challenging, especially for adolescent females. BMD values at the hip, spine, and femoral neck have been shown to be associated with suboptimal BMI values.[13]

VITAMIN D DEFICIENCY

The importance of vitamin D in normal bone metabolism cannot be overemphasized. Vitamin D is an essential component of normal bone mineralization and is necessary for intestinal calcium absorption. It is typically synthesized in the skin or absorbed from the diet, two pathways that may be limited in CF. As a fat-soluble vitamin, absorption in pancreatic insufficient CF patients is limited despite supplemental vitamin therapy. Limited body fat may prevent adequate vitamin D stores,[14] although this topic has become somewhat controversial. In addition, there is speculation that CF patients may avoid sun exposure due to photosensitivity that may result from the frequent use of antibiotics, antifungal medication, or drug–drug or drug–vitamin (vitamin A) interactions.[15–17] Thus, vitamin D conversion to the active form may be limited. Annual laboratory determination of the vitamin D level is recommended by all working groups, but the goal level remains somewhat elusive. Although 1,25-dihydroxyvitamin D $(1,25(OH)_2D)$ is the active form, 25-dihydroxyvitamin D $(25(OH)D)$ has a longer half-life and better reflects vitamin D stores. $1,25(OH)_2D$ levels should not be used to routinely screen for vitamin D deficiency, but only used for monitoring in selected conditions, such as genetic or acquired disorders of vitamin D metabolism.[18]

The Institute of Medicine (IOM)–recommended daily intake of vitamin D was set with the assumption of minimal to no sunlight due to individual variations in sun exposure.[19]

In healthy individuals, the 2011 Endocrine Society Clinical Practice Guidelines label vitamin D deficiency as 25(OH)D level less than or equal to 20 ng/mL (50 nmol/L) and insufficiency as a 25(OH)D level of 21–29 ng/mL (52.5–72.5 nmol/L),[18] one of the few societies to specify a "gray zone." The European Guidelines in CF[20] also recommend a minimum 25(OH)D level of 20 ng/mL (50 nmol/L). In contrast, the Endocrine Society of the United States, the Canadian Society of Endocrinology and Metabolism, and the National Osteoporosis Foundation define vitamin D deficiency as 25(OH)D <30 ng/mL (75 nmol/L). The most recent CFF consensus statement[21] recommends a minimum level of 30 ng/mL (75 nmol/L) based on studies largely in non-CF patients, which show that PTH levels begin to increase once 25(OH)D levels drop below 30 ng/mL (75 nmol/L).[21,22] The CFF statement was also endorsed by multiple other societies, including the Endocrine Society of the United States, Cystic Fibrosis Canada, and The Paediatric Endocrine Society so that a maximum consensus could be reached. A recently published study in CF, however, increased the target level to >35 ng/mL (87.5 nmol/L) as this was associated with the lowest percentages of patients with PTH levels >50 pg/mL.[23] Such a wide range of "normal" levels is due in no small part to differences because of latitude, season, outcome measures such as PTH level or fracture, and the multi-compartment model of pharmacokinetics. The steady state of 25(OH)D levels is not reached until several weeks or months after oral dosing. Autumn has been proposed as the optimal time for routine vitamin D assessment, since stores are likely built up during the sunny days of summer and levels are likely reduced during the winter with less solar exposure.

Despite recommendations to target higher vitamin D levels in patients with CF, the unfortunate fact remains that few patients actually achieve and maintain these goals.[21,24,25] In a 2010 study, 97 children with CF received replacement therapy with 50,000 IU of ergocalciferol daily for 4 weeks, but only <25% of the original cohort maintained serum levels >30 ng/mL (75 nmol/L) 6 months after completion of therapy, attesting to the transient nature of the replacement therapy.[26] Thus vitamin D replacement needs to be a maintenance regimen and not a one-time effort. Even though targeting higher vitamin D levels has long been a goal in preventing osteopenia-related fractures, there is actually little available data to correlate BMD with 25(OH)D levels.[13] However, it must be remembered that overall bone density is the product of years of change, whereas serum 25(OH)D levels can rise and fall repeatedly over the course of a year, so this association may be difficult to prove.

VITAMIN K DEFICIENCY

Vitamin K has a direct effect on osteocalcin activity by posttranslational carboxylation of osteocalcin glutamic acid residues, which increases the affinity for hydroxyapatite and the binding of calcium to increase bone density. It is therefore feasible that a deficiency of vitamin K may lead to diminished BMD. Numerous observational studies outside CF have linked low vitamin K levels to fractures and low bone density. Similar to vitamin D, vitamin K is poorly absorbed from the gastrointestinal (GI) tract in CF. In addition, frequent use of antibiotics decreases the native intestinal bacterial flora that is necessary for conversion of the active form of vitamin K. High levels of uncarboxylated osteocalcin have been associated with lower BMD in CF children[27] and may in fact predict BMD better than 25(OH)D levels. Supplementation of vitamin K may play a role in improvement of bone mineralization.[24] In one study, 20 children and adolescents with CF were treated with 10 mg vitamin K weekly in addition to their CF-specific fat-soluble vitamins, and although BMD scores did not change, there was a decrease in serum PTH levels and an increase in bone alkaline phosphatase, serum osteocalcin, and other markers of bone formation, indicating a possible positive effect on bone formation.[28]

CALCIUM DEFICIENCY

Medical and lay literature is replete with advice regarding increasing calcium intake, especially in high-risk groups such as postmenopausal women. However, CF patients may remain deficient in calcium, likely as a combined result from poor intake and decreased absorption from vitamin D deficiency.[29] It is unclear whether or not serum calcium levels actually correlate with BMD at any site, and at least one recent study[13] could not find an association of low serum calcium levels with reduced BMD in 55 CF patients. Regardless, guidelines for healthy adolescents and young adults recommend intake of at least 1200 mg of calcium daily, therefore CF patients should not be regarded differently.[21]

CHRONIC INFECTION, INFLAMMATION, AND LUNG DISEASE

The interplay of multiple factors, including chronic infection resulting in a heightened inflammatory state, is associated with diminished bone density. Markers of bone resorption are elevated in CF during pulmonary exacerbations, and levels fall again after treatment and resolution of pulmonary infection.[30] A study of 24 patients before, during, and after an exacerbation showed an increase in number of osteoclastic cells as measured by tartrate-resistant acid phosphatase (TRAP) stain, with a significant decrease back to baseline following antibiotic therapy.[31] The same study and others document increases in biochemical markers of bone turnover, including TNF-α, IL-6, serum type-I collagen cross-linked N-telopeptide (NTx), and receptor activator of NF-κB ligand (RANKL),[31,32] which are associated with increased bone reabsorption and decreased mineralization; however other studies have not found such an association between markers of inflammation and BMD in CF.[11,13] Chronic inflammation has been increasingly implicated as a factor in CF and worsening lung disease. FEV$_1$ percent predicted correlated strongly with BMD measured at total hip, spine, and femoral neck[13,33] when patients with severe lung disease (FEV1 <40% predicted) and those with mild lung disease (FEV1 >60% predicted) were compared. As noted previously, patients awaiting lung transplantation commonly have low BMD and increased risk of fractures.[34]

DIRECT ROLE OF CYSTIC FIBROSIS TRANSMEMBRANE CONDUCTANCE REGULATOR IN BONE

Recent studies have suggested that CFTR may directly affect bone formation; CFTR has been localized to both osteoclasts and osteoblasts,[35] although its role in this tissue is not entirely clear. Identifying which patients might be at risk for diminished BMD may be possible by examining the genotype as an independent risk factor of diminished BMD. In a study of 88 patients with CF, including 39 homozygous for the *F508del* and 36 heterozygotes, even one copy of the F508 deletion independently predicted lower BMD as evidenced by spine and femoral neck Z-scores.[36] Animal models have also been studied to understand the genetic relationship to BMD. Mice deficient in CFTR had cortical thinning and altered trabecular architecture despite no other overt signs of CF[37] and had less cortical bone even in the absence of overt nutritional deficiency compared to wild type.[38] In another study, F508del/F508del mice underwent bone densitometry and were compared to control wild type mice at 6, 10, and 14 weeks of age. CF homozygotes demonstrated reduced BMD, lower femoral bone mass, and altered trabecular bone architecture as well as a decrease in new bone formation compared to wild type.[39] A potential mechanism for this is suggested by the altered relationship between osteoprotegerin and prostaglandin (PG) E2, driven by loss or reduction in functional CFTR. The imbalance of these factors (a reduction in osteoprotegerin and increase in PGE2) promotes inflammation-driven bone reabsorption in human bone cell culture lines.[35,40] Osteoprotegerin is a protein produced by osteoblasts that decreases osteoclast-mediated bone reabsorption while increasing alkaline phosphatase activity and mineralization.[41] In a brief report of a single CF patient (genotype F508del/G542X), ankle bone fragments were collected and compared to non-CF; osteoblastic production of osteoprotegerin was reduced to 8%–10% of that produced by normal bone cells, even when stimulated with TNFα.[42]

CYSTIC FIBROSIS-RELATED DIABETES

Non-CF patients with type 1 diabetes have been proven to have diminished bone formation and mineralization with low levels of insulin leading to impaired bone health.[43,44] Abnormalities in glucose and insulin regulation resulting from CF-related diabetes (CFRD) therefore may affect bone health as well. A recent study showed a correlation between dysglycemia (either CFRD or impaired glucose tolerance) and low BMD.[45]

GLUCOCORTICOID USE

Exogenous glucocorticoid therapy has been shown to decrease bone formation and increase bone breakdown by a variety of mechanisms, including decreasing osteoblast activity, suppressing insulin-like growth factor secretion, decreasing intestinal calcium absorption and renal tubular reabsorption, and decreasing sex hormone production.[46] Steroids tend to have the greatest effect on sites with high trabecular bone (vertebrae and ribs) as opposed to those that have more cortical bone, such as long bones.[46] Increased steroid use in CF is associated with lower BMD over a year of treatment.[4,10] The cumulative use of glucocorticoids has been shown to be a predictor for low BMD in patients awaiting lung transplantation.[34] A difficult confounder is that glucocorticoids are often administered to the sickest CF patients, and so the effect of glucocorticoids on BMD may be influenced by the presence of severe lung disease and malnutrition.

EXERCISE

The benefits of weight-bearing and aerobic exercise in non-CF populations have long been clearly established,[47-49] and similarly, complete immobilization leads to increased bone resorption in the general population.[50] In CF, a routine exercise program is crucial for several reasons, including the potential partial blockade of an overactive epithelial sodium channel that contributes to dehydrated airways and chronic lung disease.[51,52] Several studies have correlated increasing physical activity with increased BMD[53] and in a study of 67 adult CF patients, VO$_2$max predicted BMD. Again, it is difficult to determine if there is selection bias in that the healthiest patients have the best exercise tolerance as well as the highest BMD.[54] In a cross-sectional study with the use of daily portable monitoring devices,[33] routine and regular exercise was associated with increased BMD in CF. The authors also noted that incremental increase of physical activity (as measured by metabolically equivalent tasks [METs]) were strongly correlated with increasing VO$_2$max on exercise studies, and %VO$_2$max was significantly associated with BMD. In another study, grip strength (a marker of muscle mass) and 6-minute walking distance correlated with BMD.[13] Interestingly, however, the authors could not find an association with presence of vertebral fracture and BMD. In addition to direct effects, exercise may mitigate the effects of other risk factors, including diabetes, lung function, overall quality of life, and increasing lean body mass.[55] Despite general acceptance that weight-bearing exercise in particular provides bone health benefits to patients with CF,[56] a systematic review[57] has been unable to clearly document data that support this outcome.

LIGHT EXPOSURE

It is unknown if patients with CF routinely avoid sun exposure, however, anecdotal evidence suggests that this may play a role, as noted above. Drugs, drug–drug interactions, or drug–vitamin interactions can all result in photosensitivity, which may lead CF individuals to avoid direct sunlight. However, skin synthesis of vitamin D during light exposure may be the easiest way for CF patients to supplement vitamin D. Recommendations for routine sun exposure need to be weighed against the potential phototoxicity of many commonly used antibiotics and the rare but real risk of skin cancer with cumulative exposure over a lifetime.

DELAYED PUBERTY AND SEX-STEROID DEFICIENCY

Adolescents with CF may enter puberty late, usually as a consequence of malnutrition. Delayed puberty can result in delayed achievement of peak bone mass, and hypogonadism in adults is likely under-recognized and may result in "old bones in young bodies."[58] Low free testosterone levels in CF adults have been correlated to low BMD[10] and to increased vertebral fractures in men.[59] Another study of 191 CF adults found low serum estradiol levels in a quarter of patients (both men and women), which was significantly associated with femur BMD in both sexes.[59] Testosterone may be administered to men with delayed pubertal growth, but it should not be given too early due to the consequence of premature epiphyseal closure. Estrogen therapy may be used for women.

BONE MINERAL DENSITY AND MEASUREMENTS

Poor bone mineralization in CF may be the result of (1) decreased substrate to lay down new bone, such as that which is suspected in vitamin deficiency; (2) increased bone reabsorption; or (3) diminished mineralization. BMD is the amount of mineralization in a certain area or volume of bone. This is most commonly assessed and compared to gender-matched controls using dual-energy x-ray absorptiometry (DXA), which measures bone mineral content at predetermined sites (usually femur and spine) and calculates a value for areal BMD (g/cm^2). In children, the spine and total body (excepting the head) are the more common sites of assessment.[60] This is typically compared to a population mean, either as Z-scores, which compare an individual to age- and sex-matched data, or T-scores (a standard deviation score comparing the BMD of the individual to the measurement of a healthy young gender-matched adult, usually aged 25–30 years). In adults, osteopenia is diagnosed when a T-score is –1 to –2.5. Osteoporosis exists when the T-score is –2.5 or lower. In children, this distinction is less clear, and the diagnosis is made when BMD is low for age and is accompanied by a history of bone fractures.[61]

SCREENING

Regular screening of at-risk patient populations is recommended to detect early disease and to monitor effects of therapy. Simple measurements of the anterior and posterior

vertebral heights on a lateral chest x-ray can clue a clinician to the loss of vertebral height often seen in osteoporosis (Figure 26.2). Although the indication for the chest film is usually to evaluate a pulmonary process, and hence, bony abnormalities may be overlooked by the radiologist, the lateral chest x-ray can provide important details about osteopenia of an individual's spine.

Current guidelines suggest screening of all adults and children above age 8 who exhibit other risk factors for low BMD, including low lung function, frequent use of steroids, low body weight, hypogonadism, or personal history of fracture.[20,21] Z-scoring should be used in children and adolescents and T scoring in adults.

DXA is the most common objective measurement of BMD. However, unlike in most scenarios where BMD is a good predictor of fracture, there is little evidence in CF that low BMD corresponds to fracture rate and complications of osteoporosis.[61,62] The reasons for this remain unclear, but may be related to poor bone quality instead of only loss of absolute bone mass. Quality of bone mineralization is difficult to evaluate with current screening measures. DXA itself has some variability in interpretation, compounded by the delayed puberty and small stature that is common among adolescents with CF. Therefore, adjustments for height, BMI, or bone age are generally necessary to correctly interpret studies and these are difficult to perform outside a research setting.[63] The recommendations for regular DXA scans to screen for BMD loss has also been called into question because of cross-sectional studies that show no correlation between screening and rates of vertebral or rib fractures.[62,64] Even more of a question exists in pediatrics, where there is scant data on the relationship between

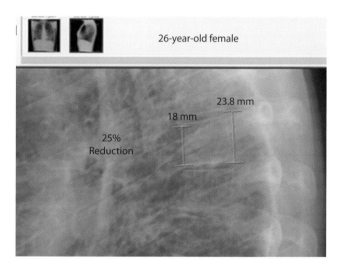

Figure 26.2 Loss of anterior vertebral height as measured on a lateral chest x-ray provides supporting evidence for osteoporosis in a CF individual. The definition of a vertebral compression fracture is >20% reduction in the anterior height of a vertebral body compared to the posterior height. Although radiologists may not always comment about fractures when interpreting lateral chest films, measuring rulers and magnifiers in imaging software packages allow for easy calculations.

pediatric fractures and BMD. Quantitative ultrasonography bone sonometry (QUS) offers an attractive alternative. This nonradiating technique, which measures sound progression through bone, and thus, bone quality, allows for portable assessment of bone density. Nonetheless, this modality has yet to be well validated either within or outside CF. The measurement of an individual's bone loss over time, rather than comparison to age-matched controls, may be a better predictor of fracture risk than a single isolated screening study.[25]

FRACTURES AND CHEST WALL DEFORMITIES

An increased fracture incidence has been noted in adults with very advanced CF, with vertebral rates more than 10 times the general population and rib fractures almost 100 times higher.[65] A meta-analysis revealed a pooled prevalence of radiologically proven vertebral fractures in 14% CF young adults, and nonvertebral fractures were present in 19.7%.[2] Patients seeking lung transplantation are at increased risk, both pre- and posttransplantation, with fracture rates posttransplant exceeding 25%.[34] Rib fractures clearly play an important role in CF, as pain induced by rib fracture may limit the person's tolerance of airway clearance maneuvers. Rib fractures have been documented in up to 15% patients.[34] Indeed, excessive coughing itself has been shown to cause rib fractures, most commonly in women with underlying osteopenia or osteoporosis.[66] Chronic effects of osteopenia include kyphoscoliosis and chest wall

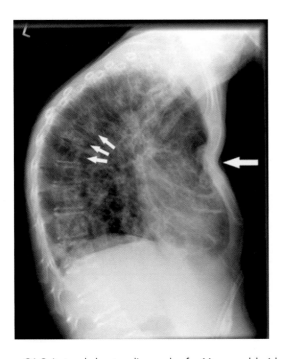

Figure 26.3 Lateral chest radiograph of a 16-year-old girl with cystic fibrosis and severe lung disease and osteoporotic fractures of the sternum (large arrow) and the vertebral bodies of B6 and B7 (small arrows). (Reproduced from Latzin, P., Griese, M., Hermanns, V., Krammer, B, *Thorax* 2005; 60: 616. With permission from BMJ Publishing Group Ltd.)

deformities (Figure 26.3), which may further impair lung function.[14,21] Interestingly, BMD does not always correlate with fracture rate as discussed above.[67,68] In a cross-sectional study of 55 adult CF patients, among 20 patients with a documented history of fractures, 25% had normal T-scores at the hip, spine, and femoral neck.[13] BMD also did not correlate with having exocrine pancreatic insufficiency or diabetes mellitus in that study.

BIOCHEMICAL MARKERS

People with CF typically demonstrate higher rates of bone turnover and lower markers of bone formation such as osteocalcin and bone alkaline phosphatase compared to controls.[21,69] Elevations in markers of bone reabsorption have also been noted, including urinary hydroxyproline and urinary *N*-telopeptide,[10,21] but to date no role exists for the measurement of these values outside the research arena.

MANAGEMENT

The goal of management of diminished BMD in CF is to prevent painful fractures and the resultant comorbidities that may result, such as worsening lung function. Although no proven association between BMD and fractures has been seen in the few CF studies published, the association is so strong outside CF that it still guides treatment principles (Figure 26.4). Ideally, prevention begins in childhood, with focus on adequate nutrition, maintenance of lung function, encouragement of regular exercise, and vitamin supplementation. Screening for low BMD should occur in all adults, and in children who demonstrate the risk factors previously discussed. If a baseline DEXA shows a T-score of <–1.0, then nutrition should be emphasized, including adequate intake of calcium, vitamin D, and vitamin K, along with targeting BMI >25th percentile, encouraging physical activity, and screening for CFRD. DEXA should be repeated every 5 years.[21] For those with an initial T-score of between –1.0 and –2.5, more aggressive treatment is recommended, including actively evaluating for pulmonary infections and screening for CFRD. An endocrine referral should be considered, and the nutritional supplementation discussed above should also be implemented. Even if the T/Z score is higher than –2.5, if fragility fractures (fractures without significant associated trauma as well as virtually all vertebral fractures) have occurred, bone loss is at a rate of greater than 3%–5%/year, or the patient is awaiting lung transplant, bisphosphonate therapy should be strongly considered and DEXA should be repeated in 2–3 years. Finally, if the initial T-score is <–2.5, these individuals require close attention to prevent morbidity and mortality. In addition to all the other measures recommended for patients with higher bone density, the patients in this group should begin therapy with bisphosphonates (oral or IV), and repeated screening with DEXA should be performed on an annual basis.[21] T-scores

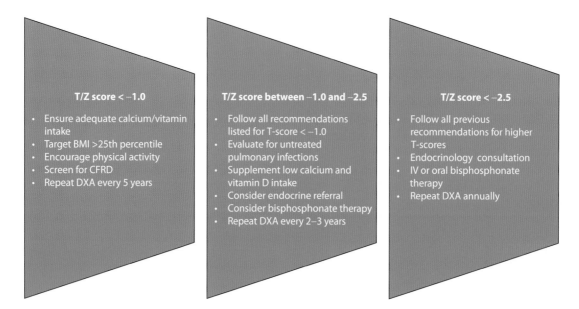

T/Z score < −1.0

- Ensure adequate calcium/vitamin intake
- Target BMI >25th percentile
- Encourage physical activity
- Screen for CFRD
- Repeat DXA every 5 years

T/Z score between −1.0 and −2.5

- Follow all recommendations listed for T-score < −1.0
- Evaluate for untreated pulmonary infections
- Supplement low calcium and vitamin D intake
- Consider endocrine referral
- Consider bisphosphonate therapy
- Repeat DXA every 2–3 years

T/Z score < −2.5

- Follow all previous recommendations for higher T-scores
- Endocrinology consultation
- IV or oral bisphosphonate therapy
- Repeat DXA annually

Figure 26.4 Metric for recommendations for individual T-scores at initial DEXA screening. While T-scores can be used for adults older than 25 years, children under the age of 18 should be addressed using Z-scores as T-scores have not been defined for this age group. Either score may be used for young adults (ages 18–25).

may lead to an over diagnosis of low BMD in children, since pediatric patients being screened may not have yet achieved peak bone mass. Therefore, use of the Z-score, comparing children to age-matched controls, is more appropriate.[21]

VITAMIN D REPLACEMENT/CALCIUM SUPPLEMENTATION

Annual measurement of serum concentration of 25(OH)D is recommended, generally in the late fall or early winter when cutaneous synthesis is low. Target levels are discussed above and are displayed in Figure 26.5. Most recent guidelines suggest supplementation with cholecalciferol (vitamin D_3) over ergocalciferol (D_2),[70] mainly due to a robust literature in non-CF patients, as well as a small study in CF patients that showed vitamin D_3 improved 25(OH)D levels greater than vitamin D_2 over a 12-week period. CF-specific vitamin supplementations generally contain the suggested amount of 800 IU of ergocalciferol daily for adults and 400 IU daily for infants. If serum concentrations of 25(OH)D levels are low, addition of extra cholecalciferol or ergocalciferol is recommended to achieve and maintain target levels. D_3 is available for purchase without a prescription in many nutrition and grocery stores. Calcitriol has also been used to increase fractional absorption of calcium and lower PTH levels in both CF and control populations, and additionally has been shown to suppress bone reabsorption in CF patients, as evidenced by measurement of urinary NTx levels.[71] Nonetheless, calcitriol is usually reserved for patients with renal failure or those who fail conventional supplementation.

Despite national and international guidelines recommending supplementation of vitamin D to various goal levels, data on outcomes with this approach remain sparse,

and the best vitamin D preparation and dosing regimen is unknown. A recent Cochrane review of three included studies to summarize the effects of vitamin D supplementation on adults and children with CF in reducing fracture risk and improving general and respiratory outcomes was inconclusive, citing a lack of published data on which to draw conclusions.[72] The authors also note that the pubertal stage, ethnicity, season, geography, severity of illness, and pancreatic enzyme replacement should be considered as potential confounders in any study that involves vitamin D supplementation. Lack of proof showing fracture reduction should not slow efforts to improve supplementation because vitamin D is inexpensive, safe in appropriate doses, and may improve non-bone endpoints such as systemic inflammation and even reduce pulmonary exacerbations.[70] If standard supplementation fails to improve low 25(OH)D levels, aggressive repletion is recommended.[21] The Consensus Conference recommends treating with 50,000 IU of ergocalciferol weekly for 8 weeks, followed by 50,000 IU twice weekly for 8 weeks if necessary for replacement.

VITAMIN K SUPPLEMENTATION

As vitamin K has a direct effect on bone mineralization and is known to be deficient in many people with CF, clinicians should strive for maintenance of normal vitamin K levels. Practically speaking, this is most commonly assessed by the detection of a prolonged prothrombin time (PT), although a high normal PT likely reflects vitamin K deficiency[73] in CF. Direct measurement of under-carboxylated prothrombin (PIVKA-II) is a sensitive marker of subclinical vitamin K deficiency and can be detected in serum earlier than changes in coagulation

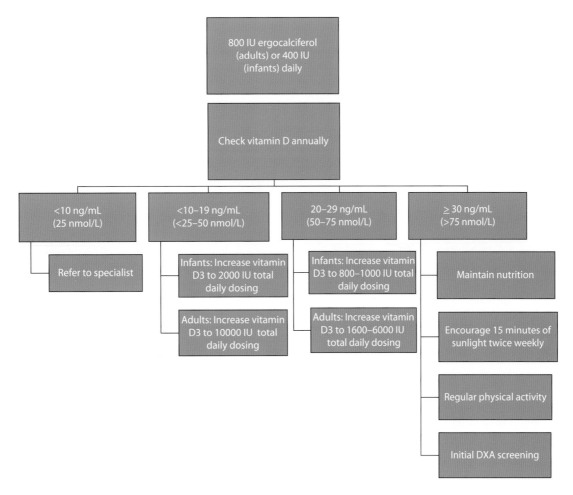

Figure 26.5 Summary of recommendations for supplementation of vitamin D at varying 25-OHD levels. 1 ng/mL is equivalent to 2.5 nmol/L.

factors, but this test is not available in many clinical laboratories and thus has limited utility for detection of vitamin K deficiency in the CF population. CF-specific fat-soluble vitamin supplements do contain vitamin K, but it is important to remember that this may need to be further accompanied by increased doses of vitamin K at baseline and more so during pulmonary exacerbations treated with antibiotics. As suggested in the study by Nicolaidou et al.,[28] 10 mg of supplemental vitamin K weekly may be a necessary supplement for children with CF.

EXERCISE

The evidence is robust that patients who are the most physically active have the greatest bone mass. Conversely, patients with the most pulmonary involvement, most sedentary lifestyle, and least aerobic capacity are the most likely to suffer from effects of diminished BMD, including fractures and kyphosis.[33] Regular weight-bearing exercise, especially if performed outside with sun exposure, is an important part of generalized bone health in all CF patients.

BISPHOSPHONATES

Bisphosphonates work by selectively inhibiting osteoclasts and thus slowing the rate of bone resorption; they have been shown to increase BMD and decrease fracture rate in postmenopausal women, men with osteoporosis, and in patients receiving long-term corticosteroids. Advances in pharmacologic therapy, including side-chain substitutions, are responsible for the different antiresorptive capacities of the various drugs. The IV preparation may be superior because of concerns over absorption in CF as well as the tendency for oral formulations to cause pill esophagitis. A common side effect of bisphosphonate therapy in CF is severe bone pain, although this can be somewhat ameliorated with the pretreatment with corticosteroids. In addition, bisphosphonates do cross the placental barrier and thus contraceptive use is recommended for all women.

Several studies have examined the effects of bisphosphonate therapy in CF patients with osteopenia and osteoporosis. A randomized, double-blind, placebo-controlled trial of 10 mg alendronate daily showed significant improvements in BMD of the spine and femur in 1 year.[74]

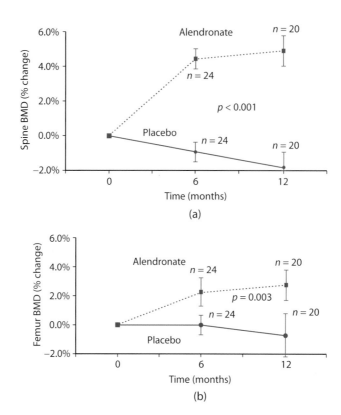

Figure 26.6 Mean ±SE change in *A* spine and *B* femur bone mineral density (BMD) (expressed as a percent of baseline) over time in subjects on alendronate plus calcium and vitamin D (dashed line) compared with placebo and calcium and vitamin D (solid line), demonstrating significantly greater improvements at the spine (*p* < .001) and femur (*p* = .003) with alendronate. (Reprinted with permission of the American Thoracic Society, Copyright 2013; Aris RM et al., *Am J Respir Crit Care Med*, 162(3 Pt 1), 941–6, 2000.)

(Figure 26.6) A Cochran review[75] of six published studies of non-transplanted CF patients concluded that while there was no change in fracture rate in 203 adult CF patients receiving bisphosphonates, there was a significantly increased gain in BMD in the spine and hip at 6, 12, and 24 months. Bone pain and flu-like symptoms were common among recipients. In one study evaluating post–lung transplant CF patients, IV pamidronate did not change the number of new fractures, despite increasing BMD at the femur and spine.[76] Notably, no patients in the posttransplant series exhibited bone pain, lending credence to the theory that corticosteroids may be helpful in reducing this complication. Larger studies are likely necessary to ascertain a true reduction in fracture rate because these previous trials were sized for BMD endpoints, not fracture assessment. The choice of bisphosphonate is not clear either, and most clinicians will initiate oral therapy and reserve IV therapy for those whose bone demineralization continue to worsen with an oral preparation.

Bisphosphonate therapy, while more controversial in children, is now routinely safely used in disorders such as osteogenesis imperfecta and cerebral palsy. To date, only one small study has looked at bisphosphonate use in CF children with persistent osteoporosis despite adequate replacement therapy with calcium and vitamin D. This study[77] showed bisphosphonates were well tolerated and significantly improved both total body and lumbar spine Z-scores. These very limited data underscore the urgent need for randomized controlled clinical trials in the pediatric CF population.

GROWTH HORMONE

A small amount of positive data exists to recommend growth hormone (GH) supplementation for prepubertal children with CF. Sixty-one children who were <25th percentile for height were treated with GH for 1 year and demonstrated a significant increase in bone mineral content. A crossover design then allowed the authors to conclude that there was ongoing bone mass accrual in the following year after cessation of GH therapy.[78] The same authors showed improvement in bone mineral content in children who were <10th percentile for height at the time of GH treatment.[79] The benefits of GH may extend beyond improvement in bone mineralization, including positive effects on weight, lean body mass, and possibly pulmonary function.[78] Should treatment with GH be considered, endocrine consultation should be sought so as to avoid potential complications such as premature closure of the epiphyseal plates.

PARATHYROID HORMONE

Teriparatide (recombinant human PTH) may prove to be a superior antiresorptive agent in people with CF, as it has been proven in those with glucocorticoid-associated osteoporosis.[80] Although this agent may offer a new avenue for treatment of CF-associated bone disease, to date there have been no randomized controlled clinical trials.

SEX STEROID REPLACEMENT THERAPY

As noted above, sex steroid replacement may help improve BMD in patients with documented hypogonadism. Routine assessment of Tanner staging in pubertal children should be performed, with consideration of referral to an endocrinologist if delayed puberty is noted. Studies have yet to be done to analyze the effects of replacement estrogen or testosterone on BMD in pubertal-delayed children.

CONCLUSIONS

CF-related bone disease is increasingly common in both the pediatric and adult CF populations, worsening with age and with advanced lung disease. As the life expectancy increases in CF patients, the prevalence of this disorder is likely to continue to increase as well. Close attention to this complication is recommended to prevent morbidity in CF. Supplementation of fat-soluble vitamins and essential minerals, encouraging physical activity, monitoring progression of puberty, and initiating therapy with antiresorptive agents may be necessary to retard deterioration of BMD. Routine screening is essentially to identify at-risk individuals prior to the occurrence of a fragility fracture.

REFERENCES

1. Doring G, Conway SP. Osteoporosis in cystic fibrosis. *J Pediatr (Rio J)* 2008; **84**(1): 1–3.
2. Paccou J, Zeboulon N, Combescure C, Gossec L, Cortet B. The prevalence of osteoporosis, osteopenia, and fractures among adults with cystic fibrosis: A systematic literature review with meta-analysis. *Calcif Tissue Int* 2010; **86**(1): 1–7.
3. Buntain HM, Schluter PJ, Bell SC et al. Controlled longitudinal study of bone mass accrual in children and adolescents with cystic fibrosis. *Thorax* 2006; **61**(2): 146–54.
4. Haworth CS, Selby PL, Horrocks AW, Mawer EB, Adams JE, Webb AK. A prospective study of change in bone mineral density over one year in adults with cystic fibrosis. *Thorax* 2002; **57**(8): 719–23.
5. Holick MF. Vitamin D deficiency. *N Engl J Med* 2007; **357**(3): 266–81.
6. Haworth CS, Webb AK, Egan JJ et al. Bone histomorphometry in adult patients with cystic fibrosis. *Chest* 2000; **118**(2): 434–9.
7. Elkin SL, Vedi S, Bord S, Garrahan NJ, Hodson ME, Compston JE. Histomorphometric analysis of bone biopsies from the iliac crest of adults with cystic fibrosis. *Am J Respir Crit Care Med* 2002; **166**(11): 1470–4.
8. Boyle MP. Update on maintaining bone health in cystic fibrosis. *Curr Opin Pulm Med* 2006; **12**(6): 453–8.
9. Grey AB, Ames RW, Matthews RD, Reid IR. Bone mineral density and body composition in adult patients with cystic fibrosis. *Thorax* 1993; **48**(6): 589–93.
10. Elkin SL, Fairney A, Burnett S et al. Vertebral deformities and low bone mineral density in adults with cystic fibrosis: A cross-sectional study. *Osteoporos Int* 2001; **12**(5): 366–72.
11. Haworth CS, Selby PL, Webb AK et al. Low bone mineral density in adults with cystic fibrosis. *Thorax* 1999; **54**(11): 961–7.
12. Gibbens DT, Gilsanz V, Boechat MI, Dufer D, Carlson ME, Wang CI. Osteoporosis in cystic fibrosis. *J Pediatr* 1988; **113**(2): 295–300.
13. Legroux-Gerot I, Leroy S, Prudhomme C et al. Bone loss in adults with cystic fibrosis: Prevalence, associated factors, and usefulness of biological markers. *Joint Bone Spine* 2012; **79**(1): 73–7.
14. Gore AP, Kwon SH, Stenbit AE. A roadmap to the brittle bones of cystic fibrosis. *J Osteoporos* 2010; **2011**: 926045.
15. Cheng MP, Paquette K, Lands LC, Ovetchkine P, Theoret Y, Quach C. Voriconazole inhibition of vitamin A metabolism: Are adverse events increased in cystic fibrosis patients? *Pediatr Pulmonol* 2010; **45**(7): 661–6.
16. Markantonis SL, Katelari A, Pappa E, Doudounakis S. Voriconazole pharmacokinetics and photosensitivity in children with cystic fibrosis. *J Cyst Fibros* 2012; **11**(3): 246–52.
17. Burdge DR, Nakielna EM, Rabin HR. Photosensitivity associated with ciprofloxacin use in adult patients with cystic fibrosis. *Antimicrob Agents Chemother* 1995; **39**(3): 793.
18. Holick MF, Binkley NC, Bischoff-Ferrari HA et al. Evaluation, treatment, and prevention of vitamin D deficiency: An Endocrine Society clinical practice guideline. *J Clin Endocrinol Metab* 2011; **96**(7): 1911–30.
19. Aloia JF. Clinical Review: The 2011 report on dietary reference intake for vitamin D: Where do we go from here? *J Clin Endocrinol Metab* 2011; **96**(10): 2987–96.
20. Sermet-Gaudelus I, Bianchi ML, Garabedian M et al. European cystic fibrosis bone mineralisation guidelines. *J Cyst Fibros* 2011; **10**(Suppl 2): S16–23.
21. Aris RM, Merkel PA, Bachrach LK et al. Guide to bone health and disease in cystic fibrosis. *J Clin Endocrinol Metab* 2005; **90**(3): 1888–96.

22. Holick MF, Siris ES, Binkley N et al. Prevalence of vitamin D inadequacy among postmenopausal North American women receiving osteoporosis therapy. *J Clin Endocrinol Metab* 2005; **90**(6): 3215–24.

23. West NE, Lechtzin N, Merlo CA et al. Appropriate goal level for 25-hydroxyvitamin D in cystic fibrosis. *Chest* 2011; **140**(2): 469–74.

24. Grey V, Atkinson S, Drury D et al. Prevalence of low bone mass and deficiencies of vitamins D and K in pediatric patients with cystic fibrosis from 3 Canadian centers. *Pediatrics* 2008; **122**(5): 1014–20.

25. Donovan DS Jr., Papadopoulos A, Staron RB et al. Bone mass and vitamin D deficiency in adults with advanced cystic fibrosis lung disease. *Am J Respir Crit Care Med* 1998; **157**(6 Pt 1): 1892–9.

26. Green DM, Leonard AR, Paranjape SM, Rosenstein BJ, Zeitlin PL, Mogayzel PJ Jr. Transient effectiveness of vitamin D_2 therapy in pediatric cystic fibrosis patients. *J Cyst Fibros* 2010; **9**(2): 143–9.

27. Fewtrell MS, Benden C, Williams JE et al. Undercarboxylated osteocalcin and bone mass in 8-12 year old children with cystic fibrosis. *J Cyst Fibros* 2008; **7**(4): 307–12.

28. Nicolaidou P, Stavrinadis I, Loukou I et al. The effect of vitamin K supplementation on biochemical markers of bone formation in children and adolescents with cystic fibrosis. *Eur J Pediatr* 2006; **165**(8): 540–5.

29. Aris RM, Lester GE, Dingman S, Ontjes DA. Altered calcium homeostasis in adults with cystic fibrosis. *Osteoporos Int* 1999; **10**(2): 102–8.

30. Aris RM, Stephens AR, Ontjes DA et al. Adverse alterations in bone metabolism are associated with lung infection in adults with cystic fibrosis. *Am J Respir Crit Care Med* 2000; **162**(5): 1674–8.

31. Shead EF, Haworth CS, Barker H, Bilton D, Compston JE. Osteoclast function, bone turnover and inflammatory cytokines during infective exacerbations of cystic fibrosis. *J Cyst Fibros* 2010; **9**(2): 93–8.

32. Manolagas SC. The role of IL-6 type cytokines and their receptors in bone. *Ann N Y Acad Sci* 1998; **840**: 194–204.

33. Tejero Garcia S, Giraldez Sanchez MA, Cejudo P et al. Bone health, daily physical activity, and exercise tolerance in patients with cystic fibrosis. *Chest* 2011; **140**(2): 475–81.

34. Aris RM, Neuringer IP, Weiner MA, Egan TM, Ontjes D. Severe osteoporosis before and after lung transplantation. *Chest* 1996; **109**(5): 1176–83.

35. Shead EF, Haworth CS, Condliffe AM, McKeon DJ, Scott MA, Compston JE. Cystic fibrosis transmembrane conductance regulator (CFTR) is expressed in human bone. *Thorax* 2007; **62**(7): 650–1.

36. King SJ, Topliss DJ, Kotsimbos T et al. Reduced bone density in cystic fibrosis: DeltaF508 mutation is an independent risk factor. *Eur Respir J* 2005; **25**(1): 54–61.

37. Haston CK, Li W, Li A, Lafleur M, Henderson JE. Persistent osteopenia in adult cystic fibrosis transmembrane conductance regulator-deficient mice. *Am J Respir Crit Care Med* 2008; **177**(3): 309–15.

38. Dif F, Marty C, Baudoin C, de Vernejoul MC, Levi G. Severe osteopenia in CFTR-null mice. *Bone* 2004; **35**(3): 595–603.

39. Le Henaff C, Gimenez A, Hay E, Marty C, Marie P, Jacquot J. The F508del mutation in cystic fibrosis transmembrane conductance regulator gene impacts bone formation. *Am J Pathol* 2012; **180**(5): 2068–75.

40. Le Heron L, Guillaume C, Velard F et al. Cystic fibrosis transmembrane conductance regulator (CFTR) regulates the production of osteoprotegerin (OPG) and prostaglandin (PG) E2 in human bone. *J Cyst Fibros* 2010; **9**(1): 69–72.

41. Grundt A, Grafe IA, Liegibel U, Sommer U, Nawroth P, Kasperk C. Direct effects of osteoprotegerin on human bone cell metabolism. *Biochem Biophys Res Commun* 2009; **389**(3): 550–5.

42. Gimenez-Maitre A, Le Henaff C, Norez C et al. Deficit of osteoprotegerin release by osteoblasts from a patient with cystic fibrosis. *Eur Respir J* 2012; **39**(3): 780–1.

43. McCabe LR. Understanding the pathology and mechanisms of type I diabetic bone loss. *J Cell Biochem* 2007; **102**(6): 1343–57.

44. Thrailkill KM, Lumpkin CK Jr., Bunn RC, Kemp SF, Fowlkes JL. Is insulin an anabolic agent in bone? Dissecting the diabetic bone for clues. *Am J Physiol Endocrinol Metab* 2005; **289**(5): E735–45.

45. Rana M, Munns CF, Selvadurai H, Briody J, Craig ME. The impact of dysglycaemia on bone mineral accrual in young people with cystic fibrosis. *Clin Endocrinol (Oxf)* 2013; **78**(1): 36–42.

46. De Nijs RN. Glucocorticoid-induced osteoporosis: A review on pathophysiology and treatment options. *Minerva Med* 2008; **99**(1): 23–43.

47. Kemmler W, von Stengel S. Dose-response effect of exercise frequency on bone mineral density in postmenopausal, osteopenic women. *Scand J Med Sci Sports* 2014; **24**(3): 526–34.

48. Nilsson M, Ohlsson C, Mellstrom D, Lorentzon M. Sport-specific association between exercise loading and the density, geometry, and microstructure of weight-bearing bone in young adult men. *Osteoporos Int* 2013; **24**(5): 1613–22.

49. Howe TE, Shea B, Dawson LJ et al. Exercise for preventing and treating osteoporosis in postmenopausal women. *Cochrane Database Syst Rev* 2011; (7): CD000333.

50. Smith E, Carroll A. Bone mineral density in adults disabled through acquired neurological conditions: A review. *J Clin Densitom* 2011; **14**(2): 85–94.

51. Schmitt L, Wiebel M, Frese F et al. Exercise reduces airway sodium ion reabsorption in cystic fibrosis but not in exercise asthma. *Eur Respir J* 2011; **37**(2): 342–8.

52. Hebestreit A, Kersting U, Basler B, Jeschke R, Hebestreit H. Exercise inhibits epithelial sodium channels in patients with cystic fibrosis. *Am J Respir Crit Care Med* 2001; **164**(3): 443–6.

53. Dodd JD, Barry SC, Barry RB, Cawood TJ, McKenna MJ, Gallagher CG. Bone mineral density in cystic fibrosis: Benefit of exercise capacity. *J Clin Densitom* 2008; **11**(4): 537–42.

54. Frangolias DD, Pare PD, Kendler DL et al. Role of exercise and nutrition status on bone mineral density in cystic fibrosis. *J Cyst Fibros* 2003; **2**(4): 163–70.

55. Dwyer TJ, Elkins MR, Bye PT. The role of exercise in maintaining health in cystic fibrosis. *Curr Opin Pulm Med* 2011; **17**(6): 455–60.

56. Hind K, Truscott JG, Conway SP. Exercise during childhood and adolescence: A prophylaxis against cystic fibrosis-related low bone mineral density? Exercise for bone health in children with cystic fibrosis. *J Cyst Fibros* 2008; **7**(4): 270–6.

57. Bradley J, Moran F. Physical training for cystic fibrosis. *Cochrane Database Syst Rev* 2008; (1): CD002768.

58. Sparks AA, McGee SJ, Boone CE, Neuringer IP, Jones SK, Aris RM. 'Old' bones in young bodies: The tale of cystic fibrosis. *Curr Opin Endocrinol Diabetes Obes* 2009; **16**(6): 407–14.

59. Rossini M, Del Marco A, Dal Santo F et al. Prevalence and correlates of vertebral fractures in adults with cystic fibrosis. *Bone* 2004; **35**(3): 771–6.

60. Gordon CM, Bachrach LK, Carpenter TO et al. Dual energy X-ray absorptiometry interpretation and reporting in children and adolescents: The 2007 ISCD Pediatric Official Positions. *J Clin Densitom* 2008; **11**(1): 43–58.

61. Baim S, Leonard MB, Bianchi ML et al. Official Positions Of The International Society for Clinical Densitometry and executive summary of the 2007 ISCD Pediatric Position Development Conference. *J Clin Densitom* 2008; **11**(1): 6–21.

62. Rossini M, Viapiana O, Del Marco A, de Terlizzi F, Gatti D, Adami S. Quantitative ultrasound in adults with cystic fibrosis: Correlation with bone mineral density and risk of vertebral fractures. *Calcif Tissue Int* 2007; **80**(1): 44–9.

63. Kelly A, Schall JI, Stallings VA, Zemel BS. Deficits in bone mineral content in children and adolescents with cystic fibrosis are related to height deficits. *J Clin Densitom* 2008; **11**(4): 581–9.

64. Stephenson A, Jamal S, Dowdell T, Pearce D, Corey M, Tullis E. Prevalence of vertebral fractures in adults with cystic fibrosis and their relationship to bone mineral density. *Chest* 2006; **130**(2): 539–44.

65. Aris RM, Renner JB, Winders AD et al. Increased rate of fractures and severe kyphosis: Sequelae of living into adulthood with cystic fibrosis. *Ann Intern Med* 1998; **128**(3): 186–93.

66. Hanak V, Hartman TE, Ryu JH. Cough-induced rib fractures. *Mayo Clin Proc* 2005; **80**(7): 879–82.

67. Hall WB, Sparks AA, Aris RM. Vitamin D deficiency in cystic fibrosis. *Int J Endocrinol* 2010; **2010**; 218691.

68. Wolfenden LL, Judd SE, Shah R, Sanyal R, Ziegler TR, Tangpricha V. Vitamin D and bone health in adults with cystic fibrosis. *Clin Endocrinol (Oxf)* 2008; **69**(3): 374–81.

69. Greer RM, Buntain HM, Potter JM et al. Abnormalities of the PTH-vitamin D axis and bone turnover markers in children, adolescents and adults with cystic fibrosis: Comparison with healthy controls. *Osteoporos Int* 2003; **14**(5): 404–11.

70. Tangpricha V, Kelly A, Stephenson A et al. An update on the screening, diagnosis, management, and treatment of vitamin D deficiency in individuals with cystic fibrosis: Evidence-based recommendations from the Cystic Fibrosis Foundation. *J Clin Endocrinol Metab* 2012; **97**(4): 1082–93.

71. Brown SA, Ontjes DA, Lester GE et al. Short-term calcitriol administration improves calcium homeostasis in adults with cystic fibrosis. *Osteoporosis Int* 2003; **14**(5): 442–9.

72. Ferguson JH, Chang AB. Vitamin D supplementation for cystic fibrosis. *Cochrane Database Syst Rev* 2012; **4**: CD007298.

73. Aris RM, Ontjes DA, Brown SA, Chalermskulrat W, Neuringer I, Lester GE. Carboxylated osteocalcin levels in cystic fibrosis. *Am J Respir Crit Care Med* 2003; **168**(9): 1129.

74. Aris RM, Lester GE, Caminiti M et al. Efficacy of alendronate in adults with cystic fibrosis with low bone density. *Am J Respir Crit Care Med* 2004; **169**(1): 77–82.

75. Conwell LS, Chang AB. Bisphosphonates for osteoporosis in people with cystic fibrosis. *Cochrane Database Syst Rev* 2012; **4**: CD002010.

76. Aris RM, Lester GE, Renner JB et al. Efficacy of pamidronate for osteoporosis in patients with cystic fibrosis following lung transplantation. *Am J Respir Crit Care Med* 2000; **162**(3 Pt 1): 941–6.

77. Ringuier B, Leboucher B, Leblanc M et al. [Effect of oral biphosphonates in patients with cystic fibrosis and low bone mineral density]. *Arch Pediatr* 2004; **11**(12): 1445–9.

78. Hardin DS, Adams-Huet B, Brown D et al. Growth hormone treatment improves growth and clinical status in prepubertal children with cystic fibrosis: Results of a multicenter randomized controlled trial. *J Clin Endocrinol Metab* 2006; **91**(12): 4925–9.

79. Hardin DS, Ahn C, Prestidge C, Seilheimer DK, Ellis KJ. Growth hormone improves bone mineral content in children with cystic fibrosis. *J Pediatr Endocrinol Metab* 2005; **18**(6): 589–95.

80. Saag KG, Shane E, Boonen S et al. Teriparatide or alendronate in glucocorticoid-induced osteoporosis. *N Engl J Med* 2007; **357**(20): 2028–39.

27

Other cystic fibrosis–related disease

KHIN MA GYI AND MARGARET HODSON

OTHER SYSTEM DISORDERS IN CYSTIC FIBROSIS

Cystic fibrosis (CF) is a multiorgan, multisystem disease. Some manifestations are due to epithelial cystic fibrosis transmembrane conductance regulator (CFTR) dysfunction in individual organs and some result from the systemic inflammatory response to chronic airway infection. There are also treatment-related complications such as aminoglycoside-induced acute and chronic kidney disease (CKD). These multisystem complications have considerable impact on quality of life, morbidity, and mortality and have become an important concern as patients with CF are living longer.[1,2] In this chapter, several multisystem complications are discussed, including vasculitis and dermatological problems; arthropathies; renal disease; electrolyte abnormalities; and neurological, hematological, ocular, and oral health issues together with deafness and vestibular dysfunction.

VASCULITIS AND DERMATOLOGICAL PROBLEMS

Vasculitis is a well recognized but uncommon complication of CF. The estimated frequency is about 2%–3%.[3–5] Although it can occur in childhood, the majority of cases occur in adult CF patients over 20 years of age. Vasculitis mainly involves the small vessels, including arterioles, capillaries, and/or venules. A common histological finding is leukocytoclastic vasculitis.[3,6] There is vascular and perivascular infiltration by neutrophils, endothelial swelling, and fibrinoid necrosis of the vessel walls. Cutaneous vasculitis is the usual presentation but systemic involvement can occasionally occur affecting the renal, gastrointestinal, and central nervous systems. In some cases of renal involvement, biopsies show changes similar to those of Henoch–Schonlein purpura.[3–5]

The etiology of vasculitis is not well understood. Circulating immune complexes have been frequently reported in CF patients with vasculitis, suggestive of an underlying immune mechanism.[4,7] Multiple factors, including chronic persistent bacterial infections and medications may provide a potential source of antigen.[3–5,7] Many cases of vasculitis have been associated with hyperglobulinemia.[4,8] Purpura due to cryoglobulinemia has been described in one patient.[9]Antineutrophilic cytoplasmic antibody (ANCA), against bacterial permeability–increasing protein (BPI), has been observed in sera of 55%–90% CF patients.[3,4,10–12] BPI is an important host defense protein with bactericidal and antiendotoxin properties. It has protective activity against lipopolysaccharide-induced vascular endothelial cells injury.[13] Therefore, it is postulated that anti-BPI antibody may predispose to vasculitis. Whether this particular mechanism is responsible for CF vasculitis is not established. Anti-BPI is correlated with pseudomonal load, severity of lung disease, and the presence of vasculitis in adult CF patients.[10,12]

Cutaneous vasculitis presents as a petechial or maculopapular rash, commonly involving the lower limbs, around the ankles, and on the dorsum of the feet (Figure 27.1). It may extend to the upper limbs, trunk, and face. It is nonblanching, sometimes palpable, painful, and can be itchy. Constitutional symptoms including fever, malaise, and myalgia may be present. Arthralgia and arthritis involving the ankles or knees occur in about 50% cases. Hematuria and proteinuria may be present in cases with renal involvement. Recurrent iron deficiency anemia and intestinal bleeding can be presenting features of vasculitis involving the gastrointestinal tract.[7,14,15] Central nervous system involvement has been described in at least one case.[4] In the majority of cases, purpura disappears within a few days to a few weeks, but in a few cases may become recurrent.

Patients should have a full history and examination with appropriate tests, such as chest x-ray, erythrocyte sedimentation rate (ESR), full blood count, electrolytes, liver function tests, antinuclear factor, ANCA, BPI, myeloperoxidase (MPO),

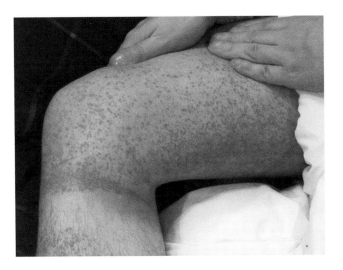

Figure 27.1 Vasculitis. CF patient with recurrent vasculitic rash.

and proteinase-3 (PR3) antibodies. Urine microscopy and creatinine clearance are essential to exclude renal involvement.

Treatment for cutaneous vasculitis without systemic involvement is symptomatic with nonsteroidal anti-inflammatory agents and antihistamine if necessary. In recurrent, severe or persistent vasculitis, and in cases with systemic involvement, corticosteroids, azathioprine, and methotrexate have been used. Recently, a dramatic response to chloroquine when added to steroid treatment was reported.[16] Treatment with plasmapheresis has been described in cases of severe hyperglobulinemic purpura.[8] Any suspected medications should be withdrawn. The majority of CF vasculitis occurs in the presence of CF lung disease. Many reported cases show increased mortality after the appearance of vasculitis. It is not certain whether the deleterious effect of vasculitis contributes to the poor prognosis, or simply reflects the severity of the underlying CF lung disease.

Other dermatological problems include diffuse dermatitis, aquagenic wrinkling of the palms (Figure 27.2), and drug-related skin reactions. In infants, diffuse nutrient deficiency dermatitis, which is an acrodermatitis enteropathica-like eruptions, may be the first presenting feature of CF before gastrointestinal and pulmonary symptoms. The rash consists of extensive dry, scaly, fissured, or itchy erythematous plaques involving the perioral area, diaper region, and extremities. It is thought to be related to deficiency of zinc, essential fatty acids, and protein.[17,18] Aquagenic wrinkling of the palms is characterized by the rapid and transient formation of edematous whitish papules and plaques on the palms and soles on exposure to water.[19] Aquagenic wrinkling of palms on exposure to alcohol gel has also been reported. It has been suggested that a mutation in CFTR causing high concentration of salt and abnormal regulation of water channels in skin may play a role in the pathogenesis.[17] There is also evidence of measurable increase in transepidermal water loss.[19]

Patients with CF have increased rates of atopy, drug allergy, and hypersensitivity. The drug reactions include urticaria, angioedema, morbilliform rash, Stevens–Johnson

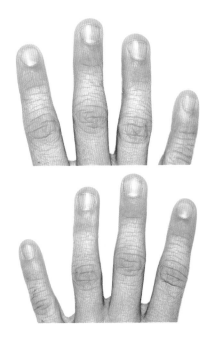

Figure 27.2 Aquagenic wrinkling of the fingers. (Courtesy of Prof. Andrew Bush.)

syndrome, and vasculitis. Drug hypersensitivity is found in approximately 30% of CF patients. This may be due to the frequent use of antibiotics. Aminoglycosides are repeatedly used, but drug reactions are rare. Ciprofloxacin tends to cause joint problems in some children, rather than rashes. A high incidence of rash after piperacillin treatment and photosensitivity due to quinolones have also been frequently reported in CF.[17,20,21] The cutaneous manifestations of CF are summarized by Bernstein et al.[17]

ARTHROPATHIES

Joint symptoms occur in up to 12% of CF patients.[6,22,23] They may be directly related to CF or a complication of drug treatment, or due to the presence of a coincidental disease. The most common arthropathies related to CF are episodic arthritis (EA) also known as CF-associated arthritis (CFAA) and hypertrophic pulmonary osteoarthropathy (HPOA). They can occur at any age, but more commonly affects adults in the second decade of life.

EPISODIC ARTHRITIS/CYSTIC FIBROSIS-ASSOCIATED ARTHRITIS

This is the most common form of arthritis in CF and affects 2%–8% of adults. It is characterized by acute onset of mono- or polyarticular arthritis affecting large joints such as the knees, ankles, wrists, hips, and shoulders. Occasionally the small joints of the hands and feet may be affected. It is usually asymmetrical and can present as arthralgia or sometimes be associated with swelling and disabling pain.

Episodes are transient and subside spontaneously within 7–10 days. Some cases may evolve into relapsing and remitting courses, which may last for weeks or years. Episodes may be associated with a flu-like illness, high fever, vasculitic rash, and erythema nodosum.[5,6,23] Characteristically, EA is nonerosive with negative rheumatoid factor, and the x-rays are normal. However, progression to erosive, chronic destructive polyarthritis has been reported in small subgroups of patients.[23]

The underlying etiology is unknown but immunological mechanisms may play a role. Chronic, persistent bacterial infection with excessive antigen load can cause immune stimulation and hyperactive immune system resulting in the formation of immune complexes.[24,25] It is speculated that arthritis may be due to a spillover of immune complexes from the respiratory tract into the circulation with subsequent deposition in the joints. High levels of circulating immune complexes are reported in CF arthropathy patients, compared with CF patients without arthropathy. Immunoglobulins and complement depositions have been found in synovial blood vessels in biopsies taken during an exacerbation of EA.[6] There is no evidence of an association with any specific HLA types.[26]

There is no consistent relationship between CFAA and the severity of underlying pulmonary disease but it can be associated with a pulmonary exacerbation. Treatment is usually symptomatic, with nonsteroidal anti-inflammatory agents. Oral corticosteroids can be used to control the inflammation. Very rarely, azathioprine, sulfasalazine, and hydroxychloroquine have been tried in combination with steroid or as steroid-sparing agents.[23,27]

HYPERTROPHIC PULMONARY OSTEOARTHROPATHY

HPOA was the first joint disease described in CF. It occurs in 2%–7% of CF patients, predominantly affecting young adults; the median age of onset is about 20, and it rarely occurs before 10 years of age.[28–30] It is characterized by clubbing and chronic periostitis of the long bones with or without periosteal new bone formation (Figure 27.3).

Most patients present with an insidious onset of asymmetrical polyarthritis with pain, swelling, and effusions involving the knees, ankles, wrists, and associated tenderness of the ends of the long bones. It rarely involves the small joints of the hands or feet. Large joint effusions can sometimes occur. Gynecomastia and mastalgia may be present.[28] In contrast to EA, HPOA is associated with more severe underlying lung disease and it accompanies or worsens during acute pulmonary exacerbations.[22,23] The etiology of HPOA is unknown. Theories have included neurogenic and humoral mechanisms and a hyperactive immune system as a result of acute infection. HPOA can regress after vagotomy and lung transplantation. Another hypothesis relates to platelet function. The hypothesis proposes that in the presence of some lung disease, megakaryocytes accumulate in the small vessels of the distal long bones, inappropriately

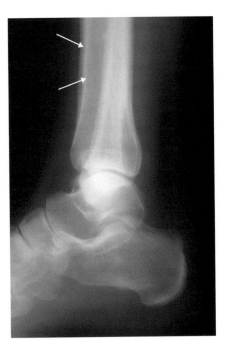

Figure 27.3 Hypertrophic pulmonary osteoarthropathy (HPOA). Arrows show new bone formation.

releasing some mediators, which can cause inflammation and new bone formation. In one study, platelet-derived growth factor (PDGF) was significantly higher in HPOA patients compared with healthy controls.[31]

Management includes intensive treatment of underlying lung disease and acute exacerbations, nonsteroidal anti-inflammatory agents for pain and occasionally corticosteroids are used. In severe, refractory cases, intravenous pamidronate can be useful.[32] The onset of HPOA is associated with an increased mortality.[27]

OTHER SYSTEMIC DISEASES INVOLVING THE JOINTS IN CYSTIC FIBROSIS

A few cases of rheumatoid arthritis (RA) have been reported in CF patients.[22,33–35] RA occurs more frequently in CF than can be attributed to chance alone. It has been postulated that CF EA may be a mild form of RA with the potential for progressing to full-blown RA after several years of antigen stimulation, related to episodes of infective exacerbations.[33] Clinical presentation includes symmetrical polyarthritis with nodules, joint erosion, and positive rheumatoid factor (Figure 27.4). Disease modifying and immunomodulatory agents, e.g., TNF-α antagonists can be safely used, which may also have a positive impact on the lung disease.[36] Before TNF-α is used, the recommendations of the British Thoracic Society (BTS) guidance should be studied if there is any suspicion of tuberculosis or atypical mycobacterial infection.[37]

Other causes of arthropathy include sarcoidosis,[38] amyloidosis,[39,40] gout secondary to hyperuricemia,[41] and adult onset Still's disease.[42] The most common group of drugs responsible for arthritis in CF patients are the quinolones, such as ciprofloxacin, causing acute tenosynovitis

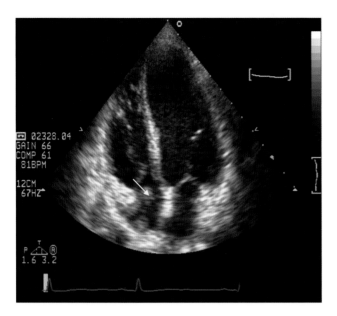

Figure 27.7 Right atrial thrombus around TIVAD (arrowed). This CF patient has PFO with right to left shunt and presented with TIA. (From Simmonds NJ et al., *J Med Case Rep*, 3, 8582, 2009.)

the underlying mechanisms may be cerebral hypoperfusion. During coughing increased intrathoracic pressure is transmitted via the valveless great veins to the intracranial compartment causing transient increased intracranial pressure, resulting in impairment of cerebral blood flow. Increased intrathoracic pressure also obstructs venous return causing reduced cardiac output and low blood pressure, resulting in cerebral hypoperfusion.[123] In addition, hypoxia can occur during prolonged episodes of coughing. In advanced lung disease, extreme pressure changes in the thoracic cavity during inspiration can cause physiological tamponade that may interfere with cardiac output and cerebral perfusion.[124]

Rao et al. described two CF patients who developed cough-induced hemiplegic migraine resulting in acute neurological symptoms and altered consciousness. The symptoms responded to treatment with verapamil.[125] Hemiplegic migraine is one of the disorders characterized under channelopathy.[126] Since CFTR is abundantly expressed in the brain[127] and is responsible for regulating other ion channels, it is suggested that it may indirectly contribute to the production of migraine.[125]

Headache is common and in one study 55% CF children had chronic headache and the main etiologies were hypercarbia or hypoxia, sinusitis, and migraine.[128] Facial palsy has been reported in association with vitamin A deficiency.[129-131] Benign intracranial hypertension in CF has been associated with hypovitaminosis A and ciprofloxacin.[131,132] Severe vitamin E deficiency can cause muscle weakness, hyporeflexia, ataxia, and reduced vibration and position sense.[133] Chiari type 1 malformation, characterized by herniation of cerebellar tonsils through the foramen magnum was reported to be more common in CF than in the general population. Neurological presentations include

swallowing dysfunction, syncopal attacks, numbness of extremities, recurrent vomiting, and headaches.[134]

Investigations of neurological symptoms include a detailed neurological history and examination, blood tests including electrolytes and vitamin levels, glucose monitoring, neurological imaging with CT and MRI brain scan, EEG, 24-hour ECG monitoring, echocardiogram with a shunt study, carotid Doppler, and overnight CO_2 and oxygen saturation monitoring.

HEMATOLOGICAL PROBLEMS

Some patients can present with hematological problems. Two cases presenting with anemia and one with pancytopenia before their CF was diagnosed have been reported.[135] The causes are uncertain, but the hypotheses include chronic disease and maldigestion, secondary to pancreatic dysfunction.[136] The anemia may be hemolytic indicating vitamin E deficiency.[137] Low levels of vitamin E are common in infants.[138] Investigations of children with anemia include peripheral blood film, hemoglobin, electrophoresis, hemolytic screen, autoantibodies, and occasionally a bone marrow aspirate.[137] Severe hemolytic anemia and clotting disorders due to vitamin E and vitamin K deficiency, respectively, may be the first presenting signs of CF in infants.[139,140]

Iron deficiency with usually normal hemoglobin is common in CF and is thought to be due to anemia of chronic disease as a result of chronic inflammation. It was found to be directly related to the increased severity of suppurative lung disease associated with *Pseudomonas aeruginosa*, poor lung function, and poor clinical status.[141] Low serum and increased sputum iron were observed in these cases. Treatment is to address the underlying inflammation rather than iron supplementation.[142] Liver disease and splenomegaly may lead to thrombocytopenia or neutropenia. Megaloblastic anemia may result from terminal ileal resection. The CF patient takes many drugs that may in some individuals cause hematological abnormalities. Thrombophilic abnormalities have been described in some CF patients but most abnormalities were inconsistent. The clinical significance is not clear but it may be relevant in totally implanted venous access device (TIVAD)-related thrombosis (Figure 27.7).[143,144]

OCULAR PROBLEMS

Endogenous endopthalmitis caused by *P. aeruginosa* rarely occurs in CF patients after lung transplantation but has been reported in patients who have not undergone a transplant. The visual prognosis is poor, and usually enucleation is necessary despite aggressive surgical intervention and appropriate antibiotic therapy.[145,146] Vitamin A deficiency can cause xeropthalmia, night blindness, and poor dark adaptation. Severe vitamin E deficiency is associated with abnormal eye movement and visual field restrictions.[133] Vitamin A levels may be low due to malabsorption, liver disease, or poor compliance with prescribed supplements. It is recommended that regular vitamin A supplements are given to patients with CF, and regular monitoring of plasma levels of vitamin A are carried out in these patients.[147] However, as the Cochrane Review states, there are no clinical trials from which to draw conclusions on the benefits (or otherwise) of regular administration of vitamin A in people with CF. However, they recommend that until further data are available vitamin A should be given.[148] Vitamin E supplements are also usually given to patients with CF.

ORAL HEALTH

A decreased prevalence of dental caries, plaque, and gingivitis was observed in CF children, and this was thought to be due to long-term antibiotic usage and pancreatic enzyme supplements. However, enamel opacities are more common in people with CF.[149–151] These enamel opacities are thought to be due to reduced pH resulting in a lack of calcium influx during maturation and hypomineralization in CF. Similar changes have been found in the teeth of CF mice. Tetracycline is known to give children a high incidence of tooth discoloration and hypoplasia, and therefore, it must be avoided. In view of these findings, it is recommended that CF patients have regular dental care.[151]

DEAFNESS AND VESTIBULAR FUNCTION

Chapter 21 focuses on the upper airways in CF, the major issue being the chronic rhinosinusitis and infection with/without nasal polyposis. However, the CF team needs the help of ENT colleagues in their area as loss of hearing and vestibular dysfunction also occur in CF patients.

Aminoglycosides, which are widely used to treat *Pseudomonas* infection in CF patients, have toxic effects that lead to hearing loss and vestibular toxicity as well as the well-known kidney toxicity discussed earlier. Studies of 70 patients from a CF clinic found an overall prevalence of hearing impairment in 17%.[152] The most straightforward measurement of hearing impairment is a pure tone audiogram.[153] Aminoglycoside ototoxicity causes degeneration of the ear cells in the organ of Corti.[154] Some mitochondrial mutations are associated with ototoxicity; the best known is the A1555G mutation.[155]

Opinions differ on the cost-effectiveness of screening all CF patients for the A1555G mutation.[156,157] However, it is advisable to perform regular audiograms on patients having frequent aminoglycosides and all patients with hearing problems.

To reduce these side effects, once daily aminoglycoside administration, the use of tobramycin rather than gentamicin, careful monitoring of drug levels, screening for mutations, and the use of aspirin or N-acetylcysteine have been suggested.[153] Another possibility in patients with ototoxicity is to treat acute exacerbations with cephalosporin, carbapenens, or beta-lactam antibiotics without an aminoglycoside, unless the infection is life threatening. The evidence that results are better when an aminoglycoside is added and two antibiotics are administered is small.

Vestibulotoxicity with aminoglycosides is due to damage of the hair cells in the vestibular system. Patients may feel dizzy and light headed, and they can partially recover if the aminoglycoside is discontinued.

REFERENCES

1. Elborn JS. How can we prevent multisystem complications of cystic fibrosis? *Semin Respir Crit Care Med* 2007; **28**(03): 303–11.
2. Schechter MS, Stecenko AA. Chronic kidney disease: A new morbidity of cystic fibrosis or an old morbidity of diabetes mellitus? *Am J Respir Crit Care Med* 2011; **184**(10): 1101–2.
3. Finnegan MJ, Hinchcliffe J, Russell-Jones D et al. Vasculitis complicating cystic fibrosis. *Q J Med* 1989; **72**(267): 609–21.
4. Hodson ME. Vasculitis and arthropathy in cystic fibrosis. *J R Soc Med* 1992; **85**(Suppl 19): 38–40.
5. Schidlow DV, Goldsmith DP, Palmer J, Huang NN. Arthritis in cystic fibrosis. *Arch Dis Child* 1984; **59**(4): 377–9.
6. Bourke S, Rooney M, Fitzgerald M, Bresnihan B. Episodic arthropathy in adult cystic fibrosis. *Q J Med* 1987; **64**(244): 651–9.
7. Parameswaran K, Keaney NP, Veale D. A case of chronic gastrointestinal blood loss in cystic fibrosis. *Respir Med* 1995; **89**(8): 577–9.
8. Nielsen HE, Lundh S, Jacobsen SV, Hoiby N. Hypergammaglobulinemic purpura in cystic fibrosis. *Acta Paediatr Scand* 1978; **67**(4): 443–7.
9. Garty BZ, Scanlin T, Goldsmith DP, Grunstein M. Cutaneous manifestations of cystic fibrosis: Possible role of cryoglobulins. *Br J Dermatol* 1989; **121**(5): 655–8.
10. Mahadeva R, Dunn AC, Westerbeek RC et al. Anti-neutrophil cytoplasmic antibodies (ANCA) against bactericidal/permeability-increasing protein (BPI) and cystic fibrosis lung disease. *Clin Exp Immunol* 1999; **117**(3): 561–7.
11. Sediva A, Kolarova I, Bartunkova J. Antineutrophil cytoplasmic antibodies in children. *Eur J Pediatr* 1998; **157**(12): 987–91.
12. Zhao MH, Jayne DR, Ardiles LG, Culley F, Hodson ME, Lockwood CM. Autoantibodies against bactericidal/permeability-increasing protein in patients with cystic fibrosis. *Q J Med* 1996; **89**(4): 259–65.

13. Arditi M, Zhou J, Huang SH, Luckett PM, Marra MN, Kim KS. Bactericidal/permeability-increasing protein protects vascular endothelial cells from lipopolysaccharide-induced activation and injury. *Infect Immun* 1994; **62**(9): 3930–6.

14. McFarlane H, Holzel A, Brenchley P et al. Immune complexes in cystic fibrosis. *Br Med J* 1975; **1**(5955): 423–8.

15. Soter NA, Mihm MC Jr., Colten HR. Cutaneous necrotizing venulitis in patients with cystic fibrosis. *J Pediatr* 1979; **95**(2): 197–201.

16. Molyneux ID, Moon T, Webb AK, Morice AH. Treatment of cystic fibrosis associated cutaneous vasculitis with chloroquine. *J Cyst Fibros* 2010; **9**(6): 439–41.

17. Bernstein ML, McCusker MM, Grant-Kels JM. Cutaneous manifestations of cystic fibrosis. *Pediatr Dermatol* 2008; **25**(2): 150–7.

18. Hansen RC, Lemen R, Revsin B. Cystic fibrosis manifesting with acrodermatitis enteropathica-like eruption. Association with essential fatty acid and zinc deficiencies. *Arch Dermatol* 1983; **119**(1): 51–5.

19. Arkin LM, Flory JH, Shin DB et al. High prevalence of aquagenic wrinkling of the palms in patients with cystic fibrosis and association with measurable increases in transepidermal water loss. *Pediatr Dermatol* 2012; **29**(5): 560–6.

20. Ramesh S. Antibiotic hypersensitivity in patients with CF. *Clin Rev Allergy Immunol* 2002; **23**(1): 123–42.

21. Stead RJ, Kennedy HG, Hodson ME, Batten JC. Adverse reactions to piperacillin in adults with cystic fibrosis. *Thorax* 1985; **40**(3): 184–6.

22. Dixey J, Redington AN, Butler RC et al. The arthropathy of cystic fibrosis. *Ann Rheum Dis* 1988; **47**(3): 218–23.

23. Rush PJ, Shore A, Coblentz C, Wilmot D, Corey M, Levison H. The musculoskeletal manifestations of cystic fibrosis. *Semin Arthritis Rheum* 1986; **15**(3): 213–25.

24. Moss RB, Lewiston NJ. Immune complexes and humoral response to *Pseudomonas aeruginosa* in cystic fibrosis. *Am Rev Respir Dis* 1980; **121**(1): 23–9.

25. Wisnieski JJ, Todd EW, Fuller RK et al. Immune complexes and complement abnormalities in patients with cystic fibrosis. Increased mortality associated with circulating immune complexes and decreased function of the alternative complement pathway. *Am Rev Respir Dis* 1985; **132**(4): 770–6.

26. Rush PJ, Gladman DD, Shore A, Anhorn KA. Absence of an association between HLA typing in cystic fibrosis arthritis and hypertrophic osteoarthropathy. *Ann Rheum Dis* 1991; **50**(11): 763–4.

27. Phillips BM, David TJ. Pathogenesis and management of arthropathy in cystic fibrosis. *J R Soc Med* 1986; **79**(Suppl 12): 44–50.

28. Braude S, Kennedy H, Hodson M, Batten J. Hypertrophic osteoarthropathy in cystic fibrosis. *Br Med J (Clin Res Ed)* 1984; **288**(6420): 822–3.

29. Cohen AM, Yulish BS, Wasser KB, Vignos PJ, Jones PK, Sorin SB. Evaluation of pulmonary hypertrophic osteoarthropathy in cystic fibrosis. A comprehensive study. *Am J Dis Child* 1986; **140**(1): 74–7.

30. Johnson S, Knox AJ. Arthropathy in cystic fibrosis. *Respir Med* 1994; **88**(8): 567–70.

31. Silveri F, De Angelis R, Argentati F, Brecciaroli D, Muti S, Cervini C. Hypertrophic osteoarthropathy: Endothelium and platelet function. *Clin Rheumatol* 1996; **15**(5): 435–9.

32. Garske LA, Bell SC. Pamidronate results in symptom control of hypertrophic pulmonary osteoarthropathy in cystic fibrosis. *Chest* 2002; **121**(4): 1363–4.

33. Botton E, Saraux A, Laselve H, Jousse S, Le Goff P. Musculoskeletal manifestations in cystic fibrosis. *Joint Bone Spine* 2003; **70**(5): 327–35.

34. Gardiner PV, Roberts SD, Bell AL. Cystic fibrosis and rheumatoid arthritis. *Br J Rheumatol* 1989; **28**(2): 179.

35. Lawrence JM III, Moore TL, Madson KL, Rejent AJ, Osborn TG. Arthropathies of cystic fibrosis: Case reports and review of the literature. *J Rheumatol Suppl* 1993; **38**: 12–5.

36. Visser S, Martin M, Serisier D. Improvements in cystic fibrosis lung disease and airway inflammation associated with etanercept therapy for rheumatoid arthritis: A case report. *Lung* 2012; **190**(5): 579–81.

37. British Thoracic Society Standards of Care Committee. BTS recommendations for assessing risk and for managing *Mycobacterium tuberculosis* infection and disease in patients due to startanti-TNF-alpha treatment. *Thorax* 2005; **60**(10): 800–5.

38. Soden M, Tempany E, Bresnihan B. Sarcoid arthropathy in cystic fibrosis. *Br J Rheumatol* 1989; **28**(4): 341–3.

39. Gaffney K, Gibbons D, Keogh B, FitzGerald MX. Amyloidosis complicating cystic fibrosis. *Thorax* 1993; **48**(9): 949–50.

40. Ristow SC, Condemi JJ, Stuard ID, Schwartz RH, Bryson MF. Systemic amyloidosis in cystic fibrosis. *Am J Dis Child* 1977; **131**(8): 886–8.

41. Horsley A, Helm J, Brennan A, Bright-Thomas R, Webb K, Jones A. Gout and hyperuricaemia in adults with cystic fibrosis. *JRSM* 2011; **104**(Suppl 1): S36–9.

42. Albersmeyer MP, Hilge RG, Schulze-Koops H, Sitter T. Adult-onset Still's disease in a patient with cystic fibrosis and its successful treatment with anakinra. *Rheumatology* 2012; **51**(9): 1730–2.

43. Warren RW. Rheumatologic aspects of pediatric cystic fibrosis patients treated with fluoroquinolones. *Pediatr Infect Dis J* 1997; **16**(1): 118–22.

44. Morales MM, Carroll TP, Morita T et al. Both the wild type and a functional isoform of CFTR are expressed in kidney. *Am J Physiol* 1996; **270**(6 Pt 2): F1038–48.

45. Riordan JR, Rommens JM, Kerem B et al. Identification of the cystic fibrosis gene: Cloning and characterization of complementary DNA. *Science* 1989; **245**(4922): 1066–73.

46. Sullivan LP, Wallace DP, Grantham JJ. Chloride and fluid secretion in polycystic kidney disease. *J Am Soc Nephrol* 1998; **9**(5): 903–16.

47. Donckerwolcke RA, Diemen-Steenvoorde R, van der LJ, Koomans HA, Boer WH. Impaired diluting segment chloride reabsorption in patients with cystic fibrosis. *Child Nephrol Urol* 1992; **12**(4): 186–91.

48. Stenvinkel P, Hjelte L, Alvan G, Hedman A, Hultman E, Strandvik B. Decreased renal clearance of sodium in cystic fibrosis. *Acta Paediatr Scand* 1991; **80**(2): 194–8.

49. Touw DJ. Clinical pharmacokinetics of antimicrobial drugs in cystic fibrosis. *Pharm World Sci* 1998; **20**(4): 149–60.

50. Abramowsky CR, Swinehart GL. The nephropathy of cystic fibrosis: A human model of chronic nephrotoxicity. *Hum Pathol* 1982; **13**(10): 934–9.

51. Scott AI, Clarke BE, Healy H, Emden D, Bell SC. Microvascular complications in cystic fibrosis-related diabetes mellitus: A case report. *JOP* 2000; **1**(4): 208–10.

52. Westall GP, Binder J, Kotsimbos T et al. Nodular glomerulosclerosis in cystic fibrosis mimics diabetic nephropathy. *Nephron Clin Pract* 2004; **96**(3): c70–5.

53. Katz SM, Krueger LJ, Falkner B. Microscopic nephrocalcinosis in cystic fibrosis. *N Engl J Med* 1988; **319**(5): 263–6.

54. Kuwertz-Broking E, Koch HG, Schulze Everding A et al. Colchicine for secondary nephropathic amyloidosis in cysic fibrosis. *Lancet* 1995; **345**: 1178–9.

55. Stirati G, Antonelli M, Fofi C, Fierimonte S, Pecci G. IgA nephropathy in cystic fibrosis. *J Nephrol* 1999; **12**(1): 30–1.

56. Nazareth D, Walshaw M. A review of renal disease in cystic fibrosis. *J Cyst Fibros* 2013; **12**(4): 309–17.

57. Soulsby N, Greville H, Coulthard K, Doecke C. Renal dysfunction in cystic fibrosis: Is there cause for concern? *Pediatr Pulmonol* 2009; **44**(10): 947–53.

58. Chidekel AS, Dolan TF Jr. Cystic fibrosis and calcium oxalate nephrolithiasis. *Yale J Biol Med* 1996; **69**(4): 317–21.

59. Hoppe B, Hesse A, Bromme S, Rietschel E, Michalk D. Urinary excretion substances in patients with cystic fibrosis: Risk of urolithiasis? *Pediatr Nephrol* 1998; **12**(4): 275–9.

60. Matthews LA, Doershuk CF, Stern RC, Resnick MI. Urolithiasis and cystic fibrosis. *J Urol* 1996; **155**(5): 1563–4.

61. Perez-Brayfield MR, Caplan D, Gatti JM, Smith EA, Kirsch AJ. Metabolic risk factors for stone formation in patients with cystic fibrosis. *J Urol* 2002; **167**(2 Pt 1): 480–4.

62. Gibney EM, Goldfarb DS. The association of nephrolithiasis with cystic fibrosis. *Am J Kidney Dis* 2003; **42**(1): 1–11.

63. Terribile M, Capuano M, Cangiano G et al. Factors increasing the risk for stone formation in adult patients with cystic fibrosis. *Nephrol Dial Transplant* 2006; **21**(7): 1870–5.

64. von der HR, Balestra AP, Bianchetti MG et al. Which factors account for renal stone formation in cystic fibrosis? *Clin Nephrol* 2003; **59**(3): 160–3.

65. Bohles H, Gebhardt B, Beeg T, Sewell AC, Solem E, Posselt G. Antibiotic treatment-induced tubular dysfunction as a risk factor for renal stone formation in cystic fibrosis. *J Pediatr* 2002; **140**(1): 103–9.

66. Hoppe B, von Unruh GE, Blank G et al. Absorptive hyperoxaluria leads to an increased risk for urolithiasis or nephrocalcinosis in cystic fibrosis. *Am J Kidney Dis* 2005; **46**(3): 440–5.

67. Holmes RP, Goodman HO, Assimos DG. Contribution of dietary oxalate to urinary oxalate excretion. *Kidney Int* 2001; **59**(1): 270–6.

68. Dobbins JW, Binder HJ. Importance of the colon in enteric hyperoxaluria. *N Engl J Med* 1977; **296**(6): 298–301.

69. Bohles H, Michalk D. Is there a risk for kidney stone formation in cystic fibrosis? *Helv Paediatr Acta* 1982; **37**(3): 267–72.

70. Sidhu H, Hoppe B, Hesse A et al. Absence of *Oxalobacter formigenes* in cystic fibrosis patients: A risk factor for hyperoxaluria. *Lancet* 1998; **352**(9133): 1026–9.

71. Lieske JC, Goldfarb DS, De SC, Regnier C. Use of a probiotic to decrease enteric hyperoxaluria. *Kidney Int* 2005; **68**(3): 1244–9.

72. Lieske JC, Tremaine WJ, De SC et al. Diet, but not oral probiotics, effectively reduces urinary oxalate excretion and calcium oxalate supersaturation. *Kidney Int* 2010; **78**(11): 1178–85.

73. Quon BS, Mayer-Hamblett N, Aitken ML, Smyth AR, Goss CH. Risk factors for chronic kidney disease in adults with cystic fibrosis. *Am J Respir Crit Care Med* 2011; **184**(10): 1147–52.

74. Al-Aloul M, Miller H, Stockton P, Ledson MJ, Walshaw MJ. Acute renal failure in CF patients chronically infected by the Liverpool epidemic *Pseudomonas aeruginosa* strain (LES). *J Cyst Fibros* 2005; **4**(3): 197–201.

75. Bertenshaw C, Watson AR, Lewis S, Smyth A. Survey of acute renal failure in patients with cystic fibrosis in the UK. *Thorax* 2007; **62**(6): 541–5.

76. Drew J, Watson AR, Smyth A. Acute renal failure and cystic fibrosis. *Arch Dis Child* 2003; **88**(7): 646.

77. Smyth A, Lewis S, Bertenshaw C, Choonara I, McGaw J, Watson A. Case-control study of acute renal failure in patients with cystic fibrosis in the UK. *Thorax* 2008; **63**(6): 532–5.

78. Kennedy SE, Henry RL, Rosenberg AR. Antibiotic-related renal failure and cystic fibrosis. *J Paediatr Child Health* 2005; **41**(7): 382–3.

Table 28.1 Prepregnancy counseling issues

Clinical
- Cystic fibrosis carrier status of partner
- Prepregnancy level of lung function
- Diabetic status, control, and screening
- Nutritional status and management throughout pregnancy
- Check current medication and potential changes
- Risk of premature delivery and the increased risk of cesarean section
- Possible deterioration and the importance of regaining lost lung function postdelivery
- Increased need for outpatient visits and admissions
- Breast-feeding

Psychosocial
- Possibility of single parenthood
- Sources of ongoing postnatal support
- Demands of parenthood
- Deterioration of health status during and after pregnancy

because it is not possible to screen for all the CF mutations, there is still a very small risk of the fetus being affected by CF. It should not be assumed that all men would wish to go down the route of assisted conception; nonetheless it is important that everyone is made aware of their options. Investigations for the male will include semen analysis, testosterone and follicular-stimulating hormone (FSH) measurements. Although in the majority of men with CF sperm production is normal, high levels of FSH are associated with an increased risk of impaired spermatogenesis (ARSM Practice Committee).[10] In addition to counseling for the various risks of assisted conception including ovarian hyperstimulation, female partners need to be screened for CF carrier status and, if necessary, preimplantation genetic diagnosis may be considered.

There are a number of methods by which sperm can be retrieved either from the epididymis or directly from the testes. Percutaneous epididymal sperm aspiration is undertaken using local anesthesia and sperm can be aspirated in nearly 90% of cases. In contrast, microepididymal sperm aspiration is normally carried out under a general anesthetic and involves a more extensive surgical technique, dissecting the epididymal tubule surgically and then aspirating the sperm.[11] Sperm has been retrieved in over 98% of cases using this technique. In some men, the epididymis may be absent or abnormal, but sperm can still be retrieved by direct testicular aspiration or biopsy.

The success of ICSI is related to the age of the mother and is approximately 35% in women less than 35 years, but falling to 5%–10% in those over 40 years. Additionally, the success of the technique does not appear to be compromised by the presence of CF mutations in the male partner.[12] Couples must be made aware that assisted conception techniques do have some specific risks. One report revealed a nearly 3% risk of an abnormal karyotype and, although nearly half of these were inherited from the father, the remainder were de novo abnormalities.[13] The rate of abnormality appears to be significantly increased in men with a reduced sperm count, which may be of relevance in some men with CF; however,

there are no reports of offspring with an abnormal karyotype in the CF literature to date. One study in the general population has demonstrated an increased risk of rare imprinting disorders, but overall there appears to be little difference between the risk of anomalies and long-term development in babies born either by ICSI or IVF.[14] ICSI therefore is a viable technique in helping to overcome male fertility issues in CF.

Fatherhood with CF presents significant challenges and men and their partners should be counseled before undergoing treatment. Many of the same issues discussed with young women with CF who wish to be mothers should also be discussed with men (Table 28.1). Important considerations include current health status, maintaining treatment regimens when there is a baby at home, admissions to hospital, deteriorating health, prognosis, and leaving a single parent behind.

FEMALE FERTILITY

The average age of menarche in the general population has been reported as 12.9 years in an American study, compared to 14.4 years for girls with CF.[15] The age of menarche is related to the general well-being of the individual, and as one might expect, those with more severe disease, frequently reflected in a low body mass index (BMI), have a later menarche, and are therefore less likely to be ovulating.[16] In a Swedish study, the average age of menarche in a CF population was 14.9 years, but even women with a good clinical status had menarchal delay, most severe in those homozygous for delta F508.[17]

In women with CF, luteinizing hormonal changes at puberty are the same as the normal population. However for reasons that are not fully understood, FSH changes appear to occur at lower levels, with pubertal levels reached 2 years later than the normal population perhaps explaining the delayed menarche. Recent studies have shown that the cystic fibrosis transmembrane conductance regulator (*CFTR*) gene is expressed in the hypothalamus and it is possible that this may have a bearing on the release of gonadotrophin-releasing hormone.[18] Additionally, CFTR is expressed in the cervix, uterus, ovary, and fallopian tubes, and it has been hypothesized that it could also be involved in two conditions associated with reduced fertility, namely polycystic ovaries and hydrosalpix.[19,20] Recent animal studies have examined the possible influence of CF on fertility. Two mouse models of CF were demonstrated to have fewer pups per litter and fewer litters over a 5-month period than wild type females.[21]

Women with CF have an anatomically normal reproductive tract and therefore it is prudent to assume everyone is fertile and all women should be given appropriate contraception advice. In some women with CF, a low BMI may be associated with anovulatory cycles and secondary amenorrhea. It is also possible that changes in the properties of cervical mucus may also inhibit fertilization. Reduced water content in the cervical mucus of women with CF as compared to controls has been demonstrated and the normal mid-cycle increase in water content of cervical mucus, leading to a more profuse cervical discharge, is not observed in patients with CF.[22] Instead, a thicker, sticky mucus plug forms which is likely to provide a greater obstruction to any sperm. However, although this data are frequently referred to it may no longer be relevant as the general health status of individuals with CF 30 years ago is not comparable with the CF population today. Earlier data also report biochemical analysis of the cervical mucus showing markedly reduced sodium content in women with CF, but there are no up-to-date specific functional studies that have formally demonstrated this.[23]

Women with CF who are unable to fall pregnant should be offered the same appropriate infertility investigation and support as women without CF. In women with severe disease it is essential that prepregnancy counseling is detailed, direct, and should involve the partner. There may be ethical debate in treating this group of women and it may be appropriate, if assisted conception is considered, to refer to the local ethics committee. Intrauterine insemination has been used successfully to overcome abnormal cervical mucus and successful assisted conception has been reported.[24,25] The majority of women with CF today are planning a life similar to their peer group and, more often than not, that includes starting a family. Although the majority of women conceive naturally, there are still a small percent who require help and in a recent series over 10% of conceptions in 48 CF pregnancies resulted from IVF.[26]

CONTRACEPTION AND CYSTIC FIBROSIS

It is not possible to predict the fertility of any one individual, irrespective of when their menarche occurred or the regularity or otherwise of their menstrual cycle. Therefore, it is vital that all young women with CF have appropriate counseling regarding contraception. The issues of education regarding reproductive and genetic knowledge among adolescents and adults with CF should provide an easy link to contraception. Although the current evidence would suggest that pregnancy does not have a detrimental effect on the progression of CF, a pregnancy undoubtedly imposes a bigger treatment burden on the individual. In addition, the responsibilities of parenthood may weigh very heavily on a young girl with an existing chronic and life-limiting condition. It is essential that the responsibility for discussing contraception falls not only on the individual's parents but also on the CF teams, pediatric and adult, responsible for her care. Despite the explosion of knowledge regarding CF, the frequent hospital visits and contacts with medical staff, understanding of the condition by patients themselves is perhaps surprisingly poor. One study reported that although 96% of female patients with CF knew they were able to have children, only 65% thought it was harder for men and over a quarter were unsure whether it was harder for men or women. Furthermore, only 26% were aware of assisted reproduction techniques. It is clear that there is much work to be done to educate the CF population about reproductive matters.[27] The human papilloma virus (HPV) vaccine aimed at reducing the risk of developing cervical carcinoma is routinely administered to all girls between the ages of 12 and 14 years. This intervention could provide an ideal opportunity to discuss contraception and its importance.

Despite the enormous changes that pregnancy may impose on a woman with CF, the uptake of contraception is depressing low. In a study from Aberdeen, only 59% of sexually active women were found to be using some form of contraception, and more worryingly this compares unfavorably with the national UK average of 65%.[2] The rate of contraceptive use was a little better in a study from United States, where 70% of women were using contraception as compared to the national American rate of 62%.[28] Sadly, a recent survey from the United Kingdom showed that although 79% of women were sexually active, only half were using contraception. None of the women had considered sterilization, the use of the progesterone implants, or intrauterine devices (IUDs). Sixty-two percent reported that they had not received any contraceptive advice specific to CF and only half of the women reported that there had been a discussion regarding the potential impact of broad-spectrum antibiotics and the combined pill. One-third had experienced pregnancies of which a quarter was unplanned. It appears that some CF teams lack the training, knowledge, or perhaps the confidence to have a detailed discussion. As these women attend hospital on a frequent basis, this is a provision that could easily be improved, the annual review is an ideal time to ensure the issue of contraception is discussed.[2,28]

There are many contraceptive options and the decisions as to which to use should be individualized. From the outset it is important to stress that all forms of contraception are reversible and if one method proves unsuitable then other options should be considered. Barrier methods remain a very effective technique as they provide both a contraceptive effect and also significantly reduce the risk of sexually transmitted disease, including HPV, which is associated with cervical cancer and genital warts.

The combined oral contraception preparation (OCP) is the commonest choice in women with CF and in a recent study one quarter of women with CF used this form of contraception.[28] The combined preparation has a number of theoretical disadvantages, but evidence is accruing to suggest that it is both a safe and effective preparation. The main issue of OCP failure in the general population is poor adherence, although this seems to improve with age, from nearly 70% in 18–19 year olds to 85% in 30–34 year olds. This serves to stress the importance of encouraging good compliance in women with CF using the OCP, irrespective of their age.[29]

Other concerns regarding the OCP include the possible worsening of preexisting diabetes, malabsorption, and liver dysfunction. Theoretically, the progesterone component of the preparation may act as both a respiratory stimulant and potentially adversely affect mucus production and viscosity. Broad-spectrum antibiotics are commonly used in CF and there have been legitimate concerns regarding possible poor absorption and a loss of efficacy. However, in Archer's study there were no contraceptive failures despite the fact that 94% of the women were pancreatic insufficient.[29] This suggests malabsorption of the preparation is unlikely to be a significant issue; however, acute gastrointestinal upset should still be regarded as a time when extra precautions may be required.

A study by Fitzpatrick et al. (2004)[30] found the use of the OCP preparation caused no significant change in women's hormonal level function or clinical status. Pharmacokinetic studies of the contraceptive steroids, estradiol and levonorgestrel, found increased bioavailability of estrogen compensated for the increased body clearance of estradiol. It appeared that there were no significant changes in the pharmacokinetics of levonorgestrel. The contraceptive effect therefore of the OCP is likely to be the same as in healthy women; however, acute changes in health status and treatment regimes, such as the introduction of new antibiotics, means that contraceptive advice may need to be constantly reviewed.[31] Further pharmacokinetic data demonstrated that OCP plasma levels were not altered by a number of commonly used antibiotics including ampicillin, ciprofloxacin, clarithromycin, doxycycline, methotrexate, ofloxacin, roxithromycin, sitafloxacin, and tetracycline. In contrast, rifampicin and rifabutin have been shown to affect plasma hormone levels, and although these are less commonly used in routine care, patients being treated for nontuberculous mycobacteria must be counseled appropriately and offered alternative contraception.

Recently, the effects of estradiol and estriol on *Pseudomonas aeruginosa* in vitro and in vivo have been reported.[32] Both hormones are able to induce mucoid conversion of *P. aeruginosa* in vitro and were associated with increased clinical exacerbations and mucoid conversion in vivo. During the luteal phase of the menstrual cycle when estradiol levels are relatively low, nonmucoid *P. aeruginosa* was predominantly isolated from sputum during exacerbations, in comparison to increased proportions of mucoid

P. aeruginosa if exacerbations occurred during a time of higher estradiol levels in the follicular phase of the cycle. A study of the Cystic Fibrosis Registry of Ireland showed that OCP use was linked to a reduced antibiotic usage; this study is likely to stimulate further evaluation of the potential prophylactic benefits of OCP usage. It is not clear yet whether this apparent effect is simply due to increased compliance with all medications or a specific benefit conferred by the OCP.

The prevalence of the use of the IUD in the general population varies enormously from 0.7% in the United States, 6% in the United Kingdom, nearly 20% in France up to 51.8% in Uzbekistan. It is a highly acceptable form of contraception for many women. The more common copper device is associated with heavier menstrual loss following its insertion for the first 2 to 3 cycles although if this were to persist at a level compromising the individual's well-being or quality of life, it can be removed. IUDs may not be suitable for women with borderline iron reserve and the small risk of infection (2%) can be reduced by prophylactic antibiotic use at the time of insertion.[33]

The other type of device is the progesterone intrauterine system, which has been a major advance for many women. It acts by releasing levonorgestrel directly into the uterine cavity causing endometrial thinning. Contraceptively, it has an excellent record and is certainly the treatment of choice for many women with heavy menstrual loss. The progestogen is released locally and therefore systemic side effects are rarely reported. It is also used beneficially in women with endometriosis and there is some evidence that the risk of pelvic inflammatory disease is also reduced. The major drawback is that for the first 2 to 6 months following insertion it may cause irregular and persistent bleeding. It may also be a little more difficult to insert into the nulliparous woman; however, with the additional use of local anesthesia, it can be safely inserted in the vast majority of cases. The progesterone intrauterine system provides excellent contraception and lightens periods for up to 5 years, although as with other devices, if the bleeding pattern becomes unacceptable it can be removed. Less commonly used techniques include the transdermal contraceptive patches; Depo-Provera preparations, which are administered every 3 months; and vaginal rings. Progesterone implants such as Nexplanon or Implanon are increasingly popular. They consist of a small rod about 4 cm long and 2 mm in diameter, which is inserted on the inner aspect of the arm in the subdermal tissue. They provide excellent contraception and the failure rate is less than 0.05%, which is less than tubal ligation. The device lasts for 3 years and can be removed earlier if necessary. It is associated with irregular bleeding and some women complain of weight gain, acne, or breast tenderness.

Sterilization (tubal ligation) may be requested and there are now hysteroscopic techniques involving the placement of a small implant (microinsert) in each fallopian tube, which can be performed under local anesthetic, bypassing the need for a potentially riskier laparoscopic procedure.

PREGNANCY

PHYSIOLOGICAL CHANGES IN PREGNANCY AND CYSTIC FIBROSIS

Normal pregnancy is associated with many physiological changes of the respiratory system (Table 28.2). Although healthy women may cope with these changes, they can impose an undue burden on women whose respiratory function is already severely compromised. Similarly, the physiological changes in the cardiovascular and metabolic systems that accompany pregnancy may also be less well tolerated in women with CF.

In pregnancy, the significant increase in resting lung volume may represent a homeostatic response to the increased oxygen consumption and carbon dioxide burden. The degree of hyperventilation observed however exceeds that required to satisfy metabolic demands and adequate gas exchange and it is possible that this may be due to the respiratory stimulant effect of circulating progesterone, which sensitizes the medulla oblongata to carbon dioxide.

Although diaphragmatic function and inspiratory lung capacity increase, overall vital capacity and total lung capacity change little due to a similar reduction in the functional residual capacity of 10%–25%. This is a result of a reduction in the residual volume and end expiratory volume.[34] It has been suggested that the reduced functional residual capacity results in closure of small airways at the lung bases during normal breathing, perhaps contributing to impaired gas exchange.[35] Pulmonary function changes may be of little significance in the normal pregnant woman; however, in a woman with CF with borderline pulmonary function they are likely to reduce the efficiency of gas exchange inducing a degree of hypoxemia and contribute to pulmonary decompensation. Chronic hypoxia is associated with fetal growth restriction and preterm delivery.

Cardiovascular changes occur early in normal pregnancy initially manifested by a fall in vascular resistance.

Table 28.2 Changes in respiratory function in normal pregnancy

Lung function	Change by term
FEV$_1$	Unchanged
Peak expiratory flow	Unchanged
Total lung capacity	4% Decreased
Expiratory reserve	200 mL Decreased
Residual volume	20% Decreased
Functional residual capacity	1%–20% Decreased
Tidal volume	40% Increased
Inspiratory capacity	300 mL Increased
Oxygen consumption	20%–33% Increased
Minute volume	30% Increased

FEV$_1$, forced expiratory volume in 1 second.

In a singleton pregnancy, the plasma volume at term is approximately 50% greater than that seen in a nonpregnant individual. The cardiac output begins to rise from 10 weeks gestation, reaching a plateau at the end of the second trimester, 30%–50% above the nonpregnant value.[36,37] This rise is a consequence of both an increased stroke volume and heart rate, the latter increasing from as early as 5 weeks gestation to 10–15 beats per minute over the baseline pulse. Once again these changes are usually well tolerated in the normal individual; however in women with CF, particularly those who have developed pulmonary hypertension, the increased cardiovascular demands may cause right ventricular decompensation and cardiovascular collapse. This phenomenon is more likely to be seen immediately following delivery due to the process of autotransfusion that occurs following the delivery of the placenta. Pulmonary hypertension associated with pregnancy is a grave condition carrying with it a maternal mortality as high as 50%. It is sometimes found in late-stage disease and although if a pregnancy occurs under these circumstances, the significant maternal risks should be clearly spelt out.

The normal weight gain in pregnancy is variable and is approximately 10–14 kg. The total energy requirement has been calculated to be between 80,000 and 124,000 kcal. The three major components of energy expenditure are fetal and reproductive tissue growth, the deposition of new maternal fat stores, and increased maternal metabolism. This represents a rise in dietary requirements of approximately 50–100 kcal/d in early pregnancy rising to 200–300 kcal/d from 36 weeks gestation. There is considerable individual variation, even in a normal healthy population. Poorly nourished women adapt by reducing their metabolic rate and fat production, although these adaptations may compromise fetal well-being.[38] As well as nutritional concerns the normal hormonal and physical changes that occur in pregnancy increase the likelihood of nausea and vomiting in the early stages. Women with a normal BMI are likely to tolerate associated weight loss more readily than those with a reduced BMI. Additionally, in late pregnancy, problems of dyspepsia and reflux are frequent and may exacerbate pre-pregnancy problems.

In a survey of North American CF centers, maternal weight gain in pregnancy was less than 4.5 kg in 41% of the patients.[39] In a UK study reporting 26 term and 22 pre-term live deliveries in women with CF, the mean maternal weight gain of those pregnancies reaching term was 8.9 kg and only 2.6 kg in those delivering prematurely.[40] Similarly, the mean maternal weight gain in pregnancy reported from the French Registry was only 5.5 kg.[41] The additional caloric requirements in women with CF can be difficult to achieve and supplemental feeding may be required. In one hospital, 6 of 15 women received total parenteral nutrition with indications including inadequate weight gain or intractable nausea and vomiting.[42]

In normal pregnancy significant changes in estrogens, progesterone, and human placental lactogen result in a degree of impaired glucose tolerance. The reduced renal threshold for glucose and an increased glomerular filtration rate in pregnancy results in glycosuria in up to 50% of pregnant women. Glucose tolerance may already be impaired in women with CF and insulin-dependent CF-related diabetes occurs in 8%–12% of patients. Therefore, the development of gestational diabetes will be more common, particularly in the second half of pregnancy when woman become increasingly resistant to insulin. In a study of 92 pregnancies in women with CF, the prevalence of gestational diabetes was 14%, considerably higher than the normal pregnant population.[43] Screening for diabetes in CF pregnancies should be vigilant, a random blood glucose at booking followed at 26 weeks gestation by a full glucose tolerance test is recommended as currently nearly one-third of pregnant mothers with CF require insulin.[26,42]

Although the consequences of impaired glucose tolerance on pregnancy are debated, insulin requiring diabetes is associated with worse pregnancy outcomes for both mother and baby. Women with preexisting diabetes should, therefore, be counseled to ensure their diabetic control is optimal prepregnancy and remains under tight control throughout the pregnancy.

PREGNANCY AND CYSTIC FIBROSIS

The first reported case of CF in pregnancy in 1960 provides a salutatory reminder of the difficulties involved in such pregnancies. A 20-year-old female who was believed to have an underlying diagnosis of bronchiectasis fell pregnant. A sweat test during pregnancy confirmed the diagnosis of CF. The patient remained well until the 34th week of gestation, she experienced worsening respiratory symptoms, labored spontaneously, and delivered a baby in good condition. The patient's symptoms failed to resolve postnatally and 6 weeks after delivery, despite active intervention she died.[44] This report was reviewed with other early cases, and although the data made scanty reference to objective respiratory function, two distinct populations appeared to emerge.[45] In 5 of 10 women, the pregnancy did not appear to have an adverse effect on the course of maternal disease. None of the mothers in this group were diabetic; in four cases, the pregnancy went to term and there was no significant decline in their lung function. However, of the other five women, two had diabetes; all delivered prematurely and suffered a loss of lung function postnatally. Additionally, one stillbirth and one neonatal death occurred, two women died in the immediate postpartum period, and two others died within 18 months of delivery. The conclusion of this review was that although pregnancy was possible in women with CF, there appeared to be both an increased risk of fetal prematurity, a loss of maternal lung function, and even loss of life, in those with a more severe preexisting disease. Similar findings were reported in small subsequent studies.[46,47]

In view of the potentially devastating consequences of an unwanted pregnancy in women with severe CF, some authors have advocated termination of pregnancy in women with poor lung function (forced expiratory volume in 1 second [FEV$_1$] of less than 50%) or progressive pulmonary deterioration.[48] Successful term pregnancies have been achieved in women with poor lung function and it has been suggested that stable prepregnancy lung function may be the key.[49]

There have been a number of subsequent reviews examining retrospective data, which have been inconsistently reported with many of the earlier ones containing nonspecific information regarding pulmonary function. Since 1990 specific data relating to the number of pregnancies and their outcomes have been collected by the US Cystic Fibrosis Registry. Thus, in 111 pregnancies reported in 1990, 48% of the pregnancies were completed, 32% of women underwent a therapeutic termination, and, at the time of reporting, 31% of the pregnancies were still progressing.[50] Of the completed pregnancies nearly a quarter were preterm and diabetes mellitus was reported in 5% of the pregnant group. A larger series described the outcomes of 217 pregnancies in 162 women.[51] The overall rate of miscarriage was 5% and the rate of termination of pregnancy was 14%, although it is possible that this figure may have been under reported. In 82% of the cases, the pregnancy progressed past 20 weeks gestation. Nearly a quarter of the pregnancies (24%) delivered preterm, as a consequence of onset of spontaneous labor, rather than of induced labor or maternal complications. It was suggested that this may be due to the effect of chronic hypoxia in the fetus or poor maternal nutrition and pancreatic insufficiency. Startlingly 8% of the mothers died within 6 months of delivery and 14% within 2 years. Once again, the study appeared to confirm the association between maternal death and poor prepregnancy lung function. The fetal perinatal death rate was 8%, with the commonest cause of fetal death being extreme prematurity.

Edenborough et al.[52] were the first to report the outcome of such pregnancies together with objective lung function measurements. Their data reinforced the earlier conclusions that patients with milder CF and good nutritional status were able to tolerate pregnancy well. In contrast those with worse lung function, hepatic or pancreatic involvement, pulmonary hypertension, and reduced BMI were at a significantly increased risk from the pregnancy. A reduction of 13% in FEV$_1$ and 11% in forced vital capacity during pregnancy were reported, although most of this was regained following delivery. In those with moderate to severe lung disease, which was defined as an FEV$_1$ < 70%, there was an increased risk of preterm delivery and increased loss of lung function as compared to those with more mild disease. The authors advised against pregnancy in severe disease (FEV$_1$ < 50%).

In the largest single-center study of 46 pregnancies that continued beyond the first trimester, fetal outcomes were extremely good with all babies surviving.[26] There was an increased risk of fetal prematurity and cesarean section. Prematurity in the majority of cases was iatrogenic due to concerns regarding maternal well-being, but neonatal expertise has given clinicians confidence that early delivery is still associated with good outcomes.

LONG-TERM EFFECT OF PREGNANCY

Seven studies have addressed the long-term effects of pregnancy on CF. As the prognosis continues to improve, the number of cases will continue to grow. Much of the data are retrospective, but it is becoming more robust and women are being matched with nonpregnant controls. Interestingly, the conclusions of five of the earlier studies were very similar. The studies provide little direct evidence for a statistically significant loss of lung function due to pregnancy as compared to nonpregnant matched controls.[41,52–57] All studies agreed that in women with good preexisting lung function, pregnancy is generally well tolerated. However, data from the French CF Registry concluded that although pregnancy probably has a slight adverse effect on the health of CF women, in the group of women with poor prepregnancy lung function, the risk of preterm delivery was significantly greater and there was a greater risk of significant loss of lung function. Fifteen percent of women still died within 3 years of their pregnancy and all three women who had an FEV_1 of less than 50% before pregnancy died within a year.[41]

The largest parallel-cohort study, by a considerable margin, studied women from the US CF Registry from 1985 to 1997. This study of 680 pregnant women with CF, matched to over 3000 control women with CF, concluded that woman with CF who became pregnant had a better 10-year survival rate than women who had not been pregnant. This was also the conclusion in the subgroups of women with poor lung function ($FEV_1 < 40\%$) and insulin-dependent diabetes.[56] The study was able to quantify that 20% of women would fail to see their child's 10th birthday and in those with severe disease, 40% would have died. In a more recent UK study, similar findings were reported with 50% of women with poor lung function ($FEV_1 < 50\%$) dying within 8 years of delivery.[26] Analysis of data from the Epidemiologic Study of Cystic Fibrosis concluded from a matched study of 119 pregnant women with a median 6-year follow-up that pregnancy and motherhood did not accelerate disease progression. However, there was an increase in pulmonary exacerbations and hospital visits.[57]

PREPREGNANCY COUNSELING

Encouraging young women with CF to feel confident in discussing their reproductive plans with the CF team is an important step in planning a safe and successful pregnancy. Where discussion and joint decision making is encouraged, pregnancy preparations are more useful. The mass of complex information relating to pregnancy requires consideration and is best undertaken prior to pregnancy with the woman's partner involved in all discussions whenever possible. Counseling needs to be individualized as each couple will have a different background, belief system, and level of knowledge (Table 28.1). The genetic implications of the disease, the risk of inheritance, and options of investigation need to be discussed. Genotyping the partner and

genetic counseling should take place as early as possible. Prenatal testing by chorionic villus sampling or amniocentesis may be offered. These discussions will be most difficult for individuals with poor lung function as couples will have to consider issues such as deteriorating disease status, life expectancy, and being left as a single parent. In addition, the potentially adverse neonatal implications of a very premature delivery, including the risk of long-term handicap should be considered.

Counseling should be honest and straightforward, but couples should be left in no doubt of the commitment they are embarking on. The pregnancy itself will require a much greater demand on their time, with additional monitoring and hospital visits. Postnatally, mothers must understand that their role as parents still needs to be balanced between caring for a baby and the considerable treatment burden of a chronic and progressive disease. Despite these conflicts, whatever decisions prospective parents may make, they must feel supported by the CF team.

OBSTETRIC MANAGEMENT

The role of the obstetrician is to become one part of the CF multidisciplinary team providing care for the individual. Coordinating the healthcare professionals involved in patient care is important to ensure good interprofessional communication between the extended team which should an obstetrician, midwives and, specialist anesthetist.

Once a woman becomes pregnant, the normal aspects of antenatal care should not be forgotten. This includes offering screening tests for maternal blood group and possible congenital infections, such as rubella, hepatitis, syphilis, and human immunodeficiency virus. Toxoplasmosis is routinely screened for in Europe and in the United States, but not in the United Kingdom. The risk of chromosomal anomalies should be discussed and offered. Diabetes should be screened for with a full glucose tolerance test and in the preexisting diabetic meticulous glucose control should be maintained. Serial ultrasound scans to look for possible evidence of fetal growth restriction, and assessment of the uterine and fetal circulation by Doppler ultrasound can help to provide information about the maternal and fetal well-being.

Regular outpatient attendance at both the CF and obstetric clinics requires additional hospital visits, but if these prove difficult where possible support at home should be provided by the CF team, particularly in the latter stages of the pregnancy. Women should be encouraged to attend antenatal classes, although any concerns related to CF should be discussed with the CF team or obstetrician. Careful liaison throughout the pregnancy with the CF team permits appropriate outpatient or inpatient management. Infective exacerbations should be aggressively treated with intravenous antibiotics; this may require liaison with the pharmacist to ensure the most appropriate antibiotic regimen. The mother should be offered the opportunity to meet the obstetric anesthetists to understand the level of

and refined anesthetic management during surgery, which can be challenging. Principles of anesthetic management include light premedication and anxiolysis in the anesthetic room, standard cardiothoracic monitoring, generally insertion of central venous and pulmonary artery catheters under anesthesia with continuous monitoring of cardiac output, and mixed venous oxygen saturation. We routinely use transesophageal echocardiography to evaluate right and left ventricular function and pulmonary artery and venous flows following anastomoses. Ventilation strategies include avoidance of dynamic hyperinflation, permissive hypercapnia according to patient's preexisting condition, and avoidance of barotrauma. During single lung ventilation, inhaled pulmonary vasodilators such as prostacyclin and nitric oxide are used routinely and an aggressive regime of inotropic and vasoconstrictor support is employed. Particular attention is placed on management of pulmonary artery clamping, adequacy of one lung ventilation, de-airing, reperfusion, and postreperfusion shunt management. Recently, we have included measurement of intracerebral oxygenation on a routine basis.

Our approach to postoperative pain control includes a standard placement of a thoracic epidural catheter, which is usually inserted in the intensive care unit once coagulation indexes are within normal limits. If at all possible, patients are extubated within the first 24 hours after surgery. Although possible, we do not advocate extubation in the operating theater, as we prefer to stabilize and assess all patients on the intensive care unit first.

PERIOPERATIVE MANAGEMENT

The aim of management in the early transplant period is to treat any primary graft dysfunction (PGD), initiate effective immunosuppression, minimize the risk of infection, protect other organ systems (such as kidneys and bowels), and rehabilitate the patient as rapidly as possible. This requires close liaison between transplant physicians, surgeons, and intensive care staff, together with experienced nursing staff and physiotherapists as well as support from microbiologists, pathologists, and radiologists, experienced in thoracic organ transplantation. Detailed information on donor management, organ retrieval and preservation, and surgical techniques is beyond the scope of this chapter.

PRIMARY GRAFT DYSFUNCTION

PGD is manifest as reduced arterial oxygen to fraction of inspired oxygen (PaO_2/FiO_2) ratio in the early postoperative period.[28] It is not only a consequence of tissue ischemia during lung retrieval, preservation process, and lung reperfusion during surgery but also an inflammatory response due to injury to the donor lung before retrieval.[29,30] It is a major cause of mortality in the first 30 days following transplantation. The presence of PGD has also been associated with an increased risk of late graft dysfunction.

Treatment is mostly supportive with ventilatory support such as in acute respiratory distress syndrome with low tidal volumes, permissive hypercapnia, care of the patient in the prone position, and maintaining a negative fluid balance as long as this does not unduly affect renal function in the presence of nephrotoxic immunosuppression and antibiotics. As well as in the preoperative situation, extracorporeal support with ECMO or Novalung can be used successfully to support gas exchange while recovery of lung function occurs.[31]

Evidence for pharmacological intervention in PGD is lacking. Nitric oxide may produce an improvement in gas exchange in those patients with PGD and elevated pulmonary artery pressure.[32–35] Surfactant used to treat lungs prior to retrieval has shown some effects on late recovery but no early effect on gas exchange,[36] and further study is required to evaluate this expensive treatment.

IMMUNOSUPPRESSION

Immunosuppression following lung transplantation is achieved with an initial induction phase followed by maintenance and therapeutic drug monitoring. Induction was previously achieved with polyclonal antithymocyte globulins. Given at the time of organ transplantation, these immunoglobulins cause profound depletion of circulating lymphocytes. Use of antithymocyte globulin has now largely been supplanted by human-murine chimeric monoclonal antibodies that inhibit T-cell proliferation by binding to the interleukin (IL)-2 receptor. These agents may reduce the risk of rejection during the first month post transplant and allow for slower introduction of other CNIs to aid in renal recovery after surgery, but this may be at the expense of increased severity of infection or later increased incidence of malignancy.[37] There is no current consensus about the routine usage of induction immunosuppression.

Patients also receive loading doses of maintenance immunosuppression with a CNI, an antimetabolite, and steroids. Tacrolimus and ciclosporin are CNIs: metabolites of these drugs bind to cytoplasmic calcineurin and therefore interfere with the transcription of various cytokines, including IL-2, -3, -4, and -5; tumor necrosis factor-α; interferon-γ; and granulocyte/macrophage colony stimulating factor and therefore inhibit T-cell stimulation.[38,39] Cell cycle inhibitors (azathioprine, mycophenolate mofetil) interfere with DNA and RNA synthesis, and purine synthesis, thereby inhibiting proliferation of T- and B-lymphocytes.

The choice of immunosuppressive regimen varies between lung transplant centers probably because immunosuppressive regimens following lung transplantation are based on trials in kidney transplant recipients and thereafter on clinical experience. There have been relatively few large trials in lung transplant recipients, and these have not shown dramatic differences in outcomes related to immunosuppressant choice. In practice, centers tailor maintenance regimen according to side effects, drug toxicity, and incidence of opportunistic infections in individuals.

INFECTION TREATMENT AND PROPHYLAXIS

Infections occurring in the perioperative period are commonly with either donor- or recipient-derived organisms,[40,41] surgical wound infections, intravenous line-associated infections, or gastrointestinal infections with *Clostriodium difficile* probably as a consequence of the intensive antibiotic therapy required to prevent systemic infections from recipient-derived organisms.

Appropriate intravenous antibiotic treatment is essential at the time of lung transplantation for CF, and these antibiotics will normally be continued until the patient is mobilizing and able to clear their secretions.[42,43] Nebulized antibiotic therapy is continued at least in the immediate post-transplant period to try to prevent reinfection of the lungs with pathogenic organisms from the upper airways.[44] This long-term treatment has become more common as there is increasing evidence of a link between chronic post-transplantation endobronchial infection with *Pseudomonas* and subsequent development of BOS.

Care must be taken when explanting lungs to guard against contamination of the thoracic cavity by airway secretions. It may be prudent at explantation to electively wash out the thoracic cavity, either with saline or with an antiseptic solution.[45] The use of antifungal prophylaxis for those known to be colonized with fungi pretransplantation can reduce the postoperative rate of fungal infections.[46] Cytomegalovirus (CMV) remains an important organism following lung transplantation due to both the systemic illness and tissue injury to the graft and also the potential consequences of the infection including acute and chronic rejection through enhanced graft recognition by host defenses. It is our practice to offer universal CMV prophylaxis for high- and moderate-risk cases with oral valganciclovir (Roche, Welwyn Garden City, United Kingdom).

INTENSIVE CARE MANAGEMENT AND REHABILITATION

The patient is invariably ventilated for a few hours post transplantation. At this time, inotropic support is also often necessary, particularly if the operation was performed on CPB. It is important at this stage to pay meticulous attention to fluid balance to on the one hand avoid pulmonary edema in the newly transplanted lungs, which unsurprisingly seem to have increased vascular permeability, and on the other hand avoid hypovolemic insults to the kidneys and other organs. Careful monitoring of renal function is necessary, particularly as the patients will be receiving a CNI and potentially nephrotoxic antibiotics on a background of subnormal renal function due to cystic-fibrosis related diabetes (CFRD) and repeated courses of aminoglycoside antibiotics.

Many patients will have a temporary paralytic ileus early post transplantation, but as soon as nasogastric feeding is being absorbed as judged by a lack of aspirates from the nasogastric tube during feeding institution of laxatives and pancreatic enzyme replacement therapy is essential to avoid progression to distal ileal obstruction syndrome. For this reason, most centers commence small volumes of enteral feeds very early post transplantation, along with stimulant and osmotic laxatives.

Many patients undergoing cadaveric organ transplantation can be extubated within the first 24 hours post transplantation. It is then essential that they begin to mobilize and, in particular, that they clear respiratory secretions. Delay in extubation can occur for a number of reasons including PGD, other difficulty in ventilation due to retained secretion or anastomotic air leak, postoperative bleeding or hemodynamic instability, or delayed neurological recovery. It is highly desirable to perform an early tracheostomy in this situation to allow the patient to be supported by the ventilator while conscious and performing active airways clearance and rehabilitation.

Following extubation, the goal is to rehabilitate the patient; reduce antimicrobial treatments to the maintenance prophylactic regimen and stabilize immunosuppression levels; monitor graft function for complications, the most common of which are lower respiratory infection and acute rejection; and finally prepare the patient for discharge. Most centers will perform at least one transbronchial biopsy and lavage prior to the patient being discharged. The typical inpatient stay following an uncomplicated transplant is about 3–6 weeks and slightly longer in subjects who have other medical conditions, or those who have particularly difficult preoperative microbiology. Clinical psychologists may be involved in effective preparation for discharge planning with patients post lung transplantation, to optimize psychological well-being.[47] Post lung transplantation, individuals may have heightened anxiety about returning home and reintegrating into home and work roles. The risk of developing posttraumatic stress disorder following intensive care has led to suggestions for continued monitoring of individuals' psychological well-being post lung transplantation, with a view to enhancing quality of life.[48] In addition, clinical psychologists help individuals post transplantation to adjust to their new health status, including identifying future goals, building a new sense of self, and acknowledging any symptoms of survivor guilt, in terms of both the donor and peers on the transplant waiting list.

POST-TRANSPLANT MANAGEMENT

The common complications following lung transplantation are the development of BOS, opportunistic infections, and other long-term side effects of immunosuppressive medications. Less frequently, anastomotic complications or malignancies, principally post-transplant lymphoproliferative disease (PTLD) and skin malignancies, occur.[1] The goal of post-transplant management is to maintain adequate immunosuppression, protect the graft from nonimmune insults, protect other organ systems from the consequences of immunosuppressive therapy (particularly renal failure), and monitor for complications.

BRONCHIOLITIS OBLITERANS SYNDROME: MANAGEMENT AND RISK FACTORS

Obliterative bronchiolitis (OB) remains the leading cause of morbidity and late mortality after lung transplantation. The 1-, 3-, and 5-year prevalences of BOS are reported as 10%, 30%, and 45%, respectively, and they progress at a very variable rate to respiratory failure.[49] True OB is diagnosed histologically with irreversible airflow obstruction by fibroproliferative cells occluding the airways. However, adequate biopsies are not always easy to obtain. It is rarely possible to get adequate tissue samples from transbronchial biopsy, and open lung biopsy is a hazardous procedure in patients who already have respiratory compromise. Therefore, the transplant community has adopted the term BOS as the clinical correlate of OB.[50,51] BOS is defined by an irreversible fall in lung function when other causes are excluded and is graded from BOS 0P to BOS 3 (Table 29.2). OB and BOS have previously been described as a form of chronic rejection. However, it is likely that there are many factors that contribute to the development of BOS. Some episodes of deterioration in lung function are reversible, and so the term chronic allograft dysfunction is being used to describe a spectrum of conditions (Table 29.3) that

can be investigated and treated rather than uniformly giving more immunosuppression for BOS when it was thought to be simply immune-mediated injury to the lung.

However, careful attention to adequate immunosuppression remains important. The great majority of lung transplant recipients remain on three maintenance immunosuppressive agents lifelong.[49] Typically, one of these will be a CNI, one will be a cell cycle inhibitor, and the third will be prednisolone. The most important side effect of these agents is that they cause a predisposition to opportunistic infections, and the incidence of malignancy is increased. In addition, however, they have a number of specific side effects, which are listed in Table 29.4.

CNIs have a narrow therapeutic window and significant side effects. Absorption after oral administration is poor and can be even poorer in patients with CF. Available CNI is given twice daily, and dosage adjustment is performed dependent on trough blood levels. However, there is increasing evidence that trough levels do not reflect systemic exposure, as assessed by a full pharmokinetic profile over 12 hours (AUC 0-12).[52,53] Once-daily preparations of tacrolimus are now available and may have advantages with compliance.[54] However, changes in drug formulations whether to slow release preparations or to generic formulations now that tacrolimus is off license can lead to differences in the dosing schedule and different formulations should not be considered equivalent and careful monitoring of drug levels is necessary when changing between formulations.[55]

In nonrandomized studies, switching from ciclosporin to tacrolimus slowed the decline in lung function[56] and switching from azathioprine to mycophenolate had a similar effect,[57] but many centers use tacrolimus and mycophenolate as first-line agents now. Sirolimus and everolimus are newer antiproliferative immunosuppressant drugs that are not used immediately post transplantation due to adverse effects on wound healing but may later arrest the decline in spirometry.[58,59] Their major advantage is a lack of nephrotoxicity, and they have a role in providing immunosuppression in patients undergoing rapid deterioration in renal function due to CNIs.[60] Total lymphoid irradiation and extracorporeal photochemotherapy[61] may slow the decline

Table 29.2 BOS grading

Grade	Definition
BOS 0	$FEV_1 > 90\%$ of baseline and $MEF_{25-75} > 75\%$ of baseline
BOS 0-p	FEV_1 81%–90% of baseline and/or $FEF_{25-75} \leq 75\%$ of baseline
BOS 1	FEV_1 66%–80% of baseline
BOS 2	FEV_1 51%–65% of baseline
BOS 3	$FEV_1 \leq 50\%$ of baseline

Note: Baseline function is defined as the average of the two highest (not necessarily consecutive) measurements of FEV_1 obtained at least 3 weeks apart MEF, mid-expiratory flow.

Table 29.3 Classification of chronic lung allograft dysfunction

Lung allograft dysfunction					
LB/NRAD	ACR	AMR	Airway injury		RAS
			Inhalation	Infection (colonization)	
		GORD	Pollution		
Rx Azithromycin	Increased immunosuppression	?	Nissen fundoplication	? Infection prophylaxis	?
		BOS			

Note: ACR, acute cellular rejection; AMR, antibody-mediacted rejection; LB, lymphocytic bronchiolitis; NRAD, neutrophilic reversible airways dysfunction; RAS, restrictive allograft syndrome; ?, uncertain.

Table 29.4 Side effects of maintenance immunosuppression

Drug	Side effect
Ciclosporin	Nephrotoxicity
	Tremor
	Paresthesia/hypersensitivity
	Hypertension
	Hypercholesterolemia
	Hypertrichosis
	Gingival hypertrophy
Tacrolimus	Nephrotoxicity
	Tremor
	Paresthesia/hypersensitivity
	Hypertension
	Hypercholesterolemia
	Neurotoxicity
	Diabetes mellitus
	Alopecia
Prednisolone	Cushing's syndrome
	Dyspepsia
	Peptic ulceration
	Osteoporosis
	Proximal myopathy
	Increased appetite
	Neuropsychiatric effects
	Glaucoma, papilledema, cataracts
	Skin atrophy, striae, bruising, acne
Azathioprine	Bone marrow suppression
	Hypersensitivity reactions
Mycophenolate mofetil	Bone marrow suppression
	Nausea, dyspepsia, diarrhea, constipation
	Hyperglycemia
	Hypercholesterolemia

Note: Only the commonest or most important side effects are listed.

in spirometry without systemic side effects. Addition of methotrexate may be helpful for some patients.[62] Nebulized ciclosporin may be helpful and is under evaluation.[63,64]

Risk factors for bronchiolitis obliterans syndrome

Acute immune-mediated injury to the lung is a strong risk factor for BOS and is the basis on which more immunosuppression is often given to patients developing BOS. Adherence to the medical regimen should always be considered when potent immunosuppressive drugs appear to be ineffective. Late or recurrent/refractory acute cellular rejection and lymphocytic bronchiolitis are both lesions associated with progression to BOS.[65] The severity of lymphocytic bronchiolitis has now been shown to predict long-term

outcomes after lung transplantation independent of acute vascular rejection.[66] It is likely that there is also a subset of patients with chronic neutrophilic airway inflammation who also go on to develop BOS. These patients often show an excess of neutrophils in bronchoalveolar lavage fluid and respond to treatment with macrolide antibiotics.[67,68]

The production of de novo donor-specific anti-HLA antibodies has recently been shown in a multivariate analysis to be a strong risk factor for BOS and death (authors' own data) and may represent a target for intervention either by antibody removal with treatments such as plasmapheresis or by pharmacological interventions with either directed therapy against plasma cells with bortezomib or nondirected therapy with rituximab and pooled immunoglobulins. Clinical efficacy of these approaches is the subject of a current evaluation.

Nonimmune insults such as gastroesophageal reflux[69] or airway infection or air pollution may lead to graft dysfunction, and aggressive intervention where possible may reverse this dysfunction or slow further decline.[70] However, prospective studies of interventions in BOS are lacking and the variable natural history of progression of OB makes evaluating treatments very difficult. Some of these patients stabilize and can continue for many years with limited lung function. Others develop steadily worsening graft dysfunction and progress to respiratory failure.[71]

Early interventions focusing on identifiable risk factors for BOS may be one of the reasons why long-term survival after lung transplantation is slowly improving. A number of centers have reported a very high prevalence of gastroesophageal reflux in transplant recipients, and a gratifying improvement in outcomes following surgical treatment of this reflux.[70] Infection prophylaxis and prompt attempts to identify infectious agents and aggressively treat them may also help to prevent progression of BOS.[72,73]

Repeat lung transplantation is rarely performed. The main reason for this is the shortage of donor organs and the potential additional risks involved in retransplantation. In particular, repeat surgery may be more difficult because of adhesions caused by the previous surgery and other systemic complications such as renal dysfunction are more prevalent. With donor shortage leading to a triage of donor organs to those with the highest expectation of the biggest benefits, transplant recipients rarely meet the criteria for a second transplantation. However, in patients without comorbidities due to long-term immunosuppression who meet the same criteria for surgery as individuals with a primary lung disease, retransplantation has been performed successfully.[74]

GRAFT MONITORING

After discharge, patients are recommended to monitor their own health and to report to the transplant center if they have any untoward symptoms. Patients are provided with portable spirometers and asked to record spirometry daily and report if their forced expiratory volume in 1 second

(FEV$_1$) falls by 10% or more. When a patient presents with acute respiratory symptoms, rapid diagnosis and treatment are essential. The clinical picture of early acute rejection is nonspecific and indistinguishable from an infection. Patients who have cough, malaise, low-grade pyrexia, or minor drop in lung function should be thoroughly evaluated.[75,76] Chest radiography may be normal in the presence of rejection, but even if changes are seen they do not distinguish between rejection and infection. Although fractional exhaled nitric oxide measurement has been proposed as a noninvasive marker of acute rejection, the sensitivity and specificity of this marker is still unclear. In most cases, urgent bronchoscopy, lavage, and transbronchial biopsy are indicated.[77–80] The biopsy is graded for the presence of rejection using a scoring system developed by the ISHLT.[81] The presence of infection on lavage should always be taken seriously.

Many transplant centers have traditionally performed surveillance bronchoscopies and biopsies in asymptomatic patients during the first year post transplantation. The value of these surveillance biopsies is uncertain. Although there is no doubt that surveillance bronchoscopy frequently shows asymptomatic mild rejection and asymptomatic mild infection, it is not yet clear whether the treatment of these abnormal findings has a positive impact on long-term outcome. In practice, there may be relatively little difference in the way patients are managed. In 1997, Tam and colleagues[82] reported a post hoc analysis of patients transplanted in the Papworth Centre. After surveillance biopsies were suspended, they described no difference in outcome for 75 patients who did not have surveillance biopsies compared with historical controls who did. However, the non-surveillance biopsy group had just as many biopsies in their first year as the historical controls, presumably because more frequent biopsies were performed during symptomatic episodes. The pickup rate of surveillance transbronchial biopsy has differed between published studies. Experience in a pediatric population at the Great Ormond Street suggests that the detection rate for infection or rejection is as high as 40% in asymptomatic subjects. The clinical significance of low-grade rejection is unknown. Hopkins et al. have prospectively analyzed 1159 transbronchial biopsies in 128 patients. Of these biopsies, 24% showed A1 rejection, of which the great majority of biopsies were in asymptomatic patients. Of these patients, 34.5% progressed to develop either high-grade acute rejection or lymphocytic bronchiolitis. In addition, 68% of patients who had multiple A1 lesions subsequently developed BOS, compared with 43% of patients who had one or fewer lesions.[83]

OPPORTUNISTIC INFECTIONS

Lung transplant recipients are in many ways surprisingly robust, and many do not even catch a cold from other members of the household. Due to lifelong immunosuppression it is often thought that infective symptoms must be due to atypical organisms, but community-acquired infections are in fact more likely to be due to common pathogens. However, the temptation to treat lung transplant recipients in the community can lead to delayed diagnosis of atypical infections and problems with drug interactions in those not experienced in prescribing immunosuppressive drugs. For these reasons, a referral back to the transplant center for evaluation of symptoms is preferable to empirical treatment in the community.

As well as the more usual bacterial pathogens, pseudomonal, fungal, and community-acquired viral infections are common. There is evidence that chronic infection of airways with Pseudomonas and Aspergillus promotes the development of BOS.[72,73] Therefore, the authors advocate continued use of nebulized antipseudomonal antibiotics (usually colistin) to prevent recolonization of transplanted lungs with Pseudomonas, which continues to colonize the sinuses. All patients receive some form of antifungal prophylaxis (either oral azole drugs or nebulized amphotericin, and oral nystatin).[84,85] Patients who are at high or medium risk for CMV activation receive prophylactic valganciclovir for approximately 3 months. Ongoing treatment with co-trimoxazole is also recommended as prophylaxis against Pneumocystis carinii pneumonia.

Community-acquired virus infections can be trivial or can be associated with severe chronic lung damage. The use of viral polymerase chain reaction (PCR) has improved diagnostic ability in a clinically relevant time frame and has brought some advantages. Recognizing a virus as the cause of graft dysfunction prevents inappropriate treatment for rejection given in the absence of a diagnosis as in the era prior to PCR availability. It also allows an opportunity for antiviral therapy in those with severe graft dysfunction. Respiratory syncytial virus and human metapneumovirus leading to a significant drop in lung function can be treated with ribavirin,[86] and adenovirus has responded to cidofovir. Influenza viruses can often be prevented with annual vaccination, which is strongly encouraged. Treatment with osetamilivir may shorten the duration of influenza infections that do occur. Viral pneumonitis diagnosed on transbronchial biopsy or computed tomography (CT) scanning of the chest can be treated with high-dose steroids and pooled immunoglobulins.[87] This approach is currently being evaluated.

The annual incidence of fungal infections in lung transplant recipients has recently been reported to be 18.8%.[88] Infections were most common in the first 6 months following transplantation and were more common in diabetic recipients and in those taking tacrolimus- or sirolimus-based immunosuppression compared with patients taking ciclosporin. More modern immunosuppressive regimens thought to be better at preventing acute cellular rejection may therefore be playing a role in increasing numbers of fungal infections. However, the high efficacy and low toxicity of oral azole drugs such as voriconazole allows early institution of treatment and has led to a very much reduced mortality compared to historical case series.[88] The necessity to monitor azole levels to improve efficacy and the differences between individuals in the metabolism of these drugs is currently being investigated at the authors' center.

NONINFECTIOUS COMPLICATIONS

Different complications exist in the early and late post-transplantation periods. Early complications are usually related to bronchial anastamosis.[89] In the absence of bronchial artery circulation, healing of the anastamosis is dependent on a retrograde blood supply from pulmonary collaterals. This healing can be further hampered by corticosteroids, or by post-transplant infections. In the early days of lung transplantation, early necrosis leading to subsequent stenosis, or even dehiscence, was an important complication. Improvement in surgical techniques, particularly performing the anastomosis more distally, has reduced the incidence of these complications. The commonest time for bronchial stenosis to develop is 2–4 months post transplantation. Treatment of choice is balloon dilatation, which often needs to be repeated to have a long-lasting effect.[89,90] If the stenosis is caused by granuloma formation, then repeated laser treatment or cryotherapy may also be of benefit.[91] If these techniques are unsuccessful, an expandable bronchial stent can be placed. This has the disadvantage of interrupting ciliary transport, and the stent itself may be a focus for infection or retention of secretions. Other early complications are damage to the phrenic nerve,[92] leading to impairment of diaphragmatic function, and damage to vagus nerve, which contributes to delayed gastric emptying.

Late complications following lung transplantation include an increased incidence of malignancy and CNI-induced renal impairment. PTLD is a heterogeneous condition that varies from a relatively benign proliferation of B-lymphocytes to monoclonal lymphoma. Although the majority of PTLD tumors are of B-cell origin, rare T-cell and other cell type tumors have been diagnosed. The incidence is higher in lung transplant recipients than in other solid organ recipients[93] and is higher in children than in adults, with a lifetime prevalence of 7% in pediatric lung transplant recipients. The majority of disorders are caused by a clonal expansion of B-cells infected with Epstein–Barr virus (EBV), because of loss of normal T-cell surveillance due to immunosuppression. Historically, PTLD has carried a high mortality, with a 1-year survival as low as 50%. With the introduction of the anti-B-cell monoclonal antibody (rituximab), outcomes have dramatically improved.[94]

Lifelong immunosuppression results in a higher incidence of other malignancies in transplant recipients and also contributes to these malignancies being more aggressive.[95] In addition to PTLD, the most common cancers in cardiothoracic transplant recipients are skin cancers, lung cancers, prostate cancer, and Kaposi's sarcoma. The usual risk factors for developing such cancers apply to transplant recipients also. Therefore, it is important to give transplant patients advice about environmental exposures that may predispose to these malignancies such as sunbathing, for example.

Renal impairment is extremely common post transplantation, because of long-term treatment with CNIs.[49] There is no difference in nephrotoxicity between ciclosporin and tacrolimus. Patients with CF are particularly at risk, because many of them have impaired renal function before they come to transplant probably due to repeated courses of aminoglycoside antibiotic treatment and the effect of diabetes on kidneys. Although this was previously seen mostly in adult CF transplant recipients, our recent experience has been that the majority of children with CF coming to transplant also have impaired renal function (author's own data). Treatment of renal failure can be extremely difficult. One approach has been to withdraw the CNI and give sirolimus or everolimus as an alternative immunosuppressant. Snell and colleagues have reported improved renal function in adult lung recipients with renal failure managed by this approach.[60] However, there are no data regarding the long-term efficacy of sirolimus in the maintenance of lung allografts, and such patients may therefore be at risk of acute rejection or BOS. Other noninfectious complications are listed in Table 29.4.

NONTRANSPLANT COMPLICATIONS

Subjects with CF who have transplants must still be monitored for all other CF-related complications. In particular, bone disease, diabetes mellitus, and growth failure are more common in transplant recipients than in the general CF population. It should also be remembered that following transplantation nonrespiratory complications, such as fat-soluble vitamin deficiency, salt depletion in hot weather, nasal polyps, CF-related diabetes, liver disease, and distal ileal obstruction, still occur.

LONG-TERM OUTCOMES

Lung transplantation brings huge improvements in functional status and a distinct survival benefit to recipients with many underlying lung diseases, but nowhere are these benefits more marked than in patients with CF-related lung disease. After the early mortality associated with lung transplantation patients transplanted for CF reach a survival benefit compared to waiting list survival after a few months.[96] This is in contrast to patients undergoing lung transplantation for other indications such as emphysema who take much longer post-transplant to reach a point where they have a survival benefit compared to waiting list survival.[97]

Despite impressive functional improvements and a survival benefit, lung transplant recipients still require lifelong medication and intensive hospital follow-up. However, bilateral lung transplantation leads to almost normal lung function at 1-year post transplant. More than 80% of survivors report no activity limitations at 3, 5, and 10 years.[1] Dramatic improvements in health-related quality of life have been noted, as measured by the St. Georges respiratory questionnaire, EQ5D, and SF-36.[98] Approximately half of lung transplant recipients under retirement age were in employment 5 years after lung transplantation.

Despite the large improvements in lung function and exercise capacity, the exercise capacity of lung transplant recipients does not return to normal. Proposed mechanisms include preoperative deconditioning and metabolic changes in muscles due to immunosuppression. Ventilatory factors do not limit exercise capacity, and this highlights the need for vigorous rehabilitation (preoperatively as well as postoperatively) to get the most from lung transplantation.[17,99,100]

SPECIFIC PEDIATRIC ISSUES

There are a number of small but important differences in how monitoring is performed in children compared to adults.

LUNG FUNCTION TESTING

Most children over the age of 4 years are able to perform spirometry successfully, provided they are given adequate training. It may be necessary to modify the outcome measures that are used (for example, by reporting $FEV_{0.75}$ rather than FEV_1). As well as performing spirometry on every clinic visit, most transplant centers provide the family with a portable spirometer that the child should use daily at home.

TRANSBRONCHIAL BIOPSY

If a child is suspected of having rejection or lower respiratory infection, then bronchoscopy and transbronchial biopsy should nearly always be performed. Preferably, this should be done as early as possible, prior to starting treatment. The technique employed varies between centers, with some preferring general anesthesia and others using sedation. General anesthesia with a laryngeal mask airway allows the use of adult-size (e.g., 4.9 mm) bronchoscopes even in preschool children. This allows adequate samples to be obtained.

RADIOLOGY

The new generation of multislice CT scanners allows rapid acquisition of high-resolution images with relatively little radiation exposure. General anesthesia is rarely necessary for this investigation, even in the youngest children. If high-resolution CT is to be used for monitoring graft structure in asymptomatic children, then it is essential that the protocol is modified from the normal adult settings so that the radiation dose is minimized.

INFECTIONS

This is one area where pediatric practice differs from adult practice. Many children will not have had previous exposure to common viruses, and the incidence of primary infection is much higher in them than in adults. It is therefore essential that immunization status is optimized prior to listing for transplantation. Following transplantation, the family should be given advice to keep their child away from outbreaks of measles, varicella, and so on and to seek advice if their child has been in contact with other children who may be infectious. PTLD is far more common in children than in adults, and in most cases it is related to reactivation of EBV infection. Although there are many centers that now monitor quantitative EBV load post transplantation, there is little evidence that viral load is related to subsequent development of PTLD.

GROWTH AND DEVELOPMENT

Many children who are referred for lung transplantation have growth failure secondary to chronic illness. Even if a transplant is successful, the use of maintenance corticosteroids post transplantation also affects linear growth. If the child has had no episodes of rejection, it is important to reduce the steroid dose to the lowest dose possible to allow catch-up growth. The use of growth hormone in these situations is controversial, as there is some laboratory evidence that it may trigger acute rejection. The transplanted lungs themselves grow as the child grows. There is some evidence from lung function testing and from CT that the airways of transplanted lungs grow with the child, but it is still unclear as to whether graft alveoli continue to multiply post transplant or whether they simply distend.

PSYCHOSOCIAL ISSUES

Many children coming for transplantation are physically and emotionally immature because of their chronic illness. A successful transplant allows a child to transform their life and catch up on many of the activities that were previously denied to them. Some children find this change in lifestyle difficult, particularly if it coincides with puberty.

Anecdotal reports from a number of centers suggest that survival rates post transplantation are steadily improving. Nonadherence to therapy is therefore becoming a proportionately greater cause of poor outcomes. This problem is particularly seen in teenage patients and appears worst in those who have a chronic illness like CF. There is limited evidence as to the best approach for assisting children in this position. However, most centers stress that adolescents should steadily take more responsibility for their own care and are given practical assistance to boost adherence to therapy. In addition, it is important to encourage adolescents to develop long-term goals and ambitions so that they have positive aims for the future.

In conclusion, monitoring of children post transplantation is broadly similar to that performed for adults. Techniques for some investigations need to be modified, and particular attention needs to be paid to viral infections, growth, and psychological development.

REFERENCES

1. Christie JD, Edwards LB, Kucheryavaya AY, Benden C, Dobbels F, Kirk R et al. The Registry of the International Society for Heart and Lung Transplantation: Twenty-eighth adult lung and heart-lung transplant report—2011. *J Heart Lung Transplant* 2011; **30**: 1104–22.

2. NHSBT. 2011. *NHSBT Transplant Activity in the UK Annual Report.* Retrieved 15/1/13, 2013, from http://www.organdonation.nhs.uk /statistics/transplant_activity_report/current _activity_reports/ukt/activity_report_2011_12.pdf.

3. Aurora P, Lynn IM. Lung transplantation and end of life issues in cystic fibrosis. *Paediatr Respir Rev* 2000; **1**: 114–20.

4. Steinman TI, Becker BN, Frost AE, Olthoff KM, Smart FW, Suki WN et al. Guidelines for the referral and management of patients eligible for solid organ transplantation. *Transplantation* 2001; **71**(9): 1189–204.

5. Aurora P. When should children be referred for lung or heart-lung transplantation? *Pediatr Pulmonol Suppl* 2004; **26**: 116–8.

6. Minai OA, Budev MM. Referral for lung transplantation: A moving target. *Chest* 2005; **127**: 705–7.

7. Audit UC. 2011. *UK Cardiothoracic Transplant Audit Annual Report.* Retrieved 15/1/13, 2013, from http://www.rcseng.ac.uk/surgeons/research /surgical-research/docs/uk-cardiothoracic-transplant -audit-report-2011/at_download/file.

8. Orens JB, Estenne M, Arcasoy S, Conte JV, Corris P, Egan JJ et al. International guidelines for the selection of lung transplant candidates: 2006 Update—a consensus report from the Pulmonary Scientific Council of the International Society for Heart and Lung Transplantation. *J Heart Lung Transplant* 2006; **25**: 745–55.

9. Egan TM, Murray S, Bustami RT, Shearon TH, McCullough KP, Edwards LB et al. Development of the new lung allocation system in the United States. *Am J Transplant* 2006; **6**: 1212–27.

10. Krinsley J. Perioperative glucose control. *Curr Opin Anaesthesiol* 2006; **19**: 111–6.

11. Zamora M, Edwards L, Weill D. Impact of cystic fibrosis related diabetes on lung transplant ourcomes. *J Heart Lung Transpl* 2004; **23**(2): S93.

12. Silverborn M, Jeppsson A, Martensson G, Nilsson F. New-onset cardiovascular risk factors in lung transplant recipients. *J Heart Lung Transplant* 2005; **24**: 1536–43.

13. Esposito C, De Mauri A, Vitulo P, Oggionni T, Cornacchia F, Valentino R et al. Risk factors for chronic renal dysfunction in lung transplant recipients. *Transplantation* 2007; **84**: 1701–3.

14. Takaoka ST, Weinacker AB. The value of preoperative pulmonary rehabilitation. *Thorac Surg Clin* 2005; **15**: 203–11.

15. Lands LC, Smountas AA, Mesiano G, Brosseau L, Shennib H, Charbonneau M et al. Maximal exercise capacity and peripheral skeletal muscle function following lung transplantation. *J Heart Lung Transplant* 1999; **18**: 113–20.

16. Pinet C, Cassart M, Scillia P, Lamotte M, Knoop C, Casimir G et al. Function and bulk of respiratory and limb muscles in patients with cystic fibrosis. *Am J Respir Crit Care Med* 2003; **168**: 989–94.

17. Wickerson L, Mathur S, Brooks D. Exercise training after lung transplantation: A systematic review. Crown 2010. Published by Elsevier, Inc. *J Heart Lung Transplant* 2010; **29**: 497–503.

18. Martinu T, Babyak MA, O'Connell CF, Carney RM, Trulock EP, Davis RD et al. Baseline 6-min walk distance predicts survival in lung transplant candidates. *Am J Transplant* 2008; **8**: 1498–505.

19. Rahman NM, Davies RJ, Gleeson FV. Pleural interventions: Management of acute and chronic pneumothorax. *Semin Respir Crit Care Med* 2008; **29**(4): 427–40.

20. Blondeau K, Mertens V, Vanaudenaerde BA, Verleden GM, Van Raemdonck DE, Sifrim D et al. Gastro-oesophageal reflux and gastric aspiration in lung transplant patients with or without chronic rejection. *Eur Respir J* 2008; **31**: 707–13.

21. Davis RD, Jr., Lau CL, Eubanks S, Messier RH, Hadjiliadis D, Steele MP et al. Improved lung allograft function after fundoplication in patients with gastroesophageal reflux disease undergoing lung transplantation. *J Thorac Cardiovasc Surg* 2003; **125**: 533–42.

22. McAnally KJ, Valentine VG, LaPlace SG, McFadden PM, Seoane L, Taylor DE. Effect of pre-transplantation prednisone on survival after lung transplantation. *J Heart Lung Transplant* 2006; **25**: 67–74.

23. Madden BP, Kariyawasam H, Siddiqi AJ, Machin A, Pryor JA, Hodson ME. Noninvasive ventilation in cystic fibrosis patients with acute or chronic respiratory failure. *Eur Respir J* 2002; **19**(2): 310–3.

24. Mason DP, Thuita L, Nowicki ER, Murthy SC, Pettersson GB, Blackstone EH. Should lung transplantation be performed for patients on mechanical respiratory support? The US experience. The American Association for Thoracic Surgery. Published by Mosby, Inc. *J Thorac Cardiovasc Surg* 2010; **139**: 765–773 e761.

25. Cypel M, Keshavjee S. Extracorporeal life support as a bridge to lung transplantation. Elsevier, Inc. *Clin Chest Med* 2011; **32**: 245–51.

26. Fuehner T, Kuehn C, Hadem J, Wiesner O, Gottlieb J, Tudorache I. Extracorporeal membrane oxygenation in awake patients as bridge to lung transplantation. *Am J Respir Crit Care Med* 2012; **185**: 763–8.

27. Egan TM, Kotloff RM. Pro/con debate: Lung allocation should be based on medical urgency and transplant survival and not on waiting time. *Chest* 2005; **128**: 407–15.

28. Christie JD, Carby M, Bag R, Corris P, Hertz M, Weill D. Report of the ISHLT Working Group on Primary Lung Graft Dysfunction part II: Definition. A consensus statement of the International Society for Heart and Lung Transplantation. *J Heart Lung Transplant* 2005; **24**: 1454–9.

29. Barr ML, Kawut SM, Whelan TP, Girgis R, Bottcher H, Sonett J et al. Report of the ISHLT Working Group on Primary Lung Graft Dysfunction part IV: Recipient-related risk factors and markers. *J Heart Lung Transplant* 2005; **24**: 1468–82.

30. de Perrot M, Bonser RS, Dark J, Kelly RF, McGiffin D, Menza R et al. Report of the ISHLT Working Group on Primary Lung Graft Dysfunction part III: Donor-related risk factors and markers. *J Heart Lung Transplant* 2005; **24**: 1460–7.

31. Hartwig MG, Appel JZ, 3rd, Cantu E, 3rd, Simsir S, Lin SS, Hsieh CC et al. Improved results treating lung allograft failure with venovenous extracorporeal membrane oxygenation. *Ann Thorac Surg* 2005; **80**: 1872–9; discussion 1879–80.

32. Date H, Triantafillou AN, Trulock EP, Pohl MS, Cooper JD, Patterson GA. Inhaled nitric oxide reduces human lung allograft dysfunction. *J Thorac Cardiovasc Surg* 1996; **111**: 913–9.

33. Garat C, Jayr C, Eddahibi S, Laffon M, Meignan M, Adnot S. Effects of inhaled nitric oxide or inhibition of endogenous nitric oxide formation on hyper-oxic lung injury. *Am J Respir Crit Care Med* 1997; **155**(6): 1957–64.

34. Murakami S, Bacha EA, Mazmanian GM, Detruit H, Chapelier A, Dartevelle P et al. Effects of various timings and concentrations of inhaled nitric oxide in lung ischemia-reperfusion. The Paris-Sud University Lung Transplantation Group. *Am J Respir Crit Care Med* 1997; **156**(2 Pt 1): 454–8.

35. Ardehali A, Laks H, Levine M, Shpiner R, Ross D, Watson LD et al. A prospective trial of inhaled nitric oxide in clinical lung transplantation. *Transplantation* 2001; **72**(1): 112–5.

36. Struber M, Fischer S, Niedermeyer J, Warnecke G, Gohrbandt B, Gorler A et al. Effects of exogenous surfactant instillation in clinical lung transplantation: A prospective, randomized trial. *J Thorac Cardiovasc Surg* 2007; **133**: 1620–5.

37. Brock MV, Borja MC, Ferber L, Orens JB, Anzcek RA, Krishnan J et al. Induction therapy in lung transplantation: A prospective, controlled clinical trial comparing OKT3, anti-thymocyte globulin, and daclizumab. *J Heart Lung Transplant* 2001; **20**: 1282–90.

38. Calne RY, Rolles K, White DJ, Thiru S, Evans DB, McMaster P et al. Cyclosporin A initially as the only immunosuppressant in 34 recipients of cadaveric organs: 32 Kidneys, 2 pancreases, and 2 livers. *Lancet* 1979; **2**: 1033–6.

39. Calne RY, Thiru S, McMaster P, Craddock GN, White DJ, Evans DJ et al. Cyclosporin A in patients receiving renal allografts from cadaver donors. 1978. *J Am Soc Nephrol* 1998; **9**(9): 1751–6.

40. Flume PA, Egan TM, Paradowski LJ, Detterbeck FC, Thompson JT, Yankaskas JR. Infectious complications of lung transplantation. Impact of cystic fibrosis. *Am J Respir Crit Care Med* 1994; **149**(6): 1601–7.

41. Avlonitis VS, Krause A, Luzzi L, Powell H, Phillips JA, Corris PA et al. Bacterial colonization of the donor lower airways is a predictor of poor outcome in lung transplantation. *Eur J Cardiothorac Surg* 2003; **24**: 601–7.

42. De Soyza A, Archer L, Wardle J, Parry G, Dark JH, Gould K et al. Pulmonary transplantation for cystic fibrosis: Pre-transplant recipient characteristics in patients dying of peri-operative sepsis. *J Heart Lung Transplant* 2003; **22**: 764–9.

43. Dobbin C, Maley M, Harkness J, Benn R, Malouf M, Glanville A et al. The impact of pan-resistant bacterial pathogens on survival after lung transplantation in cystic fibrosis: Results from a single large referral centre. *J Hosp Infect* 2004; **56**: 277–82.

44. Hodson ME, Gallagher CG, Govan JR. A randomised clinical trial of nebulised tobramycin or colistin in cystic fibrosis. *Eur Respir J* 2002; **20**(3): 658–64.

45. Perry JD, Riley G, Johnston S, Dark JH, Gould FK. Activity of disinfectants against Gram-negative bacilli isolated from patients undergoing lung transplantation for cystic fibrosis. *J Heart Lung Transplant* 2002; **21**: 1230–1.

46. Koo S, Kubiak DW, Issa NC, Dietzek A, Boukedes S, Camp PC et al. A targeted peritransplant antifungal strategy for the prevention of invasive fungal disease after lung transplantation: A sequential cohort analysis. *Transplantation* 2012; **94**(3): 281–6.

47. Barbour KA, Blumenthal JA, Palmer SM. Psychosocial issues in the assessment and management of patients undergoing lung transplantation. *Chest* 2006; **129**: 1367–74.

48. Kollner V, Schade I, Maulhardt T, Maercker A, Joraschky P, Gulielmos V. Posttraumatic stress disorder and quality of life after heart or lung transplantation. *Transplant Proc* 2002; **34**: 2192–3.

49. Christie JD, Edwards LB, Aurora P, Dobbels F, Kirk R, Rahmel AO et al. Registry of the International Society for Heart and Lung Transplantation: Twenty-fifth official adult lung and heart/lung transplantation report—2008. *J Heart Lung Transplant* 2008; **27**: 957–69.

50. Cooper JD, Billingham M, Egan T, Hertz MI, Higenbottam T, Lynch J et al. A working formulation for the standardization of nomenclature and for clinical staging of chronic dysfunction in lung allografts. International Society for Heart and Lung Transplantation. *J Heart Lung Transplant* 1993; **12**(5): 713–6.

51. Estenne M, Maurer JR, Boehler A, Egan JJ, Frost A, Hertz M et al. Bronchiolitis obliterans syndrome 2001: An update of the diagnostic criteria. *J Heart Lung Transplant* 2002; **21**: 297–310.

52. Levy G, Thervet E, Lake J, Uchida K. Patient management by Neoral C (2) monitoring: An international consensus statement. *Transplantation* 2002; **73** (Suppl 9): S12–8.

53. Nashan B, Cole E, Levy G, Thervet E. Clinical validation studies of Neoral C (2) monitoring: A review. *Transplantation* 2002; **73**(Suppl 9): S3–11.

54. Kuypers DR, Peeters PC, Sennesael JJ, Kianda MN, Vrijens B, Kristanto P et al. Improved adherence to tacrolimus once-daily formulation in renal recipients: A randomized controlled trial using electronic monitoring. *Transplantation* 2012; **95**(2): 333–40.

55. Uber PA, Ross HJ, Zuckermann AO, Sweet SC, Corris PA, McNeil K et al. Generic drug immunosuppression in thoracic transplantation: An ISHLT educational advisory. *J Heart Lung Transplant* 2009; **28**: 655–60.

56. Sarahrudi K, Estenne M, Corris P, Niedermayer J, Knoop C, Glanville A et al. International experience with conversion from cyclosporine to tacrolimus for acute and chronic lung allograft rejection. *J Thorac Cardiovasc Surg* 2004; **127**: 1126–32.

57. Speich R, Boehler A, Thurnheer R, Weder W. Salvage therapy with mycophenolate mofetil for lung transplant bronchiolitis obliterans: Importance of dosage. *Transplantation* 1997; **64**(3): 533–5.

58. Cahill BC, Somerville KT, Crompton JA, Parker ST, O'Rourke MK, Stringham JC et al. Early experience with sirolimus in lung transplant recipients with chronic allograft rejection. *J Heart Lung Transplant* 2003; **22**: 169–76.

59. Snell GI, Valentine VG, Vitulo P, Glanville AR, McGiffin DC, Loyd JE et al. Everolimus versus azathioprine in maintenance lung transplant recipients: An international, randomized, double-blind clinical trial. *Am J Transplant* 2006; **6**: 169–77.

60. Snell GI, Levvey BJ, Chin W, Kotsimbos T, Whitford H, Waters KN et al. Sirolimus allows renal recovery in lung and heart transplant recipients with chronic renal impairment. *J Heart Lung Transplant* 2002; **21**: 540–6.

61. Benden C, Speich R, Hofbauer GF, Irani S, Eich-Wanger C, Russi EW et al. Extracorporeal photopheresis after lung transplantation: A 10-year single-center experience. *Transplantation* 2008; **86**: 1625–7.

62. Dusmet M, Maurer J, Winton T, Kesten S. Methotrexate can halt the progression of bronchiolitis obliterans syndrome in lung transplant recipients. *J Heart Lung Transplant* 1996; **15**(9): 948–54.

63. Iacono AT, Johnson BA, Grgurich WF, Youssef JG, Corcoran TE, Seiler DA et al. A randomized trial of inhaled cyclosporine in lung-transplant recipients. Massachusetts Medical Society. *N Engl J Med* 2006; **354**: 141–50.

64. Groves S, Galazka M, Johnson B, Corcoran T, Verceles A, Britt E et al. Inhaled cyclosporine and pulmonary function in lung transplant recipients. *J Aerosol Med Pulm Drug Deliv* 2010; **23**(1): 31–9.

65. Sharples LD, McNeil K, Stewart S, Wallwork J. Risk factors for bronchiolitis obliterans: A systematic review of recent publications. *J Heart Lung Transplant* 2002; **21**: 271–81.

66. Glanville AR, Aboyoun CL, Havryk A, Plit M, Rainer S, Malouf MA. Severity of lymphocytic bronchiolitis predicts long-term outcome after lung transplantation. *Am J Respir Crit Care Med* 2008; **177**: 1033–40.

67. Verleden GM, Vanaudenaerde BM, Dupont LJ, Van Raemdonck DE. Azithromycin reduces airway neutrophilia and interleukin-8 in patients with bronchiolitis obliterans syndrome. *Am J Respir Crit Care Med* 2006; **174**: 566–70.

68. Vos R, Vanaudenaerde BM, Verleden SE, De Vleeschauwer SI, Willems-Widyastuti A, Van Raemdonck DE et al. A randomised controlled trial of azithromycin to prevent chronic rejection after lung transplantation. *Eur Respir J* 2011; **37**: 164–72.

69. Palmer SM, Miralles AP, Howell DN, Brazer SR, Tapson VF, Davis RD. Gastroesophageal reflux as a reversible cause of allograft dysfunction after lung transplantation. *Chest* 2000; **118**(4): 1214–7.

70. Cantu E, 3rd, Appel JZ, 3rd, Hartwig MG, Woreta H, Green C, Messier R et al. J. Maxwell Chamberlain Memorial Paper. Early fundoplication prevents chronic allograft dysfunction in patients with gastroesophageal reflux disease. *Ann Thorac Surg* 2004; **78**: 1142–51; discussion 1142–51.

71. Jackson CH, Sharples LD, McNeil K, Stewart S, Wallwork J. Acute and chronic onset of bronchiolitis obliterans syndrome (BOS): Are they different entities? *J Heart Lung Transplant* 2002; **21**: 658–66.

72. Botha P, Archer L, Anderson RL, Lordan J, Dark JH, Corris PA et al. *Pseudomonas aeruginosa* colonization of the allograft after lung transplantation and the risk of bronchiolitis obliterans syndrome. *Transplantation* 2008; **85**: 771–4.

73. Vos R, Vanaudenaerde BM, Geudens N, Dupont LJ, Van Raemdonck DE, Verleden GM. Pseudomonal airway colonisation: Risk factor for bronchiolitis obliterans syndrome after lung transplantation? *Eur Respir J* 2008; **31**: 1037–45.

74. Novick RJ, Stitt L. Pulmonary retransplantation. *Semin Thorac Cardiovasc Surg* 1998; **10**: 227–36.

75. Morlion B, Knoop C, Paiva M, Estenne M. Internet-based home monitoring of pulmonary function after lung transplantation. *Am J Respir Crit Care Med* 2002; **165**(5): 694–7.

76. De Vito Dabbs A, Hoffman LA, Iacono AT, Zullo TG, McCurry KR, Dauber JH. Are symptom reports useful for differentiating between acute rejection and pulmonary infection after lung transplantation? *Heart Lung* 2004; **33**: 372–80.

77. Gabbay E, Walters EH, Orsida B, Whitford H, Ward C, Kotsimbos TC et al. Post-lung transplant bronchiolitis obliterans syndrome (BOS) is characterized by increased exhaled nitric oxide levels and epithelial inducible nitric oxide synthase. *Am J Respir Crit Care Med* 2000; **162**(6): 2182–7.

78. Verleden GM, Dupont LJ, Delcroix M, Van Raemdonck D, Vanhaecke J, Lerut T. Exhaled nitric oxide after lung transplantation: Impact of the native lung. *Eur Respir J* 2003; **21**(3): 429–32.

79. Verleden GM, Dupont LJ, Van Raemdonck DE, Vanhaecke J. Accuracy of exhaled nitric oxide measurements for the diagnosis of bronchiolitis obliterans syndrome after lung transplantation. *Transplantation* 2004; **78**: 730–3.

80. Brugiere O, Thabut G, Mal H, Marceau A, Dauriat G, Marrash-Chahla R et al. Exhaled NO may predict the decline in lung function in bronchiolitis obliterans syndrome. *Eur Respir J* 2005; **25**: 813–9.

81. Yousem SA, Berry GI, Cagle PT, Chamberlain D, Husain AN, Hruban RH. Revision of the 1990 working formulation for the classification of pulmonary allograft rejection: Lung Rejection Study Group. *J Heart Lung Transplant* 1996; **15**(1 Pt 1): 1–15.

82. Tamm M, Sharples LD, Higenbottam TW, Stewart S, Wallwork J. Bronchiolitis obliterans syndrome in heart-lung transplantation: Surveillance biopsies. *Am J Respir Crit Care Med* 1997; **155**(5): 1705–10.

83. Hopkins PM, Aboyoun CL, Chhajed PN, Malouf MA, Plit ML, Rainer SP et al. Association of minimal rejection in lung transplant recipients with obliterative bronchiolitis. *Am J Respir Crit Care Med* 2004; **170**: 1022–6.

84. Dummer JS, Lazariashvilli N, Barnes J, Ninan M, Milstone AP. A survey of anti-fungal management in lung transplantation. *J Heart Lung Transplant* 2004; **23**: 1376–81.

85. Shitrit D, Ollech JE, Ollech A, Bakal I, Saute M, Sahar G et al. Itraconazole prophylaxis in lung transplant recipients receiving tacrolimus (FK 506): Efficacy and drug interaction. *J Heart Lung Transplant* 2005; **24**: 2148–52.

86. Glanville AR, Scott AI, Morton JM, Aboyoun CL, Plit ML, Carter IW et al. Intravenous ribavirin is a safe and cost-effective treatment for respiratory syncytial virus infection after lung transplantation. *J Heart Lung Transplant* 2005; **24**: 2114–9.

87. Carby M, Jones A, Burke M, Hall A, Banner N. Varicella infection after heart and lung transplantation: A single-center experience. *J Heart Lung Transplant* 2007; **26**: 399–402.

88. Dhar D, Dickson JL, Carby MR, Lyster HS, Hall AV, Banner NR. Fungal infection in cardiothoracic transplant recipients: Outcome without systemic amphotericin therapy. *Transpl Int* 2012; **25**(7): 758–64.

89. Choong CK, Sweet SC, Zoole JB, Guthrie TJ, Mendeloff EN, Haddad FJ et al. Bronchial airway anastomotic complications after pediatric lung transplantation: Incidence, cause, management, and outcome. *J Thorac Cardiovasc Surg* 2006; **131**: 198–203.

90. Orons PD, Amesur NB, Dauber JH, Zajko AB, Keenan RJ, Iacono AT. Balloon dilation and endobronchial stent placement for bronchial strictures after lung transplantation. *J Vasc Interv Radiol* 2000; **11**(1): 89–99.

91. Maiwand MO, Zehr KJ, Dyke CM, Peralta M, Tadjkarimi S, Khagani A et al. The role of cryotherapy for airway complications after lung and heart-lung transplantation. *Eur J Cardiothorac Surg* 1997; **12**: 549–54.

92. Sheridan PH, Jr., Cheriyan A, Doud J, Dornseif SE, Montoya A, Houck J et al. Incidence of phrenic neuropathy after isolated lung transplantation. The Loyola University Lung Transplant Group. *J Heart Lung Transplant* 1995; **14**(4): 684–91.

93. Craig FE, Gulley ML, Banks PM. Posttransplantation lymphoproliferative disorders. *Am J Clin Pathol* 1993; **99**(3): 265–76.

94. Verschuuren EA, Stevens SJ, van Imhoff GW, Middeldorp JM, de Boer C, Koeter G et al. Treatment of post-transplant lymphoproliferative disease with rituximab: The remission, the relapse, and the complication. *Transplantation* 2002; **73**(1): 100–4.

95. Kotloff RM, Ahya VN. Medical complications of lung transplantation. *Eur Respir J* 2004; **23**(2): 334–42.

96. Titman A, Rogers CA, Bonser RS, Banner NR, Sharples LD. Disease-specific survival benefit of lung transplantation in adults: A national cohort study. *Am J Transplant* 2009; **9**: 1640–9.

97. Verleden GM, Dupont LJ, Van Raemdonck DE, Vos R, Vanaudenaerde BM. Lung transplantation: A 15-year single-center experience. *Clin Transpl* 2007: 121–30.

98. Eskander A, Waddell TK, Faughnan ME, Chowdhury N, Singer LG. BODE index and quality of life in advanced chronic obstructive pulmonary disease before and after lung transplantation. A 2011 International Society for Heart and Lung Transplantation. Published by Elsevier, Inc. *J Heart Lung Transplant* 2011; **30**: 1334–41.

99. Maury G, Langer D, Verleden G, Dupont L, Gosselink R, Decramer M et al. Skeletal muscle force and functional exercise tolerance before and after lung transplantation: A cohort study. *Am J Transplant* 2008; **8**: 1275–81.

100. Langer D, Cebria i Iranzo MA, Burtin C, Verleden SE, Vanaudenaerde BM, Troosters T et al. Determinants of physical activity in daily life in candidates for lung transplantation. Elsevier, Ltd. *Respir Med* 2012; **106**: 747–54.

30

Growing old with cystic fibrosis

NICHOLAS J. SIMMONDS

INTRODUCTION

The demographics of cystic fibrosis (CF) have changed beyond recognition since it was first described as a distinct disease by the pathologist Dorothy Andersen in 1938.[1] At that time it was termed "cystic fibrosis of the pancreas" as pancreatic destruction was considered the primary defect and the respiratory manifestations were thought to be a secondary complication of malabsorption. The diagnosis was devastating as over 70% of children died within the first year of life, usually from meconium ileus, severe malnutrition, and/or respiratory failure. Since then our understanding of the pathophysiology and underlying disease mechanisms have improved vastly but the ultimate aim of a cure is yet to be realized. Death in childhood is now rare and life expectancy has improved steadily (Figure 30.1).[2] However, it has only been in the last 30 years that reaching adulthood has become a realistic prospect for the majority of individuals. We are now in an era where, in developed countries, the number of adult CF patients outnumber children.[2] Most of this is due to improvements in care in early and subsequent stages of the disease. The effective transition of patients from pediatric to adult services by a structured and cohesive approach has provided consistency of long-term treatment planning and remains an exemplar for other lifelong diseases. The recognition of CF as a wide spectrum of disease is also now well established; this is evidenced by a smaller, but not insignificant proportion (approximately 10%), of adult patients with an "atypical" phenotype, who usually present with milder clinical features and often have a better prognosis.[3–6] In this chapter, survival trends will be explored with a particular focus on long-term survival and aging with CF. The characteristics of older adult patients will be described, factors important for longevity explored, and diseases of aging (CF and non-CF related) discussed.

SURVIVAL TRENDS

Since 1938, key scientific advances—including the identification of hypertonic sweat in the 1950s and the discovery of the CF gene (cystic fibrosis transmembrane conductance regulator gene, CFTR) in 1989—have been instrumental in improving our understanding of CF pathophysiology.[7–9] However, even before these, important improvements in care had been implemented as a result of careful clinical observation and a systematic approach to the disease complications (e.g., infection and nutritional deficiency) resulting in a significant decline in mortality. Key treatment milestones included the introduction of penicillin and effective nutritional management (crude pancreatic extract and a high fat/protein diet) in the 1940s; routine physiotherapy for airway clearance and effective surgical management of meconium ileus in the 1950s; the opening of specialized CF centers and founding of many national CF organizations in the 1960s; inhaled antibiotics; lung transplant programs commencing in the 1980s; effective mucus treatment with drugs such as nebulized recombinant human deoxyribonuclease (DNase),[10] from the early 1990s; azithromycin from the 2000s[11]; and more recently, the introduction of mutation-specific, protein modulating, drugs.[12] In the United States and other developed countries, median survival rose from 14 years in 1968 to 20 years in the mid-1970s.[13] Since then median survival has improved almost by a year every year and is now approximately 40 years in most developed countries (e.g., 41.4 years; UK Registry 2010 Annual Report).[2,14] CF is no longer a disease that primarily affects children—in the United Kingdom, 55.7% of the total CF population are ≥16 years and 7.6% are aged >40 years (Figure 30.2); in the United States, 48.3% are aged ≥18 years.[2,14] Successive cohorts are living progressively longer, with children born at the turn of the twenty-first century predicted to live beyond 50 years of age.[15]

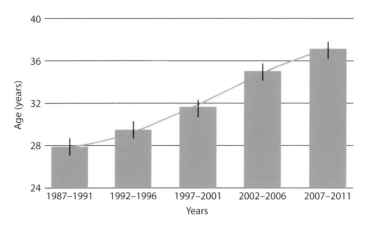

Figure 30.1 Predicted median survival, 1987 to 2011. The graph plots predicted median survival against each time period (year range) for which the prediction was made, demonstrating steady yearly improvement, with current median survival approximately 40 years of age in most developed countries. (From Cystic Fibrosis Foundation, *Patient Registry Annual Data Report*, 2011. With permission.)

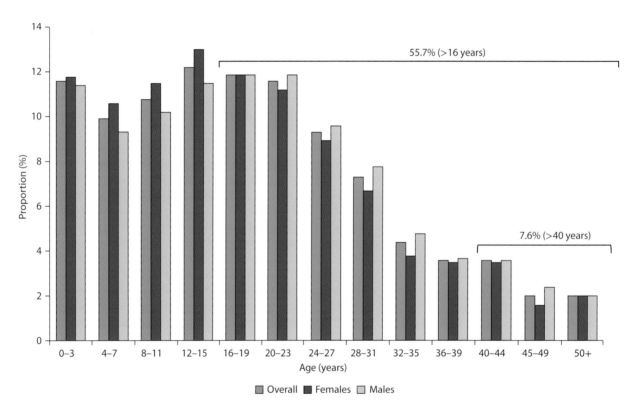

Figure 30.2 Age and sex distribution. In many developed countries, adults with cystic fibrosis (CF) now outnumber children. In the United Kingdom, 55.7% of the CF population are adults (aged >16 years) and 7.6% are aged over 40 years. (Modified from Cystic Fibrosis Trust [United Kingdom], *Annual Data Report*, 2010. With permission.)

SPECTRUM OF DISEASE

The diagnosis of CF is confirmed if an individual has at least one phenotypic feature (e.g., widespread bronchiectasis, malabsorption, or congenital bilateral absence of the vas deferens), evidence of abnormal CFTR function (e.g., by sweat test), and/or two recognized *CFTR* mutations.[16,17] Based on these criteria, in the majority of cases the diagnosis is straightforward. A high index of suspicion should also result from other clinical features such as digital clubbing and *Pseudomonas aeruginosa* growth in the sputum. However, CF disease expression is highly variable and, in some cases, reaching the diagnosis is not straightforward—this is particularly the case for adults presenting for the first time. Chapter 9 covers the diagnosis of CF in greater detail.

When the *CFTR* gene was first discovered, it was thought that disease variability would be explained by different mutations, but the correlation of genotype with phenotype has been repeatedly shown to be poor, with the exception of pancreatic status (e.g., sufficiency vs. insufficiency).[18] The most common genotype classes (groups I to III) are usually associated with more severe disease; typically, a patient carrying one of these mutations on each CF gene is diagnosed early (i.e., aged <1 year) and has pancreatic insufficiency.[19,20] Patients with at least one nonclassic mutation (classes IV to VI) are often diagnosed later and pancreatic sufficient, therefore, have better nutrition.[5,21] Some mutations associated with preservation of CFTR function manifest as milder lung disease, but for the vast majority of other mutations this does not hold true and variability may exist among two individuals with the same genotype.[19] Putative mechanisms to explain this include numerous infectious, nutritional, and environmental influences, although none are likely to fully explain the differences.[22] Non-CFTR genes or polymorphisms, acting as modifiers of disease expression (gene modifiers), probably contribute to disease heterogeneity. To date, there are a limited number of identified polymorphisms associated with lung function severity and others associated with CF-related diabetes (CFRD) and liver disease.[23–25]

Individuals with milder phenotypes may present in adulthood and are usually classified as having nonclassic (or atypical) CF as they often have single-organ involvement and normal nutritional status (Figure 30.3).[5] They can be a diagnostic challenge as they may have an equivocal (or normal) sweat chloride and only one (or even no) identifiable

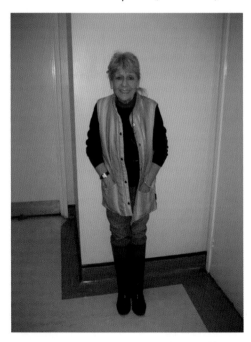

Figure 30.3 Nonclassic CF. A 71-year-old patient diagnosed as an adult. She has diffuse bronchiectasis, pancreatic sufficiency, and her airways are chronically infected with *P. aeruginosa*. Her sweat chloride was in the equivocal range and she is compound heterozygote for the *F508del* and *D1152H* mutations. (Reprinted by permission with written consent from the patient.)

CFTR mutation.[21] They are usually pancreatic sufficient and may present with extrapulmonary features; consequently, they are sometimes first seen in a clinical settings outside of respiratory medicine, such as men with azoospermia in fertility clinics. For this reason, the diagnosis is often delayed (sometimes by many years), which causes frustration and anxiety. As newborn screening is now routinely practiced in many countries, this issue will significantly decline in years to come; however, it will be replaced by a new set of challenges as it will lead to the identification of patients who are asymptomatic and could remain so for many years. The effect it will have on patients with nonclassic CF and potentially a lower risk of developing extensive disease will result in a tremendous "burden" of investigations, clinic visits, and treatments. However, if ultimately patients have better health and their survival rate is improved as suggested in studies of classic CF,[26] then newborn screening will be justified. The next 40 years or so will provide critical information on this debate.

LONG-TERM SURVIVORS

Forty years of age, although essentially an arbitrary threshold, has been used by recent studies to define "long-term survivors" or "older" CF patients.[27–29] Historically, patients surviving into middle age were regarded as medical curiosities.[6] Many of the early case reports fulfilled the criteria for nonclassic CF, as they presented later in life owing to their milder phenotype and pancreatic sufficiency. With increasing awareness of disease heterogeneity, many respiratory physicians are now considering the diagnosis in adults with diffuse "idiopathic" bronchiectasis and referring them for CF evaluation. Furthermore, as discussed already, CF treatments have vastly improved outcomes and, therefore, many more patients are surviving into middle-age despite having classic CF.

Three large observational studies have recently confirmed these findings. A single-center UK study of 112 patients who had reached 40 years of age without transplantation revealed that 30% were homozygous for the mutation *F508del*, 82% were pancreatic insufficient, and 68% were diagnosed in childhood.[28] A US study of patients aged >40 years showed that receiving a late (median age 48.8 years) compared with an early (median age 2.0 years) diagnosis defined a very different phenotype, with fewer *F508del* mutations, less pancreatic insufficiency, and better lung function, but a higher prevalence of positive isolates for nontuberculous mycobacteria (NTM).[29] The authors of a multicenter, international study reported on the characteristics of 366 CF patients aged >40 years confirming that a significant proportion had features suggestive of classic CF, but that significant geographical variation was present.[27] Patients attending the London (United Kingdom) and Minneapolis (Minnesota) CF centers were clinically and genetically similar, with low rates of pancreatic sufficiency

(16% and 21%, respectively) and high levels of homozygous *F508del* frequency (47% and 45%, respectively) compared with those attending the Verona (Italy) and Toronto (Ontario) CF centers (pancreatic sufficiency 60% and 40%, respectively, homozygous *F508del* frequency 9% and 26%, respectively). Many patients had relatively stable disease despite their age, with an average forced expiratory volume in 1 second (FEV1) of >50% predicted (Figure 30.4), and the overall median survival from the age of 40 years was 13 years suggesting that lung function decline may stabilize in later life (Figure 30.5), although a "healthy survivor effect" may also be important. However, the phenomenon of slowing of lung function decline in the modern era of

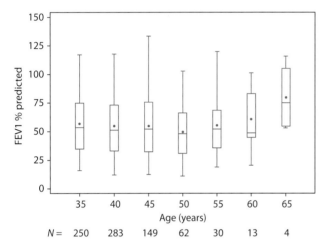

Figure 30.4 Cross-sectional lung function (FEV1 [forced expiratory volume in 1 second] and FVC [forced vital capacity]) for patients aged over 40 years. The graph shows relatively stable parameters and an average FEV1 over 50% predicted for the surviving patients. (From Hodson ME, Simmonds NJ, Warwick WJ et al., *J Cyst Fibros*, 7, 537–42, 2008. With permission.)

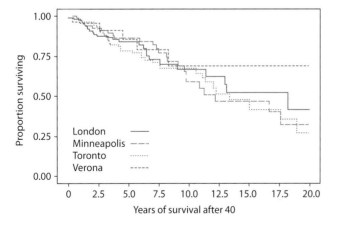

Figure 30.5 Survival after reaching 40 years of age. The survival curves are from four large CF centers across Europe and North America. The median survival of patients who have reached 40 years of age was 13 years, and no significant difference was detected between the centers. (From Hodson ME, Simmonds NJ, Warwick WJ et al., *J Cyst Fibros*, 7, 537–42, 2008. With permission.)

treatment is recognized at all stages of lung function including when FEV1 is low as median survival when FEV1 first declines below 30% of the predicted value is now at least 5.3 years compared with 2 years in the early 1990s.[30]

DETERMINANTS OF LONG-TERM SURVIVAL

The emerging older CF population provides an opportunity to evaluate key factors that are important for long-term survival. Over the decades there have been many publications on the influences of survival in CF in general.[31–33] Despite being a monogenetic disease it is well recognized that a myriad of factors are important; these broadly can be classified as genetic (CFTR and non-CFTR related, e.g., gene modifiers) and nongenetic—including environmental (e.g., pathogens, gender, tobacco smoke exposure, and climate), healthcare-related (e.g., access to specialist clinics and adherence), and socioeconomic factors.[34–39] As previously described, genotype poorly correlates with phenotype apart from a few mutations associated with pancreatic sufficiency. In most studies, female sex is a poor prognostic factor—this is poorly understood although may relate to female sex hormones, earlier *P. aeruginosa* infection, lower weight, CFRD, and psychosocial issues (e.g., body image).[40–43] Interestingly, in one study of patients aged over 40 years, females diagnosed in adulthood had better survival than their male counterparts.[44] This contrasted with the older females who were diagnosed in childhood who had a faster rate of decline in FEV1 and were less likely to reach age 40 than males. Some of this difference may relate to CFRD as some studies have reported an accelerated decline and worse survival in females, although others have challenged this by demonstrating similar outcomes if a focused and intensive management strategy is used.[45,46]

Socioeconomic factors are important in the general CF population, with less advantaged patients having worse outcomes. A recent publication has confirmed that this association still exists in the United Kingdom and remains unchanged over a 20 year period.[47] However, thus far, the evidence has been less compelling for long-term survival.[48] Among patients with severe mutations, the most important predictors of long-term survival do not specifically relate to CFTR function, but are more closely related to early clinical parameters.[49] Patients are statistically more likely to reach 40 years of age if they are not chronically infected with *P. aeruginosa* during childhood (odds ratio [OR] 0.18, 95% confidence interval [CI] 0.05–0.65; $p = .01$) and their body mass index (BMI) (OR 1.76, 95% CI 1.40–2.22; $p < .01$) and FEV1 (OR 1.54 per 5% increase, 95% CI 1.32–1.80; $p < .01$) are optimal at the time of transition to the adult clinic.[48]

For patients who are diagnosed in adulthood, it has been shown that despite the delay in onset of significant symptoms, their rate of FEV1 decline and death from respiratory complications is similar beyond 40 years of age to patients who are diagnosed in childhood.[44] The same study also demonstrated that when these patients are followed at CF centers, their FEV1 improves significantly. This finding has important implications for the older patient group and the development of services for the future, as it reinforces the need to reach a diagnosis in all patients as early as possible and to institute CF-specific care (e.g., nebulized recombinant DNase, inhaled antibiotics, and intensive nutritional management). Improved outcomes should then extend to the older population, but as we do not fully know which aspect of centre care is most important, this should be supported by careful observation and follow-up with appropriate research studies where indicated.

CHANGING DISEASE PREVALENCE AND PSYCHOSOCIAL ISSUES IN AN AGING CF POPULATION

The progressive improvement in median-predicted survival is impressive, but, importantly, it brings with it the potential for a new set of medical and psychosocial issues, which may be isolated or multiple and complex. Broadly, these can be considered as CFTR or non-CFTR related.

CFTR RELATED

As CF is a lifelong condition, longevity exposes organs to abnormal CFTR function for a longer duration; susceptible tissue will eventually be rendered diseased and may manifest as new symptoms or complications for the patient. A prime example of this is CFRD, which has an age-dependent prevalence.[50] In the first few years of life it is extremely rare,

rising to a prevalence of approximately 10% by age 10, 30% by the mid-20s, and >40% in patients aged over 40 years (Figure 30.6).[14] This rise directly relates to pancreatic glandular tissue exposure to abnormal CFTR function, which over time causes progressive damage throughout the whole gland, including endocrine tissue. By the same mechanism some patients with pancreatic sufficiency may eventually develop insufficiency over time (usually in their third or fourth decade) and, conversely, patients who are not pancreatic insufficient do not develop CFRD.

Other CFTR-related age-associated conditions include bone disease and arthropathy (Figure 30.6). The causes of CF bone disease (osteopenia and osteoporosis) are multifactorial, including vitamin D insufficiency, corticosteroid use, and inflammation-related mediators. The cumulative effect of these over time increases the risk of its development (prevalence approximately 5% at 11 years, rising to 26% by 35 years[14]) although CFTR has been identified in bone tissue itself, thus providing an age-independent risk factor and putative mechanism for the considerable variability in presentation and severity.[51] CF arthropathy is a poorly understood complication of CF, characterized by a nonerosive polyarthropathy and occasionally an associated cutaneous vasculitis.[52] Its prevalence slowly increases over age, from approximately 4% at 18 years to nearly 10% at 40 years.[14] Its course usually closely parallels pulmonary disease status, getting worse during pulmonary exacerbations, and thus probably reflects the regulation of inflammatory mediators.

Other CF-related complications are not directly related to age but worsen as a result of disease progression, of which time (or age) is a covariate. For example, as lung disease worsens, the prevalence of large volume hemoptysis and pneumothoraces increases and is therefore much higher in adults than children—in a large registry-based North

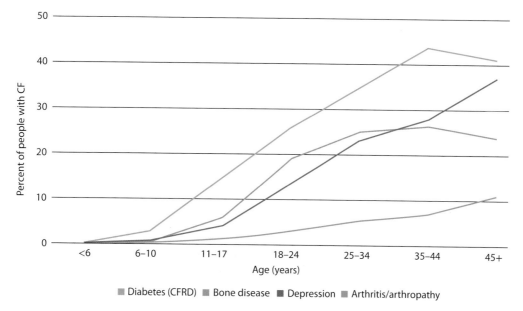

Figure 30.6 Age-related medical conditions. The graph demonstrates an increasing prevalence as age increases, with CF-related diabetes, and depression affecting a high proportion of adults, particularly over 30 years of age. (From Cystic Fibrosis Foundation, *Patient Registry Annual Data Report*, 2011. With permission.)

American study, 75% of all episodes of massive hemoptysis and 72% of all pneumothoraces occurred in patients aged over 18 years.[53,54] Sputum microbiology is also variable over the lifetime of the patient. The prevalence of chronic *P. aeruginosa* is approximately 30% at 15 years and doubles at 30 years but appears to decrease beyond this.[2] In part, this may relate to fewer patients within registries and the nonclassic phenotype in the older age group, but changing host defense mechanisms and airway microbiota diversity may also be important.[55] As already stated, NTM may also be more common in older patients, and one study demonstrated a relatively high prevalence (~10%) of allergic bronchopulmonary aspergillosis in patients aged over 40 years.[28] In addition to the changing prevalence of relatively common airway pathogens, there is the potential of selecting resistant organisms and also the emergence of new ones from a lifetime of multiple courses of antibiotics. The prevalence of less common organisms, such as *Stenotrophomonas maltophilia* and *Achromobacter xylosoxidans*, is increasing which may in part be a result of intensive antimicrobial treatment, as clearance of one organism provides an opportunity for another to overcome host defenses.[56]

An important exception to these observations is the prevalence of CF-related cirrhosis and portal hypertension, which remains relatively unchanged throughout adulthood (>16 years; prevalence 2.5%) as the main risk period for its development is during childhood and adolescence.[2]

NON-CFTR RELATED

Age-related complications of the general population are beginning to emerge in older patients with CF adding to their already burdensome treatment regimen and increasing the potential for drug-related interactions and side effects. Historically, most authorities held the opinion that the risk of cardiovascular disease (i.e., from atherosclerosis) is very low in CF as a result of lipid malabsorption.[57] Mechanistically, this is plausible, but cases of myocardial infarction in pancreatic insufficient patients have been reported and may well relate to the rising incidence of CFRD and other more dominant genetic and environmental (e.g., tobacco smoke exposure) risk factors.[58,59] However, the impact of a lifelong CF diet—with high fat and protein content—may eventually take its toll. A retrospective study of 334 adults with CF (77% pancreatic insufficient) reported that 24% of pancreatic insufficient (vs. 43% of pancreatic sufficient) patients had an abnormal total cholesterol/high-density lipoprotein ratio.[60] Importantly, this ratio and total cholesterol levels both increased with age and BMI, even after excluding pancreatic sufficient patients. Furthermore, although nutritional repletion will always remain a cornerstone of effective CF management, there is an emerging recognition of the overweight, or even obese, CF patient as survival improves. The risks in the general population (including processed fatty foods and lifestyle) are likely to be relevant in CF too and, importantly, this risk is not restricted to pancreatic sufficient patients. A study of 187 adult CF patients from a

Canadian clinic highlights this issue as 11% were categorized as overweight (BMI > 25 kg/m^2), of which 62% were pancreatic insufficient.[61]

The prevalence of systemic hypertension is very common in the general population, increasing with age, and may well become more prevalent in CF. The recent finding of increased arterial stiffness in CF,[62] although currently of uncertain clinical significance, may too influence cardiovascular outcomes in the long-term as has been suggested in other disease groups (e.g., chronic obstructive pulmonary disease).[63]

Another important area for consideration as patients with CF live longer relates to their drug use, including side effects and allergies/intolerances. Drug allergies and intolerances are more common in CF than the general population and are probably due to being exposed to repeated and high doses of IV antibiotics. Both immunoglobulin E (IgE)- and non-IgE-mediated mechanisms are responsible and CF adults are at greater risk than children with an overall reported prevalence between 2% and 25%.[64] Aminoglycosides, particular tobramycin, are highly effective against bacteria such as *P. aeruginosa* and have been instrumental in slowing pulmonary decline and controlling disease over the decades.[65] However, with high usage and a large cumulative dose over many years, the trade-off is likely to be an increasing prevalence of oto- and nephrotoxicity in older patients. A study of 80 adult CF patients who had received a median of 40 courses of aminoglycosides (range 1–130) demonstrated that 42% had evidence of abnormal renal function (creatinine clearance <80 mL/min/1.73 m^2); the number of antibiotic courses correlated with renal disease ($r = 0.59$).[66] A large US registry study ($n = 11,912$) with a median follow-up of 4 years showed an annual renal disease prevalence (glomerular filtration rate < 60 mL/min/1.73 m^2) of 2.3%, with disease prevalence doubling with every 10-year increase in age.[67] Interestingly, only CFRD, not exacerbation rate, predicted the risk of chronic kidney disease, although the authors accept exacerbation rate is only a surrogate marker for intravenous antibiotic use and this does not rule out aminoglycosides as a contributory factor. Furthermore, inhaled antibiotics may not be without risk as systemic absorption can occur, potentially exposing the kidneys to low systemic levels over the long term.[68] Ototoxicity, with high-frequency hearing loss and/or balance disturbances, is a result of degeneration of hair cells in the organ of Corti or vestibular apparatus, respectively. The reported prevalence varies dependent on the method of measurement and the definition used but in one of the largest series of adult CF patients ($n = 153$), over half had some evidence of auditory impairment (ranging from mild [42.2%] to severe [8.6%]).[69]

One final area for consideration in an aging CF population, which may be both CFTR and non-CFTR related, is the risk of developing cancer. A retrospective study of CF patients over 40 years reported an all-cause cancer prevalence of 4%.[28] Publications in the mid 1990s first reported a higher than average prevalence of gastrointestinal (GI) cancers in CF,[70,71] a finding supported by a recent study of 344,144 patient-years (nontransplant) from the US Cystic Fibrosis Foundation Registry, reporting an elevated risk of GI tract cancers with a standardized incidence ratio of 3.5 (95% CI 2.6–4.7).[72] The mechanism is unknown but speculatively could relate to CFTR ion transport abnormalities in the GI tract, alterations of the gut microbiome, prolonged enzyme exposure, or other unmeasured factors.

The psychosocial impact of improved survival is of course largely positive as the expectation for patients transitioning to adult services should be for an active and independent life with similar opportunities to their peers—e.g., further/higher education, employment, and relationships. This is being realized—registry data reported 69.7% (United Kingdom) and 68.9% (United States) of adults in work or study and 39.5% (United States) cohabiting or married.[2,14] However, burden of treatment, adherence, and the psychological stresses of living with a chronic condition should not be underestimated; they increase throughout adulthood, probably as a result of increasing comorbidity and personal responsibilities. Depression, for example, has a prevalence of 20% in adolescence rising to 40% at 40 years (Figure 30.6).[14] This, and other psychological conditions, are therefore not uncommon and require a careful multidisciplinary team approach.

CONCLUSIONS

The demographics of CF have changed considerably over the last few decades with a rising adult population. Current survivorship models suggest this will continue for at least another 10 years with children born today with CF expected to live into their sixth decade. However, with new drug developments—including CFTR protein modulators and gene therapy—median survival may continue beyond this prediction. The ultimate aim, short of a cure, is of course to significantly modify the disease course and maintain excellent health parameters from an early age. If this is achievable, adults of the future may well have a life expectancy approaching normal and live with a chronic condition, perhaps dominated by the GI and pancreatic complications. However, this is still speculative and at the current time the focus must remain on the management of multisystem pathologies by early, effective, and intensive treatment to reduce lung function decline and optimize nutrition. The present challenge is to ensure that adult burden of treatment is reduced by judicious and targeted treatment whenever possible, and effective support is provided to enable independent, active, and successful lives throughout adulthood.

REFERENCES

1. Andersen DH. Cystic fibrosis of the pancreas and its relation to celiac disease. A clinical and pathological study. *Arch Dis Child* 1938; **56**: 344–99.
2. Cystic Fibrosis Trust. *Cystic Fibrosis Data Report 2010.* Kent, United Kingdom: Cystic Fibrosis Trust; 2011.
3. Gilljam M, Ellis L, Corey M, Zielenski J, Durie P, Tullis DE. Clinical manifestations of cystic fibrosis among patients with diagnosis in adulthood. *Chest* 2004; **126**: 1215–24.
4. Gilljam M, Bjorck E. Cystic fibrosis diagnosed in an elderly man. *Respiration* 2004; **71**: 98–100.
5. Nick JA, Rodman DM. Manifestations of cystic fibrosis diagnosed in adulthood. *Curr Opin Pulm Med* 2005; **11**: 513–8.
6. Hunt B, Geddes DM. Newly diagnosed cystic fibrosis in middle and later life. *Thorax* 1985; **40**: 23–6.
7. di Sant'Agnese PA, Darling P, Perera G, Shea E. Abnormal electrolyte composition of sweat in cystic fibrosis of the pancreas; clinical significance and relationship to the disease. *Pediatrics* 1953; **12**: 549–63.
8. Riordan JR, Rommens JM, Kerem B, et al. Identification of the cystic fibrosis gene: Cloning and characterization of complementary DNA. *Science* 1989; **245**: 1066–73.
9. Rommens JM, Iannuzzi MC, Kerem B, et al. Identification of the cystic fibrosis gene: Chromosome walking and jumping. *Science* 1989; **245**: 1059–65.
10. Fuchs HJ, Borowitz DS, Christiansen DH, et al. Effect of aerosolized recombinant human DNase on exacerbations of respiratory symptoms and on pulmonary function in patients with cystic fibrosis. The Pulmozyme Study Group. *N Engl J Med* 1994; **331**: 637–42.
11. Saiman L, Marshall BC, Mayer-Hamblett N, et al. Azithromycin in patients with cystic fibrosis chronically infected with Pseudomonas aeruginosa: A randomized controlled trial. *JAMA* 2003; **290**: 1749–56.
12. Ramsey BW, Davies J, McElvaney NG, et al. A CFTR potentiator in patients with cystic fibrosis and the G551D mutation. *N Engl J Med* 2011; **365**: 1663–72.
13. Warwick WJ, Pogue RE, Gerber HU, Nesbitt CJ. Survival patterns in cyctic fibrosis. *J Chronic Dis* 1975; **28**: 609–22.
14. Cystic Fibrosis Foundation. *Patient Registry Annual Data Report 2011.* Bethesda, MD: Cystic Fibrosis Foundation; 2012.
15. Dodge JA, Lewis PA, Stanton M, Wilsher J. Cystic fibrosis mortality and survival in the UK: 1947–2003. *Eur Respir J* 2007; **29**: 522–6.
16. De Boeck K, Wilschanski M, Castellani C, et al. Cystic fibrosis: Terminology and diagnostic algorithms. *Thorax* 2006; **61**: 627–35.
17. Farrell PM, Rosenstein BJ, White TB, et al. Guidelines for diagnosis of cystic fibrosis in newborns through older adults: Cystic Fibrosis Foundation consensus report. *J Pediatr* 2008; **153**: S4–14.
18. The Cystic Fibrosis Genotype-Phenotype Consortium. Correlation between genotype and phenotype in patients with cystic fibrosis. *N Engl J Med* 1993; **329**: 1308–13.

19. McKone EF, Emerson SS, Edwards KL, Aitken ML. Effect of genotype on phenotype and mortality in cystic fibrosis: A retrospective cohort study. Lancet 2003; **361**: 1671–6.

20. McCloskey M, Redmond AO, Hill A, Elborn JS. Clinical features associated with a delayed diagnosis of cystic fibrosis. *Respiration* 2000; **67**: 402–7.

21. Augarten A, Kerem BS, Yahav Y, et al. Mild cystic fibrosis and normal or borderline sweat test in patients with the 3849 + 10 kb C—>T mutation. *Lancet* 1993; **342**: 25–6.

22. Schechter MS. Non-genetic influences on cystic fibrosis lung disease: The role of sociodemographic characteristics, environmental exposures, and healthcare interventions. *Semin Respir Crit Care Med* 2003; **24**: 639–52.

23. Drumm ML, Konstan MW, Schluchter MD, et al. Genetic modifiers of lung disease in cystic fibrosis. *N Engl J Med* 2005; **353**: 1443–53.

24. Bartlett JR, Friedman KJ, Ling SC, et al. Genetic modifiers of liver disease in cystic fibrosis. *JAMA* 2009; **302**: 1076–83.

25. Blackman SM, Hsu S, Ritter SE, et al. A susceptibility gene for type 2 diabetes confers substantial risk for diabetes complicating cystic fibrosis. *Diabetologia* 2009; **52**: 1858–65.

26. Farrell PM, Kosorok MR, Laxova A, et al. Nutritional benefits of neonatal screening for cystic fibrosis. Wisconsin Cystic Fibrosis Neonatal Screening Study Group. *N Engl J Med* 1997; **337**: 963–9.

27. Hodson ME, Simmonds NJ, Warwick WJ, et al. An international/multicentre report on patients with cystic fibrosis (CF) over the age of 40 years. *J Cyst Fibros* 2008; **7**: 537–42.

28. Simmonds NJ, Cullinan P, Hodson ME. Growing old with cystic fibrosis—The characteristics of long-term survivors of cystic fibrosis. *Respir Med* 2009; **103**: 629–35.

29. Rodman DM, Polis JM, Heltshe SL, et al. Late diagnosis defines a unique population of long-term survivors of cystic fibrosis. *Am J Respir Crit Care Med* 2005; **171**: 621–6.

30. George PM, Banya W, Pareek N, et al. Improved survival at low lung function in cystic fibrosis: Cohort study from 1990 to 2007. *BMJ* 2011; **342**: d1008.

31. Courtney JM, Bradley J, Mccaughan J, et al. Predictors of mortality in adults with cystic fibrosis. *Pediatr Pulmonol* 2007; **42**: 525–32.

32. Corey M, Farewell V. Determinants of mortality from cystic fibrosis in Canada, 1970–1989. *Am J Epidemiol* 1996; **143**: 1007–17.

33. Corey M, McLaughlin FJ, Williams M, Levison H. A comparison of survival, growth, and pulmonary function in patients with cystic fibrosis in Boston and Toronto. *J Clin Epidemiol* 1988; **41**: 583–91.

34. Collaco JM, McGready J, Green DM, et al. Effect of temperature on cystic fibrosis lung disease and infections: A replicated cohort study. *PLoS ONE* 2011; **6**: e27784.

35. Schechter MS, Shelton BJ, Margolis PA, Fitzsimmons SC. The association of socioeconomic status with outcomes in cystic fibrosis patients in the United States. *Am J Respir Crit Care Med* 2001; **163**: 1331–7.

36. Schechter MS, Margolis PA. Relationship between socioeconomic status and disease severity in cystic fibrosis. *J Pediatr* 1998; **132**: 260–4.

37. Mahadeva R, Webb K, Westerbeek RC, et al. Clinical outcome in relation to care in centres specialising in cystic fibrosis: Cross sectional study. *BMJ* 1998; **316**: 1771–5.

38. Collaco JM, Vanscoy L, Bremer L, et al. Interactions between secondhand smoke and genes that affect cystic fibrosis lung disease. *JAMA* 2008; **299**: 417–24.

39. Daniels T, Goodacre L, Sutton C, Pollard K, Conway S, Peckham D. Accurate assessment of adherence: Self-report and clinician report vs electronic monitoring of nebulizers. *Chest* 2011; **140**: 425–32.

40. Demko CA, Byard PJ, Davis PB. Gender differences in cystic fibrosis: Pseudomonas aeruginosa infection. *J Clin Epidemiol* 1995; **48**: 1041–9.

41. Rosenfeld M, Davis R, FitzSimmons S, Pepe M, Ramsey B. Gender gap in cystic fibrosis mortality. *Am J Epidemiol* 1997; **145**: 794–803.

42. Chotirmall SH, Smith SG, Gunaratnam C, et al. Effect of estrogen on pseudomonas mucoidy and exacerbations in cystic fibrosis. *N Engl J Med* 2012; **366**: 1978–86.

43. Willis E, Miller R, Wyn J. Gendered embodiment and survival for young people with cystic fibrosis. *Soc Sci Med* 2001; **53**: 1163–74.

44. Nick JA, Chacon CS, Brayshaw SJ, et al. Effects of gender and age at diagnosis on disease progression in long-term survivors of cystic fibrosis. *Am J Respir Crit Care Med* 2010; **182**: 614–26.

45. Milla CE, Billings J, Moran A. Diabetes is associated with dramatically decreased survival in female but not male subjects with cystic fibrosis. *Diabetes Care* 2005; **28**: 2141–4.

46. Moran A, Dunitz J, Nathan B, Saeed A, Holme B, Thomas W. Cystic fibrosis-related diabetes: Current trends in prevalence, incidence, and mortality. *Diabetes Care* 2009; **32**: 1626–31.

47. Barr HL, Britton J, Smyth AR, Fogarty AW. Association between socioeconomic status, sex, and age at death from cystic fibrosis in England and Wales 1959 to 2008.: Cross sectional study. *BMJ* 2011; **343**: d4662.

48. Simmonds NJ, Macneill SJ, Cullinan P, Hodson ME. Cystic fibrosis and survival to 40 years: A case-control study. *Eur Respir J* 2010; **36**: 1277–83.

49. Simmonds NJ, D'Souza L, Roughton M, Alton EW, Davies JC, Hodson ME. Cystic fibrosis and survival to 40 years: A study of cystic fibrosis transmembrane conductance regulator function. *Eur Respir J* 2011; **37**: 1076–82.

50. Marshall BC, Butler SM, Stoddard M, Moran AM, Liou TG, Morgan WJ. Epidemiology of cystic fibrosis-related diabetes. *J Pediatr* 2005; **146**: 681–7.

51. Shead EF, Haworth CS, Condliffe AM, McKeon DJ, Scott MA, Compston JE. Cystic fibrosis transmembrane conductance regulator (CFTR) is expressed in human bone. *Thorax* 2007; **62**: 650–1.

52. Hodson ME. Vasculitis and arthropathy in cystic fibrosis. *J R Soc Med* 1999; **85** (Suppl 9): 38–40.

53. Flume PA, Yankaskas JR, Ebeling M, Hulsey T, Clark LL. Massive hemoptysis in cystic fibrosis. *Chest* 2005; **128**: 729–38.

54. Flume PA, Strange C, Ye X, Ebeling M, Hulsey T, Clark LL. Pneumothorax in cystic fibrosis. *Chest* 2005; **128**: 720–8.

55. Stressmann FA, Rogers GB, van der Gast CJ, et al. Long-term cultivation-independent microbial diversity analysis demonstrates that bacterial communities infecting the adult cystic fibrosis lung show stability and resilience. *Thorax* 2012; **67**: 867–73.

56. LiPuma JJ. The changing microbial epidemiology in cystic fibrosis. *Clin Microbiol Rev* 2010; **23**: 299–323.

57. Figueroa V, Milla C, Parks EJ, Schwarzenberg SJ, Moran A. Abnormal lipid concentrations in cystic fibrosis. *Am J Clin Nutr* 2002; **75**: 1005–11.

58. Perrin FM, Serino W. Ischaemic heart disease—A new issue in cystic fibrosis? *J R Soc Med* 2010; **103** (Suppl 1): S44–8.

59. Onady GM, Farinet CL. An adult cystic fibrosis patient presenting with persistent dyspnea: Case report. *BMC Pulm Med* 2006; **6**: 9.

60. Rhodes B, Nash EF, Tullis E, et al. Prevalence of dyslipidemia in adults with cystic fibrosis. *J Cyst Fibros* 2010; **9**: 24–8.

61. Coderre L, Fadainia C, Belson L, et al. LDL-cholesterol and insulin are independently associated with body mass index in adult cystic fibrosis patients. *J Cyst Fibros* 2012; **11**: 393–7.

62. Hull JH, Garrod R, Ho TB, et al. Increased augmentation index in patients with cystic fibrosis. *Eur Respir J* 2009; **34**: 1322–8.

63. Maclay JD, McAllister DA, Mills NL, et al. Vascular dysfunction in chronic obstructive pulmonary disease. *Am J Respir Crit Care Med* 2009; **180**: 513–20.

64. Parmar JS, Nasser S. Antibiotic allergy in cystic fibrosis. *Thorax* 2005; **60**: 517–20.

65. Smyth A, Tan KH, Hyman-Taylor P, et al. Once versus three-times daily regimens of tobramycin treatment for pulmonary exacerbations of cystic fibrosis—The TOPIC study: A randomised controlled trial. *Lancet* 2005; **365**: 573–8.

66. Al-Aloul M, Miller H, Alapati S, Stockton PA, Ledson MJ, Walshaw MJ. Renal impairment in cystic fibrosis patients due to repeated intravenous aminoglycoside use. *Pediatr Pulmonol* 2005; **39**: 15–20.

67. Quon BS, Mayer-Hamblett N, Aitken ML, Smyth AR, Goss CH. Risk factors for chronic kidney disease in adults with cystic fibrosis. *Am J Respir Crit Care Med* 2011; **184**: 1147–52.

68. Ring E, Eber E, Erwa W, Zach MS. Urinary N-acetyl-beta-D-glucosaminidase activity in patients with cystic fibrosis on long-term gentamicin inhalation. *Arch Dis Child* 1998; **78**: 540–3.

69. Conrad DJ, Stenbit AE, Zettner EM, Wick I, Eckhardt C, Hardiman G. Frequency of mitochondrial 12S ribosomal RNA variants in an adult cystic fibrosis population. *Pharmacogenet Genomics* 2008; **18**: 1095–102.

70. Sheldon CD, Hodson ME, Carpenter LM, Swerdlow AJ. A cohort study of cystic fibrosis and malignancy. *Br J Cancer* 1993; **68**: 1025–8.

71. Neglia JP, Fitzsimmons SC, Maisonneuve P, et al. The risk of cancer among patients with cystic fibrosis. Cystic Fibrosis and Cancer Study Group. *N Engl J Med* 1995; **332**: 494–9.

72. Maisonneuve P, Marshall BC, Knapp EA, Lowenfels AB. Cancer risk in cystic fibrosis: A 20-year nationwide study from the United States. *J Natl Cancer Inst* 2013; **105**: 122–9.

FURTHER READING

Bombieri C, Claustres M, De BK, et al. Recommendations for the classification of diseases as CFTR-related disorders. *J Cyst Fibros* 2011; **10** (Suppl 2): S86–102.

Dequeker E, Stuhrmann M, Morris MA, et al. Best practice guidelines for molecular genetic diagnosis of cystic fibrosis and CFTR-related disorders—Updated European recommendations. *Eur J Hum Genet* 2009; **17**: 51–65.

PART 5

Monitoring

31

Quality improvement: Using databases to improve cystic fibrosis care

CHRISTOPHER H. GOSS, BRADLEY S. QUON, AND DIANA BILTON

OVERVIEW

DEFINITION OF QI

Quality improvement (QI) in health care has been defined as "an interdisciplinary process to raise the likelihood of the delivery of best practices for preventive, diagnostic, therapeutic, and rehabilitative care to maintain, restore, or improve health outcomes of individuals and populations."[1] Continuous quality improvement (CQI) in health care can be described as an iterative approach to improving processes to reduce unexpected variation in health outcomes. CQI represents one model to achieve QI and has long been recognized as a key to success in the manufacturing industry with companies like Toyota leading the way. The role of QI and CQI has been less well adopted in the healthcare profession but is clearly increasing in prominence in this setting.[2] A review of the number of articles cited on PubMed on October 19, 2012 with the search term "quality improvement" in the title or abstract yielded over 13,000 articles, with over 1,300 publications since January 1, 2012. Health care, and specifically the care of chronic lung diseases like cystic fibrosis (CF), represents ideal settings for the application of QI and CQI.

HOW DO WE DO IT?

One of the key goals of QI is to improve care—this is often done by changing physician and care provider behavior.[3] QI work focuses on ensuring more consistent and efficient use of proven efficacious treatments. The classic scenario occurs when an efficacious intervention (i.e., the use of inhaled dornase alfa in CF patients with moderate lung impairment) is not used in CF patients who should by all accounts be receiving this treatment. Not uncommonly, practitioners in a specific clinical setting will fail to prescribe recommended treatments; the reasons for underutilization of recommended efficacious therapies are often site specific and relate to barriers that are either structural or based on practitioner education. Through an iterative process of QI, one can begin to identify and intervene on the barriers to effect change in care (Table 31.1).

Local QI projects can vary considerably in scope and some will narrowly focus on physician behavior to improve quality of care. For example, improving aspirin use in the treatment of an acute myocardial infarction in and of itself represents an important end point.[3,6] An iterative project to improve documentation of the method of contraception used by CF women might be one CF-specific example of a local QI initiative. The ultimate goal of this project would be to ensure documentation of whether birth control is used; such health information may improve patient care. This intervention may provide hypothesis generating ideas regarding how to ensure CF providers discuss sexual behaviors with their female patients and lead to further educational opportunities (i.e., the discussion of sexually transmitted diseases, fertility in CF women). Merely improving documentation of the method of birth control may meet the needs of the project. Further studies could try to evaluate the content of conversations related to reproductive health and the success or failure of knowledge transfer to the patient. Long-term outcomes would not be needed at this early stage to judge the value of a QI program that succeeded in improving documentation.

If the goal of the proposed research is to generate generalizable results to affect change in care in many settings, rigorous scientific methodology is needed to ensure bias and confounding have been adequately addressed. This can be achieved either via randomization (i.e., cluster randomization) or in the analytical phase of the project (adjusting for confounders including temporal effects unrelated to the intervention). As noted above, merely demonstrating change in physician behavior may be an appropriate

Table 31.1 Tools and methods to achieve quality improvement[4,5]

- Delineate healthcare process
- Collect data over time to document variation in care practices and clinical outcomes
- Document unwanted and unnecessary variation
- Collect information regarding customer/beneficiary knowledge (i.e., measurements of illness burden, functional status, quality of life, recipients' assessment of the quality of their care)
- Adopt widespread public sharing of information
- Improve communication by building teams and enhancing group learning using specific skills (i.e., Situation, Background, Assessment, and Request [SBAR])
- Create a leadership plan acknowledging, leading, following, and making changes in health care
- Build knowledge (locally useful), then take initiative, and use adaptive action, reviewing, and reflecting
- Make small tests of change (i.e., Plan-Do-Study-Act [PDSA] cycles)

Sources: Batalden PB, Davidoff F, *Qual Saf Health Care* 16(1), 2–3, 2007; Institute for Healthcare Improvement, *Improvement Methods: Getting Started*, Cambridge, MA, Institute for Healthcare Improvement, 2011.

outcome. Other interventions will need to demonstrate change in physician behavior that in turn leads to a desirable outcome. In CF, improving the use of oral azithromycin in persons with CF who are culture negative for *Pseudomonas aeruginosa* may represent a good intermediary end point,[7] but this therapy has not been widely accepted as an efficacious treatment in CF as noted by a recent Cochrane review on the subject.[8] Thus, in QI research directed at improving use of azithromycin in this population, outcome measures deemed of high value to CF patients like exacerbation rate, lung function over more than 6 months, and annual rate of lung function decline should be included to support the contention that such an effort would be of value in the CF community.

To begin work in QI, it is necessary to have a measure of the scope of the problem. Thus, one of the key components of QI is access to high-quality data regarding patient characteristics, treatments, and clinical outcomes. In the words of management guru Peter Drucker, "if you can't measure it, you can't manage it." As with all data sources in clinical research, it is necessary to know how the data were collected, how complete they are (degree of missingness), whether a data edit or validation system was in place, and whether the data included key variables of interest for the research question at hand.

The first step in any QI project or research is to fully understand the healthcare process of the problem at hand. Next, it is necessary to document variation in care where variation would not be anticipated. CF is ideally suited for evaluation of QI research because of the existence in many countries of comprehensive patient registries with data regarding the management of people with CF.[9–14] The US CF Foundation (CFF) recognized the critical role of data collection and measurement in QI early on and thus created a patient registry in 1966, the CFF Patient Registry (CFFPR).[15] This registry has evolved over the years from a few variables on vital status to allow for a better understanding of the natural history of disease to a comprehensive database that gives healthcare providers and researchers the information they need to develop care guidelines, improve delivery of

care, and identify eligible patients for clinical trials. The US CFFPR now includes detailed annual and encounter-based data on over 300 unique variables running the gamut from active pulmonary therapies to sputum microbiology to pulmonary function test results to CF-related comorbidities for each of its more than 26,000 participants.[16] The CFFPR has been used to evaluate survival and temporal changes in survival,[17,18] predictors of survival,[19–22] impact of sputum microbiology,[23–26] and complications related to CF.[27–29] To support international improvements in care, the CFF facilitated the development of the UK CF Registry with the donation of the software platform to the UK CF Trust to allow web-based data collection from the UK cohort now numbering just over 9000 patients. That development fostered publications along similar lines in particular identifying use of gentamicin as a particular risk factor for renal failure in CF[30] and highlighting the relationship between diabetes control and survival.[31,32] Thus, the presence of a robust dataset in a specialist condition generates research and enquiry aimed at improving future management ahead of any definitive QI initiative.

More recent publications from the United States have addressed issues related to process of care and access to care representing the beginning of the use of registry data in CF for QI.[33–37] Several additional examples of such assessments have been performed in CF. In the first example, the use of oral ibuprofen (a therapy with grade B level evidence-based on a recent systematic review) was documented to have been used in only 3.5% of CF patients in 2010. The authors used observational data to demonstrate that use of oral ibuprofen was associated with reduced lung function decline as demonstrated in two randomized clinical trials.[36,38,39]

Two studies have used registry data to address specific components of process of care.[35] In the first of these studies using data from the Epidemiologic Study in CF (ESCF), Johnson et al. evaluated US CF centers that cared for at least 50 persons with CF, ranking these centers based on the median forced expiratory volume in 1 second (FEV1) within each of three age groups (6–12 years, 13–17 years, and ≥18 years). They found that those centers that saw

39. Konstan MW, Byard PJ, Hoppel CL, Davis PB. Effect of high-dose ibuprofen in patients with cystic fibrosis. *N Engl J Med* 1995; **332**(13): 848–54.

40. Padman R, McColley SA, Miller DP, Konstan MW, Morgan WJ, Schechter MS, et al. Infant care patterns at epidemiologic study of cystic fibrosis sites that achieve superior childhood lung function. *Pediatrics* 2007; **119**(3): e531–7.

41. Moher D, Schulz KF, Altman D. The CONSORT statement: Revised recommendations for improving the quality of reports of parallel-group randomized trials. *JAMA* 2001; **285**(15): 1987–91.

42. von Elm E, Altman DG, Egger M, Pocock SJ, Gotzsche PC, Vandenbroucke JP. The Strengthening the Reporting of Observational Studies in Epidemiology (STROBE) statement: Guidelines for reporting observational studies. *Ann Intern Med* 2007; **147**(8): 573–7.

43. Moher D, Cook DJ, Eastwood S, Olkin I, Rennie D, Stroup DF. Improving the quality of reports of meta-analyses of randomised controlled trials: The QUOROM statement. Quality of Reporting of Meta-analyses. *Lancet* 1999; **354**(9193): 1896–900.

44. Ogrinc G, Mooney SE, Estrada C, Foster T, Goldmann D, Hall LW, et al. The SQUIRE (Standards for Quality Improvement Reporting Excellence) guidelines for quality improvement reporting: Explanation and elaboration. *Qual Saf Health Care* 2008; **17** (Suppl 1): i13–32.

45. Davidoff F, Batalden P, Stevens D, Ogrinc G, Mooney S. Publication guidelines for improvement studies in health care: Evolution of the SQUIRE Project. *Ann Intern Med* 2008; **149**(9): 670–6.

46. Davidoff F, Batalden P, Stevens D, Ogrinc G, Mooney SE. Publication guidelines for quality improvement studies in health care: Evolution of the SQUIRE project. *BMJ* 2009; **338**: a3152.

47. Moss F, Thompson R. A new structure for quality improvement reports. *Qual Health Care* 1999; **8**(2): 76.

48. Berwick DM. The science of improvement. *JAMA* 2008; **299**(10): 1182–4.

49. Auerbach AD, Landefeld CS, Shojania KG. The tension between needing to improve care and knowing how to do it. *N Engl J Med* 2007; **357**(6): 608–13.

50. Scales DC, Dainty K, Hales B, Pinto R, Fowler RA, Adhikari NK, et al. A multifaceted intervention for quality improvement in a network of intensive care units: A cluster randomized trial. *JAMA* 2011; **305**(4): 363–72.

51. Curtis JR, Levy MM. Improving the science and politics of quality improvement. *JAMA* 2011; **305**(4): 406–7.

52. Goss CH, Mayer-Hamblett N, Kronmal RA, Ramsey BW. The cystic fibrosis therapeutics development network (CF TDN): A paradigm of a clinical trials network for genetic and orphan diseases. *Adv Drug Deliv Rev* 2002; **54**(11): 1505–28.

53. Schechter MS, Gutierrez HH. Improving the quality of care for patients with cystic fibrosis. *Curr Opin Pediatr* 2010; **22**(3): 296–301.

54. Kraynack NC, Gothard MD, Falletta LM, McBride JT. Approach to treating cystic fibrosis pulmonary exacerbations varies widely across US CF care centers. *Pediatr Pulmonol* 2011; **46**(9): 870–81.

55. Kraynack NC, McBride JT. Improving care at cystic fibrosis centers through quality improvement. *Semin Respir Crit Care Med* 2009; **30**(5): 547–58.

56. Cystic Fibrosis Center News. [10]. 2004. Chicago, IL: Children's Memorial Hospital.

57. Stern M, Wiedemann B, Wenzlaff P. From registry to quality management: The German Cystic Fibrosis Quality Assessment project 1995–2006. *Eur Respir J* 2008; **31**(1): 29–35.

58. Stern M, Niemann N, Wiedemann B, Wenzlaff P. Benchmarking improves quality in cystic fibrosis care: A pilot project involving 12 centres. *Int J Qual Health Care* 2011; **23**(3): 349–56.

59. Stern M. The use of a Cystic Fibrosis Patient Registry to assess outcomes and improve cystic fibrosis care in Germany. *Curr Opin Pulm Med* 2011; **17**(6): 473–7.

60. Corey M, McLaughlin FJ, Williams M, Levison H. A comparison of survival, growth, and pulmonary function in patients with cystic fibrosis in Boston and Toronto. *J Clin Epidemiol* 1988; **41**(6): 583–91.

61. Martin B, Schechter MS, Jaffe A, Cooper P, Bell SC, Ranganathan S. Comparison of the US and Australian cystic fibrosis registries: The impact of newborn screening. *Pediatrics* 2012; **129**(2): e348–55.

62. Goss CH, Macneill SJ, Quinton H, Marshall B, Elbert A, Petren K, et al. Children and young adults in the US have improved lung function compared to the UK. *Pediatr Pulmonol* 2012; **35**: 378.

32

Infant and preschool lung function

SARATH RANGANATHAN

BACKGROUND

Improvements in outcomes for those with cystic fibrosis (CF) that are evident by school-age point to the period of early life as crucial in determining long-term outcomes (Figure 32.1). This is unsurprising given that the early years are a time of rapid lung development. Measurement of lung function is a central part of the clinical assessment of older children and adults with CF. Serial tests provide longitudinal information about the extent of abnormality, progression of disease, and individual response to treatment. As evidence accumulates that chronic pulmonary disease commences in infancy, the need to evaluate lung function early is self-evident. Neutrophil-dominated inflammation similar to that seen in older subjects has been identified in the lungs of affected infants[1,2] and understanding of how airway pathology evolves during the first years of life is improving. Recent studies add to knowledge as to how useful lung function testing in the preschool years could be, and also the nature of functional changes in CF. The limiting factors, however, remain that infant lung function is technically difficult to perform, expensive, time consuming, and requires sedation, which makes it difficult to recruit healthy subjects as controls. Furthermore, between infancy and school age, toddlers are too old to sedate and too young to cooperate with most testing.

Many of the prior studies of lung function in infants with CF were difficult to interpret due to the small numbers of subjects, lack of appropriate control data from prospectively studied healthy infants, and the use of relatively insensitive techniques.[3] Recent studies are just beginning to bridge the "silent years" of lung function testing before children are old enough to perform spirometry. Functional lung disease in CF is characterized by airway obstruction, peripheral airway disease leading to ventilation inhomogeneity, and air trapping. Based on this pathophysiology, tests of forced expiration, gas mixing, and lung volumes are the most appropriate to adapt for use in infants and preschool

children with CF.[4] Commercially available tests that interrogate all these facets of lung function are now available in infants and, to a lesser extent, in preschool children with CF.

In older subjects with CF, measurements from spirometry, for example, forced expiratory volume in 1 second (FEV_1) and maximal expiratory flow at low lung volumes (e.g., MEF_{25}), are most frequently used to assess airway function. Methods to assess forced expiration over an extended volume range in infants were described nearly 20 years ago.[5,6] This raised volume rapid thoracoabdominal technique (raised volume technique, RVRTC) involves using a pump or augmented manual inflations to increase the volume of inspiration to near total lung capacity prior to forcing expiration (see Video 32.2). From the RVRTC flow-volume curves, it is possible to derive parameters comparable to those obtained in older subjects such as forced expiratory volume in 0.4 or 0.5 second ($FEV_{0.4}$ or $FEV_{0.5}$) and MEF_{25}.[7] $FEV_{0.5}$ is most frequently reported but, due to rapid lung and airway growth during the first 2 years of life, changes rapidly and so may not reflect lung function from the same airway generations in an individual measured at different ages. The commercialization of the equipment for this technique and the standardization of the test[8] has contributed to its take-up by more than 100 centers worldwide with at least 50% of such centers claiming to utilize such tests for clinical, in addition to research, purposes.[9] Measurements from the RVRTC are more repeatable than those obtained using spirometry in older subjects. Forced expired volumes are generally less variable compared with flows (within test coefficient of variation for $FEV_{0.5}$ of 3.6% compared with MEF_{25} of 8.9%).[7]

The multiple-breath washout test (MBW) is used to detect inhomogeneous lung disease. It can be performed during tidal breathing and essentially determines how efficiently the lungs are able to ventilate exogenous (for example, sulfur hexafluoride) or endogenous (for example, nitrogen) inert gases during the breathing cycle (usually exhalation) (Figure 32.2 and Video 32.3). The most commonly reported

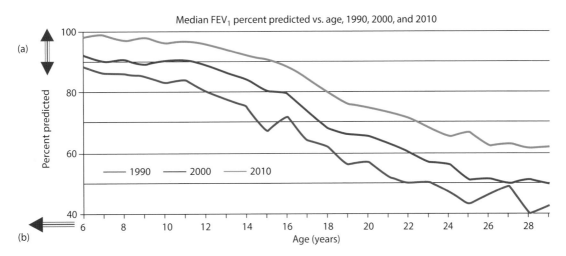

Figure 32.1 Lung function in those with cystic fibrosis (CF) has improved significantly over the last 20 years with increased forced expiratory volume in 1 second evident for each cohort by the time of the first recorded school-age spirometry (arrow b). This indicates that changes in clinical management during the infant and preschool years is critical (arrow b) and also highlights the importance of monitoring lung function during this period. (Adapted from US Cystic Fibrosis Foundation, *2011 Annual Report of the National Patient Registry*, Bethseda, MD: US Cystic Fibrosis Foundation, 2011. With permission.)

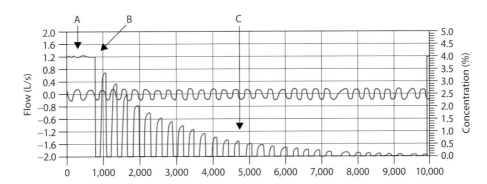

Figure 32.2 Expired gas concentration during multiple-breath inert gas washout performed during tidal breathing. During the wash-in phase (A) a steady-state gas concentration (in this example, 4%) indicates that wash-in is complete at which time the subject is disconnected from the test gas and breathes air (B). Subsequently, the concentration of test gas in expired air decreases exponentially (C). The lung clearance index is calculated as the cumulative expired volume, expressed as a ratio to functional residual capacity, required to reduce the concentration of the inert gas 40-fold, arbitrarily, from a starting concentration of 4% to 0.1%.

measurement is the lung clearance index (LCI), which is calculated as the cumulative expired volume required to decrease the starting concentration of the inert gas 40-fold divided by functional residual capacity (FRC) calculated by the Fowler method.[10] This MBW-determined ventilation inhomogeneity appears to be a sensitive marker of early and mild lung disease,[11,12] and in older children, it appears to be a good surrogate for structural lung changes determined by chest computed tomography (CT).[13,14] Lung volumes, for example, FRC can be measured by plethysmography (see Video 32.1). The first report of FRC_{pleth} was published more than 40 years ago by Phelan et al. who identified hyperinflation as an early functional feature of CF.[13–15]

STUDIES IN INFANTS

EVIDENCE FOR DIMINISHED AIRWAY FUNCTION IN INFANTS WITH CF AFTER A CLINICAL DIAGNOSIS

Two papers in infants diagnosed with CF after a clinical presentation were published as part of the London Collaborative Cystic Fibrosis Study.[16,17] Airway function was measured to test the hypothesis that lung function is diminished shortly after diagnosis independent of clinically recognized lower respiratory illness. The RVRTC was used to assess the airway function of 47 infants newly diagnosed with CF and 137 healthy infants. The lung function of infants with CF was compared with that of healthy infants and expressed as standard deviation (SD) scores (z-scores). The respiratory status of the CF infants was assessed by their specialist physicians who were blinded to the results of airway function.

Multiple linear regression was used to assess the influence of CF on $FEV_{0.4}$ after accounting for differences in body size, gender, and exposure to maternal smoking measured by salivary cotinine level. On average, the decrement in $FEV_{0.4}$ in those with CF was 40 mL ($p < .001$) when their median (range) age was 30 (6–93) weeks (Figure 32.3). This was irrespective of clinical evidence of prior lower respiratory illness as this particular subgroup of infants (of median age 12 weeks) had a similar decrement in airway function.

Approximately a third of infants with CF had an $FEV_{0.5}$ below the 2.5th centile.[17] In 17 CF infants assessed as having normal clinical respiratory status by their specialist, the mean z-score for $FEV_{0.5}$ was −1.1 and there were four infants whose airway function was below the 2.5th centile for healthy infants.

Therefore, lung function was diminished early in the course of disease in those with CF irrespective of clinical evidence of prior lower respiratory illness and even when specialist physicians identified infants with CF as having normal respiratory status. Infants were diagnosed with CF following a clinical presentation of the disease and those without clinical evidence of prior lower respiratory illness usually had presented with meconium ileus in the newborn period or had evidence of significant failure to thrive when airway function was assessed, and so might not be considered truly asymptomatic individuals.

The ability of LCI measured by MBW to identify diminished lung function was compared with the RVRTC by Lum et al.[18] MBW was done using a mass spectrometer as tests were undertaken prior to validation of commercially available equipment. Compared with controls, infants with CF had a significantly higher LCI (8.4 vs. 7.2) and significantly lower values for all forced expiratory flow-volume parameters compared with controls. Girls had significantly lower $FEV_{0.5}$ and MEF_{75-25} than boys: mean (95% confidence interval [CI] girls–boys) was −1.2 (−2.1 to −0.3) for $FEV_{0.5}$ z-score. When using both the MBW and RVRTC techniques, abnormalities were detected in 72% of the infants, with abnormalities detected in 41% using both techniques and a further 15% by each of the two tests performed. These findings support the view that monitoring of early lung disease and functional status in infants and young children with CF may be enhanced by using both MBW and the RVRTC.

EVIDENCE FOR DIMINISHED AIRWAY FUNCTION IN INFANTS WITH CF AFTER NEWBORN SCREENING

Linnane et al. measured lung function using the RVRTC in infants with CF shortly after a diagnosis by newborn screening and healthy controls without CF. Measurements

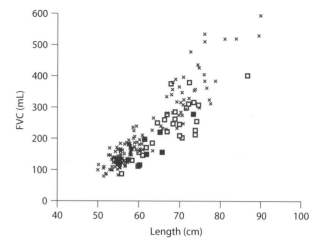

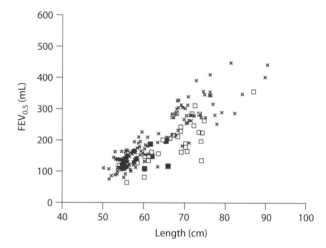

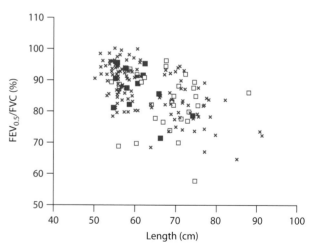

Figure 32.3 Forced vital capacity (FVC), forced expiratory volume in 0.5 second ($FEV_{0.5}$), and $FEV_{0.5}/FVC$ plotted against length. Crosses indicate airway function of healthy infants. The open and closed squares indicate infants with CF with and without prior lower respiratory illness, respectively. Infants with CF have evidence of diminished airway function.

commenced prior to the standardization of the RVRTC and before widespread availability of commercial equipment. An inflation pressure of 20 cmH_2O (rather than the current recommendation of 30 cmH_2O inflation pressure) was used to raise and standardize lung volume prior to forced expiration. The study did not identify diminished lung function in those with CF compared with the controls during the first 3–6 months of life, but older children with CF appeared to have a significant reduction in z-scores for $FEV_{0.5}$ and flows.[19] In contrast, Hoo et al.[20] identified significant impairment in lung function at approximately 3 months of age compared with controls. In their study, lung function was done using commercial equipment and the recommended inflation pressure of 30 cmH_2O. The difference between these two studies may be explained by the higher inflation pressure used in the latter study. It is known that increasing lung volume (by increasing the inflation pressure) improves the sensitivity of the test compared with forced expiratory maneuvers done at tidal lung volumes[17] and so it is possible that using 30 cmH_2O (Hoo et al.) compared with 20 cmH_2O (Linnane et al.) was responsible for the contrasting findings in lung function measured soon after diagnosis.

In the study by Hoo et al., the reduction in lung function was approximately 1 z-score for $FEV_{0.5}$ (Table 32.1). The RVRTC identified more infants with diminished lung function than MBW (25% vs. 21%, respectively). Again, combining the tests increased sensitivity to detect diminished lung function. Use of LCI and $FEV_{0.5}$ identified diminished lung function in 35% of infants. FRC measured by plethysmography (FRC_{pleth}) was less sensitive, identifying abnormality in 18% of infants, but when all three tests were combined, 44% of infants had some detectable abnormality outside the normal range compared with controls. It is unclear how these functional findings related to neutrophilic pulmonary inflammation or early structural lung disease as these were not assessed.

Table 32.1 Comparison of outcomes between infants with CF and controls at 3 months

Lung function measurement	Difference in z-score between CF and controls	Proportion with abnormal lung function (%)
LCI	0.51	21
FRC_{MBW}	0.38	
FRC_{pleth}	0.85	18
$FRC_{pleth} \times FRC_{MBW}$	0.48	20
$FEV_{0.5}$	−0.92	25
MEF_{25-75}	−0.66	24
LCI + $FEV_{0.5}$		35
LIC + $FEV_{0.5}$ + FRC_{pleth}		44

Source: Adaped from Hoo HF, Thia LP, Nguyen TT, Bush A, Chudleigh J, Lum S et al., Thorax, 67(10), 874–81, 2012. With permission.

$FEV_{0.5}$, forced expiratory volume in 0.5 second; FRC, functional residual capacity; LCI, lung clearance index; MEF, maximal expiratory flow; MBW, multiple-breath washout.

DOES INITIAL IMPAIRMENT IN AIRWAY FUNCTION NOTED IN INFANTS FOLLOWING CLINICAL DIAGNOSIS OF CF PERSIST DESPITE TREATMENT IN SPECIALIST CENTERS?

The evolution of airway function in the London cohort was assessed by measuring $FEV_{0.5}$ using RVRTC soon after diagnosis (median age 28 weeks), 6 months later in subjects with CF, and on two occasions 6 months apart (median age 7.4 and 33.7 weeks) in healthy infants. Repeated measurements were successful in 34 CF and 32 healthy subjects. After adjustment for age, length, sex, and exposure to maternal smoking, mean $FEV_{0.5}$ was significantly lower in infants with CF both shortly after diagnosis and at second test, with no significant difference in rate of increase in $FEV_{0.5}$ with growth between the two groups. When compared with published reference data, $FEV_{0.5}$ was reduced by an average of 2 z-scores on both test occasions in those with CF. Subjects with CF experienced a mean (95% CI) reduction in $FEV_{0.5}$ of 20%[21]

Data from the London Collaborative study, therefore, suggest that airway function is diminished soon after diagnosis in infants with CF and does not catch-up (or deteriorate) over a 6-month period during infancy and early childhood despite treatment in centers specializing in the management of CF.

In a large US study, mean z-scores for many parameters also differed significantly from historical control values. Mean (95% CI) z-scores were the following: −0.52 (−0.78 to −0.25) for MEF_{25}; 1.92 (1.39–2.45) for FRC; 1.22 (0.68–1.76) for residual volume; 0.87 (0.60–1.13) for FRC/total lung capacity; and 0.66 (0.27–1.06) for residual volume/total lung capacity.[22] These data confirm that lung function is clearly diminished in children with CF who were diagnosed following clinical presentations.

WHAT IS THE ASSOCIATION BETWEEN EARLY LUNG FUNCTION AND MARKERS OF INFLAMMATION OR INFECTION?

Few investigators have combined bronchoscopy with bronchoalveolar lavage (BAL) and infant lung function in the same study. In one study, specific respiratory system compliance was measured using the single breath occlusion technique and lung volumes by nitrogen washout in 22 children with CF of median age 23 months.[23] Diminished lung function correlated with BAL markers of both inflammation (interleukin-8 and neutrophil percentage) and infection. However, for the majority of subjects, lung function remained within the normal range and only very little of the variability in lung function was explained by either inflammation or infection. In another study, recruitment commenced in infancy but measurements in 40 subjects were made initially at a mean of 13 months of age.[24] No association between lung function and IL-8 concentration, neutrophil density, or pathogen load was demonstrated. However, due to the invasive nature of the assessments, not all parameters were measured simultaneously; BAL being performed annually and infant lung function every 6 months. An association of borderline significance between $FEV_{0.5}$ measured using RVRTC and infection (defined as at least 10^5 colony forming units of bacterial respiratory pathogens per milliliter of BAL fluid) and no association between $FEV_{0.5}$ and pulmonary inflammation was identified in a third study in 36 CF children during the second year of life.[25]

Recent data from the Australian Early Respiratory Surveillance Team identified lower lung function in those with evidence of free neutrophil elastase on BAL done contemporaneously with assessments of lung function.[26] Z-scores for $FEV_{0.5}$ were lower by 0.96 in those with such neutrophilic inflammation compared with those without. Longitudinal analyses identified an association between lower respiratory infection with *Staphylococcus aureus* or *Pseudomonas aeruginosa* and with decline in lung function that was not identified by cross-sectional analyses.

WHAT IS THE ASSOCIATION BETWEEN EARLY LUNG FUNCTION AND EARLY LUNG STRUCTURAL CHANGES?

Recent studies evaluating MBW as a surrogate for structural airway damage detected by CT have been favorable.[13,14,27] In a study by Owens et al., chest CT abnormalities correlated better with LCI than spirometry in school-age children. Eighty-four percent of subjects with CF had abnormal LCI, whereas only 58% and 47% had abnormal FRC values and spirometric indices, respectively.[13] These data, obtained in school-age children with CF, were not, however, replicated using MBW in infants.[28] Hall et al. studied 49 infants with CF, 13 of whom had bronchiectasis and 24 air trapping on chest CT, respectively. The second moment ratio, but not LCI, was associated with these structural changes, but the identified associations were weak, suggesting that in infants with CF, MBW was not an adequate surrogate for structural changes identified by chest CT.

Associations between forced expiratory volumes and flows and structural changes on chest CT have also been identified. Martinez et al.[29] identified lower lung function measured by the RVRTC in those with bronchial wall thickening relative to the airway luminal diameter in a small study of 13 infants with CF compared with 10 control subjects. Preliminary data have also been published describing the association between functional measurements of air trapping measured by calculating the difference between trapped (FRC_{pleth}) and communicating (FRC_{MBW}) lung volumes[30] and its relationship to trapped gas as determined by expiratory chest CT scans.[31] The rationale for making such comparisons is that air trapping is the commonest manifestation of structural lung changes identified by chest CT in infants with CF.[32,33] Statistically significant associations were identified between these functional and structural

assessments of air trapping although functional measurements of trapped gas did not appear to be physiologically plausible as measured FRC_{MBW} was larger than FRC_{pleth} in some subjects, indicating that further studies are needed to determine how trapped gas can be measured accurately in young children using the new commercial devices. Although, as proof of principle, these studies together indicate that early lung structure and function assessments are associated, there are insufficient data currently to show that monitoring of lung function offers a radiation-free surrogate to chest CT in infants and young children with CF. In the case of measuring air trapping, calculating differences between measurements from two techniques that each have their own inherent variability may lead to large percentage errors.

LUNG FUNCTION IN MULTICENTER STUDIES IN INFANTS WITH CF

Multicenter studies are required to assess the benefit of early interventions in CF and so if infant lung function is going to be used as an outcome measure in such studies they must be feasible in this setting. Even though guidelines for the performance of the RVRTC have been published, the incorporation of this test into multicenter studies is difficult. Considerable effort is required to develop standard operating procedures and quality assurance. Even though centers experienced in performing infant lung function tests are likely to contribute greater numbers of higher quality data,[22] multicenter studies are feasible, as demonstrated by a 10 center study reported on by Davis et al.[22] In this study, 100 infants with CF were assessed using the RVRTC and plethysmography every 6 months with reproducibility assessed by repeating lung function in 74 infants on two occasions 1 month apart. Lung function appeared to be reproducible with intraclass correlation coefficients of 0.9 for $FEV_{0.5}$ and 0.93 for FRC, respectively. Overall, feasibility of obtaining successful lung function data in the study was 75% but varied from below 40% to near 100% depending on the experience of the center.[22] These data have informed the use of the RVRTC as a lung function outcome measure in intervention studies in infants with CF (see later). The use of LCI as an outcome measure in multicenter trials is discussed in Chapter 39.

EARLY LUNG FUNCTION IN RECENT INTERVENTION STUDIES

The RVRTC was used to determine if lung function improved following a course of hospitalization for intravenous antibiotics in infants with CF.[34] Lung function improved significantly with treatment. For example, mean z-score for $FEV_{0.5}$ improved from −3.06 before treatment to −1.1 on completion of intravenous antibiotics, indicating that RVRTC was sensitive to change and could be used to monitor response to treatment in a similar way to the routine use of spirometry in older subjects with CF, albeit with the greater burden of requiring sedation and the increased technical requirements.

RECENT STUDIES IN PRESCHOOL CHILDREN

Too old to sedate routinely, considered fickle and noncooperative by many, the years between two and six provide several challenges to those wishing to measure lung function. In many centers, preschool children with CF do not undergo lung function until they are able to perform reproducible forced expiratory maneuvers. To bridge the "silent years," recent studies have focused on preschool subjects with CF by skillfully using tests requiring minimal passive cooperation or by using incentives to effectively coerce the subject. By following infants with CF through the preschool years, studies are beginning to highlight the longer-term implications of diminished lung function identified early in life. Although demanding in its own right, obtaining preschool lung function is still easier than infant lung function. Lung function at this age should be considered a means to monitor progress and response to interventions rather than an opportunity to detect the earliest lung disease, which is best detected during the first 2 years of life. With this caveat in mind, a number of techniques have been assessed in preschool children with CF.

RESISTANCE INTERRUPTER TECHNIQUE

The resistance interrupter technique (Rint) requires minimal cooperation and can be performed in the ambulatory setting in preschool children.[36] Rint is a noninvasive method of measuring airway resistance first described in 1927. It is based on the assumption that during an imperceptibly brief interruption of airflow during tidal breathing, the pressure changes at the airway opening can be used to determine the alveolar pressure (P) at the moment of interruption, and, hence, knowing the flow immediately prior to interruption (V'), resistance can be calculated as P/V'. Resistance measured by this technique was significantly elevated (Z-score of 1.31 compared with 0.19 in healthy controls) in 40 subjects with CF aged between 3 and 8 years.[37] Those with a history of prior lower respiratory illness or exposure to environmental tobacco smoke had significantly elevated expiratory resistance. Although measurements in those with CF were no more variable than those made in healthy subjects, the overall variability of the resistance measurements was high. Expiratory resistance measured by the interrupter technique depends on the proximal airways and so physiologically it would not appear to be the ideal test to measure peripheral airway function associated with early pulmonary disease. Furthermore, as with plethysmography (above), alveolar pressure cannot be assumed to track mouth pressure in the presence of airflow obstruction. Most studies have shown that Rint measurements in preschool children do not distinguish health from disease[38] and two longitudinal studies in 21[39] and 30[40] preschool children with CF, respectively, showed no deterioration in Rint despite evidence of progressive worsening of radiological changes. Rint is now considered to be of limited value in preschool children with CF.[38]

INCENTIVE SPIROMETRY

In recent years, computer animation programs have been developed to instruct and stimulate young children in maximal forced expiratory maneuvers. Children are asked to blow out candles, to make airplanes fly, or to blow up balloons on the computer screen. These programs help children to focus on the task and provide a visual motivation to accomplish an optimal maneuver. A wide range of such programs is now available. The type of incentive software and the age and experience of the subject determine the reproducibility of measurements obtained in this way.[41] Tracking of lung function is likely to persist through the preschool years (that is, those with the lowest airway function in infancy maintain this position with growth). When infants who had undergone lung function were retested at a mean age of 3.9 years, mean (SD) z-scores were -0.55 (0.85) for $FEV_{0.5}$, with only one child with CF still having an abnormal $FEV_{0.5}$.[42] This could either suggest that airway function may improve through the preschool years or alternatively that incentive spirometry is less able to identify diminished airway function in preschool subjects than the RVRTC in infants.

Contrary to popular notions, skilled pediatric pulmonary function technicians, who regularly work with preschool children, may find greater success using conventional spirometry if the subject is appropriately coached. In a recent study, 33 of 38 children with CF (including 4 of 6 three-year olds and 9 of 11 four-year olds) were able to perform either two or three conventional spirometry maneuvers (without incentive) and fulfill study acceptability and reproducibility criteria.[43] Children with CF had significantly lower forced vital capacity (FVC), FEV_1, and MEF_{75-25} than healthy subjects. Those homozygous for $\Delta F508$ had significantly lower FVC and FEV_1 than heterozygotes. Subjects were well at the time of lung function and so the feasibility and variability of performing spirometry during exacerbations is not known.

RVRTC had been performed previously in 14 subjects during infancy in this study and again tracking of lung function occurred through to the preschool assessments.[43] In those with lung function in the normal range as infants (z-score for $MEF_{75-25} \geq -2$), there was no significant change in z-score for the same parameter measured using spirometry. However, z-scores increased significantly between infancy and childhood in four subjects with diminished MEF_{75-25} as infants. Similarly, these data would suggest that either airway function genuinely improves with age or that the RVRTC is better able to detect diminished airway function in infants than spirometry in preschool children. The reasons for improvement could include the result of treatment, normal lung development, or an increase in airway luminal diameter such that obstruction is less severe in older subjects. The process of augmenting inflations, the effects of sedation, and testing in the supine opposed to upright position in infants may alter airway and lung mechanics, increasing detection of functional abnormalities by the RVRTC when compared with older children tested using spirometry.

Several studies have now been published using spirometry in preschool children[38,40,42-44] and these suggest that abnormalities in lung function, although mild, are already present at this age and commonly detected. The reliability of measurements of forced expiration depends on strict quality control. Recently, quality control recommendations for spirometry have been published for preschool children,[45] which have enhanced the standardization of testing protocols with this technique.

MULTIPLE-BREATH WASHOUT

This exciting technique is performed during tidal breathing and therefore requires minimal cooperation. Several parameters can be measured, the commonest being measures of the efficiency of expiration such as the LCI and the moment ratios.[10]

As reductions in flow from obstructed lung regions appear to be compensated by increases in flow from unobstructed regions (a concept known as "kinematic interdependence of regional expiratory flows"), during measurements of forced expiration upstream (peripheral) nonuniformities may be masked.[46] For this reason, the maximum forced expiratory flow-volume curve is not considered as the ideal tool for the detection of early non-uniform airway disease while the multiple-breath inert gas washout technique should be more sensitive at detecting such inhomogeneities.

Measurements using the technique have been made in CF subjects of all ages. Inert gas washout disclosed airway dysfunction in the majority of children with CF aged 3 to 18 years who had normal lung function assessed by spirometry, suggesting that multiple-breath inert gas washout is indeed of greater value than spirometry in detecting early CF lung disease.[47] Increased LCI measurements are a consistent finding in CF. These findings have recently been confirmed in younger subjects.[12] MBW indices are better predictors of subsequent abnormal FEV_1 in school-age children than spirometry.[48] Although multiple-breath inert gas washout appears to be a sensitive test of early functional dysfunction in those with CF, it is not known if it will be more or less useful than parameters of forced expiration to monitor lung function longitudinally or the response to therapeutic interventions and so further studies are required to determine its role. As measurements in infants have so far been incorporated into studies with protocols including more invasive and complex tests, they

have been performed following sedation of the infant. It is possible that when used alone, a period of natural sleep without sedation would be sufficient to enable successful performance of the test. This would significantly enhance the ability of investigators to obtain longitudinal data during the first months of life.

Recommendations for the methodological conduct of the MBW test have been developed recently and will enhance standardized testing.[10] Commercial devices have been developed and efforts are ongoing to evaluate the role of these, utilizing a nitrogen washout protocol, in both infants and preschool children with CF.

FORCED OSCILLATION TECHNIQUE (FOT)

The FOT requires minimal cooperation and is easy to perform in preschool children using commercially available equipment (Figure 32.4).

In one longitudinal study in which FOT, Rint, and plethysmographic airway resistance were measured serially in preschool children with CF, only resistance was abnormal in the CF group.[40] Elevated respiratory system resistance and decreased respiratory system reactance have been reported in the past using the FOT[49] but have not been confirmed by more recent studies.[40,44] Gangell et al.[50] reported worse lung function using FOT in those children who had been symptomatic in the preceding month compared with asymptomatic children. However, in longitudinal studies using FOT, no association was identified between FOT parameters and the presence of infection in the airways or cough symptom score.[40,44,51] These studies suggested that FOT may be too insensitive to use routinely for monitoring lung disease in preschool children.

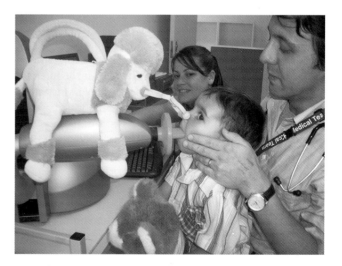

Figure 32.4 Forced oscillation technique performed during tidal breathing in a preschool child aged 2 years. The child is able to maintain a seal around the mouthpiece. The cheeks and chin are supported by the investigator to decrease the influence of upper airway shunt impedance. A second observer is vigilant for technical problems, such as glottic closure and leaks, and any signs of distress in the child.

procedure. Low-pressure suction either manually or using wall suction is recommended. Whether to pool all samples for subsequent analysis or to use the first sample from two lobes for microbiology only is still being debated. The first sample is of more bronchial origin, contains a higher percentage of neutrophils and, in older children, has been shown to better differentiate CF from healthy individuals; however, the relevance of this finding for clinical and research purposes is still unclear.

CLINICAL USE

Diagnostic and therapeutic bronchoscopy

As in any other patient group, flexible bronchoscopy can be utilized to diagnose lower airway abnormalities. Although recent data from the pig model of CF have suggested primary abnormalities in airway cartilage, the relevance of this finding for infants with CF is unclear and there is currently no evidence that CF infants have a higher incidence of bronchial malformations or a higher incidence of tracheobronchomalacia.

As in any age group, infants with CF can develop atelectasis, and bronchoscopy can be used to mobilize secretions by either suction alone or in combination with instillation of mucolytics such as dornase alfa. For a more detailed description see Chapter 18.

Bronchoalveolar lavage

BAL is currently the only technique that enables sampling of the lower respiratory tract to detect infection and inflammation in children and adults who are unable to produce sputum. The clinical alternative to collection of lower respiratory tract samples has been the use of oropharyngeal (OP) samples or induced sputum collection. Induced sputum samples are thought to have at least as good if not a higher diagnostic yield compared with gastric lavage in infants and young children for the diagnosis of tuberculosis.[6] Culture and inflammatory parameters in induced sputum and BAL from infants and young children with CF have not yet been compared although comparison of airway inflammatory parameters in induced sputum and BAL from mild adult asthmatics would suggest that they sample different compartments. Induced sputum is thought to sample the larger airways while BAL is thought to be more a peripheral airway sample.[7] To date, induced sputum has not widely been used in young children with CF, and further research is required. OP cultures are widely used as a proxy for lower respiratory tract infection although these samples are not suitable for providing inflammatory data. Unfortunately, it has been recognized that when OP and BAL cultures are compared at the same time point when patients are stable clinically, OP cultures have a poor sensitivity and positive predictive value for lower respiratory tract infection with *Pseudomonas aeruginosa* particularly in younger children (Table 33.1).[8] On the other hand, the specificity and negative predictive value is better; indicating that OP cultures are useful to exclude (or lower the likelihood of) lower airway infection with *P. aeruginosa*. In children with CF, where lower respiratory tract infection and inflammation are recognized to occur even in the first few months of life, early pulmonary infection, particularly with *P. aeruginosa*, is associated with increased morbidity and mortality[10] the use of bronchoscopy and BAL would therefore seem logical. Theoretically, the clinician, armed with knowledge of what is cultured from the lower respiratory tract and the inflammatory status of their patient, would be able to choose appropriate antibiotic therapy and consider approaches to managing inflammation, and this should lead to improved long-term outcomes. On the other hand, flexible bronchoscopy and BAL are semi-invasive procedures and are usually performed under general anesthesia. If bronchoscopy and BAL are to be used clinically, then when should they be performed? Some CF centers have elected to perform bronchoscopy and BAL at around 3 months of age and then on an annual surveillance basis at times of stability up until children can expectorate sputum and have demonstrated

Table 33.1 Comparison of BAL and OP cultures collected at the same time for the detection of *P. aeruginosa* and *Staphylococcus aureus* in young children with CF.

Diagnostic accuracy of OP cultures for detection of *P. aeruginosa (Pa)*						
	Pa Prevalence	Mean age	Sens (%)	Spec (%)	PPV (%)	NPV (%)
Rosenfeld[8]	8%	8 mo	44	95	44	95
Armstrong[9]	11%[a]	17 mo	71	93	57	96
Rosenfeld[8]	23%	26 mo	68	94	76	91
Diagnostic accuracy of OP cultures for detection of *S. aureus (Sa)*						
	Sa Prevalence	Mean age	Sens (%)	Spec (%)	PPV (%)	NPV (%)
Rosenfeld[8]	34%	8 months	80	77	64	88
Armstrong[9]	19%[a]	17 months	86	61	33	95
Rosenfeld[8]	37%	26 months	73	71	59	82

Notes: Data from the Armstrong cohort were also included in the Rosenfeld study. Sens, sensitivity; Spec, specificity; PPV, positive predictive value; NPV, negative predictive value.

[a] ≥10⁵ cfu/mL.

the presence of infection and inflammation in infants and young children (Video 33.2).[11,12] Others have suggested that BAL might be more useful in symptomatic patients with higher diagnostic yield.[13]

To examine the benefits or otherwise of bronchoscopy and BAL in infants and young children with CF, a randomized controlled trial (ACFBAL study) was designed and conducted in eight CF centers across Australia and New Zealand.[14] A total of 170 infants aged <6 months with a confirmed diagnosis of classical CF were randomized to either BAL-directed therapy or standard management. Those randomized to standard care received care according to clinical status and OP culture results. Infants randomized to the BAL group underwent BAL (1) before 6 months of age when well, (2) when hospitalized for pulmonary exacerbations, (3) if *P. aeruginosa* was cultured from OP specimens, and (4) following *P. aeruginosa* eradication therapy. At 5 years of age, 157 children who completed the trial underwent BAL, chest high-resolution computed-tomography scan and pulmonary function testing. There were no statistically significant differences in this well-powered study between groups for any clinical, microbiologic or radiographic outcome at age 5 years and only 12% of children had *P. aeruginosa* cultured in their final BAL at age 5 years. Chronic infection was defined as failure to clear infection on BAL in the BAL group and OP culture in the standard group despite two consecutive *P. aeruginosa* eradication courses of treatment. Prior to the final outcome BAL, one child in the BAL group and four receiving standard management had met the study definition for chronic *P. aeruginosa* infection. Therefore, the prevalence of chronic infection was very low in both groups. However, of these five children only the one child from the BAL group had *P. aeruginosa* detected at their final BAL.

If OP cultures have poor sensitivity and poor positive predictive value for detection of *P. aeruginosa*, as suggested by previous work, then why was there no difference between groups after 5 years? In a previous study, Rosenfeld et al combined data from three different CF centers and examined the relationship between one OP culture and BAL taken at one specific time point which was not during exacerbation. However, this study did not examine the utility of using OP cultures over a period of time or taken during exacerbations when they might provide greater sensitivity and positive predictive value. In the ACFBAL study, patients averaged around three OP cultures per year per child and this strategy was associated with low rates of *P. aeruginosa* in BAL at age 5 years (12% children).

While others have suggested the greatest benefit of BAL might be in stable children with negative OP cultures, the ACFBAL trial used BAL at the times when clinicians are most likely to want answers i.e. at times when patients are unwell. In this setting two potential scenarios can be envisioned: firstly, the patient has a negative OP culture and BAL could help to detect one or more pathogens to guide treatment, or secondly, the patient has a positive OP culture and the clinicians might be wondering if the organism was really present in the lower respiratory tract (because of low

positive predictive value of OP culture). Finally, the study used BAL in another clinical scenario: after eradication treatment to check for clearance. Each scenario has its own complexity and the lack of difference between the BAL and control group should not be seen as evidence that BAL is not potentially useful in any of these settings on an individual patient basis.

An alternative strategy not assessed in this study and utilized by some centers is to perform a surveillance BAL either after initial diagnosis and/or at routine intervals (usually on an annual basis). The boundaries between clinical utility and research are not always clearly defined in this setting. An annual BAL surveillance program over the first 5 years of life has previously reported finding *P. aeruginosa* in 28.4% children which is less than the ACFBAL study over the first 5 years of life.[15] While the number of children was rather small, an annual surveillance strategy reported the cross sectional prevalence of bronchiectasis at age 5–6 years of 60%. While a direct comparison is not feasible, the prevalence of bronchiectasis at age 5 years was similar in the ACFBAL study (58%)[16] suggesting no apparent large benefit to the surveillance bronchoscopy strategy to date.

Therefore, at the present time, the available data do not suggest a clinical benefit of routine bronchoscopy and BAL in infants with CF. On the other hand, a "low-threshold" approach seems warranted to avoid missing the opportunity to treat an otherwise missed lower airway infection. There is consensus amongst CF clinicians that in a child not responding to empiric antibiotic treatment guided by clinical assessment and OP culture results, then bronchoscopy and BAL should be strongly considered.

RESEARCH USE

As outlined in a recent review on outcome measures for clinical trials in infants and young children, BAL is unlikely to become a primary outcome measure in interventional studies in this age group.[17] However, BAL can provide important mechanistic information in interventions that affect the balance if infection and inflammation. Examples are the COMBAT CF study (AZI001; ACTRN12610001072000; NCT01270074) assessing the effect of azithromycin on lung disease progression in CF infants where BAL will provide important information on treatment efficacy on airway inflammation, bacterial and potentially viral infection as well as being a safety measure assessing the evolution of macrolide resistance of bacterial organisms. BAL can therefore support or define potential mechanisms of action that could not otherwise be clarified. In addition, BAL plays an important role in cross-validating other less-invasive biomarkers that could potentially be used as outcome measures derived from blood and urine that could be sampled more frequently in an interventional trial. In trials of CFTR pharmacotherapy, while not essential for defining safety, BAL is currently the only way to demonstrate effects of therapy on the progression of airway inflammation in young children. BAL could also give valuable information on therapy-induced changes in the airway microbiome, potentially positive or negative, during interventional studies.

While definition of the mechanism of action is usually part of early phase studies, it is unlikely that full development programs will happen in infants and young children and there could only be one pivotal study for any given drug in this age group. It may be important to integrate BAL into these trials, potentially in subgroups of patients to better understand how an intervention affects or impacts on the progression of infection and inflammation. There could potentially be a disadvantage of performing BALs only at times of clinical stability as infection and inflammation and potential effects of interventions on these processes could be underestimated with this strategy. BAL at times of clinical instability may increase its yield, but is also associated with a higher risk of procedure-related side effects. However, it is unlikely that a sampling strategy on BALs performed more frequently than once in a year is realistic. Cross-validated systemic markers of inflammation and other culture techniques to capture infection may help to close the gap as they allow for more frequent sampling.

SAFETY AND ADVERSE EVENTS

In general, flexible bronchoscopy and BAL are well tolerated in the pediatric population.[18] The most comprehensive assessment of safety of flexible bronchoscopy in children was reported in 2002 by de Blic et al.[19] and included 1328 procedures in 1153 children with a mean age of 4.5 years. The majority of procedures were conducted under conscious sedation using intravenous midazolam, passing

the bronchoscope through an endoscopic face mask and BAL was performed in just under half of the procedures. Complications were seen in 6.9% procedures with 1.7% classified as major and 5.2% as minor. The most common major complication was transient desaturation to less than 90% particularly in younger children and the most common minor complication was cough during the procedure seen only in children having conscious sedation. Following the procedure, the most common complication was fever, which was seen more often when BAL was performed and occurred in 9% of procedures involving BAL and only 1.9% when BAL was not performed. Picard et al. reported fever within 24 hours postoperatively in 44/91 children (48%) and again more commonly when BAL was performed (52.2%).[20] Fever was seen more commonly in younger children. Contamination of the bronchoscope with pathogens such as *P. aeruginosa* and mycobacterial species has also been reported.

The safety of bronchoscopy and BAL in infants and preschool children with CF taking part in the ACFBAL study was reported by Wainwright et al. in 2008 and 2011.[14,21] There were 524 bronchoscopy and BAL procedures in 160 children all conducted under general anesthesia using a laryngeal mask. In 25 procedures (4.8%), there was a substantial clinical deterioration recorded either intraoperatively or within 24 hours of the procedure (Table 33.2). Fever within 24 hours of the procedure and transient worsening of cough were relatively common adverse events. In addition, there are increasing concerns related to potential neurobehavioral consequences of exposure of young children in the first few years of life to general anesthetic agents[22] and the results of randomized controlled studies are awaited. While, in general, the procedure was well tolerated in young children with CF, there are potential adverse events that should be carefully considered and families appropriately counseled.

Table 33.2 Adverse events associated with 524 BAL procedures in ACFBAL study

	No (%)
Substantial clinical deterioration during and within 24 h of BAL	25 (4.8)
Haemoglobin desaturation <90% requiring intervention during procedure	7
Ventricular tachyarrhthmia	1
Stridor post-BAL	3
Supplemental oxygen required >2 hours postoperatively	6
Noninvasive ventilation postoperatively	1
Respiratory distress postoperatively with no supplemental oxygen use	2
High fever ≥38.5°C and systemically unwell (febrile seizure, n = 1)	3
Other likely unrelated to procedure (UTI, malfunction central venous line)	2
Unplanned hospital admission post-BAL (6 with high fever, 6 substantial clinical deterioration)	12 (2.3)
Contaminated bronchoscope (*Enterobacter cloacae* from one procedure and coagulase-negative *Staphylococcus*, *Corynebacterium* and α-hemolytic *Streptococcus* species from another)	2 (0.4)
Fever ≥38.5°C within 24 hours of BAL	40 (7.6)
Fever <38.5°C within 24 hours of BAL	52 (9.9)
Transient worsening of cough post-BAL	151 (29)

SUMMARY

Flexible bronchoscopy and BAL have contributed enormously to our understanding of early CF lung disease and continue to provide unique research insights. Clinical benefit, however, may be more restricted partly due to the limited treatment options currently available to use as targeted therapies in infants and young children. It is likely that unless specific anti-inflammatory therapies become available, in clinical practice, bronchoscopy and BAL may best be reserved for young children whose condition is deteriorating despite parenteral antibiotic therapy, when unusual or antibiotic resistant pathogens are suspected.

VIDEOS

- *Video 33.1 (http://goo.gl/qB87PR)*: Flexible bronchoscopy in a well child with cystic fibrosis and a BAL that cultured no recognized pathogens.
- *Video 33.2 (http://goo.gl/ofltvT)*: Flexible bronchoscopy in an infant with cystic fibrosis with no respiratory symptoms and current airway infection with *P. aeruginosa*.

REFERENCES

1. Khan TZ, Wagener JS, Bost T, Martinez J, Accurso FJ, Riches DWH. Early pulmonary inflammation in infants with cystic fibrosis. *Am J Respir Crit Care Med* 1995; **151**: 1075–82.
2. Armstrong DS, Grimwood K, Carzino R, Carlin JB, Olinsky A, Phelan PD. Lower respiratory infection and inflammation in infants with newly diagnosed cystic fibrosis. *BMJ* 1995; **310**: 1571–2.
3. De Blic J, Midulla F, Barbato A, Clement A, Dab I, Eber E, Green C et al. ERS Task Force on bronchoalveolar lavage in children. *Eur Respir J* 2000; **15**: 217–231.
4. Gutierrez J, Grimwood K, Armstrong D et al. Interlobar differences in bronchoalveolar lavage fluid from children with cystic fibrosis. *Eur Respir J* 2001; **17**: 281–6.
5. Gilchrist FJ, Salamat S, Clayton S, Peach J, Alexander J, Lenney W. Bronchoalveolar lavage in children with cystic fibrosis: How many lobes should be sampled? *Arch Dis Child* 2011; **96**(3): 215–7.
6. Zar HJ, Hanslo D, Apolles P, Swingler G, Hussey G. Induced sputum versus gastric lavage for microbiological confirmation of pulmonary tuberculosis in infants and young children: A prospective study. *Lancet* 2005; **365**(9454): 130–4.
7. Pizzichini E, Pizzichini MM, Kidney JC et al. Induced sputum, bronchoalveolar lavage and blood from mild asthmatics: Inflammatory cells, lymphocyte subsets and soluble markers compared. *Eur Respir J* 1998; **11**(4): 828–34.
8. Rosenfeld M, Emerson J, Accurso F et al. Diagnostic accuracy of oropharyngeal cultures in infants and young children with cystic fibrosis. *Pediatr Pulmonol* 1999; **28**: 321–8.
9. Armstrong D, Grimwood K, Carlin J, Carzino R, Olinsky A, Phelan P. Bronchoalveolar lavage or oropharyngeal cultures to identify lower respiratory pathogens in infants with cystic fibrosis. *Pediatr Pulmonol* 1996; **21**(5): 267–75.
10. Gibson R, Burns J, Ramsey B. Pathophysiology and management of pulmonary infections in cystic fibrosis. *Am J Respir Crit Care Med* 2003; **168**(8): 918–51.
11. Armstrong DS, Hook SM, Jamsen KM et al. Lower airway inflammation in infants with cystic fibrosis detected by newborn screening. *Pediatr Pulmonol* 2005; **40**(6): 500–10.
12. Sly PD, Brennan S, Gangell C et al. Lung disease at diagnosis in infants with cystic fibrosis detected by newborn screening. *Am J Respir Crit Care Med* 2009; **180**(2): 146–52.
13. Furness JC, Habeb A, Spencer DA, O'Brien CJ. To the editor: Bronchoalveolar lavage (BAL) in pediatric cystic fibrosis (CF): Its clinical use modified by audit in a regional CF center. *Pediatr Pulmonol* 2002; **33**(3): 234.
14. Wainwright CE, Vidmar S, Armstrong DS et al. Effect of bronchoalveolar lavage-directed therapy on *Pseudomonas aeruginosa* infection and structural lung injury in children with cystic fibrosis: A randomized trial. *JAMA* 2011; **306**(2): 163–71.
15. Douglas T, Brennan S, Gard S et al. Acquisition and eradication of *P. aeruginosa* in young children with cystic fibrosis. *Eur Respir J* 2009; **33**(2): 305–11.
16. Stick SM, Brennan S, Murray C et al. Bronchiectasis in infants and preschool children diagnosed with cystic fibrosis after newborn screening. *J Pediatr* 2009; **155**(5): 623–8 e1.
17. Stick S, Tiddens H, Aurora P, Gustafsson P, Ranganathan S, Robinson P, Rosenfeld M, Sly P, Ratjen F. Early intervention studies in infants and preschool children with cystic fibrosis: Are we ready? *Eur Respir J* 2013 Aug; **42**(2): 527–38. doi: 10.1183/09031936.00108212. Epub 2013 Mar 21.
18. Nussbaum E. Pediatric fiberoptic bronchoscopy: Clinical experience with 2,836 bronchoscopies. *Pediatr Crit Care Med* 2002; **3**(2): 171–6.
19. de Blic J, Marchac V, Scheinmann P. Complications of flexible bronchoscopy in children: Prospective study of 1,328 procedures. *Eur Respir J* 2002; **20**(5): 1271–6.
20. Picard E, Schwartz S, Golderg S, Glick T, Villa Y, Kerem E. A prospective study of fever and bacteremia after flexible fibreoptic bronchoscopy in children. *Chest* 2000; **117**: 573–7.
21. Wainwright C, Grimwood K, Carlin J et al. Safety of bronchoalveolar lavage in young children with cystic fibrosis. *Pediatr Pulmonol* 2008; **43**(10): 965–72.
22. Istaphanous GK, Loepke AW. General anesthetics and the developing brain. *Curr Opin Anaesthesiol* 2009; **22**(3): 368–73.

Table 34.2 Guidelines for routine chest CT in CF

Scan mode	Helical
Scan parameter	Under 9 kg: 80 kVp, 60 ref mAs 10 kg and above: 100 kVp, 30–48 ref mAs
Tube rotation	0.5 seconds
Tube collimation	0.6 mm
Pitch	1
Scan slice width	0.6 mm
Recon slice width	1 m
Recon kernel—medium	Soft B30 and high resolution B60
Contrast media	Omnipaque 300, 2 mL/kg to a maximum of 100 mL
Scan delay	Using pressure injector, 25 seconds from start of injection

modulation futile. Iterative reconstruction is also widely available on modern CT scanners. It allows use of lower exposure factors with significant reduction in image noise, without loss of diagnostic information, with a reported dose reduction of 35% noted in chest CT.[55]

PATIENT CARE

Because of the speed of present-day CT scanners, children over 3 years of age are usually compliant for their procedure provided they are properly prepared through play therapy beforehand, using a mock-up toy of the scanner to take the child and their parents through the scanning process. It is also a good opportunity to assess the child's ability to respond to breath-holding instructions; otherwise, gentle respiration is encouraged. A range of suitable sedatives may be prescribed to younger children, which include the light-acting sedative chloral hydrate at a dose of 50 mg/kg, or the short-acting midazolam hydrochloride at 0.1 mg/kg body weight. Some centers prefer the quicker acting sedative propofol, but this must be administered in the presence of an anesthesiologist. The use of general anesthesia is generally reserved only for those noncompliant patients or in cases where sedation is not successful.

NEW TECHNIQUES

PROJECTION RADIOGRAPHY

The development of digital imaging within plain film radiography is very advantageous in children. First introduced to computed radiography (CR) and later in direct read-out radiography (DR) systems (utilizing flat-panel detector [FD] technology), this technology helped provide greater efficiency in converting incident x-ray energy into image signal. This has greatly improved resultant image quality, when compared with conventional screen-film-based systems, when equivalent exposure parameters were used. This technique is important as it has the potential for lowering radiation dosage to the patient and reducing the risk of non-diagnostic exposure. Using postprocessing computer techniques, both bone and soft-tissue anatomy are optimally displayed on the same image, thus eliminating the need for repeated radiation exposure.[56-58] In general, FD technology is an efficient method of obtaining high-quality image data, enabling immediate image preview, storage, and distribution over local-area networks for viewing by clinicians, thus enhancing efficiency and productivity within high-workflow radiology departments.

Other applications of FD technology include digital tomosynthesis (or digital tomography) providing quasi-3-dimenional images, adapted for use in chest imaging. As a chest radiograph is a two-dimensional image, sensitivity may be reduced when detecting underlying pathology because of overlapping anatomy. This is overcome by CT applications but with an inherent increased radiation dose. Tomosynthesis evolved from conventional geometric tomography and was introduced as a low-dose alternative for chest radiographic examination, in monitoring children with CF, and in the detection of pulmonary nodules.[59,60] This technique, involving the acquisition of a number of projection images at different angles during a single vertical motion of the x-ray tube (between a given angular range of −17.5 and +17.5 degrees) directed at a stationary digital FD, results in up to 60 coronal sectional images at an arbitrary depth.[59-61] Anatomical structures within each image section are sharply depicted, whereas structures located anteriorly and posteriorly are blurred. Spatial resolution is higher in tomosynthesis when compared to CT in the acquired imaging plane, but depth resolution is inferior, due to the limited angles used.

Further limitations to this imaging technique include the necessity of a 10-second acquisition time, increasing the likelihood of respiratory motion artefacts in noncompliant patients, and so will exclude younger children who are unable to breath-hold. Although the radiation dose for tomosynthesis is much reduced compared with CT, it is three times higher than a frontal chest radiograph.

OTHER TECHNIQUES

MAGNETIC RESONANCE IMAGING

Hyperpolarised noble-gas magnetic resonance imaging (MRI) of the lung is a relatively new, versatile imaging modality that depicts both lung function and morphology.[62] With this technique, it is possible to acquire images of the lung with relatively high temporal and spatial resolution. Helium (^{3}He) and xenon (^{129}Xe) are the two nonradioactive isotopes of noble gases that can be hyperpolarized, but ^{3}He has been primarily used for hyperpolarized MRI of the lungs in humans.[62,63] Mucus plugging and airway obstruction result in ventilation inhomogeneity in CF lungs and hyperpolarized^3 He MRI of the lung reflects these functional changes as shown in older children and adults.[64,65] HRCT is the imaging modality of choice to assess structural CF lung disease, but its ability to assess lung function is limited. The other major limitation is the level of radiation exposure, particularly for longitudinal assessment of disease progression, which requires repeated scans.[3] He MRI involves no ionizing radiation, which makes it an ideal imaging tool in children.[66]

^{3}He MRI has the potential to serve as a biomarker for assessment of severity of lung disease and to follow disease progression in children with CF. However, this technique is still in its relative infancy and has yet to be evaluated in preschool children, the current major limitation being that the technology to polarize noble gases is not widely available, and the gases themselves are very expensive. The other potential limitation is that MRI in children under 5 years of age requires either sedation or a general anesthetic and the scanner can be claustrophobic.

MOLECULAR IMAGING TECHNIQUES

Molecular imaging is distinct from structural or functional imaging and aims to noninvasively characterize and quantify cellular and subcellular events. These techniques include optical imaging and radionuclide-based methods such as planar gamma scintigraphy, single-photon emission computed tomography (SPECT), and positron emission tomography (PET). These modalities offer the possibility of monitoring and quantifying molecular and cellular processes noninvasively. However, they are still limited to the research laboratory and the potential impact on clinical research and practice is yet undetermined.[67]

REFERENCES

1. Brody AS, Molina PL, Klein JS, Rothman BS, Ramagopal M, Swartz DR. High-resolution computed tomography of the chest in children with cystic fibrosis: Support for use as an outcome surrogate. *Pediatr Radiol* 1999; **29**(10): 731–35.

2. de Jong PA, Nakano Y, Lequin MH et al. Progressive damage on high resolution computed tomography despite stable lung function in cystic fibrosis. *Eur Respir J* 2004; **23**(1): 93–7.

3. Cystic Fibrosis Foundation guidelines for patient services, evaluation, and monitoring in cystic fibrosis centers. The Cystic Fibrosis Foundation Center Committee and Guidelines Subcommittee. *Am J Dis Child* 1990; **144**(12): 1311–2.

4. Kerem E, Conway S, Elborn S, Heijerman H. Standards of care for patients with cystic fibrosis: A European consensus. *J Cyst Fibros* 2005; **4**(1):7–26.

5. Wood BP. Cystic fibrosis: 1997. *Radiology* 1997; **204**(1):1–10.

6. Oikonomou A, Hansell DM. Recent advances in imaging. In: Bush A, Alton EWFW, Davies JC, Griesenbach U, Jaffe A (Eds). *Progress in Respiratory Research*, volume 34: *Cystic Fibrosis in the 21st Century*, Volume 34, *Progress in Respiratory Research* Cape Town, South Africa: Karger; 2006.

7. Tomashefski JF Jr., Bruce M, Stern RC, Dearborn DG, Dahms B. Pulmonary air cysts in cystic fibrosis: Relation of pathologic features to radiologic findings and history of pneumothorax. *Hum Pathol* 1985; **16**(3): 253–61.

8. Shwachman H, Kulczycki LL. Long-term study of one hundred five patients with cystic fibrosis; studies made over a five- to fourteen-year period. *AMA J Dis Child* 1958; **96**(1): 6–15.

9. Tiddens HA. Detecting early structural lung damage in cystic fibrosis. *Pediatr Pulmonol* 2002; **34**(3): 228–31.

10. Chrispin AR, Norman AP. The systematic evaluation of the chest radiograph in cystic fibrosis. *Pediatr Radiol* 1974; **2**(2): 101–5.

11. van der Put JM, Meradji M, Danoesastro D, Kerrebijn KF. Chest radiographs in cystic fibrosis. A follow-up study with application of a quantitative system. *Pediatr Radiol* 1982; **12**(2): 57–61.

12. Brasfield D, Hicks G, Soong S, Peters J, Tiller R. Evaluation of scoring system of the chest radiograph in cystic fibrosis: A collaborative study. *AJR Am J Roentgenol* 1980; **134**(6): 1195–8.

13. Weatherly MR, Palmer CG, Peters ME et al. Wisconsin cystic fibrosis chest radiograph scoring system. *Pediatrics* 1993; **91**(2): 488–95.

14. Conway SP, Pond MN, Bowler I et al. The chest radiograph in cystic fibrosis: A new scoring system compared with the Chrispin–Norman and Brasfield scores. *Thorax* 1994; **49**(9): 860–2.

15. Jacobsen LE, Houston CS, Habbick BF, Genereux GP, Howie JL. Cystic fibrosis: A comparison of computed tomography and plain chest radiographs. *Can Assoc Radiol J* 1986; **37**(1): 17–21.

16. Greene KE, Takasugi JE, Godwin JD, Richardson ML, Burke W, Aitken ML. Radiographic changes in acute exacerbations of cystic fibrosis in adults: A pilot study. *AJR Am J Roentgenol* 1994; **163**(3): 557–62.

17. de Jong PA, Ottink MD, Robben SG et al. Pulmonary disease assessment in cystic fibrosis: Comparison of CT scoring systems and value of bronchial and arterial dimension measurements. *Radiology* 2004; **231**(2): 434–9.

18. Stick SM, Brennan S, Murray C et al. Bronchiectasis in infants and preschool children diagnosed with cystic fibrosis after newborn screening. *J Pediatr* 2009; **155**(5): 623–8.

19. Mott LS, Park J, Gangell CL et al. Distribution of early structural lung changes due to cystic fibrosis detected with chest computed tomography. *J Pediatr* 2013; **163**(1): 243–8.

20. Thia LP, Calder A, Stocks J, Bush A, Owens CM, Wallis C, Young C, Sullivan Y, Wade A, McEwan A, Brody AS; London Cystic Fibrosis Collaboration. Is chest CT useful in newborn screened infants with cystic fibrosis at 1 year of age? *Thorax* 2014; **69**(4): 320–7.

21. Hansell DM, Bankier AA, MacMahon H, McLoud TC, Muller NL, Remy J. Fleischner Society: Glossary of terms for thoracic imaging. *Radiology* 2008; **246**(3): 697–722.

22. Mott LS, Park J, Murray CP et al. Progression of early structural lung disease in young children with cystic fibrosis assessed using CT. *Thorax* 2012; **67**(6): 509–16.

23. Brody AS, Klein JS, Molina PL, Quan J, Bean JA, Wilmott RW. High-resolution computed tomography in young patients with cystic fibrosis: Distribution of abnormalities and correlation with pulmonary function tests. *J Pediatr* 2004; **145**(1): 32–8.

24. Lindblad A, de Jong PA, Brink M, Tiddens HA, Gustafsson P. Measurements of ventilation inhomogeneity correlates better to structural changes on high resolution CT than conventional spirometry. *Pediatr Pulmonol* 2005; **40**(S28): 310–1.

25. Demirkazik FB, Ariyurek OM, Ozcelik U, Gocmen A, Hassanabad HK, Kiper N. High resolution CT in children with cystic fibrosis: Correlation with pulmonary functions and radiographic scores. *Eur J Radiol* 2001; **37**(1): 54–9.

26. Shah RM, Sexauer W, Ostrum BJ, Fiel SB, Friedman AC. High-resolution CT in the acute exacerbation of cystic fibrosis: Evaluation of acute findings, reversibility of those findings, and clinical correlation. *AJR Am J Roentgenol* 1997; **169**(2): 375–80.

27. Robinson TE, Leung AN, Northway WH et al. Spirometer-triggered high-resolution computed tomography and pulmonary function measurements during an acute exacerbation in patients with cystic fibrosis. *J Pediatr* 2001; **138**(4): 553–9.

28. de Jong PA, Mayo JR, Golmohammadi K et al. Estimation of cancer mortality associated with repetitive computed tomography scanning. *Am J Respir Crit Care Med* 2006; **173**(2): 199–203.

29. Mayo JR, Jackson SA, Muller NL. High-resolution CT of the chest: Radiation dose. *AJR Am J Roentgenol* 1993; **160**(3): 479–81.

30. Copley SJ, Padley SP. High-resolution CT of paediatric lung disease. *Eur Radiol* 2001; **11**(12): 2564–75.

31. Garcia-Pena P, Lucaya J. HRCT in children: Technique and indications. *Eur Radiol* 2004; **14** Suppl 4: L13–30.

32. Lucaya J, Piqueras J, Garcia-Pena P, Enriquez G, Garcia-Macias M, Sotil J. Low-dose high-resolution CT of the chest in children and young adults: Dose, cooperation, artifact incidence, and image quality. *AJR Am J Roentgenol* 2000; **175**(4): 985–92.

33. Owens C. Radiology of diffuse interstitial pulmonary disease in children. *Eur Radiol* 2004; 14 Suppl 4: L2–12.

34. Brody AS. Thoracic CT technique in children. *J Thorac Imaging* 2001; **16**(4): 259–68.

35. Kuhn JP, Brody AS. High-resolution CT of pediatric lung disease. *Radiol Clin North Am* 2002; **40**(1): 89–110.

36. Donnelly LF, Frush DP. Pediatric multidetector body CT. *Radiol Clin North Am* 2003; **41**(3): 637–55.

37. Long FR, Castile RG, Brody AS et al. Lungs in infants and young children: Improved thin-section CT with a noninvasive controlled-ventilation technique—initial experience. *Radiology* 1999; **212**(2): 588–93.

38. Robinson TE, Leung AN, Moss RB, Blankenberg FG, al Dabbagh H, Northway WH. Standardized high-resolution CT of the lung using a spirometer-triggered electron beam CT scanner. *AJR Am J Roentgenol* 1999; **172**(6): 1636–8.

39. Helbich TH, Heinz-Peer G, Eichler I et al. Cystic fibrosis: CT assessment of lung involvement in children and adults. *Radiology* 1999; **213**(2): 537–44.

40. Robinson TE, Goris ML, Zhu HJ et al. Dornase alfa reduces air trapping in children with mild cystic fibrosis lung disease: A quantitative analysis. *Chest* 2005; **128**(4): 2327–35.

41. Long FR, Castile RG. Technique and clinical applications of full-inflation and end-exhalation controlled-ventilation chest CT in infants and young children. *Pediatr Radiol* 2001; **31**(6): 413–22.

42. Bhalla M, Turcios N, Aponte V et al. Cystic fibrosis: Scoring system with thin-section CT. *Radiology* 1991; **179**(3): 783–8.

43. Nathanson I, Conboy K, Murphy S, Afshani E, Kuhn JP. Ultrafast computerized tomography of the chest in cystic fibrosis: A new scoring system. *Pediatr Pulmonol* 1991; **11**(1): 81–6.

44. Maffessanti M, Candusso M, Brizzi F, Piovesana F. Cystic fibrosis in children: HRCT findings and distribution of disease. *J Thorac Imaging* 1996; **11**(1): 27–38.

45. Santamaria F, Grillo G, Guidi G et al. Cystic fibrosis: When should high-resolution computed tomography of the chest be obtained? *Pediatrics* 1998; **101**(5): 908–13.

46. Helbich TH, Heinz-Peer G, Fleischmann D et al. Evolution of CT findings in patients with cystic fibrosis. *AJR Am J Roentgenol* 1999; **173**(1): 81–8.

47. Kroft LJ, Roelofs JJ, Geleijns J. Scan time and patient dose for thoracic imaging in neonates and small children using axial volumetric 320-detector row CT compared to helical 64-, 32-, and 16- detector row CT acquisitions. *Pediatr Radiol* 2010; **40**(3): 294–300.

48. Graser A, Johnson TR, Chandarana H, Macari M. Dual energy CT: Preliminary observations and potential clinical applications in the abdomen. *Eur Radiol* 2009; **19**(1): 13–23.

49. Hoey ET, Gopalan D, Ganesh V et al. Dual-energy CT pulmonary angiography: A novel technique for assessing acute and chronic pulmonary thromboembolism. *Clin Radiol* 2009; **64**(4): 414–9.

50. Johnson TR, Krauss B, Sedlmair M et al. Material differentiation by dual energy CT: Initial experience. *Eur Radiol* 2007; **17**(6): 1510–7.

51. Goo HW. Initial experience of dual-energy lung perfusion CT using a dual-source CT system in children. *Pediatr Radiol* 2010; **40**(9): 1536–44.

52. Goo HW, Yang DH, Hong SJ et al. Xenon ventilation CT using dual-source and dual-energy technique in children with bronchiolitis obliterans: Correlation of xenon and CT density values with pulmonary function test results. *Pediatr Radiol* 2010; **40**(9): 1490–7.

53. Kim JE, Newman B. Evaluation of a radiation dose reduction strategy for pediatric chest CT. *AJR Am J Roentgenol* 2010; **194**(5):1188–93.

54. Paterson A, Frush DP. Dose reduction in paediatric MDCT: General principles. *Clin Radiol* 2007; **62**(6): 507–17.

55. Pontana F, Duhamel A, Pagniez J et al. Chest computed tomography using iterative reconstruction vs filtered back projection (Part 2): Image quality of low-dose CT examinations in 80 patients. *Eur Radiol* 2011; **21**(3): 636–43.

56. Korner M, Weber CH, Wirth S, Pfeifer KJ, Reiser MF, Treitl M. Advances in digital radiography: Physical principles and system overview. *Radiographics* 2007; **27**(3): 675–86.

57. Spahn M. Flat detectors and their clinical applications. *Eur Radiol* 2005; **15**(9): 1934–47.

58. Seibert JA. Flat-panel detectors: How much better are they? *Pediatr Radiol* 2006; **36**(Suppl 2): 173–81.

59. Vult von SK, Bjorkman-Burtscher I, Geijer M. Tomosynthesis in pulmonary cystic fibrosis with comparison to radiography and computed tomography: A pictorial review. *Insights Imaging* 2012; **3**(1): 81–9.

60. Vikgren J, Zachrisson S, Svalkvist A et al. Comparison of chest tomosynthesis and chest radiography for detection of pulmonary nodules: Human observer study of clinical cases. *Radiology* 2008; **249**(3): 1034–41.

61. Dobbins JT III, Godfrey DJ. Digital x-ray tomosynthesis: Current state of the art and clinical potential. *Phys Med Biol* 2003; **48**(19): R65–106.

62. Altes TA, de Lange EE. Applications of hyperpolarized helium-3 gas magnetic resonance imaging in pediatric lung disease. *Top Magn Reson Imaging* 2003; **14**(3): 231–6.

63. Kauczor HU. Hyperpolarized helium-3 gas magnetic resonance imaging of the lung. *Top Magn Reson Imaging* 2003; **14**(3): 223–30.

64. Koumellis P, Van Beek EJ, Woodhouse N et al. Quantitative analysis of regional airways obstruction using dynamic hyperpolarized 3He MRI-preliminary results in children with cystic fibrosis. *J Magn Reson Imaging* 2005; **22**(3): 420–6.

65. Mentore K, Froh DK, de Lange EE, Brookeman JR, Paget-Brown AO, Altes TA. Hyperpolarized HHe 3 MRI of the lung in cystic fibrosis: Assessment at baseline and after bronchodilator and airway clearance treatment. *Acad Radiol* 2005; **12**(11): 1423–9.

66. Puderbach M, Kauczor HU. Assessment of lung function in children by cross-sectional imaging: Techniques and clinical applications. *Pediatr Radiol* 2006; **36**: 192–204.

67. Richard JC, Chen DL, Ferkol T, Schuster DP. Molecular imaging for pediatric lung diseases. *Pediatr Pulmonol* 2004; **37**(4): 286–96.

68. de Jong PA, Tiddens HA. Cystic fibrosis specific computed tomography scoring. *Proc Am Thorac Soc* 2007; **4**(4): 338–42.

35

Physiological monitoring of older children and adults

MARK ROSENTHAL

INTRODUCTION

In 2009, cystic fibrosis (CF) officially became a disease of adults in the United Kingdom when the numbers of adults with CF exceeded that of children for the first time. So, monitoring in childhood to affect what happens in adulthood assumes ever greater importance. Data collection is not an end in itself; its purpose is to enhance the clinicians' understanding of the state of an individual patient. This chapter therefore deals with lung function testing at two different levels; the first is how lung function should be monitored and interpreted on a day-to-day basis in the clinic and used for routine decision making, for example, whether a course of intravenous antibiotics is warranted. Second, how lung function declines as the CF patient gets older and the relationship between conventional lung function tests such as spirometry and newer measures such as lung clearance index (LCI) and their rates of change with time until death. The final parts deal with other physiological tests and how to assess the safety of air travel in CF subjects. The use of lung function in databases as a quality improvement (QI) measure is discussed in Chapter 31.

THE OUTPATIENT CLINIC

As 95% of people with CF die of respiratory failure, monitoring lung function and responding to decrements as far as is possible is crucial. A short-term decline in forced expired volume in 1 second (FEV_1) of >10% is a key part of the definition of a pulmonary exacerbation (below). A slower decline but over a longer period demands close attention, including consideration of additional diagnoses such as allergic bronchopulmonary aspergillosis (ABPA), the requirement for new treatments such as a trial of recombinant human deoxyribonuclease (rhDNase),

hypertonic saline (HS) or azithromycin, and the management of adherence to current and future treatment. A precipitous decline in lung function demands immediate attention, hospital admission, diagnostic endeavor, and aggressive treatment. Forced vital capacity (FVC) is far less sensitive to both acute and indeed chronic change. The terms "slower decline" and "precipitous decline" though eloquent are meaningless without some definition. Opinions differ. Objectively, the variability in spirometry in subjects with CF can be considerable. Cooper et al.[1] found that FEV_1 varied by 10% and mid-expiratory flow (MEF) by 20% in stable CF subjects, and Fuchs et al.[2] used a >10% decline in FEV_1 as part of the definition of a pulmonary exacerbation. Chavasse et al.[3] found that within occasion FEV_1 variability was less than the data given by Cooper et al[1] in CF children (5%) and reduced further when using nose clips (3.2%). So an absolute reduction of >10% in FEV_1 or 20% in MEF whether over a short (1 month) or longer (6 months) period certainly merits close attention, and indeed a decline in FEV_1 is part of most if not all definitions of a pulmonary exacerbation in school-age children and adults. Clearly other measurements have a role in outpatient assessment, including oxygen saturation. Subjectively, our clinic has regularly seen subjects whose lung function is "a little down," who are trying to minimize their symptoms but their oxygen saturation is <94%. Other factors such as weight loss are also important. Clinical geneticists use the German term "gestalt" meaning form or face and unquestionably the biggest service a regular CF clinic with stable personnel, serving patients over a long period, can do is to detect that indefinable quality that "all is not right with the patient's gestalt" and a slavish adherence to lung function measurements is as wrong as ignoring them. CF care still remains a mixed art/science with *all* measurements as well as gestalt determining the correct course of action. As with all chronic diseases (e.g., asthma/leukemia), adherence to treatment is rarely above 60% and doctors are usually the worst healthcare group at assessing it.[4]

Despite widespread recommendations that annually, plethysmographic measures of lung volume (total lung capacity, residual volume and functional residual capacity, FRC), airway resistance, specific airway conductance, and carbon monoxide transfer should be measured, the evidence of any value with the possible exception of FRC is small. There is no published evidence to support their value for either short-term—as these measurements are too complex and time consuming to perform at every clinic visit, especially in children—or long-term predictive benefit. I reviewed all the Royal Brompton Hospital annual assessment lung function data in middle childhood[5] to see if there was any predictive effect for death or lung transplantation 10–15 years on. This is summarized in Figures 35.1 and 35.2 showing that the predictive effect was worse even than tossing a coin, an FEV_1 even 1 year hence could only have 66% of its variance explained by the FEV_1 1 year in the past. Nonetheless, maintaining FEV_1 as normal as possible remains a major

goal of CF care, and FEV_1 is used as a benchmark of clinic performance in the US Cystic Fibrosis Foundation QI program.

RESPONSIVENESS OF FEV_1 TO ACUTE CHANGES IN TREATMENT

The response of an acute deterioration in FEV_1 with a pulmonary exacerbation is discussed in Chapter 17, and the failure to return FEV_1 to baseline in a significant number of exacerbations is a major concern. Clinically, despite the shortcomings of this measure as a long-term prognostic feature, change in FEV_1 is often used to assess the response to new interventions such as azithromycin and rhDNase, conventionally 10% being thought to translate into worthwhile benefit. However, reduction in numbers of pulmonary exacerbations may be a better marker. In general, the rate of decline of FEV_1 is so slow (below) that its use as a clinical trial end point is called into question (see Chapter 39). However, the extraordinary 1–2 year effects of the G551D-specific treatment ivacaftor on FEV_1 demonstrate that for

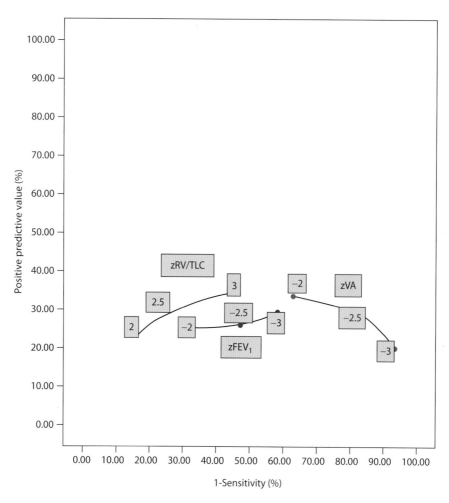

Figure 35.1 The relationship of positive predictive value and sensitivity for death/transplantation for $zFEV_1$, zRV/TLC, and zVA for children aged 10 years relating positive predictive value and sensitivity at various z-score cut-offs. FEV_1, forced expired volume in 1 second; RV/TLC, residual volume to total lung capacity; VA, alveolar volume. (From Rosenthal M, *Pediatr Pulmonol* 43, 945–52, 2008. With permission.)

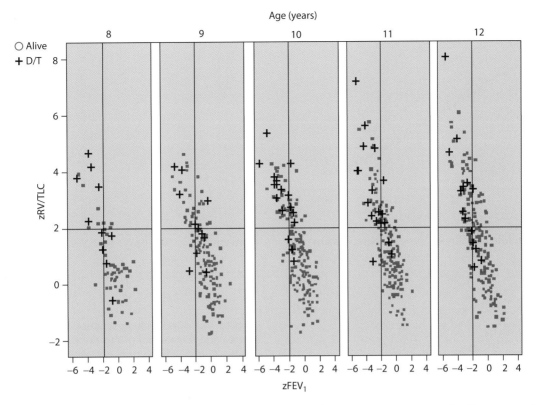

Figure 35.2 The relationship between $zFEV_1$ and zRV/TLC at each year from ages 8 to 12 years. Gridlines set at the limits of normality (−2 for $zFEV_1$ and +2 for zRV/TLC). + = Patients destined to die or have lung transplants early (D/T); O = those still alive. (From Rosenthal M, *Pediatr Pulmonol* 43, 945–52, 2008. With permission.)

really powerful treatments, FEV_1 improvements over baseline are still demonstrable. It is important, however, to note that the survival curves are now so flat that no percentage change with treatment in FEV_1 has been demonstrated to associate with improved survival, nor is this ever likely to be possible.

LONGITUDINAL STUDIES OF LUNG FUNCTION AND PREDICTION OF SURVIVAL

It is necessary at the outset to summarize the difficulties involved in such data; although longitudinal analysis is a mathematician's paradise, the reality of prediction is very difficult indeed. This is illustrated by Figure 35.3 showing the remarkable decrease in childhood mortality with each succeeding birth cohort.[6] The effect is that any data linking childhood parameters to life expectancy is essentially irrelevant by the time of its publication due to the inexorable change in disease management over the period. Those who live longer may not be representative of the whole group (for example, their genotype) and may skew the data, an example of survivor bias. To avoid this problem, authors use proxies for death such as for example FEV_1 <30%, but as will be illustrated, the significance of this finding has also changed with time and generally improved disease management. It

also needs emphasizing that publications may use terms such as median age at death which is concrete, based on actual deaths but is always out of date and also median survival, which is based on prior mortality statistics applied to a hypothetical population projected into the future[7] with all the inaccuracies that brings, especially in small populations. Furthermore, the application of population data, for example, from registries to an individual, is also fraught with hazard as will be illustrated.

LUNG FUNCTION

Before looking at how lung function changes and declines in CF, it is necessary to give a brief overview of how spirometry at least changes during life in the healthy individual. To summarize, spirometric variables rise in a linear manner with height in younger children until the pubertal years when marked rises occur and the previous, very similar but not identical lung function between the sexes, diverges. Longitudinal studies have shown that the preschool years are key determinants of long-term lung function. Thus, lung function tracks from ages 4–6 into late middle age, both in the general population and in children with wheeze. No comparable studies have been performed in CF, but it seems likely that the same will be true and that the very early years are a crucial time in determining outcome in CF. Peak lung function occurs at around 20 years, perhaps slightly earlier in females[8] and then slowly declines (Figure 35.4) so that by

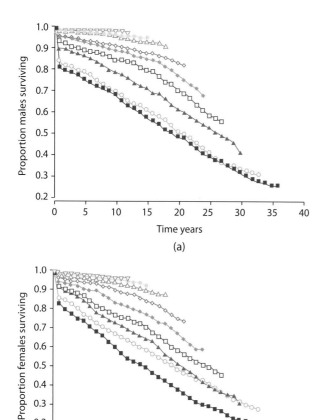

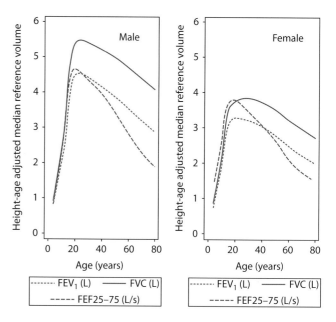

Figure 35.4 Median lung function data for Caucasian males and females following the pooling of many studies by the Global lung initiative. Note the relatively higher FEF$_{25-75}$ in females compared with males. FEF, forced expiratory flow. (From Stanojevic S et al., *Am J Respir Crit Care Med* 177, 253–60, 2008. With permission.)

Figure 35.3 The ever-decreasing cystic fibrosis mortality by 2003 with each succeeding cohort of births from 1970 to 1994. **(a)** Males, **(b)** females. (From Dodge JA et al., *Eur Respir J* 29, 522–6, 2007. With permission.)

age 80 years, spirometry is now back to the level of a 10-year old.[9] This work by the Global lung initiative (GLI) is the first to provide continuous data from age 3 years to >80 years. The GLI does not assume a normal or indeed symmetrical distribution of values around the 50th centile and the LMS system is used to calculate z scores, where L is a measure of spread of values, M is the median, and S is a measure of the skew. The general formula for calculating any z score for a particular value x is $((x/M)^L - 1)/(L \times S)$.

Prepubertal girls have shorter and wider airways as manifest by greater MEF rates per unit lung volume. The reason spirometry diverges so markedly between males and females during puberty even in those with identical heights is probably due to the way the pubertal thoracic cage grows. In males, the cage during puberty grows in all three dimensions, length, width, and depth; in females, it only increases in two dimensions, length and depth but not width.[10] Boys of differing pubertal stages but similar heights could have lung function 1 to 2 z scores different and girls 0.75 to 1 z score different. However, as pubertal stage is infrequently assessed, the GLI used an age/height

interaction, which will be an approximation for the effects of puberty (Figure 35.5). Lung function is not completely consonant with pubertal growth. For example, MEF peak change is 1–1.5 years after peak height velocity. This may be due to the contribution of muscle power to spirometry, which is also not consonant with the growth spurt. Thus, it is clear that growth, pubertal development, and muscle power all play a role in at least spirometry any or all of which can be compromised by CF.

However, valuable spirometry is in the individual clinic setting, the evidence that spirometry is a reliable indicator of long-term health, prognosis, and life expectancy, which is much more doubtful, whereas the LCI has not been used for long enough to know its true clinical, as opposed to research, role. Three vignettes illustrate the problem. A 16-year-old girl who had spent the last 2 months in hospital receiving intensive treatment and who had an FEV$_1$ resolutely fixed at 18% predicted survived 8.5 years. An undernourished 10-year old who initially refused a gastrostomy and had an FEV$_1$ of 37% predicted became a strapping 27-year old with a gastrostomy whose FEV$_1$ was still 37%. A girl who at 13 years had an FEV$_1$ of 85% and a body mass index on the 50th centile received a lung transplant 15 months later. Having said all this, it is clearly better to have a normal rather than a very abnormal FEV$_1$. Clinical state and survival are likely to be better, and the patient is likely to have fewer pulmonary exacerbations.[11] Certainly UK registry data suggest that good lung function at transition and in the thirties predicts a group with a good long-term outlook and reduced need for hospital stays. However, there are no formal analyses of the

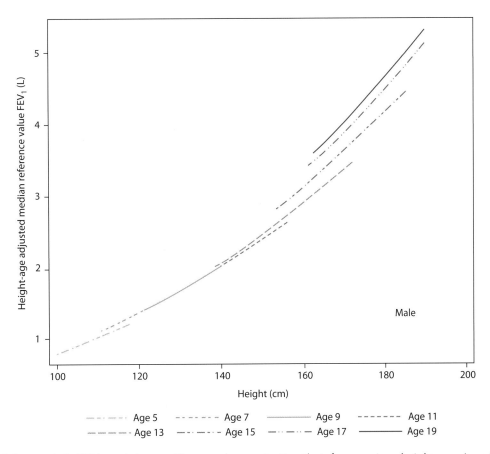

Figure 35.5 Height trends in FEV$_1$ at eight specific ages demonstrating that, for any given height, age is as important to consider in determining reference ranges, especially during puberty where it is essentially a proxy for pubertal stage. In contrast to adulthood where there is a decline with age, throughout childhood at any given height an older subject can be expected to have higher values of lung function. This effect is most marked during puberty. (Reproduced and modified from Stanojevic S et al., *Am J Respir Crit Care Med*, 177, 253–60, 2008. With permission.)

predictive value of FEV$_1$ at these time points on survival in the current literature (see also Chapter 30).

An important issue is what lung function parameter to measure and what constitutes a relevant change. Although FEV$_1$ is unquestionably the commonest single measure of lung function used and is discussed extensively below, FVC, MEF, transfer factor (DL$_{CO}$), and the ratio of residual volume to total lung capacity have also all been studied.[5] Newer measures such as the LCI (which is discussed more extensively in the context of infants and preschool children in Chapter 32) are also being used. Kraemer et al.[12] in a longitudinal cohort study extending throughout childhood has demonstrated that abnormalities in LCI occur some 2 to 3 years earlier than changes in FEV$_1$ and that an abnormal LCI was present in 52% of children with a normal FEV$_1$, whereas for the converse (normal LCI, abnormal FEV$_1$) the rate was only 0.5%, confirming the reports in the preschool child. The next most useful measure was forced expired flow at 50% of FVC (MEF$_{50}$) and third was plethysmographically measured FRC. It is also true that computed tomography scanning appears to be more sensitive to change in structure than spirometry (the role of high-resolution computed tomography [HRCT] is discussed in Chapter 38); this is hardly surprising given the well-known insensitivity of spirometry to distal airway disease.

The factors that may be relevant to the absolute lung function and rate of change over time include: gender; genotype (at the cystic fibrosis transmembrane conductance regulator [CFTR] locus and modifier genes); pancreatic status; CF-related diabetes (CFRD) and prediabetic insulin deficiency; microbiology; markers of nutrition such as weight for age or body mass index, education, social class, and psychological factors.

GENDER

Gender is important because of the long-standing evidence of reduced female life expectancy. As an example, Aurora's 2-year survivorship study of 181 children referred for transplant demonstrated that female gender consistently led to a reduced 2-year survivorship by 15%, irrespective of FEV$_1$. Unfortunately, as with so many such models, it has not been validated in a second population. It could be that there is something about the effect of CFTR dysfunction or absence *per se* in girls which makes them die earlier, or it could be that they are more prone to particular complications, or it could be (see earlier) that as they gain much less lung function in puberty per unit height, they have less reserve and thus run into problems sooner. Hence, two individuals one male and one female of identical height and identical relative lung function (say, FEV$_1$ 30%) will have markedly different absolute lung function, thus accounting for the earlier onset of those pulmonary complications which shorten life. Demko et al.[13] showed that acquisition of mucoid *Pseudomonas* in children <6 years of age led to a greater rate of death over the next 10 years (40%) in girls than boys (20%) implying that girls are more vulnerable to the effects of infection with *Pseudomonas aeruginosa*, although it must be pointed out that a 40% death rate before ages 16–18 years is extraordinarily high and probably indicates the era in which the data were collected (1954–1990) as this century's UK total child CF deaths before 16 years is at most 5%. However, this difference might disappear if effective antipseudomonal treatment was in place (assuming equal efficacy in both genders). The subject of gender differences is discussed in more detail in Chapter 2.

Although epidemiological studies have always demonstrated that life expectancy for girls with CF was consistently worse than boys,[14] multicenter studies by definition involve centers with likely different treatment policies, which may make interpretation difficult. Verma et al.[15] have shown in a large single center longitudinal study that since 1993, if anything lung function in girls (an unsafe proxy for survival) is now superior to boys. Thus, female sex, at least in childhood (including the teenage years), does not seem necessarily to convey a worse prognosis as regards lung function. However, whether this will translate into a life expectancy that does not differ between the sexes remains to be seen. Australian data still suggest excess female deaths in childhood,[16] but Italian longitudinal data from 1988 found no difference. However, they subtly point out that in the general population more girls survive throughout childhood than boys so equal survival in CF still implies a 15% excess death rate in girls. In London, United Kingdom, from 2000 to 2009 inclusive, out of 1022 CF children, there were 11 deaths (9 female) and 8 transplants (6 female) at median age of 14 years.[17] So while lung function is equalizing between males and females in children, this is not yet translating into equal risks of death.

DIABETES MELLITUS

It is clear that CFRD is the single-most important new determinant of CF outcome this century. Data have, however, been appearing in this regard since the 1980s. Finkelstein et al.[18] demonstrated that only 25% of CF patients with CFRD were alive aged 30 years compared with 60% of the nondiabetics and that the clinical decline predated diagnosis by at least 2 years. This underscores the need for active detection strategies of the early phases of insulin deficiency (Chapter 24). Clinicians should certainly perform a glucose tolerance test in any subject with an unexplained clinical deterioration, and if this is normal,

undertake a period of home glucose monitoring using a subcutaneous system (continous glucose monitoring system). Koch et al.'s[19] analysis of the European CF database demonstrated that in every age cohort CFRD subjects had an FEV$_1$ 10% lower than non-CFRD subjects. Schaedel et al.[20] studied the entire CF Swedish population alive in 1998 and born prior to 1993 and in addition included 25 patients who died in the 1990s, 9 from the 1980s, and 21 (16 alive) who had been transplanted to minimize bias. Table 35.1 shows the significant association of in particular, chronic infection with *P. aeruginosa* and the diagnosis of diabetes mellitus, such that in the 19- to 24-year age group, the relative risk of an FEV$_1$ <60% was increased 2.6 (95% confidence interval (CI) 1.1–6.5) times if the patient was pancreatic insufficient (PI), 1.7 (CI 1.1–2.8) times if chronically infected with *P. aeruginosa*, and 1.5 (1.1–2.2) times if a diagnosis of diabetes had been given (CFRD). The authors do not state whether these factors are additive, but the implication from Table 35.1 is that diabetes in a PI CF patient had increased the rate of FEV$_1$ decline by an extra 50%.

What was not analyzed in the previous studies but is clear in the studies of Milla et al.[21] and Sims et al.[22] that the differential effect of CFRD on females. Milla et al. studied the 1081 patients from a single US clinic, which performed annual oral glucose tolerance tests, with complete follow-up data from 1987 to 2002 or death. The median survival for male subjects without and with CFRD was 49.5 and 47.4 years, respectively, whereas for females it was 47.0 and 30.7 years, respectively ($p < .001$), not confounded by genotype, microbiology, nutrition, pregnancy, or steroid usage. This difference accounted for 89% of the excess female mortality over males. In the cross-sectional part of a study from the UK database, Sims et al. showed that female subjects were 12 (3–59) times more likely to have CFRD than males. Females with CFRD but without *P. aeruginosa* had an FEV$_1$ 20% (95% CI 12–28%) lower than non-CFRD females, and in chronically infected subjects, the FEV$_1$ difference was 14% (95% CI 8–19). Interestingly, the FEV$_1$ decline in female CFRD subjects did *not* occur in the first year after diagnosis suggesting an opportunity for intervention, though this is at odds with the observation of lung function decline before CFRD diagnosis.[23] However, it should be stated that the completeness and quality of the UK data, in terms of ascertainment of the diagnosis of CFRD at least, is below that of the American study.

Most importantly, earlier diagnosis and aggressive management has eliminated the gender gap and almost eliminated the difference between diabetics and nondiabetics (Figure 35.6) in terms of mortality.[24] It is clear that diagnostic criteria which remain too rigid and related to old style type I and II diabetes will change and thus more CF patients will be diagnosed with CFRD or at least insulin deficiency. The inevitable effect on predicting outcomes from retrospective data during a period of changes in attitude, diagnostic criteria, and therapy for diabetes in CF is obvious.

Table 35.1 Annual rate of decline of FEV_1 in Swedish CF population ($n = 420$) up to 40 years of age

	Rate of decline of FEV_1 (%/yr)	Significance of difference compared to top line of each box
ΔΔ508/ΔF508 del	0.8	
2 Severe mutations	0.9	.6
1 or 2 Missense mutations	0.04	.01
Male	0.6	
Female	0.9	.16
PS	0.2	
PI	0.9	.01
Dead/transplanted	2.0	
Alive/not transplanted	0.6	.00001
PI/PA	1.0	
PI/No PA	0.5	.03
PS/PA	0.3	
PS/No PA	0.2	.83
PI/Diabetes	1.2	
PI/No Diabetes	0.7	.02
PI/Cirrhosis	0.8	
PI/No cirrhosis	0.8	.84

Source: Data adapted from Schaedel C et al., *Pediatr Pulmonol* 33, 483–91, 2002. With permission.
Notes: Confidence intervals were not stated. CF, cystic fibrosis; FEV_1, forced expired volume in 1 second; PA, chronically infected with
P. aeruginosa (three positive in 6 months); PI, pancreatic insufficient; PS, pancreatic sufficient.

THE EFFECT OF TIME ON EPIDEMIOLOGY AND THE ASSUMPTIONS OF LINEAR CHANGES IN SPIROMETRY

An important point is that as clinicians we are interested in the prognosis for an individual, but the data on which the prognosis is based comes from large mixed longitudinal cohorts. Epidemiological data may help us understand mechanisms of disease, but as is well known when considering the prognosis in a given individual, it is not good for guiding decision making, for example, transplant referral. Kerem et al.[25] looking at survival when FEV_1 <30% predicted showed a median 2-year survival effectively saying that the chance of surviving 2 years for an individual was the same as tossing a coin. To beautifully illustrate the effect of improved disease management and the danger of extrapolating excellent but old data, a repeat study of 276 patients[26] showed that with an FEV_1 <30%, median survival steadily increased from 1.2 years in 1991 (less than Kerem's study) to 5.3 years in the 2003 group (2.5 times more than Kerem's study) especially after 1994, a date that coincides with the introduction of deoxyribonuclease (DNase).

This is also illustrated by Zemel et al.'s[27] longitudinal data in children from the US national CF patient registry which demonstrates the curvilinear reduction in FEV_1 (more rapid in girls compared with boys) and the negative interaction with weight (nutritional status as judged by weight z score and percent weight for height influences lung function decline). Interestingly those with the best

initial lung function declined more quickly than those with a lower initial lung function. Whether this illustrates the phenomenon of regression to the mean or is a biological phenomenon cannot be determined from this study alone. However, in either case, children in mid childhood had a decline in lung function that settled to a very slow rate (c1%/year).

The second paper, only published in abstract form, reviewed the 30 deaths occurring in Melbourne, Australia, in a single center and in particular the lung function in the years before death.[28] Table 35.2 shows the median FEV_1 2 years prior to death. At least one-third of subjects had an FEV_1 >75% 2 years before death demonstrating that even a normal FEV_1 cannot be absolutely reassuring as a precipitate and seemingly unstoppable decline remains a real if small threat. The London data[21] showed an FEV_1 5 years before death of 62% but 1 year before death, the FEV_1 was the same as the last recorded at 32%.

This chimes in with the data of Milla and Warwick,[29] which tried to determine whether an FEV_1 of <30% occurring on at least three occasions within 12 months predicted mortality. This hypothesis at that time was based on the previous observation that an FEV_1 <30% predicted >50% mortality within 2 years.[25] Of the 49/56 deceased patients with an FEV_1 <30% close to death, only 17/49 had entered this range in the previous 2 years, the rest having had similar lung function for 2 to 14 years. Gender, nutrition (< or >85% weight for height), presence of diabetes treated with insulin or decade (1975–1984 or 1985–1994) in which the lung

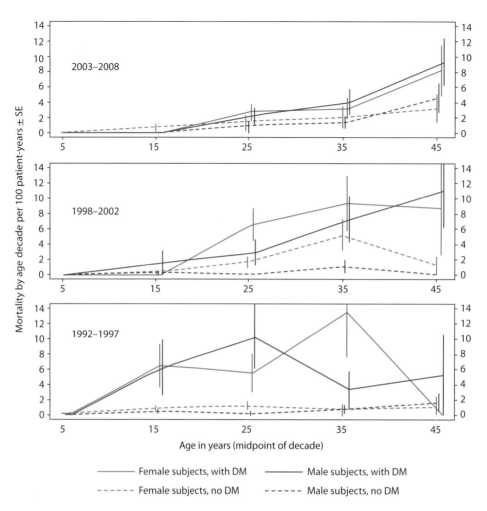

Figure 35.6 Survival curves for male cystic fibrosis (CF) subjects with (blue solid) and without diabetes (blue hatched) and female CF subjects with (red solid) and without diabetes (red hatched) over three 5-year time periods. Note the gender and mortality differences progressively disappearing with each successive time period. (From Moran A, et al. *Diabetes Care* 32, 1626–31, 2009. With permission.)

Table 35.2 Data from Robinson et al. showing very wide range of FEV$_1$, 2 years prior to death in Melbourne, Australia

	Number	Median age at death in months (range)	Median FEV$_1$ 2 years before death% predicted (range)
Male	13	176 (62–233)	69 (31–90)
Female	17	171 (89–225)	47 (24–102)
Total	30	172 (62–233)	52.5 (24–102)

Source: Robinson PJ et al., *Pediatr Pulmonol* Suppl 19, A452, 1999. With permission.

function first reached 30% had no effect on outcome, and rate of decline of FVC was no different between survivors and nonsurvivors. The conclusion was that patients who had an FEV$_1$ that continued to decline rapidly had a greater risk of death than those whose FEV$_1$ was low (<30%) but declined slowly. Looking at young adults as a whole, Que et al.[30] demonstrated the steady slowing of FEV$_1$ decline over time at one institution so that for those born between 1985 and 1989 the rate of decline was now 0.8%/year (Table 35.3) when aged 18 to 22 years. They also tabulated the rates of decline from other studies (placebo arm) and cohorts and

these are summarized and added to in Table 35.4. It clearly demonstrates the variability depending on institution, year of birth, and study, much of the largest and most up to date being Vandenbranden et al.,[41] where >2000 adolescents and young adults from the US CF database were evaluated and in contrast to Que's report there was still a fairly brisk decline in FEV$_1$ in young adults aged 18–22 years, which was unexpectedly greater than that occurring in contemporaneous adolescents aged 14–17 years (Table 35.4).

A large study on the decline of lung function comes from the European CF database,[42] which examined 12,500

Table 35.3 Lung function decline in young adults aged 18–22 years

	Birth cohort					
	1960–4	1965–9	1970–4	1975–80	1980–4	1985–9
Follow-up to	1978	1983	1988	1993	1998	2003
Study (n)	132	120	114	90	90	108
FEV$_1$ slope/yr	−2.1	−2.6	−2.5	−1.8	−1.1	−0.8

Source: Que C et al., Thorax 61, 155–7, 2006. With permission.

Table 35.4 Published rates of decline in percentage predicted FEV$_1$ in CF from cohort studies or the placebo arms of clinical trials

Reference	Pt No	Age (years)	Follow-up (years)	Annual decline in %FEV$_1$	
				Mean	SE
Ref. [31]	132	5–27	7	−1.87 (Male)	NS
				−2.71 (Female)	NS
Ref. [32]	39	7–40	2	−2.2	1.67
Ref. [33]	325	4–28	15	−1.25	0.14
Ref. [34]	43	5–39	4	−3.6	0.55
Ref. [35]	95	6–14	4	−1.5	NS
Ref. [36]	366	18–32 (born 1960–1974)	15	−2.72	NS
Ref. [37]	215		2–5	−2.3	0.28
Ref. [38]	152		4	−0.8	NS
Ref. [39]	52	Children	3.9	−2.2	NS
Ref. [40]	53	Children	3.8	−1.8	NS
Ref. [30]	98	18–22	5	−0.8	0.8
Ref. [41]	2267	14–22	Minimum 1	−1.1 (14–18 years)	0.12
				−2.7 (18–22 years)	0.11

Source: Modified from Que C et al., Thorax 61, 155–7, 2006. With permission.

subjects between 1993 and 1997, mainly to examine the effects of ABPA. Figure 35.7 is a reproduction of their mixed longitudinal data depending on the initial entry FEV$_1$ and the initial age group at measurement. What it illustrates is that regardless of the starting FEV$_1$, the rate of subsequent decline was remarkably similar (and largely unaffected by ABPA) and independent of age. The crucial conclusion of this is that the starting FEV$_1$ is determined much earlier in childhood and that once a low FEV$_1$ is established, although the rate of decline appears similar, inevitably the ones with the low initial FEV$_1$ run into trouble sooner. These observations tie in with the studies in infancy and preschool children (Chapter 32), which suggests that lung function tracks from diagnosis until school age at least.

As time has gone, increasingly sophisticated mathematics is being brought to bear on longitudinal data. Two relevant studies illustrate this. The first[43] looked at the 21,000 patients in the US epidemiological study in cystic fibrosis and examined both population data and crucially, individual year to year changes in FEV$_1$. Two conclusions emerge. First as has

always been the case, lung function decline is never linear (Figure 35.8) and demonstrates a good example of survival bias, where the FEV$_1$ after age 36 years appears to rise again as the most severely affected patients die! Second that certainly after age 15 years, individual changes in lung function do not match the overall population data again demonstrating the maxim that moving from the general to the particular and vice versa is always wrong (Figure 35.9). What it emphasizes and in agreement with Que et al.[30] is that the decline in lung function certainly slows on entering adulthood. None of these studies explain this phenomenon. Is it a physiological effect of puberty or more likely a consequence of adolescent rebellion when treatment adherence reaches a nadir which then improves once relative sanity is restored in their twenties?

The apogee of mathematical modeling is the study of Danish longitudinal lung function data from 1969 to 2010.[44] Very elegant mathematics is applied to the 70,000 data points available. Close modeling of an individual's actual data is achieved (Figure 35.10). This is used to claim that it "could be used in real time to guide the interpretation of sudden changes in lung function." The authors suggest, for

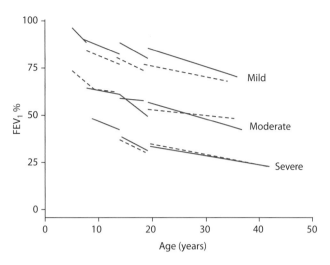

Figure 35.7 Mixed model regression lines of FEV₁% predicted versus age for allergic bronchopulmonary aspergillosis (ABPA) (hatched line) and non-ABPA CF patients (solid line). The data are divided into three groups (mild, moderate, and severe) based on the FEV₁ at enrollment in the European CF database and at four age groups: <6 years, 6–12 years, 13–17 years, and >17 years) This indicates that lung function at enrollment is the key determinant and that subsequent decline is very similar irrespective of initial FEV₁. (Reproduced and modified from Mastella G, et al. *Eur Respir J* 16, 464–71, 2000. With permission.)

instance (Figure 35.10) "the sudden drop to under 30% indicated by the arrow is not mirrored in the model trace suggesting that this may be recoverable random fluctuation"—not a chance any practicing clinician will take!

What these two studies and clinical observation demonstrates is that linear modeling of FEV₁ is always wrong and papers using this linear decline assumption should be treated most cautiously.

One unexpected consequence of the slowing rate of decline in FEV₁ is that new treatments are becoming increasingly difficult to evaluate as the use of the end point: change in rate of decline of FEV₁ is now so low that a trial is going to require each arm to have more than 200 patients to establish a significant difference.

OTHER MEASURES

Other potential ways of predicting long-term outcomes are currently HRCT, magnetic resonance imaging, and surveillance bronchoscopy. None have been used longitudinally for long enough to accurately determine their utility. HRCT has been used most, but what it signifies remains unclear. The recent London CF collaborative study concluded in children aged 7 years that although the correlation was best between LCI and HRCT changes with about 55% of the variance explained compared with spirometry (18% variance explained), it may be that HRCT reveals information that

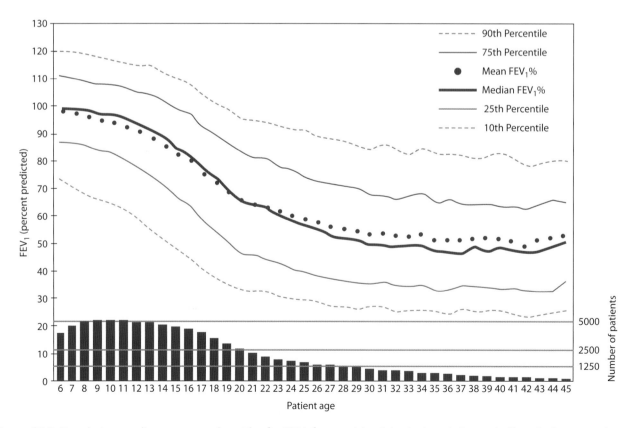

Figure 35.8 Population median, mean, and centiles for FEV₁ from epidemiological study in cystic fibrosis data together with bar chart showing number of observations at each age point. Note: a good example of survival bias from ages 36 years onwards where FEV₁ appears to rise again. (From Liou TG et al., *J Cyst Fibros* 9, 250–6, 2010. With permission.)

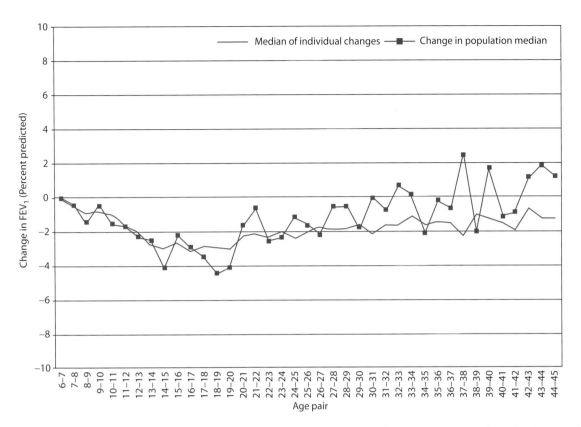

Figure 35.9 Median of individual FEV_1 changes in CF subjects year to year (bold line) superimposed on the CF population median of year to year changes (light line with with squares). Note: good matching until age 15 years, then an increasing deviation away after that. (From Liou TG et al., *J Cyst Fibros*, 9, 250–6, 2010. With permission.)

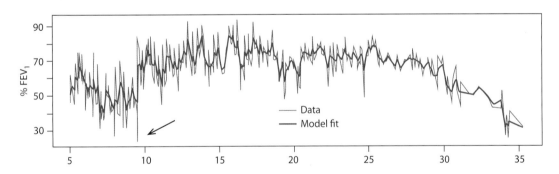

Figure 35.10 Sophisticated modeling of an individual's data showing FEV_1 against age in years. The arrow is shown as an example of where a sudden drop in lung function is outside the model data and represents a potentially recoverable situation. (From Taylor Robinson D et al., *Thorax* 67, 860–6, 2012. With permission.)

lung function cannot and vice versa.[45] In addition, exercise testing provides information that HRCT and lung function does not.[46] The only study on longitudinal bronchoscopy as surveillance did not reduce the incidence of *P. aeruginosa* isolation at aged 5 years.[47]

COMPOSITE MODELS PREDICTING SURVIVAL

The ideal study from a statistical standpoint should have at least 2000 subjects of varying ages followed for a minimum of 8 and ideally 15 years all being treated in a uniform way. The results should be then validated on a second matched contemporaneous cohort preferably from a different continent. Inevitably by the time such results have been produced, treatments and their applications have changed and together with secular trends, the results lose much of their future applicability as has been illustrated above.

Liou et al.[48] produced a validated 5-year survivorship model built from 5810 patients in 1993 from the US CF registry and tested on a further 5810 patients from the same registry. The model is shown in Table 35.5. It emphasizes the persisting survivor disadvantage of female gender and

Table 35.5 Predictive 5-year survivorship model for CF

Covariate[a] (X_{0-10})	Coefficient		Odds ratio	FEV$_1$% equivalence[b]
	β_{1-10}	SE		
Intercept	1.93	027	6.88	50
Age (per year)	−0.028	0.0060	0.97	−0.7
Gender (male = 0, female = 1)	−0.23	0.10	0.79	−6
FEV$_1$% (per%)[c]	0.038	0.0028	1.04	1
Weight-for-age z score	0.40	0.058	1.50	10
PS (0 or 1)	0.45	0.81	1.58	12
Diabetes mellitus (0 or 1)[c]	−0.49	0.15	0.61	−13
S. aureus (0 or 1)[c]	0.21	0.12	1.24	6
B. cepacia (0 or 1)[c]	−1.82	0.80	0.16	−48
No. of acute exacerbations (0–5)[c]	−0.46	0.031	0.63	−12
No. of acute exacerbations × B. cepacia	0.40	0.12	1.49	10

Source: Liou TG et al., Am J Epidemiol 153, 345–52, 2001. With permission.

Note: Hosmer–Lemeshow p value = .54; no significant difference between predicted and actual survivorship of the validated group of patients (31).

[a] The conditional probability of 5-year survival by logistic regression analysis is $\pi = \exp (XY(1 + \exp (X)$, where the logit X is:

$X = \beta_0 + \beta_1 \times$ Age $+ \beta_2 \times$ Gender $+ \beta_3 \times$ FEV$_1$% $+ \beta_4 \times$ z score $+ \beta_5 \times$ PS $+ \beta_6 \times$ Diabetes $+ \beta_7 \times$ S. aureus $+ \beta_8 \times$ B. cepacia $+ \beta_9 \times$ Exacerbations $+ \beta_{10} \times$ (Exacerbations × B. cepacia)

For a covariate X_1 and its coefficient β_1, the term $\exp (\beta_1 \times X_1)$ gives the incremental odds ratio for that covariate. Coefficients for each covariate are unitless unless specified.

[b] FEV$_1$% equivalence was calculated as β_1/βFEV$_1$%. Except for age, values are rounded to the nearest integer. For age, weight-for-age z score and acute exacerbations, the equivalences are per year, per z score point, and per exacerbation, respectively.

[c] FEV$_1$% was calculated by using raw FEV$_1$ results reported to the Cystic Fibrosis Foundation Patient Registry in 1993 for patients who did not undergo transplantation. PS was defined as not using pancreatic enzyme supplementation. Diabetes was defined as the need for insulin during or before 1993. Values for S. aureus and B. cepacia infections are from reported microbiologic data. Number of acute exacerbations is the number of episodes of acute pulmonary exacerbations of CF requiring treatment in 1993, up to a maximum of five. FEV$_1$%, forced expiratory volume in 1 second as a percentage of predicted normal; SE, standard error.

the relatively low contribution from FEV$_1$. It is interesting to note the factors *not* significant for the model included *rate* of decline of FEV$_1$, height, presence of *P. aeruginosa*, or presence/absence of the ΔF508 mutation. Liou did not analyze other measures of lung function such as FVC, but these are unlikely related to outcome. It has been argued that the reason FEV$_1$ appears to play a comparatively minor role in prognosis may be due to its insensitivity in detecting changes in particular in distal airway resistance until more than 90% distal airways are occluded. For this reason, more sensitive techniques such as LCI are becoming increasingly important. However, until these methods become more generally available, there are unlikely to be sufficient data to build them into survival models, let alone validate them in a second population. Longitudinal data are now available up to about 10 years, but this clearly has no use *yet* for true outcome data.

Whether these models even if validated translate into other settings (countries, treatment practices, or indeed into the future) is debatable. Using Liou's data on a cohort of our patients where data was available from the 1993 era (minimum of 4 years lung function data, $n = 126$, 69 males, 67 with previously isolated *P. aeruginosa*, 54 with *Staphylococcus aureus*, 4 with *Burkholderia cepacia*, 7 pancreatic sufficient, and 10 taking insulin), there were 5 deaths (3 male, none with *B. cepacia*) in patients where the *lowest* prior recorded

probability of surviving 5 years was calculated at 71% and there were 12 living patients whose lowest recorded probability of surviving 5 years had been <71% in the preceding years. One possible reason for the discrepancy may be socioeconomic. Although Liou's data showed that education was not significant, there was insufficient data to test either employment, insurance status (United States), and marital status. Schechter et al. looked at the US CF database from 1986 to 1994. The adjusted (race, age, sex, pancreatic enzyme usage) relative risk of death if on Medicaid (a proxy for poverty) was 3.65 (95% CI 3.03–4.40) times than that of insured patients. However, when the *initial* FEV$_1$ on entry to the database was included, the effect of Medicaid disappeared. Again, the importance of early life events is emphasized. The average FEV$_1$ of Medicaid patients was 9.1% (95% CI 7.2–11.0) lower than insured patients and was present from age 5 years and they were 2.3 (95% CI 2.0–2.5) times more likely to have a weight for age <fifth centile. However, they did not have fewer outpatient attendances and if anything were diagnosed earlier (median 131 days) than non-Medicaid patients (median 157 days). The influence of socioeconomic class is discussed further in Chapter 9.

The only study to satisfy the criteria (2000 patients tested on another contemporaneous cohort from a different continent) is Jackson et al.,[49] where using the data from the US CF

Dahl M, Nordestgaard BG, Lange P, Tybjaerg-Hanson A. Fifteen year follow up of pulmonary function in individuals heterozygous for the cystic fibrosis phenylalanine-508 deletion. *J Allergy Clin Immunol* 2001; **107**: 818–23.

Davis PB, Byard PJ, Konstan MW. Identifying treatments that halt progression of pulmonary disease in cystic fibrosis. *Pediatr Res* 1997; **41**: 161–5.

Kalish LA, Waltz DA, Dovey M, Potter-Bynoe G, MacAdam AJ, LiPuma JJ, Gerard C, Goldman D. Impact of Burkholderia dolosa on lung function and survival in cystic fibrosis. *Am J Respir Crit Care Med* 2006; **173**: 421–5.

Keens TG, Mansell A, Krastins IR, Levison H, Bryan AC, Hyland RH, Zamel N. Evaluation of the single breath diffusing capacity in asthma and cystic fibrosis. *Chest* 1979; **76**: 41–44.

Kosorok MR, Zeng L, West SE, et al. Acceleration of lung disease in children with cystic fibrosis after Pseudomonas aeruginosa acquisition. *Pediatr Pulmonol* 2001; **32**: 277–87.

Ramsey BW, Dorkin HL, Eisenberg JD, et al. Efficacy of aerosolized tobramycin in patients with cystic fibrosis. *N Engl J Med* 1993; **328**: 1740–6.

Robinson W, Waltz DA. FEV_1 as a guide to lung transplant referral in young patients with cystic fibrosis. *Pediatr Pulmonol* 2000; **30**: 198–202.

Rosenbluth DB, Wilson K, Ferkol T, et al. Lung function decline in cystic fibrosis patients and timing for lung transplantation referral. *Chest* 2004; **126**: 412–9.

Rosenfeld M, Pepe MS, Longton G, Emerson J, FitzSimmons S, Morgan W. Effect of choice of reference equation on anlysis of pulmonary function in cystic fibrosis patients. *Pediatr Pulmonol* 2001; **31**: 227–337.

Steinkamp G, Wiedemann B. Relationship between nutritional status and lung function in cystic fibrosis: Cross sectional and longitudinal analyses from the German CF quality assurance (CFQA) project. *Thorax* 2002; **57**: 596–601.

Wall MA, LaGesse PC, Istvan JA. The "worth" of routine spirometry in a cystic fibrosis clinic. *Pediatr Pulmonol* 1998; **25**: 231–7.

Xu W, Subbarao P, Corey M. Changing patterns of lung function decline in children with cystic fibrosis. *J Cyst Fibros* 2004; **3**: S116.

36

Exercise: Testing and use in therapy

HIRAN SELVADURAI AND DAVID ORENSTEIN

WHY DO EXERCISE TESTING?

Exercise testing is an important tool in quantifying the functional capacity of a patient with cystic fibrosis (CF). Assessment of the exercise tolerance of patients with CF provides important information about disease severity[1] and the overall well-being of the patient.[2] Exercise testing can not only help ascertain if exercise capacity is reduced but also determine the etiology of the reduced exercise capacity. During the course of an exercise test, the pulmonary system is placed under stress and subtle deficits in lung function may be identified that were not apparent during conventional static pulmonary function testing. Although spirometry, lung volumes, and lung clearance index have traditionally been useful in the diagnosis and guidance of management for patients with lung disease, these tests measure only resting lung function and do not reliably predict functional and exercise capacity.[3] Peak aerobic capacity measured during an exercise test may also predict structural lung damage as seen on high-resolution computed tomography of the chest.[4] Given these observations, exercise testing is an important diagnostic tool in the assessment of the cardiorespiratory status of the subject with CF. Subjects with CF may have reduced exercise capacity due to primary respiratory limitation and be negatively associated with chronic *Pseudomonas aeruginosa* infection but independent of static pulmonary function.[5] During a formal exercise test, subjects with a respiratory limitation will be identified by a reduced breathing reserve and even hypoxia at peak exercise (Table 36.1). Subjects with CF may have reduced exercise capacity due to secondary causes such as deconditioning.[5] During a formal laboratory-based exercise test, subjects who are deconditioned will be identified by a reduced peak aerobic capacity despite a normal breathing reserve and normal cardiac function (Table 36.2). A negative feedback loop may be created where reduced habitual activity leads to further deconditioning, prompting a further reduction in exercise capacity. Formal exercise tests

will help to determine if the etiology of reduced exercise capacity in subjects with CF is due to cardiorespiratory limitation or deconditioning.

Importantly, exercise testing has been shown to provide prognostic information for subjects with CF (Table 36.3).[6–8] Nixon et al. demonstrated that subjects with CF and with higher oxygen consumption at peak exercise (peakVO$_2$) (i.e., VO$_2$ 82% predicted normal) were more than three times as likely to survive for 8 years than those with low peakVO$_2$, (VO$_2$ less than 58% predicted). Pianosi et al.[9] demonstrated that patients with a peakVO$_2$ less than 32 mL/min/kg had a dramatic increase in mortality compared to those with peakVO$_2$ above 45 mL/min/kg. Others have demonstrated the value of assessing for carbon dioxide (CO$_2$) retention during exercise. Subjects with CO$_2$ retention during exercise testing had a significantly greater decline in forced expiratory volume in 1 second (FEV$_1$) in the ensuing years compared to their counterparts who did not retain CO$_2$.[8] Other measures such as the breathing reserve index at ventilatory threshold (defined by the point during an exercise test when the relative CO$_2$ production exceeds O$_2$ consumption) has been evaluated in patients with CF awaiting lung transplantation and demonstrated to be robust predictors of risk for mortality.[10]

BASIC EXERCISE PHYSIOLOGY IN CF

A discussion of exercise testing requires a basic understanding of exercise physiology. For an in-depth presentation of exercise physiology in non-CF subjects, we refer the readers to the work of Wasserman et al.[11]

At the onset of exercise, subjects increase their ventilation by increasing tidal volume (Vt) until it reaches approximately 60% of the subject's vital capacity.[12] With progressive exercise, subsequent increases in minute ventilation (VE) are achieved through increases in respiratory rate. However, in patients with CF, as the severity of lung disease progresses,

Table 36.1 Criteria for diagnosing respiratory limitation as a cause for reduced exercise tolerance

- PeakVO$_2$ <82% predicted
- VE/MVV is >85%
- SaO$_2$ <90%

MVV, maximal voluntary ventilation; peakVO$_2$, oxygen consumption at peak exercise; SaO$_2$, oxygen desaturation; VE, minute ventilation.

Table 36.2 Criteria for diagnosing deconditioning as a cause for reduced exercise tolerance

- PeakVO$_2$ <82% predicted
- VE/MVV at peak exercise <80%
- Normal cardiac rhythm

Table 36.3 Indications for exercise testing

In clinical practice, exercise testing may be performed for one or more of the following indications in patients with CF:

1. Evaluation of functional capacity
2. Evaluation of etiology of exercise limitation
3. Detection of exercise-induced airway obstruction
4. Detection of exercise-induced hypoxemia
5. Detection of exercise-induced arrhythmia
6. Assessment for response to specific intervention, treatment, exercise prescription, or rehabilitation program
7. Evaluation before specific treatment for baseline status or suitability for treatment, e.g., lung transplantation

there is a limited ability to increase V$_t$. Thus, in patients with moderate to severe lung disease, the respiratory rate is increased to higher levels to compensate for the inability to increase the V$_t$.[13] In spite of the increased respiratory rate, dynamic hyperinflation and a limited Vt result in relative alveolar hypoventilation and increased dead space[14,15] Furthermore, patients with CF may have a decreased ventilatory response to CO$_2$.[16] This reduced chemosensitivity may further accentuate the relative alveolar hypoventilation during exercise.[17] CO$_2$ retention during exercise has been shown to have prognostic implications in CF.[8]

Reduced oxygenation is not usually the limiting factor for exercise in subjects with CF. However, some patients will experience lower oxygen saturations during exercise. There is a greater likelihood of oxygen desaturation (SaO$_2$) in subjects whose FEV$_1$ is <50%[18] or diffusing capacity of carbon monoxide is <60%.[19] In healthy subjects, end tidal CO$_2$ levels gradually increase with the onset of exercise, plateau, and then begin to decrease by maximal exercise. It has been noted that in subjects with CF and significant lung disease

there is no decrease in CO$_2$ levels after the plateau. Patients with CF utilize a larger proportion of their total oxygen consumption on respiratory muscles when exercising than do controls.[20] Thus, there is less reserve for use by the exercising peripheral muscles and therefore exercise tolerance may be limited. Despite SaO$_2$ during exercise, the fact that supplemental oxygen prevents desaturation but does not increase maximal exercise capacity[21] suggests that reduced oxygenation is not the primary limiting factor for exercise.

There is some evidence for an intrinsic skeletal muscle defect in subjects with CF[22,23] with abnormal proton handling and reduced mitochondrial function. These studies have demonstrated mild abnormalities in oxidative work performance and recovery. Cystic fibrosis transmembrane conductance regulator chloride channel gene has been demonstrated to be expressed in human skeletal muscle,[24] and studies have demonstrated some genotype relationship with exercise tolerance.[25] However, further details on the exact localization in the muscle cell are awaited.

Cardiac function during exercise is not usually a limiting factor in CF until there is severe lung disease.[26] Stroke volume is reduced in severe airflow limitation due to the reduced inspiratory time to total respiratory time duty cycle ratio.

MODALITIES, MEASUREMENTS, AND PROTOCOLS IN EXERCISE TESTING

There is agreement that annual exercise tests should be performed in subjects with CF.[27] There are quite a few modalities and protocols that are available to perform exercise tests. Exercise testing can be done formally as a cardiopulmonary exercise test (CPET) in a laboratory on a treadmill or cycle ergometer with metabolic measurements during the exercise test. Given the problem of limited access to a laboratory that offers exercise tests,[28] a range of field tests have been validated and utilized in the care of subjects with CF (Table 36.4).

FORMAL LABORATORY-BASED EXERCISE TESTS

A formal, laboratory-based exercise test facilitates airflow, peak oxygen consumption (VO$_2$), CO$_2$ production (VCO$_2$), and heart rate measurements during exercise. Numerous variables may be computed, including VO$_2$, anaerobic threshold (AT), and VE. These indices may be useful in evaluation of the cause of a subject's exercise limitation. VO$_2$ is the best index of aerobic fitness and corresponds to the plateau in oxygen consumption, during maximal exercise in adults. In children, however, oxygen consumption does not always reach a plateau during an incremental exercise test. Therefore, the term peakVO$_2$ is used to define the maximal oxygen consumption achieved during a function limited, incremental exercise test. The AT is an estimate of the point at which CO$_2$ production exceeds oxygen uptake. This indicates the upper limit of exercise intensity that can

Table 36.4 A comparison of field tests and laboratory tests

Field test	Laboratory test
Affordable	High cost of equipment
Easy to perform	Expertise necessary to conduct and interpret test
Subject has control so less threatening	Potentially more threatening
Useful in large population studies	Difficult to perform in large research studies
Limited long-term use	Valid assessment short and long term
Diagnostic limitations	Useful diagnostic test

be achieved predominantly through the aerobic metabolic pathway. In reality, both the aerobic and anaerobic pathways of energy acquisition for skeletal muscle function run concurrently. Nevertheless, the AT is a useful point at which comparisons can be made within as well as between subjects. In healthy subjects, the AT normally occurs at 55% to 65% of the VO_{2max}. Because AT is a submaximal measurement, it is relatively independent of effort and may be useful in making comparisons in long-term follow-up assessments where the measurement of VO_{2max} is difficult.[11] The Dyspnea Index (DI) is the ratio of peakVE during exercise to the maximal voluntary ventilation (MVV) and a DI of greater than 85% is suggestive of some respiratory limitation. MVV should be determined using the 12-second sprint technique.[3] Alternatively, MVV can be estimated in healthy subjects by multiplying the FEV_1 by 35. However, while this formula can be used to estimate the measured MVV in subjects with normal lung function, it does not hold true for children with abnormal lung function.[29] In addition to the usual indices, simultaneous assessment of exercise tidal breathing flow-volume loops in relation to the maximal flow-volume loop may be done with a formal exercise test to provide information on operating lung volumes and flows during exercise.

There are several protocols available when performing exercise tests in subjects with CF. The Godfrey cycle ergometer protocol[30] is a continuous incremental cycle protocol to exhaustion and has been used extensively in clinical assessments,[31] as well as research studies.[32] This protocol is reproducible and valid.[33] It requires the subject to maintain a rate of 60 revolutions per minute (rpm) while the load is increased at a predetermined level every minute until volitional exhaustion (the point where the subject can no longer maintain a pedaling rate of 60 rpm). The aim of the study is to complete the exercise test and reach volitional exhaustion within 12 minutes of starting the test. There have been several center-dependent modifications to the Godfrey protocol and for the original protocol there are prediction equations. Subsequently, Orenstein published gender-specific prediction equations.[34] The limitation of this exercise protocol is the need for children whose standing height is less

than 125 cm to use an extension crank on the ergometer or on a pediatric-specific cycle ergometer.

The Bruce protocol[35] that is used in many adult cardiac treadmill exercise tests is also widely used in clinical assessment and research studies. It is reliable in adults and children[36,37] and sensitive to change with interventions in children with CF.[38] The Bruce protocol requires the subject to walk initially and run subsequently on a treadmill, where both the speed and the gradient of incline are increased every 3 minutes. A modification of this protocol is to increase the speed and gradient of incline every 2 minutes. Since this is a weight-bearing test, the peakVO_2 obtained in the treadmill test is greater than that obtained during a cycle ergometer test. However, estimating peak work output during an exercise test is less precise compared to when a cycle ergometer is used.

FIELD TESTS

Field tests are exercise tests that can be performed without the need for specialized exercise equipment or gas analysis. The main advantages of field tests are that they require inexpensive and portable equipment and that they are simple to perform. They are often used in the evaluation of responses to treatment or intervention, in situations that preclude the use a formal exercise test. The measurements taken during field tests include baseline and highest pulse rate, baseline and lowest oxygen saturation, subjective and objective measures of breathlessness[39,40] before and after the test, distance or steps achieved, and muscle fatigue. Field tests that have been validated in CF include the 6-minute walk test (6MWT)[41] and the 3-minute step test.[42]

The step test is a quick, simple, and portable field test. The subjects are required to step up and down a step of 15 cm height at a rate of 30 steps per minute for 3 minutes. Being externally paced, it has the additional benefit of not being dependent on patient motivation. The test is reproducible,[43] but does not measure a maximal functional capacity and the workload will vary according to the weight and height of the subject. The test is, therefore, not suited to longer term clinical intervention trials.[44]

The 6MWT is reproducible and has a significant correlation with peakVO_2.[45] It requires the subject to walk back and forth along an appropriate course of known length for 6 minutes. Normative values for healthy children performing the 6MWT are available.[46] However, as the test is self-paced, the patient's attitude and motivation are a major factor in determining the distance walked and therefore may have limited application in clinical interventional trials in patients with CF.

The 20 m, 10 m, and modified shuttle tests are maximal field tests that has been validated in subjects with CF.[47,48] The shuttle test requires the subject to walk and subsequently run up and down a 10 m or 20 m course (depending on the chosen test) keeping time with an externally paced audio signal, at incremental speeds until the subject either fails to make the shuttle distance or chooses to stop. The shuttle test

61. Hebestreit H, Kieser S, Ridiger S, et al. Physical activity is independently related to aerobic capacity in cystic fibrosis. *Eur Respir J* 2006; **28**: 734–9.

62. Schneiderman-Walker J, Wilkes D, Strug L, et al. Sex differences in habitual activity and lung function decline in children with cystic fibrosis. *J Pediatr* 2005; **147**: 321–6.

63. Schmitt L, Wiebel M, Frese F, et al. Exercise reduced airway sodium ion absorption in cystic fibrosis but not in exercise asthma. *Eur Respir J* 2011; **37**: 342–8.

64. Salh W, Bilton D, Dodd M, Webb A. Effect of exercise and physiotherapy in aiding sputum expectoration in adults with CF. *Thorax* 1989; **44**: 1006–8.

65. Paccou J, Zeboulon N, Combescure C, et al. The prevalence of osteoporosis and osteopenia and fractures among adults with CF: A systematic literature review with meta analysis. *Cacif Tissue Int* 2010; **86**: 1–7.

66. Gronowitz E, Garemo M, Lindblad A, Mellstrom D, Strandvik B. Decreased bone mineral density in normal growing patients with CF. *Acta Pediatr* 2003; **92**: 688–93.

67. Frangolias D, Pare P, Kendler D, Davidson A, et al. Role of exercise and nutrition status on bone mineral density in CF. *J Cyst Fibrosis* 2003; **2**: 163–70.

68. Britto M, Garrett J, Konrad T, Majure J. Comparison of physical activity in adolescents with cystic fibrosis versus* age matched controls. *Pediatr Pulmonol* 2000; **30**: 86–91.

69. Garcia S, Sanchez M, Cejudo P, Gallego E, et al. Bone health, daily physical activity and exercise tolerance in patients with cystic fibrosis. *Chest* 2011; **14**: 475–81.

70. Mackelvie K, Petit M, Khan K, Beck T, Mckay H. Bone mass and structure are enhanced flowing a 2 year randomised controlled trial of exercise in prepubertal boys. *Bone* 2004; **34**: 755–64.

71. Cystic Fibrosis Trust. Bone mineralization in cystic fibrosis. Working group consensus statement. February 2007. http://www.cftrust.org.uk/aboutcf/publications/consensusdoc (accessed September 12, 2012).

37

Outcome of clinical trials: Electricity, induced sputum, and breath

MICHAEL WALLER, ERIC W.F.W. ALTON, AND JANE C. DAVIES

EPITHELIAL POTENTIAL DIFFERENCE

Defective cystic fibrosis transmembrane conductance regulator (CFTR) function produces abnormal epithelial chloride (Cl^-) and sodium (Na^+) ion movement, which produces a characteristic, measurable potential difference (PD) across cell membranes and allow a direct and dynamic assessment of ion channel function. As a bioelectric assay of CFTR function, PD has developed as a clinical trial outcome particularly for therapies targeting the *CFTR* gene or protein, where activity of the protein is interrogated over and above the more standard and surrogate cystic fibrosis (CF) indices.

In vivo assessment of the airway epithelial PD can be made from both the nasal mucosa and the lower airway with the former often used as a surrogate for the latter. The nose is more easily accessible meaning measurements are less invasive and carry few complications; given the cellular similarities, such assumptions may be reasonable, but there are no data comparing PD at the two sites directly.[1]

NASAL POTENTIAL DIFFERENCE

Nasal PD (nPD) measurements have developed from the methods of Knowles et al.[2] and Alton et al.,[3] and despite some variations in equipment and technique used between operators in different CF centers, the basic principle of the procedure remains the same (Figure 37.1) (see Chapter 10). Variations exist in the method, equipment, and solutions used, and despite standardization within the Cystic Fibrosis Foundation Therapeutics Development Network (CFFTDN)[4] and European Cystic Fibrosis Society (ECFS) Diagnostic Network Working Group,[5] some differences remain.

The operator must possess a degree of technical expertise and patience while locating the optimal position for the initial PD reading; most protocols are based on the site with the highest basal PD. Operators differ in placing the catheter, varying between blind and visualized insertion along the nasal floor until the maximal negative voltage has been located, or resting under the inferior nasal turbinate, which possibly relates to some reported differences between groups; a direct comparison concluded no superiority of either method[6]; however, the authors favor the "blind" nasal floor approach. It is important to note that (1) values measured from under the inferior turbinate are more negative than those from the floor and (2) CF patients generally have a maximal basal PD at a site more distal from the external nares than non-CF subjects.

Ionic solutions are perfused in strict sequence, independently reflecting Na^+ and Cl^- movement: (1) custom Ringer's solution is used to provide a basal, unstimulated PD, which predominantly reflects Na^+ absorption[7]; (2) 0.1 mM amiloride (in Ringer's) solution which blocks Na^+ absorption via epithelial sodium channels; (3) a zero or low-chloride solution inducing Cl^- movement across the apical epithelial membrane down a concentration gradient into the luminal airway (passive chloride transport); (4) a zero or low-chloride solution containing isoprenaline (isoproterenol) to stimulate cyclic adenosine monophosphate (cAMP) production and activate CFTR (stimulated chloride transport). Perfusion of Cl^--depleted solutions aims to move Cl^- through a functional CFTR protein—in the non-CF epithelium, the PD increases (more negative), but in patients with CFTR dysfunction little or no response is seen; indeed there is often a small decrease. It is changes in these parameters, in particular Cl^- movement, that are of interest as a bioelectric measure of CFTR function in response to new therapies. Debate exists as to whether solutions should be warmed[5]; the CFFTDN recommends warming to enhance total chloride response,[8] but the ECFS Cinical Trials

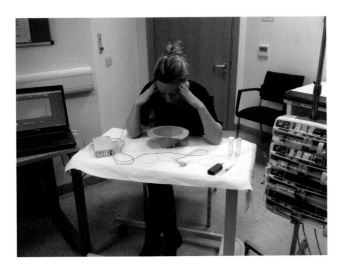

Figure 37.1 Demonstration of nasal potential difference (nPD) measurements being taken and displaying equipment used.

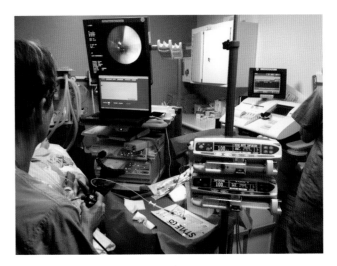

Figure 37.2 Lower airway PD measurements being made via bronchoscopy under general anesthesia.

Network (CTN) considers that the challenges inherent in this and the likely variability introduced outweigh the very small effect on ion transport and have not included warming in their protocol.[5]

LIMITATIONS OF NASAL POTENTIAL DIFFERENCE

As with all techniques, attention to detail is important. Nasal epithelial inflammation from rhinosinusitis, polyps, and previous surgery generally produce low readings and blunted responses likely related to squamous metaplasia, limiting the usefulness of the technique in patients with nasal disease. The technique has a relatively low coefficient of variability (~5%–15%) for intrasubject measurements.[9] It is crucial to note that the technique is measuring a constantly changing physiological response, not a static parameter. Operator performance, with attention to technique detail, is likely the greatest cause of variability of results. The key is the ability to achieve a constant catheter position in the nose. Further issues include rotation of the catheter and placement on the floor or inferior turbinate. These are important issues for multicenter trials[10]; developing standardized operating procedures (SOPs) is logical to reduce this variance,[11] but the key issue is standardized "in-person" operator training. Centralized data interpretation may also reduce variability.

POTENTIAL DIFFERENCE OF THE LOWER AIRWAY

The behavior and response of the CF lower airway is of greater interest as an outcome in clinical trials, although the technique is rarely used due to its invasive and technically challenging nature. No standardized technique has been developed and only few research groups perform this procedure. With the emergence of new treatments directly

targeting CFTR, electrophysiological assessment of the airways is likely to be a ever more important (Figure 37.2).

Bronchial PD poses additional challenges over and above those of nasal measurements. To limit interference in the recording measurement from the patient such as movement and coughing, and to avoid local and volatile anesthetic agents[12] that affect ion channel function, the procedure is generally performed under total intravenous (IV) general anesthesia. The single operating channel within most fiberoptic bronchoscopes limits the size of the PD catheters used. Although some systems allow for a double-lumen PD catheter to pass through this port, our group has designed a single-lumen technique; however, this method has the challenge of making measurements through a moving fluid column which is prone to bubbles and thus results in a loss of PD connection.[13] The techniques permit basal and stimulated measurements; the pooling of solutions in the airway, which then dilute subsequent perfusate, needs to be carefully avoided. We have shown clear separation between CF and non-CF basal PD in the proximal airways although in both groups, PD falls with distal progression and a disease-specific difference is not seen in the most peripheral sites measured (Figure 37.3).[13] As expected, chloride secretory responses are also significantly different between CF and non-CF.

CLINICAL CORRELATIONS WITH POTENTIAL DIFFERENCE

No definite relationship between nPD response and respiratory function has been demonstrated.[14] A correlation between CF disease severity and basal nPD[3] has been identified, with milder respiratory disease being associated with lower (less negative) basal nPD and vice versa, irrespective of genotype.[14] A study of 79 adult CF patients demonstrated relationships between residual epithelial Cl⁻ secretion and preserved pancreatic status, and a more abnormal Na⁺ transport (as indicated by a higher amiloride response) with an

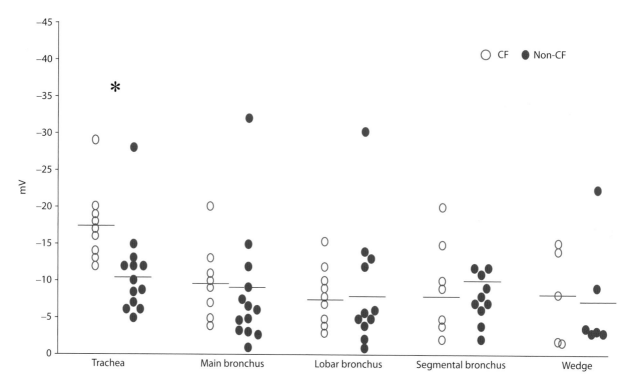

Figure 37.3 Baseline PD measurements at various sites in the lower airways of children with and without cystic fibrosis (*$p < .001$). (From Davies JC et al., *Am J Respir Crit Care Med* 171(9), 1015–9, 2005. With permission.

increased severity of lung disease.[15] One study of older CF patients did not demonstrate a correlation with survival and residual CFTR function in patients with severe CF mutations,[16] but others have reported that residual Cl^- secretion on nPD was associated with greater lung function regardless of the genotype,[17] with a good correlation between the response to isoprenaline and a higher forced expiratory volume in 1 second (FEV_1) being demonstrated in men but not in women.[18]

CLINICAL TRIALS USING POTENTIAL DIFFERENCE AS AN OUTCOME

Because of the complexity of the technique and its time-consuming nature for operator and patient, airway PD has been used most commonly and is likely to be most useful, in early stage, proof of mechanism trials.[19] Its inclusion in large, multicenter, or multinational trials will require rigorous training and standardization; indeed, as discussed below, problems with such processes were likely responsible for unacceptable variability and thus loss of power in previous reports. We next discuss illustrative trials using PD as an end point.

CPX

CPX (8-cyclopentyl-1,3-dipropylxanthine), a protein repair therapy developed to directly interact with the CFTR protein by antagonizing the A1 adenosine receptor, resulted in improved trafficking of CFTR to the plasma membrane and stimulation of chloride channel activity in F508del cells in

vitro.[20] However, a phase-1 clinical study using a single escalating oral dose protocol demonstrated no significant effect on nPD.[21] Although 9% of subjects had a significant response (defined as a total response of greater than −5 mV following perfusion with a low chloride ± isoproterenol solutions), no difference between the treatment groups was seen. The nPD measurements were independently made at each of the four study sites, without a universal trial nPD SOP. A post hoc analysis found significant variability between each of the study sites that may have contributed to this negative result.

Gentamicin

Following Bedwell's findings that the aminoglycoside gentamicin can suppress premature stop mutations and activate CFTR in vitro,[22] clinical studies tested this agent using nPD to assess CFTR function. A pilot study of nasal dosing in CF patients with premature stop mutations found significant restoration of Cl^- transport, with a response being toward that of the non-CF control group in seven out of nine subjects.[23] The effect on sodium transport was less prominent.

Similar results were seen in a double-blind, placebo-controlled, crossover trial of patients with nonsense mutations (homozygous and heterozygous) and with the F508del mutation.[24] About 11 out of 19 patients studied were homozygous for a premature stop mutation, with all subjects possessing at least one W1282X mutation. The basal PD measurements after 14 days treatment with nasal gentamicin was significantly reduced in the nonsense mutation group, with a quarter of subjects displaying levels within

was obtained by both procedures, suggesting IS may be feasible as a less invasive alternative to help investigate the lower airway flora but that more studies are needed.

BIOMARKER RESPONSE TO INTRAVENOUS ANTIBIOTICS

Inflammatory and microbiological biomarkers in IS were measured as an outcome in a clinical trial investigating the response of IV antibiotic therapy for a pulmonary exacerbation of CF, in addition to the typical surrogate end points such as FEV_1 and days in hospital.[55] The study demonstrated improvements in FEV_1 following treatment that were associated with changes in biomarkers in IS, in particular reductions in the bacterial density of *Pseudomonas aeruginosa* and *Staphylococcus aureus*, reductions in neutrophil count, IL-8 concentration, and neutrophil elastase activity. Although the authors concluded that sputum induction is relatively safe during a pulmonary exacerbation in CF, 6% of IS procedures experienced a fall of >20% FEV_1, with the greatest fall being 46%, indicating that caution and close monitoring are imperative.

Despite its potential as a validated and reproducible tool in sputum assessment in CF, few studies have reported IS as a clinical trial outcome with the majority still relying on measurements from expectorated sputum. As CF lung disease is heterogeneous with respect to anatomy, severity, and airflow limitation, reliance on spontaneous sputum production to reliably measure changes in inflammatory markers from this diverse population is perhaps suboptimal. More encouragement may be necessary to promote the use of IS in larger randomized controlled trials particularly when investigating inflammatory markers as a measureable trial outcome in response to new therapies, discussing with patients the aims, benefits, and safety of the procedure, although highlighting the short-lived yet unpleasant side-effects (coughing, bronchoconstriction) experienced.

BREATH AND BREATH CONDENSATE

Although sputum analysis is convenient, the disease heterogeneity limits this method, and measurement of exhaled compounds in the patient's breath may have potential. Recently the analysis of biomarkers in exhaled breath (EB) and its condensate have developed widespread interest as a noninvasive technique for the assessment of airways inflammation that is both acceptable to patients and easily repeatable; these fields however remain in their infancy.

Exhaled breath condensate (EBC)

Collection of EBC is a safe and noninvasive technique for sampling biomarkers in the fluid lining the lower airway, which can be performed repeatedly with minimal intervals required between sample measuring. The method is simple—a subject breathes tidally through a mouthpiece into a condenser and the cooled condensate is collected. A variety of commercial systems for EBC are available, varying in the method used to cool the EB but all aim to adhere to the following global recommendations to optimize sample and analysis:[72] the condensers must possess a one-way valve as a safety measure to prevent inspiration of cooled air to the patient and to prevent sample contamination, saliva must be prevented from entering the condensate, the patient should wear a nose-clip to avoid nasally produced compounds being measured (and similarly EB lost through the nose), and the condensing surface should be inert to prevent cross-reaction with the biomarkers. The consistency of sampling between commercial devices has not yet been established, making it important to report the device used alongside findings. Similarly, no standardization exists for the time EBC is collected nor the temperature the specimen should reach on cooling; a linear relationship exists between the volume expired and the volume of EBC, suggesting a predefined volume of EB rather than time should be used for clinical trials.[73]

EB is saturated with at least 90% water vapor, which contributes to the predominant component of the EBC;[74] the molecules of interest from the airway lining liquid form only a small fraction of the condensate collected. Two mechanisms for how the airways surface liquid (ASL) is aerosolized and thus exhaled have been proposed: one suggests that turbulence in the airway generates sufficient energy to aerosolize the ASL,[75] whereas an alternative hypothesis suggests aerosolization occurs from the popping-open of closed respiratory bronchioles and alveoli.[76] The EBC is analyzed, usually by enzyme-linked immunosorbent assay, chromogenic substrate analysis, or mass spectrometry (MS) techniques; however, it is essential that these assays be validated for the likely low concentrations of each biomarker in EBC.[77] Accurate measurement of these compounds, however, is limited by the fact that the exhaled compounds are in very low concentration, highly variable, and difficult to quantify dilution from respiratory droplets as.[78]

AIRWAY BIOMARKERS IN EXHALED BREATH CONDENSATE

Compounds of airways inflammation and oxidative stress can be measured from the EBC fraction, as can the pH of the airway lining liquid. Longitudinal studies have demonstrated increased levels of distinct biomarkers measured in EBC in patients with CF during acute respiratory exacerbations, including elevated levels of the prostaglandin isomer, 8-isoprostane,[79] likely reflecting oxidative stress on the CF airway. An increase in the inflammatory mediators, LTB4, and IL-6 has similarly been measured from EBC in CF, with higher concentrations being seen in patients infected with *P. aeruginosa*.[80] Likewise, raised nitrite and IL-8 levels have been demonstrated supporting the role of EBC as a tool for assessing airway inflammation and excessive neutrophil presence,[81] with IL-8 levels decreasing following antibiotic treatment[82]; the usefulness of nitrite as a long-term marker in CF lung disease has recently been questioned following a longitudinal study in children with mild CF, which concluded that increased levels of this biomarker did not predict pulmonary exacerbations.[83] Levels of hydrogen peroxide[84] and nitric oxide (NO)[85] have not been found to be elevated in EBC from patients with CF and are therefore deemed unsuitable as biomarkers. EBC pH from stable CF patients has been demonstrated to be chronically acidic possibly resulting from impaired CFTR-mediated bicarbonate transport, with a further reduction in pH occurring during an acute exacerbation and increase in response to antibiotic treatment.[86,87] This was recently confirmed by the UK CF Gene Therapy Consortium on an observational study (Tracking Study) measuring a series of biomarkers in CF lung disease in response to a pulmonary exacerbation[88]; significant improvement in FEV_1 and EBC pH were recorded in response to IV antibiotics, although no direct correlation between the two was made; no significant change in EBC nitrite or ammonium levels were detected. Thus, the pH of EBC may be a useful biomarker when evaluating airway inflammation and the response to antibiotic treatment.

Adenyl purines, including adenosine and adenosine monophosphate, are released from airway epithelial and inflammatory cells onto airway surfaces in response to inflammatory processes.[89] A strong negative correlation between EBC adenosine (as assessed by an EBC adenosine : urea ratio) has been demonstrated with lung function measures over time in children with CF, supporting evidence that adenosine and related purinergic signaling pathways play a role in the inflammatory component of airways disease in CF. EBC adenosine may, therefore, have a role as a longitudinal biomarker in CF pulmonary disease.[90]

No studies to date, including those of novel agents targeting CFTR function, have published EBC results as a measure of outcome. The technical difficulties and variability of measuring a biomarker at such low concentrations, along with lack of standardization and validated biomarker analysis of this technique may be key in restricting these assessments. At present, most published literature on EBC has reported longitudinal findings in small numbers of patients to address this methodological quandary in advance of pharmaceutical trials utilizing EBC as an acceptable outcome measure; a few analyze the inflammatory response of the CF airway following antibiotic and nonpharmacological treatment regimes for a pulmonary exacerbation.

Exhaled breath

The use of EB itself in CF offers a simple and noninvasive method to sample the lower airway, with several volatile and nonvolatile markers of inflammation and oxidative stress having being identified.[54] Samples are either analyzed in real time or by collection for indirect analysis; both techniques involve a patient performing a single vital capacity exhalation through a one-way valve. Collection of the specimen in a reservoir or sample container is simple, quick, and easily transferable, which allows for repeated sampling away from hospital or laboratory. The sample of EB can be analyzed by methods including sensitive MS, selected ion flow tube (SIFT)-spectrometry, gas chromatography (GC), GC/MS,[91] or electrochemical or chemiluminescence sensors.

NITRIC OXIDE

Endogenous airway NO is involved in smooth muscle relaxation, bronchodilatation and inflammation.[92] The fraction of exhaled nitric oxide (FE_{NO}), in contrast to other inflammatory airway diseases, is lower in CF compared to controls[93] and remains suppressed during a pulmonary exacerbation.[94] Defective L-arginine pathways, responsible for production of NO by NO synthases, have been proposed as the likely mechanism for this phenomenon in CF.[95]

A study measuring the response of FE_{NO} (measured by chemiluminescence analyzer) to routine IV antibiotics in 14 children with CF demonstrated a significant improvement in FEV_1 and a significant increase in FE_{NO} following treatment although no correlation between these parameters was detected.[96] A subgroup analysis found no significant change in FE_{NO} from patients chronically infected with *P. aeruginosa*, which may result from the small subgroup sample size.

FE_{NO} was analyzed in small subgroup of patients during a randomized controlled trial of the mucolytic agent dornase alfa and increased in parallel with changes in the forced vital capacity in treated patients ($n = 6$), but again no statistical association with FEV_1 was demonstrated.[97]

A recent interventional study assessing the safety and efficacy of inhaled L-arginine, in a double-blind, randomized, placebo-controlled crossover trial of 19 patients with CF measured FE_{NO} as secondary outcome measure.[98] After 14 days of treatment, a small but nonsignificant improvement in FEV_1 was detected but a significant increase in FE_{NO} compared to placebo was measured.

CARBON MONOXIDE AND ETHANE

Carbon monoxide (CO) and ethane are by-products of cellular oxidation and proinflammatory cytokine response in airway tissue damage, and are measureable in EB.[99] Levels of exhaled CO from the breath of CF patients were raised at baseline in stable lung disease[100] and increased significantly during a mild or moderate respiratory exacerbation.[101]

Similarly, elevated levels of ethane have been reported in stable CF patients, which correlated with levels of CO and lung function measurements of airways obstruction (residual volume/total lung capacity).[99]

MICROBE-DERIVED VOLATILE ORGANIC COMPOUNDS (VOCs)

Culturing bacterial species using standard techniques from nonexpectorating patients can be difficult; alternative methods of identifying the presence of pathogens, in particular *P. aeruginosa* in the lower airways from EB have been sought.

Levels of hydrogen cyanide (HCN) measured by SIFT-MS from the EB of children with CF have been demonstrated to be elevated in patients infected with *P. aeruginosa* when compared to children with asthma. However, although both mucoid and nonmucoid strains have been shown to produce HCN, the greatest concentrations were seen in mucoid strains, which may reduce the sensitivity of this biomarker.[102] Interestingly, this did not seem to be the case when HCN was measured in a sputum study, where similar levels were seen in patients with mucoid and nonmucoid strains.[103] There is also the possible confounding factor that, as HCN may also be produced by host inflammatory cells, an impression of an association with *P. aeruginosa* infection could be spurious. Further data on the utility of this biomarker are clearly needed.

Exploration of other VOCs from sputum containing *P. aeruginosa* has identified 2-nonanone as a potential biomarker, but this is so far untested in human EB.[104] 2-Aminoacetophenone (2-AA), the compound responsible for the distinctive grape-like smell produced by *P. aeruginosa*,[105] has shown promise as breath biomarker for *P. aeruginosa* in the CF lung.[106] Using GC/MS, 2-AA was measured above the limit of detection in CF patients colonized with *P. aeruginosa* significantly higher than compared to healthy controls and CF non-colonized subjects.

2-Pentylfuran (2PF) has been identified as a potential VOC in CF patients colonized with *Aspergillus fumigatus*. In a small study, EB 2PF was detected by GC/MS–MS in all studied CF patients colonized with *A. fumigatus* ($n = 4$), but in no healthy controls ($n = 10$); however, three of seven CF patients not colonized with *A. fumigatus* also had detectable levels of 2PF from their breath.[107] Although there is potential for this fungal biomarker, other confounding factors may need analysis to gain understanding of the compound's specificity and clinical application.

Although the collection of breath is easy and repeatable, concerns regarding the validity and sensitivity of the measurements may limit its use as a viable clinical trial outcome. The volatile compounds CO and ethane have proved successful as markers of a pulmonary CF exacerbation, with both HCN and 2-AA being specific breath biomarkers for infection with *P. aeruginosa*; the microbe-derived biomarkers 2-nonanone and 2PF show promise but need further development and understanding in the in vivo CF lung. Although of limited use to define an exacerbation, changes in EB FE$_{NO}$ correlate well with improvements in the airway epithelium and lung function. More studies are, however, necessary before larger interventional trials can use EB compounds as a reliable outcome measure.

HOW MIGHT SUCH CLINICAL TRIAL OUTCOME MEASURES BE OPTIMIZED FOR FUTURE USE?

As highlighted above, standardization for any of these techniques is crucially important; this is particularly the case for measurements with inherent variability such as those outlined. Many techniques have been developed independently by research groups with, until recently, little consideration paid to the resultant inability to compare data and thereby learn optimally from results. Encouragingly, both the CFFTDN and the ECFS CTN have recognized this problem and are addressing it: SOPs with widespread utility drawn up after expert consensus; training and certification procedures for sites wishing to participate in trials; and centralized reading and analysis laboratories. Adhering to such processes will improve the quality of trial data and allow us to pool results from across trials, thereby aiding in the rational design of future research programs.

REFERENCES

1. De Boeck K, et al. Cystic fibrosis: Terminology and diagnostic algorithms. *Thorax* 2006; **61**(7): 627–35.
2. Knowles M, Gatzy J, Boucher R. Increased bioelectric potential difference across respiratory epithelia in cystic fibrosis. *N Engl J Med* 1981; **305**(25): 1489–95.
3. Alton EW, et al. Nasal potential difference: A clinical diagnostic test for cystic fibrosis. *Eur Respir J* 1990; **3**(8): 922–6.
4. Standaert TA, et al. Standardized procedure for measurement of nasal potential difference: An outcome measure in multicenter cystic fibrosis clinical trials. *Pediatr Pulmonol* 2004; **37**(5): 385–92.
5. De Boeck K, et al. New clinical diagnostic procedures for cystic fibrosis in Europe. *J Cyst Fibros* 2011; **10** (Suppl 2): S53–66.
6. Vermeulen F, et al. Nasal potential measurements on the nasal floor and under the inferior turbinate: Does it matter? *Pediatr Pulmonol* 2011; **46**(2): 145–52.
7. Middleton P, Alton EWFW. In vivo measurement of airway potential difference to assess CFTR function in man. *Prog Respir Res* 2006; **34**: 102–8.
8. Boyle MP, et al. A multicenter study of the effect of solution temperature on nasal potential difference measurements. *Chest* 2003; **124**(2): 482–9.
9. Delmarco A, et al. Nasal potential difference in cystic fibrosis patients presenting borderline sweat test. *Eur Respir J* 1997; **10**(5): 1145–9.
10. Ahrens RC, et al. Use of nasal potential difference and sweat chloride as outcome measures in multicenter clinical trials in subjects with cystic fibrosis. *Pediatr Pulmonol* 2002; **33**(2): 142–50.
11. Rowe SM, Accurso F, Clancy JP. Detection of cystic fibrosis transmembrane conductance regulator activity in early-phase clinical trials. *Proc Am Thorac Soc* 2007; **4**(4): 387–98.
12. Smuszkiewicz P, et al. Comparison of the influence of halothane and isoflurane on airway transepithelial potential difference. *Pharmacol Rep* 2006; **58**(5): 736–45.

13. Davies JC, et al. Potential difference measurements in the lower airway of children with and without cystic fibrosis. *Am J Respir Crit Care Med* 2005; **171**(9): 1015–9.

14. Fajac I, et al. Relationships between nasal potential difference and respiratory function in adults with cystic fibrosis. *Eur Respir J*, 1998; **12**(6): 1295–300.

15. Fajac I, et al. Nasal airway ion transport is linked to the cystic fibrosis phenotype in adult patients. *Thorax* 2004; **59**(11): 971–6.

16. Simmonds NJ, et al. Cystic fibrosis and survival to 40 years: A study of cystic fibrosis transmembrane conductance regulator function. *Eur Respir J* 2011; **37**(5): 1076–82.

17. Ho LP, et al. Correlation between nasal potential difference measurements, genotype and clinical condition in patients with cystic fibrosis. *Eur Respir J* 1997; **10**(9): 2018–22.

18. Thomas SR, et al. Pulmonary disease severity in men with deltaF508 cystic fibrosis and residual chloride secretion. *Lancet* 1999; **353**(9157): 984–5.

19. De Boeck K, et al. CFTR biomarkers: Time for promotion to surrogate endpoint? *Eur Respir J* 2012: **41**(1): 203–16.

20. Arispe N, et al. Direct activation of cystic fibrosis transmembrane conductance regulator channels by 8-cyclopentyl-1,3-dipropylxanthine (CPX) and 1,3-diallyl-8-cyclohexylxanthine (DAX). *J Biol Chem* 1998; **273**(10): 5727–34.

21. McCarty NA, et al. A phase I randomized, multi-center trial of CPX in adult subjects with mild cystic fibrosis. *Pediatr Pulmonol* 2002; **33**(2): 90–8.

22. Bedwell DM, et al. Suppression of a CFTR premature stop mutation in a bronchial epithelial cell line. *Nat Med* 1997; **3**(11): 1280–4.

23. Wilschanski M, et al. A pilot study of the effect of gentamicin on nasal potential difference measurements in cystic fibrosis patients carrying stop mutations. *Am J Respir Crit Care Med* 2000; **161** (3 Pt 1): 860–5.

24. Wilschanski M, et al. Gentamicin-induced correction of CFTR function in patients with cystic fibrosis and CFTR stop mutations. *N Engl J Med* 2003; **349**(15): 1433–41.

25. Clancy JP, et al. No detectable improvements in cystic fibrosis transmembrane conductance regulator by nasal aminoglycosides in patients with cystic fibrosis with stop mutations. *Am J Respir Cell Mol Biol* 2007; **37**(1): 57–66.

26. Du M, et al. PTC124 is an orally bioavailable compound that promotes suppression of the human CFTR-G542X nonsense allele in a CF mouse model. *Proc Natl Acad Sci USA* 2008; **105**(6): 2064–9.

27. Kerem B, Chiba-Falek O, Kerem E. Cystic fibrosis in Jews: Frequency and mutation distribution. *Genet Test* 1997; **1**(1): 35–9.

28. Kerem E, et al. Effectiveness of PTC124 treatment of cystic fibrosis caused by nonsense mutations: A prospective phase II trial. *Lancet* 2008; **372**(9640): 719–27.

29. Wilschanski M, et al. Chronic ataluren (PTC124) treatment of nonsense mutation cystic fibrosis. *Eur Respir J* 2011; **38**(1): 59–69.

30. Kerem E, Konstan MW, et al. Ataluren for the treatment of nonsense-mutation cystic fibrosis: A randomised, double-blind, placebo-controlled phase 3 trial. *Lancet Resp Med* 2014; **2**(7): 539–47.

31. Cystic Fibrosis Foundation. *Patient Registry 2011 Annual Data Report.* Bethesda, MD: Cystic Fibrosis Foundation; 2012.

32. Cystic Fibrosis Trust. *UK CF Registry Annual Data Report 2011.*, Bromley, United Kingdom: Cystic Fibrosis Trust; 2013.

33. Van Goor F, et al. Rescue of CF airway epithelial cell function in vitro by a CFTR potentiator, VX-770. *Proc Natl Acad Sci USA* 2009; **106**(44): 18825–30.

34. Accurso FJ, et al. Effect of VX-770 in persons with cystic fibrosis and the G551D-CFTR mutation. *N Engl J Med* 2010; **363**(21): 1991–2003.

35. Ramsey BW, et al. A CFTR potentiator in patients with cystic fibrosis and the G551D mutation. *N Engl J Med* 2011; **365**(18): 1663–72.

36. Leonard A, et al. A randomized placebo-controlled trial of miglustat in cystic fibrosis based on nasal potential difference. *J Cyst Fibros* 2012; **11**(3): 231–6.

37. Leal T, et al. Modified method to measure nasal potential difference. *Clin Chem Lab Med* 2003; **41**(1): 61–7.

38. Davies JC, Alton EW. Gene therapy for cystic fibrosis. *Proc Am Thorac Soc* 2010; **7**(6): 408–14.

39. Caplen NJ, et al. Liposome-mediated CFTR gene transfer to the nasal epithelium of patients with cystic fibrosis. *Nat Med* 1995; **1**(1): 39–46.

40. Hyde SC, et al. Repeat administration of DNA/liposomes to the nasal epithelium of patients with cystic fibrosis. *Gene Ther* 2000; **7**(13): 1156–65.

41. Alton EW, et al. Cationic lipid-mediated CFTR gene transfer to the lungs and nose of patients with cystic fibrosis: A double-blind placebo-controlled trial. *Lancet* 1999; **353**(9157): 947–54.

42. Konstan MW, et al. Compacted DNA nanoparticles administered to the nasal mucosa of cystic fibrosis subjects are safe and demonstrate partial to complete cystic fibrosis transmembrane regulator reconstitution. *Hum Gene Ther* 2004; **15**(12): 1255–69.

43. Gill DR, et al. A placebo-controlled study of liposome-mediated gene transfer to the nasal epithelium of patients with cystic fibrosis. *Gene Ther* 1997; **4**(3): 199–209.

44. Davies G, et al. T4 Safety and expression of a single dose of lipid-mediated CFTR gene therapy to the upper and lower airways of patients with cystic fibrosis. *Thorax* 2011; **66** (Suppl 4): A2.

45. Crawford I, et al. Immunocytochemical localization of the cystic fibrosis gene product CFTR. *Proc Natl Acad Sci USA* 1991; **88**(20): 9262–6.

46. Berschneider HM, et al. Altered intestinal chloride transport in cystic fibrosis. *FASEB J* 1988; **2**(10): 2625–9.

47. Veeze HJ, et al. Ion transport abnormalities in rectal suction biopsies from children with cystic fibrosis. *Gastroenterology* 1991; **101**(2): 398–403.

48. Taylor CJ, Hardcastle J, Southern KW. Physiological measurements confirming the diagnosis of cystic fibrosis: The sweat test and measurements of transepithelial potential difference. *Paediatr Respir Rev* 2009; **10**(4): 220–6.

49. Derichs N, et al. Intestinal current measurement for diagnostic classification of patients with questionable cystic fibrosis: Validation and reference data. *Thorax* 2010; **65**(7): 594–9.

50. Hug MJ, Tummler B. Intestinal current measurements to diagnose cystic fibrosis. *J Cyst Fibros* 2004; **3** (Suppl 2): 157–8.

51. Clancy JP, et al. multicenter intestinal current measurements in rectal biopsies from CF and non-CF subjects to monitor CFTR function. PLoS ONE 2013; **8**(9): e73905.

52. De Jonge HR, et al. Ex vivo CF diagnosis by intestinal current measurements (ICM) in small aperture, circulating Ussing chambers. *J Cyst Fibros* 2004; **3** (Suppl 2): 159–63.

53. Amaral MD, Kunzelmann K. Molecular targeting of CFTR as a therapeutic approach to cystic fibrosis. *Trends Pharmacol Sci* 2007; **28**(7): 334–41.

54. Sagel SD. Noninvasive biomarkers of airway inflammation in cystic fibrosis. *Curr Opin Pulm Med* 2003; **9**(6): 516–21.

55. Ordonez CL, et al. Inflammatory and microbiologic markers in induced sputum after intravenous antibiotics in cystic fibrosis. *Am J Respir Crit Care Med* 2003; **168**(12): 1471–5.

56. Armstrong DS. In celebration of expectoration: Induced sputum indices as outcome measures in cystic fibrosis. *Am J Respir Crit Care Med* 2003; **168**(12): 1412–3.

57. Suri R, et al. Safety and use of sputum induction in children with cystic fibrosis. *Pediatr Pulmonol* 2003; **35**(4): 309–13.

58. Pizzichini E, et al. Indices of airway inflammation in induced sputum: Reproducibility and validity of cell and fluid-phase measurements. *Am J Respir Crit Care Med* 1996; **154**(2 Pt 1): 308–17.

59. Spanevello A, et al. Induced sputum to assess airway inflammation: A study of reproducibility. *Clin Exp Allergy* 1997; **27**(10): 1138–44.

60. De Boeck K, Alifier M, Vandeputte S. Sputum induction in young cystic fibrosis patients. *Eur Respir J* 2000; **16**(1): 91–4.

61. Pin I, et al. Use of induced sputum cell counts to investigate airway inflammation in asthma. *Thorax* 1992; **47**(1): 25–9.

62. Vignola AM, et al. Standardised methodology of sputum induction and processing. Future directions. *Eur Respir J Suppl* 2002; **37**: 51s–5s.

63. Paggiaro PL. et al. Sputum induction. *Eur Respir J Suppl* 2002; **37**: 3s–8s.

64. Pavord ID, et al. The use of induced sputum to investigate airway inflammation. *Thorax* 1997; **52**(6): 498–501.

65. Popov TA, et al. Some technical factors influencing the induction of sputum for cell analysis. *Eur Respir J* 1995; **8**(4): 559–65.

66. Gershman NH, et al. Fractional analysis of sequential induced sputum samples during sputum induction: Evidence that different lung compartments are sampled at different time points. *J Allergy Clin Immunol* 1999; **104**(2 Pt 1): 322–8.

67. Wooten OJ, Dulfano MJ. Improved homogenization techniques for sputum cytology counts. *Ann Allergy* 1978; **41**(3): 150–4.

68. Woolhouse IS, Bayley DL, Stockley RA. Effect of sputum processing with dithiothreitol on the detection of inflammatory mediators in chronic bronchitis and bronchiectasis. *Thorax* 2002; **57**(8): 667–71.

69. Sagel SD, et al. Induced sputum inflammatory measures correlate with lung function in children with cystic fibrosis. *J Pediatr* 2002; **141**(6): 811–7.

70. Sagel SD, Kapsner RK, Osberg I. Induced sputum matrix metalloproteinase-9 correlates with lung function and airway inflammation in children with cystic fibrosis. *Pediatr Pulmonol* 2005; **39**(3): 224–32.

71. Blau H, et al. Induced sputum compared to bronchoalveolar lavage in young, non-expectorating cystic fibrosis children. *J Cyst Fibros* 2013; **13**: 106–10.

72. Horvath I, et al. Exhaled breath condensate: Methodological recommendations and unresolved questions. *Eur Respir J* 2005; **26**(3): 523–48.

73. Gessner C, et al. Factors influencing breath condensate volume. *Pneumologie* 2001; **55**(9): 414–9.

74. Effros RM, et al. Dilution of respiratory solutes in exhaled condensates. *Am J Respir Crit Care Med* 2002; **165**(5): 663–9.

75. Papineni RS, Rosenthal FS. The size distribution of droplets in the exhaled breath of healthy human subjects. *J Aerosol Med* 1997; **10**(2): 105–16.

76. Hunt J. Exhaled breath condensate: An evolving tool for noninvasive evaluation of lung disease. *J Allergy Clin Immunol* 2002; **110**(1): 28–34.

77. Bayley DL, et al. Validation of assays for inflammatory mediators in exhaled breath condensate. *Eur Respir J* 2008; **31**(5): 943–8.

78. Effros RM, et al. A simple method for estimating respiratory solute dilution in exhaled breath condensates. *Am J Respir Crit Care Med* 2003; **168**(12): 1500–5.

79. Montuschi P, et al. Exhaled 8-isoprostane as a new non-invasive biomarker of oxidative stress in cystic fibrosis. *Thorax* 2000; **55**(3): 205–9.

80. Carpagnano GE, et al. Increased leukotriene B4 and interleukin-6 in exhaled breath condensate in cystic fibrosis. *Am J Respir Crit Care Med* 2003; **167**(8): 1109–12.

81. Cunningham S, et al. Measurement of inflammatory markers in the breath condensate of children with cystic fibrosis. *Eur Respir J* 2000; **15**(5): 955–7.

82. Bodini A, et al. IL-8 and pH values in exhaled condensate after antibiotics in cystic fibrosis children. *Int J Immunopathol Pharmacol* 2007; **20**(3): 467–72.

83. Horak F Jr., et al. Longitudinal monitoring of pediatric cystic fibrosis lung disease using nitrite in exhaled breath condensate. *Pediatr Pulmonol* 2007; **42**(12): 1198–206.

84. Ho LP, et al. Expired hydrogen peroxide in breath condensate of cystic fibrosis patients. *Eur Respir J* 1999; **13**(1): 103–6.

85. Ho LP, Innes JA, Greening AP. Nitrite levels in breath condensate of patients with cystic fibrosis is elevated in contrast to exhaled nitric oxide. *Thorax* 1998; **53**(8): 680–4.

86. Tate S, et al. Airways in cystic fibrosis are acidified: Detection by exhaled breath condensate. *Thorax* 2002; **57**(11): 926–9.

87. Carpagnano GE, et al. Breath condensate pH in children with cystic fibrosis and asthma: A new non-invasive marker of airway inflammation? *Chest* 2004; **125**(6): 2005–10.

88. Horsley AR, et al. Changes in physiological, functional and structural markers of cystic fibrosis lung disease with treatment of a pulmonary exacerbation. *Thorax* 2013; **68**(6): 532–9.

89. Chen Y, et al. ATP release guides neutrophil chemotaxis via P2Y2 and A3 receptors. *Science* 2006; **314**(5806): 1792–5.

90. Esther CR Jr., et al. Exhaled breath condensate adenosine tracks lung function changes in cystic fibrosis. *Am J Physiol Lung Cell Mol Physiol* 2013; **304**(7): L504–9.

91. Wilson HK, Monster AC. New technologies in the use of exhaled breath analysis for biological monitoring. *Occup Environ Med* 1999; **56**(11): 753–7.

92. Ricciardolo FL, et al. Nitric oxide in health and disease of the respiratory system. *Physiol Rev* 2004; **84**(3): 731–65.

93. Grasemann H, et al. Decreased concentration of exhaled nitric oxide (NO) in patients with cystic fibrosis. *Pediatr Pulmonol* 1997; **24**(3): 173–7.

94. Linnane SJ, et al. Total sputum nitrate plus nitrite is raised during acute pulmonary infection in cystic fibrosis. *Am J Respir Crit Care Med* 1998; **158**(1): 207–12.

95. Grasemann H. et al. Decreased systemic bioavailability of L-arginine in patients with cystic fibrosis. *Respir Res* 2006; **7**: 87.

96. Jaffe A, et al. Exhaled nitric oxide increases following admission for intravenous antibiotics in children with cystic fibrosis. *J Cyst Fibros* 2003; **2**(3): 143–7.

97. Grasemann H, et al. Dornase alpha and exhaled NO in cystic fibrosis. *Pediatr Pulmonol* 2004; **38**(5): 379–85.

98. Grasemann H, Tullis E, Ratjen F. A randomized controlled trial of inhaled L-arginine in patients with cystic fibrosis. *J Cyst Fibros* 2013; **12**(5): 468–74.

99. Paredi P, et al. Exhaled ethane is elevated in cystic fibrosis and correlates with carbon monoxide levels and airway obstruction. *Am J Respir Crit Care Med* 2000; **161** (4 Pt 1): 1247–51.

100. Yamaya M, et al. Increased carbon monoxide in exhaled air of subjects with upper respiratory tract infections. *Am J Respir Crit Care Med* 1998; **158**(1): 311–4.

101. Antuni JD, et al. Increase in exhaled carbon monoxide during exacerbations of cystic fibrosis. *Thorax* 2000; **55**(2): 138–42.

102. Enderby B, et al. Hydrogen cyanide as a biomarker for Pseudomonas aeruginosa in the breath of children with cystic fibrosis. *Pediatr Pulmonol* 2009; **44**(2): 142–7.

103. Ryall B, et al. Pseudomonas aeruginosa, cyanide accumulation and lung function in CF and non-CF bronchiectasis patients. *Eur Respir J* 2008; **32**(3): 740–7.

104. Savelev SU, et al. Volatile biomarkers of Pseudomonas aeruginosa in cystic fibrosis and noncystic fibrosis bronchiectasis. *Lett Appl Microbiol* 2011; **52**(6): 610–3.

105. Cox CD, Parker J. Use of 2-aminoacetophenone production in identification of Pseudomonas aeruginosa. *J Clin Microbiol* 1979; **9**(4): 479–84.

106. Scott-Thomas AJ, et al. 2-Aminoacetophenone as a potential breath biomarker for Pseudomonas aeruginosa in the cystic fibrosis lung. *BMC Pulm Med* 2010; **10**: 56.

107. Syhre M, Scotter JM, Chambers ST. Investigation into the production of 2-Pentylfuran by Aspergillus fumigatus and other respiratory pathogens in vitro and human breath samples. *Med Mycol* 2008; **46**(3): 209–15.

38

Chest computed tomography and clinical trials in cystic fibrosis

HARM A.W.M. TIDDENS, MARCEL VAN STRATEN, ARLETTE ODINK, AND
STEPHEN M. STICK

INTRODUCTION

Progressive lung disease starts in most children with cystic fibrosis (CF) in infancy and progresses throughout life.[1,2] The most important components of CF lung disease are bronchiectasis, which is an irreversible widening of bronchi, and trapped air which reflects small airways disease.[3,4] Imaging techniques that can be used to monitor CF lung disease in clinical trials are chest radiography, computed tomography (CT), and magnetic resonance imaging. Of these modalities CT is currently the most sensitive and feasible modality to diagnose and monitor bronchiectasis and trapped air in clinical trials. CT has been recognized as the gold standard for the detection of bronchiectasis since the mid-90s.[5,6] Bronchiectasis as detected on inspiratory chest CT scans has been well validated as clinical outcome measure over the last decades.[7,10] In more recent years, it has become clear that trapped air is also an early and important feature of CF lung disease. Trapped air can be detected on expiratory CT scans.[11] Other structural findings that can be observed on chest CT in CF and that are of interest in clinical trials are airway wall thickness and mucus impaction.[12–14] It is now recognized that inclusion of chest CT-related outcome measures can be of importance in clinical trials as primary or secondary end point to determine the efficacy of an investigational drug treatment on progression of CF lung disease and or to characterize the patient population.[15] To use chest CT in clinical trials, safe low-dose well-standardized protocols and reproducible sensitive image analysis of the structural changes of interest are needed. The aim of this chapter is to describe the importance of chest CT-related outcome measures, how CTs can be used in clinical trials, and how images can be analyzed.

STRUCTURE AND FUNCTION

Spirometry-related outcome measures have been used in most therapeutic trials in CF to date as an indirect method to detect and monitor structural lung changes. However, thanks to major improvements in CF therapy, spirometry parameters have become less sensitive to evaluate the treatment effect of an investigational drug in clinical studies.[2,16,17] In addition, it has been recognized that spirometry is not very sensitive to detect early and localized structural lung abnormalities. Hence, a more sensitive technique is needed in clinical trials to measure the therapeutic effect of interventional drugs for CF lung disease. Chest CT as outcome measure for CF lung disease has important advantages over spirometry. First, it is substantially more sensitive compared to functional measurements to detect localized structural lung disease.[2,16,17] Second, chest CT is the current gold standard technique to detect and monitor the presence of bronchiectasis in which clinical significance as outcome measure has been well established.[5,6] Third, chest CT can be used throughout life starting in infancy into adulthood.[1,2] Methods to standardize chest CT from infancy into adulthood are well defined and are used for multicenter trials. This can be done since virtually all CF centers are equipped with modern multislice CT scanners.

More recently, the multiple-breath washout (MBW) test has been suggested as a functional screenings test to identify those patients with structural lung disease. However, to date, there are no longitudinal data comparing the sensitivity of the MBW and chest CT in monitoring CF lung disease. Depending on the questions of a clinical study the most appropriate spectrum of modalities should be selected to answer those questions.[18] Inclusion of chest CT-related outcome measures should be considered in intervention studies that aim to slow down or stop progression of structural abnormalities related to CF lung disease such as bronchiectasis and trapped air.

PHENOTYPING STRUCTURAL LUNG DISEASE

It has been shown recently that the spectrum of structural abnormalities can vary widely between patients. In end-stage lung disease on the one hand there are patients who have predominantly structural abnormalities associated with inflammation or infection and on the other hand there are patients who have predominantly trapped air.[4] It is most likely that the response for individual patient to various treatments will be dependent on the spectrum of abnormalities in the lungs of that individual. For chronic obstructive pulmonary disease, it has been advocated that phenotyping of a patient at baseline using chest CT is helpful to improve our understanding and to predict the course of disease for individual patients.[19] Similarly, for understanding the individual response to treatments for CF lung disease such as mucolytics phenotyping structural lung abnormalities using chest CT at baseline could be very beneficial, although definitive data are currently lacking.

INSPIRATORY AND EXPIRATORY CT

For most treatments that target CF lung disease, acquisition of both inspiratory and expiratory chest CTs will be relevant (Figure 38.1). An inspiratory CT scan is needed for the detection of bronchiectasis. To diagnose bronchiectasis, the diameter of the airway is compared to the diameter of the adjacent or nearby pulmonary artery. When the bronchoarterial ratio exceeds one bronchiectasis or at least abnormal airway, dilatation may be diagnosed. However, it has been suggested that for younger children a lower ratio should be used.[20] This needs to be further investigated including standardizing for lung volume.[19] In addition to an abnormal diameter, the airway wall of a bronchiectatic airway is thickened and irregular (Figure 38.1). Furthermore, there may be a lack of the normal tapering of the airway diameter with each successive generation. It has been shown that the airway artery ratio is dependent on the inspiration level. Current consensus is that the diagnosis of bronchiectasis can best be made on an inspiratory CT near total lung capacity (TLC). At lower lung volumes, the diameter of the airway is reduced more relative to that of the adjacent artery.[21] Hence, at lower lung volumes, the bronchoarterial ratio can be below 1 even for a bronchiectatic airway. In addition, at low lung volumes the length of airways is reduced as well, making identification of abnormal widened airways cut in cross-section more

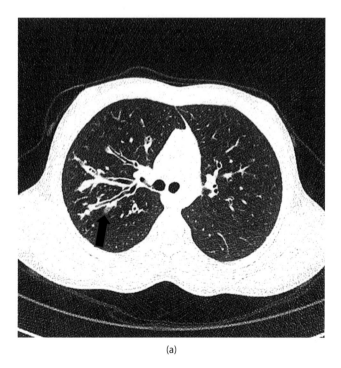

(a)

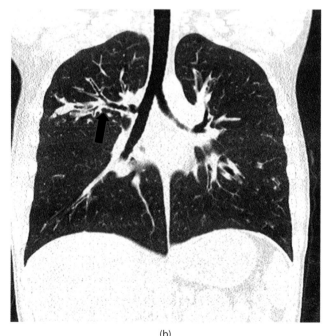

(b)

Figure 38.1 In this axial (see arrow) and coronal slice, severe bronchiectasis in the right upper lobe is present. The different characteristics of bronchiectasis can be observed. First, the airways in this lobe show considerable widening. Second, the airway wall is irregular. Third, there is lack of tapering. The latter means that despite branching of the airway, the diameter remains more or less the same over various generations. Hence, change in cross-sectional area is more severe in the more peripheral airways relative to the more central airways.

53. Stick SM, Brennan S, Murray C, Douglas T, von Ungern-Sternberg BS, Garratt LW, et al. Bronchiectasis in infants and preschool children diagnosed with cystic fibrosis after newborn screening. *J Pediatr* 2009; 155: 623–8.

54. Nasr SZ, Sakmar E, Christodoulou E, Eckhardt BP, Streetman DS, Strouse PJ. The use of high resolution computerized tomography (HRCT) of the chest in evaluating the effect of tobramycin solution for inhalation in cystic fibrosis lung disease. *Pediatr Pulmonol* 2010; **45**(5): 440–9.

55. Moss RB, Rodman D, Spencer LT, Aitken ML, Zeitlin PL, Waltz D, et al. Repeated adeno-associated virus serotype 2 aerosol-mediated cystic fibrosis transmembrane regulator gene transfer to the lungs of patients with cystic fibrosis: A multicenter, double-blind, placebo-controlled trial. *Chest* 2004; **125**(2): 509–21.

56. Niimi A, Matsumoto H, Amitani R, Nakano Y, Sakai H, Takemura M, et al. Effect of short-term treatment with inhaled corticosteroid on airway wall thickening in asthma. *Am J Med* 2004; **116**(11): 725–31.

39

Outcomes of clinical trials: Multiple breath washout tests in cystic fibrosis

PADMAJA SUBBARAO AND FELIX RATJEN

INTRODUCTION

Sensitive measures of lung function are important for the assessment of chronic diseases such as cystic fibrosis (CF). In CF, lung disease is known to be present in early childhood, and, if left untreated, leads to a progressive spiral of infection and inflammation, resulting in lung damage and ultimately pulmonary insufficiency. Spirometry derived parameters, such as the forced expiratory volume in 1 second (FEV_1), are used extensively in the assessment and follow-up of CF patients. Not only are they used to classify severity of disease but also to predict outcomes as FEV_1 has been linked to mortality. However, it is common for children with CF to maintain FEV_1 within the normal range well into the second decade of their lives.[1] This is despite evidence of progression of lung disease when assessed by other techniques such as high-resolution computed tomography (CT) scans.[2,3] With the advent of newborn screening and the recognition that CF lung disease begins in early life, there has been increased attention on developing noninvasive methods to detect these early abnormalities. These new objective assessment methods are critical to perform interventional trials in early childhood. Sensitive noninvasive tests of lung function replacing spirometry are, therefore, needed both for the clinical setting and research studies.

Multiple-breath washout (MBW) is one such methodology that holds promise as a pulmonary function test that would fit this need. An old technology that has been revisited in recent years, MBW measures the efficiency with which the lungs perform their ventilatory function especially in the distal airways. Multiple parameters can be calculated from MBW tests, one that has been extensively studied is the lung clearance index (LCI). Not only is the measurement of LCI feasible in all age groups, from infants to adulthood, it becomes abnormal much earlier than

FEV_1 detecting early airway disease in CF.[4] Furthermore, abnormalities in LCI persist from preschool to school-age years preceding the appearance of abnormalities in FEV_1,[5] suggesting that LCI is not an epiphenomenon but an early marker of lung dysfunction and may be an alternative to track early lung disease in CF (reviewed in detail in Chapter 32). Currently, most of the studies have been performed using a customized respiratory mass spectrometer which limits its use to a few specialized centers. Within the last decade, advances in technology and interest have led to the introduction of commercially available systems to perform MBW tests. This has led to a number of studies applying this technology in CF lung disease. To fully understand the role MBW tests play in the armamentarium of lung function tests, a basic understanding of the test is important. Although this will be covered in this chapter, advanced knowledge of the available commercial options and requirements for an adequate test is addressed in recently published standards and guidelines papers.[6,7]

MULTIPLE-BREATH WASHOUT

MBW and single-breath washout are two commonly used gas washout techniques. First introduced for the measurement of lung volumes with helium (He) dilution, gas washout technology is reputed to be first described by Sir Humphrey Davy's book *Researches Chemical and Philosophical* published in 1799. Advances in the middle of the last century (1949) through the introduction of fast-response gas analyzers such as respiratory mass spectrometers have allowed the measurement of many inert tracer gases including nitrogen (N_2) to measure lung volumes. Using this technology in 1952, Fowler[8] described a method to measure N_2 clearance curves of single breaths in healthy subjects and those with cardiorespiratory disease to quantify the "unevenness of gas distribution." MBW methods were further refined with the development of faster computers to integrate gas and volume signals in the late 1980s allowing the measurement of ventilation distribution and gas clearance curves during tidal breaths. One major advantage of MBW over the single-breath technique is that it can be completed during tidal breathing requiring only passive cooperation, thus permitting measurements in young patients. The two most common parameters described from MBW tests include LCI and moment ratios (MRs). MBW in its current form can be performed using a variety of tracer gases and methodologies. The main requirements for a tracer gas are: it needs to be inert, that is, it is not involved in gas exchange; it is measurable at respirable concentrations; and it is safe for inhalation. The most commonly used tracer gases are: (1) external inert gases, sulfur hexafluoride (SF$_6$), and He and (2) native inert gases, N$_2$. Tracer gases can be measured with the use of respiratory mass spectrometers, infrared analyzers, and ultrafast sensors. Washout systems determine inspired and expired tracer gas volumes by continuously measuring gas concentration synchronized with respiratory flow

measurements. Flow is measured by pneumotachographs or alternative flow meters (including ultrasonic flow meters, mass flow sensors, and turbines). It is critically important that the flow signal and gas concentration signal is meticulously synchronized to calculate the necessary parameters. The standards paper should be referred to for equipment specifications and limitations.[6]

MBW WITH EXTERNAL INERT TRACER GASES (SF$_6$, HE)

Figure 39.1 describes the procedure using external (nonresident) inert gases. During the wash-in phase of an inert gas washout test, the subject inhales a gas mixture containing the gas of interest, i.e., SF$_6$. This is continued until gas concentration is stable in the lungs and the subject's exhaled gas concentration has equilibrated with the gas concentration of the supplied inert gas. At this point, the gas supply is removed during exhalation and the washout phase is begun. During the washout, the remaining tracer gas in the lung is exhaled until it reaches 1/40th of the initial tracer gas concentration (Figure 39.2). The flow

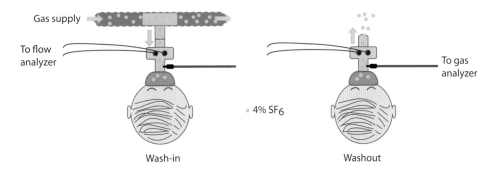

Figure 39.1 Arrows denote the flow of gases during testing phase. During washout the bias flow is removed and the tracer gas is exhaled.

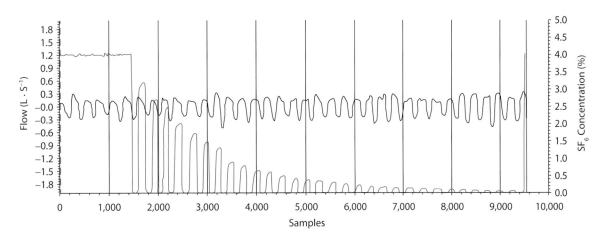

Figure 39.2 Typical tracing for multiple-breath washout for a 4-year-old boy. The green tracing represents the falling sulfur hexafluoride (SF$_6$) concentrations (as measured by a respiratory mass spectrometer) with each tidal breath and shows the monitoring is stopped when the concentration has fallen below 1/40th or 0.1% of the initial starting concentration (4%). The black tracing represents the flow signal from an integrated pneumotachograph.

measured by pneumotachograph is integrated and aligned with the gas signal for each washout maneuver. In healthy subjects, each MBW trial takes approximately 5–7 minutes to complete. Pediatric trials are currently performed in triplicate and at least two technically acceptable trials should be attained.

Combinations of external gases can be used with respiratory mass spectrometers since different densities of gases offer some insights into physiological assessments of the location of pathology. The two most commonly used gases are SF_6 and He. One advantage of SF_6 is that it is a heavy gas and thus does not leak easily compared to lighter gases such as He, where leaks from the mouthpiece or face mask are more common. Another main advantage of SF_6 is that since it is not present in appreciable quantities in ambient air, washout can be achieved simply by removing the gas source. In addition, it does not influence respiratory patterns so can easily be used in all age groups. The main disadvantages to the use of SF_6 are that it is costly, cumbersome (reliant on tanks), and a potent "greenhouse" gas, thus limiting its availability and practicality of use. He as a lighter gas is prone to leaking and thus is technically more challenging to use.

MBW WITH RESIDENT TRACER GASES

Early MBW testing used N_2 as the resident gas and a respiratory mass spectrometer as the gas analyzer. This is currently revisited as an alternative to using external tracer gases. Because N_2 is present and stable in the atmosphere and the lung at 80% fractional concentraion, the use of N_2 as a tracer gas obviates the need for a wash-in period. Thus, during an N_2 washout test, subjects simply establish a stable tidal breathing rate and then inhale 100% oxygen during tidal breathing. Over a series of tidal breaths, the resident N_2 gas is "washed out." Once the gas concentration reached 1/40th of the initial tracer gas concentration (e.g., 2% N_2), the test is stopped.

However, one potential disadvantage to the use of N_2 which led to the shift to using other external inert tracer gases is that 100% oxygen during washout can change the respiratory pattern in some individuals, particularly in infants. Second, small amounts of N_2 dissolve within the tissue of the lung and may contribute to the fractional exhaled concentration of exhaled N_2 during prolonged washouts necessitating the development of accurate correction factors. The main advantages to using N_2 are that it precludes the need for a wash-in thus potentially shortening the testing procedure, the use of oxygen is cheaper, and more readily available (medical oxygen from wall in hospital-based settings). Currently available commercial devices can be sought using either inert tracer gases or N_2 and the physiological principles of measurement are not vastly different.

During the washout test, two major categories of parameters can be calculated to describe the ventilation inhomogeneity of the lung. The first category gives an estimate of the overall ventilation homogeneity in the whole lung. The two most commonly reported parameters from this category are LCI and MR.

The other major category of parameters can be calculated when individual breaths in the washout are examined (Figure 39.3).

This tracing can be constructed for each breath during the washout test. Normalized phase III slope (SnIII) for each breath, achieved by compensating for the inert gas dilution, allows for the comparison of multiple phase III slopes during the washout. SnIII calculation is performed by dividing the phase III slope by the expired tracer gas concentration. The SnIII slopes are plotted against its corresponding breath number or turnover (TO) value. The SnIII represents ventilation inhomogeneity throughout the MBW and is mainly due to two mechanisms: convection-dependent inhomogeneity (CDI) and diffusion–convection-dependent inhomogeneity (DCDI).[9] Verbanck et al.[10] introduced the indices S_{cond} and S_{acin} to represent the CDI and DCDI components of ventilation inhomogeneity, respectively. S_{cond} is defined as the calculated SnIII increase between 1.5 and 6 TOs, whereas S_{acin} is calculated by subtracting the estimated CDI contribution to the first-breath SnIII. These parameters are based

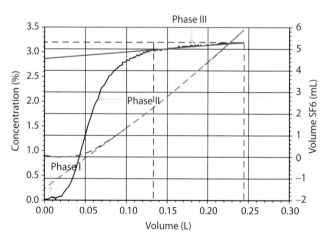

Figure 39.3 This figure shows a tracing of an individual breath from a 4-year-old boy. The black tracing is the SF_6 concentration during the first breath from a washout test. The phases of the breath are thus delineated. Phase I where the concentration of SF_6 is almost zero represents the absolute dead space of the respiratory tract. Phase II represents the bronchiolar phase. Phase III represents the alveolar phase.

26. Singer F, Kieninger E, Abbas C, Yammine S, Fuchs O, Proietti E, Regamey N, Casaulta C, Frey U, Latzin P. Practicability of nitrogen multiple-breath washout measurements in a pediatric cystic fibrosis outpatient setting. *Pediatr Pulmonol* 2012.

27. Robinson PD, Stocks J, Aurora P, Lum S. Abbreviated multi-breath washout for calculation of lung clearance index. *Pediatr Pulmonol* 2013; **48**: 336–43.

28. Yammine S, Singer F, Abbas C, Roos M, Latzin P. Multiple-breath washout measurements can be significantly shortened in children. *Thorax* 2013; **68**: 586–7.

29. Singer F, Houltz B, Latzin P, Robinson P, Gustafsson P. A realistic validation study of a new nitrogen multiple-breath washout system. *PLoS ONE* 2012; **7**: e36083.

30. Jensen R, Stanojevic S, Gibney K, Salazar JG, Gustafsson P, Subbarao P, Ratjen F. Multiple breath nitrogen washout: A feasible alternative to mass spectrometry. *PLoS ONE* 2013; **8**: e56868.

40

What have we learned over the last 5 years?

J. STUART ELBORN, JANE C. DAVIES, AND DIANA BILTON

Within the last 5 years, over 130 clinical trials have been published, ranging from interventions targeting the basic defect in cystic fibrosis transmembrane conductance regulator (CFTR) through osmotic treatments and mucolytics, novel anti-infectives, anti-inflammatories, and airway clearance techniques. Alongside these trials, there have been numerous more publications describing the development and validation of biomarkers and outcome measures. The CF Foundation (CFF) drug development pipeline (http://www.cff.org/research/drugdevelopmentpipeline/) currently has 12 agents listed as in development on its website and the newer European Cystic Fibrosis Society (ECFS) Clinical Trials Network (CTN) (https://www.ecfs.eu/ctn/clinical-trials), eight agents, or combinations. The scope and quality of this activity in a disease affecting only around 100,000 people worldwide is testament to the drive, determination, and tenacity of the clinicians, scientists, allied professionals, and pharma companies seeking to alleviate symptoms, improve quality of life, and extend survival for cystic fibrosis (CF) patients, and of course, to the willingness of the CF community to engage in research and volunteer for trials, many of which are unlikely to provide any direct benefit to themselves. So what have we learned from these trials about outcome measures? We consider there are a number of key themes.

BIOMARKERS OF CFTR FUNCTION PROVIDE USEFUL PROOF OF MECHANISM BUT MAY NOT CORRELATE WITH CLINICAL OUTCOMES

The advent of the first effective CF treatment directed at the basic defect is regarded as heralding a new era for CF research, proving the principle that CFTR is a drugable target. Trials of ivacaftor have also provided us with a unique opportunity to learn more about biomarkers of CFTR function and how they correlate with clinical outcomes.[1–3] Postregistration observational studies such as the G551D

Observational Study (GOAL; NCT01521338) will hopefully provide further insight in due course.

As discussed earlier in this chapter, the major CFTR biomarkers include sweat chloride concentration, airway potential difference measurements, and short circuit current measurements on intestinal epithelium most commonly obtained by rectal biopsy. The latter has not, to date, been used as a clinical trial outcome measure but the first two of these were used in the phase 2 trials of ivacaftor and sweat chloride also in both of the pivotal phase 3 studies. The following appear clear:

1. The degree of correction of biomarkers of CFTR function may be *organ specific*. Phase 2 trials of ivacaftor[1] reported large changes in sweat Cl^- (which have since been recapitulated in phase 3 trials)[2,3] but smaller and less consistent changes in nasal epithelial chloride secretion; changes in basal PD or amiloride response, reflecting sodium hyperabsorption, were even less consistent. Conversely, the class I targeted oral compound, ataluren, reported significant changes in nPD in phase 2 trials, but the compound did not lead to changes in sweat chloride.[4]

2. Correction of biomarkers may *correlate poorly or not at all with clinically relevant outcomes*. While within groups in the large phase 3 trials, ivacaftor led to impressive changes in clinical outcomes (lung function, exacerbation rate, weight, and quality of life), and those patients demonstrating the greatest clinical improvements were not those with the highest degree of apparent CFTR correction based on sweat, and vice versa.[2,3] More recently, combination trials of correctors with ivacaftor in patients with the *Phe508del* mutation (NCT01225211) have reported very small changes in sweat Cl^- in the presence of what appear to be statistically and clinically significant improvements in forced expiratory volume in 1 second (FEV_1). We still cannot answer the question therefore "how much CFTR correction is sufficient for clinical benefit?"

3. The third issue is the importance of *standardization* in generating good quality outcome data in the context of large trials with multiple sites. This is particularly true for complex and difficult interventions such as nPD; a lack of standardized protocols/training has been proposed as potentially leading to a negative outcome in at least one clinical trial.[5] In recognition of this, the ECFS and the CFF have been active in designing and publishing standard operating procedures (SOPs) and protocols.

4. It may also be important to tailor inclusion criteria on the basis of *preintervention measures*; the trial of the drug, miglustat, reported that a high proportion of participants displayed chloride secretion both prior to dosing and in the placebo arm on nPD.[6] Theoretically, documenting improvements in the presence of residual endogenous chloride secreting capacity could be challenging and this should be considered.

OUTCOME MEASURES NEED TO BE TAILORED TO THE POPULATION BEING STUDIED

It is becoming more and more apparent that "one size does not fit all" when it comes to trial outcome measures. Whereas this was always clear for the different types of interventions being studied, it was perhaps less well appreciated in the context of the "patient group." Examples of this are highlighted in the sections above, but the concept is well exemplified with tests of airway physiology. Standard spirometry, in particular FEV_1, is still the only outcome of CF clinical trials accepted by regulators and is the basis on which most of the currently prescribable treatments were approved. However, its potential as a trial outcome measure is likely greatest in a population with existing lung disease and decreased lung function and/or for therapeutic agents capable of leading to large improvements. Spirometry has significant limitations including (1) being difficult for preschool children and impossible for babies outside a small number of research laboratories with techniques reliant on sedation; (2) insensitivity in early disease; (3) declining so slowly in current populations receiving center care that powering for a *change in rate of decline* is virtually impossible; (4) statistically significant but small changes may turn out to be clinically unimportant or inconsistent, such as was seen in the denufosol program[7,8]; (5) there is a lack of consistency worldwide in the application of reference ranges, the majority of which are not applicable for the lifetime of a growing patient. The excellent initiative of the Global Lungs group seeks to address this significant issue (http://www.lungfunction.org/).

In this context, the increasing focus on alternative techniques, in particular the lung clearance index, is extremely welcome. The data discussed earlier in this chapter confirm its superior sensitivity at early stages of lung disease, suggest that it may possess enhanced sensitivity as an outcome measure in this group, and provide encouragement that it is being more widely considered in a clinical trial context. However, it is unlikely to be so useful in later stages of disease, when mucus shifts can decrease repeatability and *completely* obstructed airways will go undetected. As for other new or complex techniques, standardization will be key; many different techniques are available, the results of which are clearly not interchangeable.[9] The ECFS is establishing an SOP within its trial centers, with centralized collection of data which should make a significant contribution. However, for outcome measures to be most useful, they need also to be accepted as valid by regulatory agencies. There does appear to be a willingness to learn more about alternatives as illustrated by the European Medicines Agency workshop on CF Trial Outcome Measures in the latter half of 2012, which is extremely encouraging (http://www.ema.europa.eu/docs/en_GB/document_library/Report/2012/12/WC500136159.pdf).

THE IMPORTANCE OF EXACERBATIONS IS BEING INCREASINGLY RECOGNIZED; HOW USEFUL ARE THEY AS TRIAL OUTCOME MEASURES?

Pulmonary exacerbations (PEx) are far from benign, and their frequency being positively correlated with longer-term rate of decline and up to 25% of patients failing to regain baseline lung function. Given their relevance, it is unsurprising that CF investigators have considered using these events as outcomes in clinical trials. Inherent in such use, however, is an assumption that there is a standard, validated, and widely agreed definition. Multiple definitions and scoring systems have been proposed, but problems still exist: often treatment is initiated (by either clinician or patient) before sufficient symptoms/signs have accrued to fulfill a protocol-defined PEx; definitions may need to be tailored to different ages or disease severity stages; there is still a degree of subjectivity involved; finally, should we best assess *number* of PEx over a fixed period, *severity* of the event (and if so, on what do we base this, treatment required? Regaining of lung function? Time to do so?), or *time to next* PEx (likely linked to overall number). Despite these limitations a significant impact on PEx has been reported in a small number of recent trials. In certain of these, the change in PEx mirrors other significant improvements,[2] but there have been other instances where the inclusion of PEx has added substantial value to the interpretation of the results: this is perhaps most clearly demonstrated by a recent Canadian study comparing two types of physiotherapy techniques (positive expiratory pressure versus high-frequency chest wall oscillation—the "vest")[10] in which there were no differences in lung function or quality of life scores, but the PEP group had significantly fewer PExs and a shorter "time to next event." Had it not been for the inclusion of this outcome measure the two techniques would likely have been considered equivalent, with important ramifications.

IMAGING TECHNIQUES ARE MAKING PROGRESS, BUT STILL HAVE LIMITATIONS

The section on computed tomography (CT) above highlights the increasing interest in using this methodology as a trial outcome measure, particularly in childhood. There is evidence that structural changes may be observed early in life, although groups do not completely concur on the timing and severity of these changes.[11] Despite improvements in technology, valid concerns over radiation dose remain, and these are particularly acute in the young population for whom the technique may hold the most promise; the issue is compounded in the context of therapies targeting the basic defect, which may possess genuine transforative potential and therefore extend life expectancy. Pre- and poststudies using CT may enable us to understand which components of lung disease are reversible, for example, airway wall thickening, and facilitate targeted, lower radiation, limited scans. Novel, radiation-free, techniques such as hyperpolarized gas magnetic resonance imaging scanning is currently available in only a small number of centers worldwide, but may, in time, become a valid alternative and provide information on function in addition to structure.[12]

SPUTUM AND BREATH INFLAMMATORY MARKERS: NOT YET READY FOR PRIME TIME?

Multiple small studies have looked at inflammatory markers in sputum, exhaled breath condensate, and breath, and many of them reporting clear differences between CF and non-CF populations and some showing correlations with other clinically meaningful measures. Relatively few have used them as trial outcome measures and even fewer in large multicenter trials. They, therefore, have yet to earn their place in the armamentarium of valid trial outcome measures in our opinion. Sputum is limited by a high degree of variability reflecting both true geographical differences and methodological inconsistencies.

PRODUCTS STILL FAIL IN LATE-STAGE TRIALS

The current level of clinical trial activity in CF is extremely encouraging, with multiple approaches progressing through the pipeline. However, recent successes have raised expectations, particularly among the patients and their families, so it is important that these are managed appropriately. Even those drugs which have shown significant promise at early phase may still fail later either because of side effects (the leukotriene antagonist, BIIL284, NCT00060801) or lack of efficacy (adeno-associated virus-mediated *CFTR* gene therapy,[13] denufosol[8]). One should be cautious of confusing *statistical* significance with *clinical* significance, when it comes to small changes in outcomes. The current approaches of both the CFF and ECFS to spread the net wide and not focus purely on one area is one of the ways that the risks of failure can be mitigated.

SIGNIFICANT PROGRESS CAN BE MADE: MODELS OF COLLABORATION

For a relatively small population disease, the rate of progress and degree of organization of our national and international trial networks are held up globally as examples of successful collaboration. From all stages through from design, protocol review, approvals, and trial implementation, pace can be improved by such widespread collaborations. Investigators have increasingly been involved in outcome measure choice and optimization, even for large pharma-led trials and this is to be encouraged and improved further. The ECFS CTN Standardization Committee seeks to develop SOPs for outcome measures used both in the clinical and trial context and increasingly is working with the CFF Therapeutics Development Network to share protocols and expertise.

ACCEPTANCE OF RESEARCH BY THE CF COMMUNITY IS HIGH, BUT NUMBERS PARTICIPATING COULD BE IMPROVED FURTHER

Patients and families have long been considered both accepting and altruistic in their willingness to participate in research, even when it is unlikely to help them personally, either because of disease stage or enrollment into a placebo arm. With regard to the latter, the inclusion of an open-label extension phase, a feature of several recent phase 3 studies, is extremely helpful, affording patients an opportunity to experience clinical benefit no matter to which arm they are initially randomized. However, there may still be a degree of reluctance on the part of clinical teams to "burden" patients with requests to participate in research.[14] This is often quite counter to the opinions of the patients themselves, who are more likely to consider such discussions "opportunities" and to wish to at least be fully informed. A shift in the mindset of CF multidisciplinary team members is needed, not just in the large centers where research and drug trials are much more commonplace but also in the smaller or shared care centers. TORPEDO, a trial comparing methods of pseudomonas eradication, has successfully opened almost 70 sites within the United Kingdom, including many which were relatively research-naive (http://www.torpedo-cf.org.uk/). Clearly, such an approach requires resources and training, but much of the skills accrued are generic and can be applied to future trials. For trials to be conducted successfully and to high standards, resources need to be made available in terms of manpower, funding, regulatory expertise, which unfortunately in today's climate, are often lacking or suboptimal. Currently, it is estimated that a minority of the CF community in developed countries and receiving center-based care is involved in research of some sort. This contrasts with the majority of UK patients with hematological malignancies in the United Kingdom, largely thanks to huge collaborative networks, but also an expectation that every patient will be offered the opportunity to participate and move the field forward.

TRIALS ARE NEEDED FOR NOVEL THERAPIES IN VERY YOUNG CHILDREN AND INFANTS

Parents of very young children are largely willing to agree to research, even, as has been recently reported, if it involves invasive tests such as bronchoscopy or a radiation burden with CT.[15] Even the clinically available CF drugs have a poor evidence base (or none at all) in this age group, but trials are considered complex and treatments are largely extrapolated down from older patients. This evidence gap needs urgently to be addressed if we are to provide these young patients with the best possible treatments. Early studies confirm that pathology begins early in life, and there may be a window of opportunity for intervention before changes become irreversible. Nowhere is this perhaps more pertinent than in the field of CFTR-modulating agents. In the phase 3 pediatric trial of ivacaftor, children aged 6–11 years, who had a mean FEV_1 of 84% at baseline,[3] manifested the same magnitude of improvement as did the older patients, who entered the trials with lung function in the mid-60s.[2] The approximate 10% absolute improvement led the younger children to have FEV_1 within the range considered "normal," whereas there was still the older group were still substantially less than this. Is this possibly evidence of more "reversible" disease in this age group, the drugs treating airway surface mucus more easily than later effects such as remodeling, fibrosis, and bronchiectasis? Clearly any new drugs need a rigorous safety assessment, and long-term safety data are unlikely to come from trials, rather from postmarketing surveillance or phase 4 studies, but the complexity of designing trials in this young age group should not act as a deterrent.

To conclude, the design of clinical trials and choice of outcomes is evolving as we learn more about biomarkers and measures of true relevance, making clear the distinction between statistical and clinical significance of any changes observed. We are at an exciting stage in the development of new treatments for CF, and need to take all available opportunities to further refine and optimize such measures. The willingness of the CF clinical, research, and patient communities to work together collaboratively and learn from each other is held as an exemplar by other disease groups and is a resource to be valued and built upon in future years.

REFERENCES

1. Accurso FJ, Rowe SM, Clancy JP, Boyle MP, Dunitz JM, Durie PR, Sagel SD, Hornick DB, Konstan MW, Donaldson SH, Moss RB, Pilewski JM, Rubenstein RC, Uluer AZ, Aitken ML, Freedman SD, Rose LM, Mayer-Hamblett N, Dong Q, Zha J, Stone AJ, Olson ER, Ordoñez CL, Campbell PW, Ashlock MA, Ramsey BW. Effect of VX-770 in persons with cystic fibrosis and the G551D-CFTR mutation. N Engl J Med 2010; 363(21): 1991–2003.
2. Ramsey BW, Davies J, McElvaney NG, Tullis E, Bell SC, Dřevínek P, Griese M, McKone EF, Wainwright CE, Konstan MW, Moss R, Ratjen F, Sermet-Gaudelus I, Rowe SM, Dong Q, Rodriguez S, Yen K, Ordoñez C, Elborn JS; VX08-770-102 Study Group. A CFTR potentiator in patients with cystic fibrosis and the G551D mutation. N Engl J Med 2011; 365(18): 1663–72.
3. Davies JC, Wainwright CE, Canny GJ, Chilvers MA, Howenstine MS, Munck A, Mainz JG, Rodriguez S, Li H, Yen K, Ordoñez CL, Ahrens R; VX08-770-103 (ENVISION) Study Group. Efficacy and safety of ivacaftor in patients aged 6 to 11 years with cystic fibrosis with a G551D mutation. Am J Respir Crit Care Med 2013; 187(11): 1219–25.
4. Kerem E, Hirawat S, Armoni S, Yaakov Y, Shoseyov D, Cohen M, Nissim-Rafinia M, Blau H, Rivlin J, Aviram M, Elfring GL, Northcutt VJ, Miller LL, Kerem B, Wilschanski M. Effectiveness of PTC124 treatment of cystic fibrosis caused by nonsense mutations: A prospective phase II trial. Lancet 2008; 372(9640): 719–27.
5. McCarty NA, Standaert TA, Teresi M, Tuthill C, Launspach J, Kelley TJ, Milgram LJ, Hilliard KA, Regelmann WE, Weatherly MR, Aitken ML, Konstan MW, Ahrens RC. A phase I randomized, multicenter trial of CPX in adult subjects with mild cystic fibrosis. Pediatr Pulmonol 2002; 33(2): 90–8.
6. Leonard A, Lebecque P, Dingemanse J, Leal T. A randomized placebo-controlled trial of miglustat in cystic fibrosis based on nasal potential difference. J Cyst Fibros 2012; 11(3): 231–6.
7. Deterding RR, Lavange LM, Engels JM, Mathews DW, Coquillette SJ, Brody AS, Millard SP, Ramsey BW; Cystic Fibrosis Therapeutics Development Network and the Inspire 08-103 Working Group. Phase 2 randomized safety and efficacy trial of nebulized

denufosol tetrasodium in cystic fibrosis. *Am J Respir Crit Care Med* 2007; **176**(4): 362–9.

8. Ratjen F, Durham T, Navratil T, Schaberg A, Accurso FJ, Wainwright C, Barnes M, Moss RB; TIGER-2 Study Investigator Group. Long term effects of denufosol tetrasodium in patients with cystic fibrosis. *J Cyst Fibros* 2012; **11**(6): 539–49.

9. Kent L, Reix P, Innes A et al. Lung clearance index: Evidence for use in clinical trials in cystic fibrosis. *J Cyst Fibros* 2014; **13**: 123–38.

10. McIlwaine MP, Alarie N, Davidson GF, Lands LC, Ratjen F, Milner R, Owen B, Agnew JL. Long-term multicentre randomised controlled study of high frequency chest wall oscillation versus positive expiratory pressure mask in cystic fibrosis. *Thorax* 2013; **68**: 746–51.

11. Thia LP, Calder A, Stocks J, Bush A, Owens CM, Wallis C, Young C, Sullivan Y, Wade A, McEwan A, Brody AS; on behalf of the London Cystic Fibrosis Collaboration (LCFC). Is chest CT useful in newborn screened infants with cystic fibrosis at 1 year of age? *Thorax* 2014; **69**: 320–7.

12. Kirby M, Coxson HO, Parraga G. Pulmonary functional magnetic resonance imaging for paediatric lung disease. *Pediatr Respir Rev* 2013; **14**(3): 180–9.

13. Moss RB, Milla C, Colombo J, Accurso F, Zeitlin PL, Clancy JP, Spencer LT, Pilewski J, Waltz DA, Dorkin HL, Ferkol T, Pian M, Ramsey B, Carter BJ, Martin DB, Heald AE. Repeated aerosolized AAV-CFTR for treatment of cystic fibrosis: A randomized placebo-controlled phase 2B trial. *Hum Genet Ther* 2007; **18**(8): 726–32.

14. Shilling V, Williamson PR, Hickey H, Sowden E, Beresford MW, Smyth RL, Young B. Communication about children's clinical trials as observed and experienced: Qualitative study of parents and practitioners. *PLoS ONE* 2011; **6**(7): e21604.

15. Nguyen TT, Thia LP, Hoo AF, Bush A, Aurora P, Wade A, Chudleigh J, Lum S, Stocks J; on behalf of the London Cystic Fibrosis Collaboration (LCFC). Evolution of lung function during the first year of life in newborn screened cystic fibrosis infants. *Thorax* 2014; **69**: 910–7.

PART 6

Multidisciplinary care

41

Cystic fibrosis center care

SUSAN MADGE, JACKIE FRANCIS, AND DIANA BILTON

WHAT IS CF CENTER CARE?

Cystic fibrosis (CF) is a multisystem disease, which requires a holistic approach to care by a multidisciplinary team (MDT) of CF specialist health professionals.[1] The aim of CF care is to

- Prevent chronic infection
- Minimize deterioration
- Maintain independence
- Optimize quality of life
- Maximize life expectancy

The importance of specialist CF center care cannot be overemphasized and has been recognized by a number of professional organizations.[2,3] Additionally, the Cystic Fibrosis Foundation (United States) and the European Cystic Fibrosis Society also strongly endorse the principle and importance of specialist CF center care.

To ensure an optimum and comprehensive package of care, all patients must be under the direct supervision of an adequately resourced designated specialist CF center, sometimes in partnership with a network CF clinic.[4–7] The level of expertise required to treat the complex multisystem symptoms and complications can only be attained by an MDT of trained, experienced, specialist health professionals who routinely see a critical mass of patients at a specialist CF center.

Recent standards of care for CF recommend that a specialist CF center treats a minimum of either 100 adults or children.[1] It is recognized that in exceptional circumstances, the geographical location of a specialist CF center may mean that the number of patients is less than 100 although it should not be less than 50; this, however, may not be possible in areas of low populations with large distances to cover. This recommendation relates to the need for each professional in the team to maintain and develop expertise in this highly complex condition.

Patients and parents should be aware of the options for treatment that are available to them. Children with CF may be offered the option of networked care where the specialist CF center supervises CF care at a more local hospital, although parents should be aware of their options and be able to choose full care from a specialist CF center if they wish. It is necessary to balance the need for specialist care with the problems of a young child being admitted to a hospital some distance away on a regular basis. Thus, a local hospital can effectively deliver certain aspects of care under direction of the specialist team.

With the increasing complexity of CF in adulthood, full care delivered by a specialist CF center should be routine although this does not mean that patients always need to be seen in the center clinic. The challenge of remote populations in Australia has spurred the development of telemedicine with the MDT carrying out a virtual clinic online. As survival increases and young adults remain well and in full-time work, we recognize the need to provide more responsive and innovative center care, which may mean exploring newer, smarter technological advances allowing contact, tracking, reminders, and information storage.

With specific CF center care comes the importance and necessity of strict adherence to exacting infection control protocols to minimize the risk of cross-infection. Protection from known and unknown bacteria and fungi is mandatory as previous understanding of cross-infection is constantly being challenged. It is interesting that a comparison of outcomes of patients receiving center care versus those who were not revealed better lung function and nutritional status for those in center care despite higher rates of *Pseudomonas* infection.[8]

Although sharing care with a local hospital can make day-to-day disease management easier for families, the often-complicated nature of care makes close supervision from the specialist CF center essential. Specialist CF centers are staffed by professionals with experience in CF. As well as ongoing research, attending meetings, and keeping up-to-date with the literature, the CF teams maintain their experience through their day-to-day involvement with a large number of patients with CF. Staff at local hospitals are involved with the care of patients with varied problems and should not expect to become expert in all of them. Additionally, many specialist CF centers, due to the number of patients and particular expertise of staff are able to use and maintain specialist equipment. Resourcing such equipment, maintaining it, and training operators may not be a priority in local hospitals. However, good communication and liaison between both services ensures that the patient receives the best of both services.

When the specialist CF center is in a large area, it is essential that support be provided by the local hospital, sometimes referred to as the Network CF clinic in the United Kingdom. This local service must meet the same requirements and standards as a specialist CF center and must be supported and supervised in liaison with staff from the specialist CF center. It is critical for the center team to demonstrate that the recommended CF standards of care are being adhered to in order to ensure that the best quality of care is maintained. For example, in the United Kingdom, the specialist CF center must participate in the program of peer-review run in partnership by the Cystic Fibrosis Trust, the British Thoracic Society, and British Paediatric Respiratory Society. Standards required include:

- Access to diagnostic facilities (e.g., sweat testing, lung function, bronchoscopy, and radiology) and microbiology services fulfilling the CF Trust laboratory standards for processing microbiological samples.[9]
- Access to their CF center for routine and emergency care and advice. Patients should be reviewed regularly with a frequency appropriate to their individual needs, but routine appointments for a stable patient should be for every 2 to 3 months depending on the severity of their disease. Newly diagnosed infants should be seen more frequently (initially every 1 to 2 weeks).
- There must be sufficient capacity in clinics for outpatients to be seen urgently with sufficient space to ensure optimal infection control.
- There must be sufficient inpatient beds so that patients do not wait unnecessarily for an admission. Beds in a ward suitable for CF care (adhering to cross-infection policies) should always be available for an emergency admission. There needs to be capacity to ensure elective and urgent admissions can be managed appropriately.
- An urgent course of treatment should be implemented within a maximum of 24 hours of the decision being made, and a nonurgent admission within 7 working days of the planned date. Hospital ward nurses must have sufficient knowledge and experience to provide CF care.
- Patients should be seen by a consultant with specialist knowledge in CF at least twice a week; when an inpatient, additionally the consultant must be kept updated every day.

In the US centers providing care for CF patients receive accreditation from the US Cystic Fibrosis Foundation based on data completed for the registry and detailed information regarding service delivery and facilities provided at the center. In Germany, centers are engaged in cycles of quality improvement to ensure the best quality of care delivery.

THE MULTIDISCIPLINARY TEAM

CF is complex and multisystem; it is inevitable therefore that care should only be provided by a team of specialists. The staffing requirements of specialists involved in CF MDTs have been developed by working parties in the United Kingdom, Europe, Australasia, and North America; however, no two CF teams will be the same. Most teams will adapt the recommendations to meet the local needs of their patient group such as patient ages and patient numbers. Unfortunately, most CF teams around the world are subject to a limitation of resources and therefore have to work within imposed boundaries.

As multidisciplinary care is accepted as essential in the management of long-term chronic diseases, all children and adults with CF must have access to specialist advice and care from their CF centers at all times.[10] As well as access to the specialist MDT for routine or urgent care, other specialists who are familiar with the complications of CF should also be available.

Communication is a key function of a CF MDT and it is crucial that all the members of the team meet at a regular weekly meeting to discuss the patients seen both as inpatients and in outreach care. This meeting not only functions to ensure best quality of care for patients but also facilitates careful monitoring of each team member to ensure education and support and prevention of burnout. The senior members of the team are able to guide those with less experience and ensure knowledge is disseminated for best patient benefit. It can also be helpful for the CF team to meet less regularly to discuss service development, staffing, and more practical issues unrelated to direct patient care.

Several chapters are devoted to aspects of care delivered by nurses, physiotherapists, dietitians, and psychologists as part of the MDT. Although the aim of this chapter is to describe the function of the MDT, the role of other members of the team not emphasized in other chapters will be highlighted, namely the pharmacist, occupational therapist, and social worker.

THE CF MULTIDISCIPLINARY TEAM

- Consultant
- Staff grade/specialist registrar/resident
- Specialist nurse
- Specialist physiotherapist
- Specialist dietitian

- Specialist psychologist
- Pharmacist
- Social worker
- Occupational therapist
- Secretary
- Play therapist/school teacher
- Data manager

THE MEDICAL TEAM

The consultant leading a CF MDT (the Clinical Director or Lead Clinician for CF) must have a major commitment to CF care. It is useful for the consultant to have at least one senior colleague with knowledge of CF who is able to take over during periods of absence. A junior team will support the consultant, with one or more specialist registrars/residents fulfilling a more dedicated role such as that of CF Fellow. These doctors will manage the day-to-day needs of the patients and work closely with the specialist nurses. It is critical that the doctors communicate regularly about individual patient management to ensure continuity of care.

THE SPECIALIST NURSE

The specialist nurse provides a clinical, educational, and support service for patients and their families. Living with a life-limiting disease impacts on all areas of life as balancing treatment regimens with school, employment, social and family life can become overwhelming. Parents of young children find living with CF intrusive, isolating, and time consuming. Adolescents and young adults share those feelings as well as finding it differentiating at a time when they want to fit in with a peer group. Through the provision of both practical and emotional support and advice, the nurse aims to help minimize adherence issues, maintain independence, and improve quality of life.

THE SPECIALIST PHYSIOTHERAPIST

Assisting, teaching, and supporting patients and their families in airway clearance techniques is the primary role of the physiotherapist. There are however many other areas that the physiotherapist has become involved in, such as osteoporosis and posture management, urinary incontinence, exercise programs, pregnancy care (pre- and postnatal), nebulizer therapy (including the newer devices available in each country), oxygen therapy, and noninvasive ventilation.

THE SPECIALIST DIETITIAN

As with the physiotherapist, the role of the dietitian has developed over the years. Although the primary role is ensuring good nutritional status in patients, dietitians have also found themselves offering advice and support in a number of different areas. The expanded role of the dietitian includes areas such as feeding problems (often jointly with a clinical psychologist [CP]), CF-related diabetes (CFRD), distal intestinal obstructive syndrome (DIOS) and other gastrointestinal (GI) problems, enteral feeding, and pregnancy. Good communication and referral within the team is essential in this as in all other areas as the role of the dietitian often overlaps with other team members such as the nurse, physiotherapist, and psychologist.

THE SPECIALIST CLINICAL PSYCHOLOGIST

The provision of clinical psychological services to the management of CF is essential.[11] CPs work closely with the CF team supporting colleagues in psychological aspects of care and providing advice and opinion on particular issues. Areas generally covered by a CP include adherence to treatment, quality of life, management of procedural distress, management of feeding and behavioral difficulties, learning to live with a secondary diagnosis (e.g., CFRD), and end of life issues. Typically, the CP identifies patient needs through referral from team members, issues arising at MDT meetings, or during psychological assessment carried out at annual review. Problems are identified and then in discussion with the team the most appropriate methods of resolving these problems are planned. The clinical psychological service is often run in parallel with the CF service, with the CP working as a gatekeeper for the onward referral of patients to the local mental health services.

THE PHARMACIST

The specialist pharmacist plays a major part in the MDT in the care of both inpatients and outpatients. The overall role of the pharmacist in the CF team is to ensure safe, appropriate, and cost-effective drug treatment and this falls into four main areas—advice to the team, advice to the patient, organization of centrally prepared intravenous drugs (where appropriate), and managing the availability of medicines.

Pharmacists offer advice to the team around issues such as the appropriateness of therapies, adverse drug reactions including interactions between drugs, and alternative choices. The pharmacist is also involved with discharge planning ensuring liaison with the primary healthcare team and providing an accurate discharge drug summary. Liaison with other members of the CF team is important and the pharmacist works closely with the CF nurse in the provision of home intravenous antibiotics and the equipment needed for administration.

The pharmacist also works behind the scenes, taking responsibility for issues such as the procurement of unlicensed and named-patient medicines as appropriate and ensuring the managed entry of new drug therapies. The introduction of new therapies can cause problems in a resource-stressed service, and the pharmacist is involved with collaborating in finding funding and the commissioning of new therapies.

Many services have introduced self-medication schemes and the pharmacist helps with these initiatives by supporting ward staff in the introduction and maintenance of the scheme and empowering patients to take control of their treatment. Pharmacists offer medication counseling and meet with individual patients to enhance knowledge and understanding of their treatment regimens. This is done through completion of an accurate drug history at admission or annual review and then, through reviewing the medication with the patient, the pharmacist provides education and support often recommending changes where necessary such as a change in formulation or method of administration. This also helps patients with adherence issues and the pharmacist often works in partnership with the nurse and psychologist to address these problems.[1]

SOCIAL WORKER

The hospital-based social worker works closely with all members of the CF team, taking referrals directly from colleagues. The role will differ between Centers depending on availability, need, and particular patient groups. Although social workers are commonly used as a resource for their knowledge of benefits and government allowances, in most CF Centers the social worker is available both for patients attending outpatients and for those who are admitted. In some Centers, the social worker will visit patients in their homes to undertake an assessment of needs.

Recommendations for the social worker role include:

- Maintain up-to-date knowledge on all significant welfare and benefit changes and understand and apply relevant current legislation to support patients.
- Have knowledge of chronic illness and how this impacts on patients and their families both day to day and long term. Increase understanding among local and national government departments regarding these hidden consequences of CF.
- Act as a gatekeeper and liaison for the onward referral of patients to social services, housing services, and other relevant agencies.
- Follow child protection procedures and ensure effective information sharing and referral and liaison to home authority team where appropriate.
- Liaise with schools/colleges/universities to access suitable support, e.g., arrangements for getting work to students, home access to laptop computers, time extensions for coursework, and special arrangements for examinations.
- Provide information and advice on employment rights and arrange access to Disability Employment Advisors if appropriate.
- Advocate on behalf of individuals and educate government and local authority agencies regarding the possible impact of CF on access to appropriate benefits and suitable housing.
- Provide support to patients' carers as needed and provide bereavement support/end of life support to patients and families.

- Contribute to research in all areas of CF either through developing individual projects or participating in research carried out by the MDT.
- Take part in audit carried out on behalf of the CF service.

Most countries offer a benefit system for people struggling with disease or disability; unfortunately, these systems are often difficult to access and subject to delays and bureaucracy. The social worker can be helpful in negotiating the system and advocating on behalf of the patients. The social worker is often the link person in organizing packages of care provided through social services by collating relevant assessments and letters from other professionals and liaising with the local authorities. As health deteriorates, there is often a need for adaptations in the home; the social worker and the occupational therapist will assess housing needs and organize support—financial or practical—to help with this.

When young people start school or college, the social worker will often work with the nurse specialist in liaising with schools and colleges about potential problems such as access, travel, computer use, time extensions for course work, etc. Likewise the social worker can also liaise with employers to discuss short- or long-term needs for individuals.

Social workers may also be involved with assessing a patient for transplantation. Unlike other aspects of transplant assessment, the social worker does not make recommendations as to suitability; instead coping strategies, emotional, financial, and practical supports are identified. Preparing the patient for the results of the assessment is also important. Some will be accepted for transplantation and have to deal with an uncertain waiting period, and some will not be accepted and have to deal with loss of hope. Both groups will have deteriorating health and an increasing need for support.

As with other members of the CF team, the social worker can offer psychological support, particularly around issues such as acceptance of CF and the emotional and practical implications of the disease, adherence to treatment, relationship issues, and end of life issues. Medical advances are improving the lives of people with CF; however, to maximize quality of life patients must be supported in living life as independently as possible.

THE OCCUPATIONAL THERAPIST

Occupational therapy (OT) is focused on enabling the continued occupations of everyday life through adaptation, while living with an illness or disability. This may involve problem solving new ways of carrying out activities of daily living or utilizing adaptive equipment to assist with independence and decrease energy requirements for the task—particularly for those with deteriorating disease and increasing limitation in accessing things in the home, for example, stairs, bathrooms, and kitchens.

The purpose of the OT role is to work together with patients and their families by identifying any areas of difficulty within the realm of work, self-care, and leisure tasks that are currently impacting on daily life. The timing of intervention is important when working with a population with CF which at times can be a challenge; it can be difficult for young adults to accept the need for adaptations in the home environment to enable an increased quality of life. Although a young adult with normal lung function will not require the services of an OT, it is crucial that adults with lower lung function and breathlessness have access to the OT's skills.

Introduction of OT is often during an admission where information on the role of the occupational therapist as a member of the CF team is provided. This allows the patient to address any concerns they have, as they are already aware of what OT has to offer.

Assessment is carried out on the ward and an individualized treatment plan is devised in consultation with the patient that focuses on their current goals. Two of the main goals from this initial meeting include trial and practice of adaptive and new techniques. To start with, patients are encouraged to practice personal and domestic activities of daily living to enhance confidence and learn adaptive techniques. Alternatively or parallel to this they are also encouraged in the trial of adaptive equipment that can aid in independence and decrease the endurance required for the task. In some places, the OT is involved in supporting patients using home oxygen, particularly around delivery, device, and interface issues. However, this is usually a role carried out in partnership with the physiotherapists, doctors, and oxygen delivery companies.

Advocacy is another key part of the OT role through liaison with local authorities and social service occupational therapists. This includes providing a detailed functional assessment report that will include information on the disease process and the demands of daily treatment regimens. This will provide the community therapists with sufficient information to meet the needs of the patient when they return home.

The occupational therapist is an active member of the CF MDT. Although all members of the CF team make referrals, most are made through the clinical nurse specialists who bridge the gap between hospital and home. As the adult CF population increases, so will their demands for more home support, it is essential that the role of the occupational therapist in CF constantly evolves to meet needs of the patients, the CF team, and the organization.[12,13]

SECRETARY

Secretaries working in CF teams often find themselves the hub of communication for the service, with the CF team, patients and families all finding themselves making contact throughout the day. As well as the usual secretarial duties (e.g., typing clinic letters/summaries, collating clinic lists,

test results, etc.) the secretary will get to know patients and families, perhaps be involved in database management and liaison between different services.

PLAY THERAPIST/SCHOOL TEACHER

Both the play therapist and the school teacher play a central role in maintaining a link with home life and hospital. For young children, the familiarity of playing with toys, watching television, or engaging in other activities with someone who is not a member of the clinical team can provide reassurance and make an admission to hospital more acceptable. The play therapist will also often help prepare children for procedures (such as venepuncture) in a safe and nonthreatening environment. The school teacher can liaise with the child's school during an admission providing support for homework or continuation with school work that is being missed. There is a key role in interpreting the illness to the local school, who may not understand how CF can impact on education. Unfortunately, some older children need to be in hospital during examinations; the school teacher can arrange for these to be done in hospital.

DATA MANAGER

To support audit and research, it is necessary to record individual patient clinical data from all CF Centers. In many countries around the world specialist CF services are requested to contribute to their national registries. These data are usually collected from annual reviews or outpatient attendances; however, entry of such complex data can be complicated and time consuming. Many Centers have found it invaluable to use a data entry manager who becomes an essential member of the CF team.

ADDITIONAL MULTIDISCIPLINARY TEAM MEMBERS

It is often necessary to involve other specialist health professionals to manage the range of disorders that can develop over the disease course, for example, liver disease or diabetes. This may be viewed as a second tier of the MDT; access to these team members will be by referral only. Their knowledge of CF is important as it is frustrating to patients if they are referred to professionals who have no knowledge of the disease and have to spend time explaining basic facts about CF rather than tackle the problem with which they have been referred. It is beneficial if these professionals liaise closely with the primary CF team. It is the combination of the primary and secondary MDT working collectively that ensures the patient with CF receives the best care. Health professionals such as those from laboratory services are key to ensuring specific investigations that are carried out for patients with

CF; e.g., extensive microbiology and sensitivity testing on sputum cultures using appropriate culture media. When some of these specialized services are unavailable, there can sometimes be delays in treatment, which may ultimately lead to suboptimal care. The roles of the extended MDT will now be briefly described.

THE EXTENDED CF MULTIDISCIPLINARY TEAM (ALPHABETICAL ORDER)

- Chaplain/other faith leaders
- Diabetologist/Endocrinologist
- Ear, Nose, and Throat (ENT) Specialist
- Gastroenterologist and Liver Specialist
- Geneticist
- Gynecologist
- Obstetrician/Fertility Specialist
- Palliative Care Specialist
- Radiologist (including interventional radiology)
- Rheumatologist
- Specialized Laboratory Services (Microbiology including mycology and mycobacteria, Molecular Biology, Biochemistry, Immunology)
- Transplant Team/Thoracic Surgeon

SPECIALIZED LABORATORY SERVICES

In addition to routine hematology and biochemistry services, laboratories that offer specialized testing (nonroutine) for patients with CF are paramount to accurate treatment plans being instigated. This should include sputum cultures performed on multiple selective media as described in previous chapters. Biochemistry services should provide CF-related investigations such as levels of fat-soluble vitamins (A, D, and E), analysis of fecal fats, and fecal elastase in determining pancreatic function. Immunology provides services such as identifying *Pseudomonas* antibodies, *Aspergillus* precipitins, radioallergosorbent test, and total immunoglobulin E.

THE GENETICIST (INCLUDING GENETIC COUNSELORS)

The geneticist has an important role to play within the CF MDT, not only for an individual patient but also for the wider community. Collaboration with the genetics laboratory is essential for planning screening programs, particularly where a national program may have to be individualized for areas with specific ethnic and racial groups. More commonly, the geneticist confirms the diagnosis through correct identification of the genetic mutations responsible, thus assisting the clinician with planning treatment. However, genetic counseling and identification of the gene carried by individuals with CF also helps with their own or other family member's reproductive choices and decision making.

THE GASTROENTEROLOGIST

Individuals with CF present with a multitude of GI issues such as gastroesophageal reflux, liver disease, pancreatitis, and DIOS, all requiring specialist gastroenterologist intervention. Additionally, less common complications such as Crohn's disease and GI cancers are managed more successfully if a gastroenterologist with knowledge of CF works closely with the CF team. Gastroenterology services also carry out endoscopic investigations and placement of gastrostomy tubes for supplementary feeding. Close liaison with the specialist dietitian and medical team is paramount. In larger centers, joint CF gastroenterology clinics have proved useful in providing optimum management for CF patients.

DIABETOLOGIST/ENDOCRINOLOGIST

Most CF specialists have knowledge of CFRD, which is commonly managed day-to-day with a CF Specialist Dietitian. However, regular review with a Diabetologist (with specialist expertise in CF) is recommended. Manipulation of different insulin preparations and specialist monitoring for diabetes-related complications are essential in a population who are growing older. The endocrinologist can also help in the management of growth and puberty issues in the growing child as well as iatrogenic complications such as adrenal failure following prolonged steroid therapy.

EAR, NOSE, AND THROAT SPECIALIST

ENT complications such as rhinosinusitis, nasal obstruction, and nasal polyps are common in CF and may require specialist medical intervention or surgery. The CF team should, therefore, have an active working relationship with the ENT Department for the investigation and management of severe sinus disease, including mucocele. This is particularly important when surgical techniques such as polypectomy and endoscopic submucus resection are indicated.

OBSTETRICIAN/GYNECOLOGIST/ FERTILITY SPECIALIST

The CF team should be able to provide contraceptive advice and preconception support. This should be provided to both adolescents and adults. Close liaison with an obstetrician and team with experience in CF is essential throughout pregnancy. Successful outcomes for both the mother with CF and the fetus are achieved with good multidisciplinary care and excellent communication between the CF team and the obstetric team.[14]

Male infertility in CF has been transformed with the introduction of sperm aspiration from the epididymis and intracytoplasmic injection into eggs.[15] Men with CF should have access to expert advice about fertility assessment and management.

- Information about the process and about the adult center available to the adolescent and their parent.
- Evidence of good communication between pediatric and adult teams

Without this structure and commitment from professionals, parents and adolescents find themselves reluctant to accept the inevitable, what should be welcomed as recognition of adulthood becomes something that is feared and avoided.[18] Problems in this process can be due to a number of issues:

- No formal plan of transition agreed between the pediatric and adult services
- No coordinator
- Pediatric teams with concerns about the process
- Patient/family's reluctance to move
- Patient/parents perceptions about entering an adult world with CF
- No obvious adult service to liaise with
- Concern about the availability of adult services

The process of transition does not end after the transition clinic. Follow-up during the change over period must be handled carefully between the pediatric and adult teams, with an agreement as to which team takes responsibility at any given time. During the first few outpatient visits to the adult clinic, familiarity is important and the patient and their family must meet the CF team members who were introduced to them during the transition clinic. Likewise, if the patient requires an admission soon after moving the ward staff needs to be informed of their status as newly transitioned patients so that the admission can be handled sensitively.

A well-planned transition program, with good coordination and communication between the pediatric and adult teams will ensure a successful move from pediatric to adult care for most patients.[19] There will be some young people, however, who cannot be managed within guidelines. These include siblings who are close in age, the terminally ill, and those who do not attend appointments. Parents of siblings who are close in age often ask if they can go through the transition process together when they are both near an appropriate age. This often means keeping the older past the guideline age and moving the younger at an early age. Although this may be convenient for the family it may not always be right for the individual patient as they become independent adults. Over the years, a close relationship develops between patients, families, and CF teams, especially as disease deteriorates. Although childhood death is now rare in CF, moving the young person and their family to an unknown team and unknown surroundings at such a vulnerable time should be carefully considered. Finally there are group of patients who, despite everyone's best efforts, fails to attend transition clinics. Unfortunately, this group of young people misses out on the process and usually find that their next outpatient appointment is with the adult team. The adult team in this instance must be particularly aware of the individual and spend time acquainting them with the changes.

CF OUTREACH

From diagnosis parents are encouraged to learn procedures such as chest physiotherapy, how to administer oral and inhaled medication, and pay attention to diet so that children can be at home living as normal a life as possible. As children grow older, they are supported in becoming independent in all aspects of their treatment including how to manage their airway clearance and diet. Support in the home environment therefore helps both children and young adults to fully participate in school, work, and family life while maintaining their health.

The treatment demands of CF are burdensome and stressful; when a child or adult with CF is in good health, this may take up to an hour a day; however, when they become more unwell, treatment times will increase substantially. With decreasing health comes increasing needs—nebulizer therapy, home intravenous therapy, enteral feeding, oxygen therapy, physiotherapy aids, wheelchairs, and noninvasive ventilation, for example. Arranging delivery or collection, storage, and maintenance of this extra equipment also places enormous practical and psychosocial demands on parents, carers, and patients. Parents of children with CF may have other children, work, or care for other family members. Adults with CF may themselves have a family, be in employment or full-time education or care for other family members. Leading a busy and active life while maintaining a strict CF treatment regimen is a major undertaking.

Most specialist CF services in the United Kingdom offer an outreach service. The CF clinical nurse specialists usually provides this service, but in some places CF specialist physiotherapists and dietitians are also involved (Table 41.3) A comprehensive service therefore can often make a difference with adherence to treatment, hospital admissions, and coping with the day-to-day demands of CF.[20]

Much of the equipment needed in home care today is readily available, easy to use, and often disposable, for example, physiotherapy adjuncts, intravenous delivery systems, or nebulizer consumables. Technological advancements make communication with the CF team much easier. Developments such as webcams, online monitoring, telephone messaging, and SMS texting means that the patient and the professional can discuss problems and check clinical measurements such as lung function in real time. Patients today live in a technology-driven society and have no problem in adapting their knowledge in using clinical equipment.

ADVANTAGES AND DISADVANTAGES OF HOME VISITING

Although a home visiting service may appear as an obvious model of offering care, CF teams need to evaluate its usefulness in relation to each patient at every exacerbation and be sensitive to the needs of the carers. For some families

Table 41.3 Provision of CF specialist care in the home

Nurses	Physiotherapists	Dietitians
• Clinical assessments at home • Support for patients/family • Health education • Blood tests during an intravenous course of antibiotics • Maintaining intravenous access during a course of intravenous antibiotics • Lung function/oxygen saturation monitoring • Flushing of implantable venous access devices • Liaison with multidisciplinary hospital team including doctors, nurses, physiotherapists, dietitians, occupational therapists, social worker • Liaison with GP/local healthcare providers • Liaison with community services such as social services and housing departments • Support to women planning pregnancy and during pregnancy • Postnatal support • Support to patients waiting for a transplant • Bereavement support to family members	• Optimizing airway clearance techniques • Problem solving with noninvasive ventilation and liaising with respiratory support services • Lung function/oxygen saturation monitoring • Encouraging exercise programs when well and after long hospital admissions • Discussing posture • Discussing continence issues • Problem solving with nebulizers • Support for patients and family • Liaison with multidisciplinary hospital team including doctors, nurses, physiotherapists, dietitians, occupational therapists, social worker	• Monitoring and advising on feeding problems • Advice on adherence issues • Advice on oral supplements • Advice on vitamins • Problem solving and giving advice with the administration of pancreatic enzyme therapy • Problem solving and giving advice with managing CFRD • Problem solving and giving advice on the management of enteral feeding • Advising on pre- and postpregnancy nutrition including breast-feeding • Problem solving and advice about distal intestinal obstructive syndrome
• All professionals providing care in a multidisciplinary home care team must be able to cross cover for each other so that patient does not receive multiple visits, e.g., phlebotomy and spirometry skills		

CFRD, cystic fibrosis-related diabetes; GP, general practitioner.

admitting a patient to hospital is important as a respite for carers, to prevent home becoming hospital, employment pressures of the carer, isolation of the adult patient, issues with nonadherence, or because of demands from other family members. In some centers, resources will dictate and perhaps limit the level of service available. It is essential in these instances that the outreach offered is appropriate for each patient. For the CF team an admission can provide an opportunity to monitor treatment closely, especially if there has been a problem with previous treatment in the home.

On a clinical level home care may not always be suitable, but reports indicate that treatment for exacerbations is more effective in hospital than at home although more expensive for the health service.[21] Equally, when treated in the home there are economic savings for the patients in terms of being able to continue at work (for both parents and adults with CF). There is no doubt that patients and families prefer treatment at home and much of the literature supports the psychosocial benefits of home care such as ability to sleep,

mood, and overall energy levels. As with all CF treatment, care has to be individualized not only for clinical reasons but also for personal and intellectual needs. In exploring methods to improve outcome for home treatment, patient and family preference must be balanced between home visiting and hospital attendance.

MANAGING A HOME VISITING TEAM

Paying for a home visiting service can often stretch the financial restrictions of many of CF centers; however, for managers of the service it is essential to make sure that it is properly resourced and include funding for extras such as secretarial support, professional development, and basics such as computer/printers. Individuals providing a home visiting service can find their work rewarding however, an understanding of each others' roles allows for flexibility, ensuring patients do not experience an "over-load" of home visits. Meeting families in their own homes leads to a greater understanding of disease management and how families have adapted their lives to cope. Nevertheless, the role can also be isolating and dangerous, especially when travel is over large areas. Safety is an issue, many professionals carrying out this role are women who are driving through busy traffic or visiting families in remote or dangerous areas. It is important therefore that planning a visiting program so that the visiting timetable is known by team members based in the hospital, keeping in contact throughout the day using mobile phones and carrying personal alarms can reduce many of the problems.

THE CYSTIC FIBROSIS PROFESSIONAL

From diagnosis onwards parents and the young person are involved in a collaboration of care with the CF Team. Treatment decisions are planned with the involvement of parent and patient, and their views and comments are important in final decision making. It is inevitable, therefore, that an often close and trusting relationship develops between parents, patient, and CF team members. Where the CF team member is involved with providing home care, this relationship may become stronger and over many years can become difficult to manage on an emotional level. Crossing professional boundaries can become a risk for the patient, their family, and the professional and the CF team have a responsibility to be aware of colleagues and their workload.

The term "burnout" is commonly used to describe the overloading of an emotional and physical burden. It is almost inevitable that professionals involved over many years with children, distraught parents, and young adults—often peers, who have a life-limiting disease, can become "burnt-out." CF care is palliative with no cure; working with a patient population that will die may unavoidably lead to emotional involvement. This may not be a problem in itself, overinvolvement, however it will lead to serious problems, and individuals must be conscious of their working relationships and be alert to potential issues.

SUMMARY

CF center care is important as it aims to prevent complications for as long as possible through the minimization of risks and optimization of health status.[2,3,22] The members of a CF MDT work together with often overlapping roles; however, communication between all professionals within the team ensures that patients receive optimum care with a good quality of life. Children and adults with CF would like to have all the resources of a specialist CF center at their local hospital, unfortunately this will never be possible. Consensus throughout the world is for CF center care; however, shared care strategies have been adopted in some places.[23]

CF is not the only disease to have benefited from a more vigorous approach to treatment by specialized teams—particularly in pediatrics; however, the initial success of these specialist pediatric teams has led to increased survival over the years and the adoption of this model in the provision of adult care.[24,25]

Individuals with CF are surviving well into adulthood; this improving prognosis can without a doubt be attributed to medical and scientific advances. Nevertheless, the attention to detail in day-to-day management, the evaluation and introduction of more effective treatment regimens, and the specialist knowledge of professionals working in large centers has also made a significant contribution to increasing survival.

REFERENCES

1. Cystic Fibrosis Trust. *Standards for the Clinical Care of Children and Adults with Cystic Fibrosis.* London, United Kingdom: Cystic Fibrosis Trust; 2011.
2. Royal College of Physician. *Cystic Fibrosis in Adults: Recommendations for Care of Patients in the United Kingdom.* London, United Kingdom: Royal College Physicians; 1990.
3. British Paediatric Association. Cystic fibrosis in the United Kingdom 1977-85: An improving picture. *Br Med J* 1988; **297**(6663): 1599–602.
4. Neilsen OH, Schoitz PO. Cystic fibrosis in Denmark in the period 1945-81: Evaluation of centralised treatment. *Acta Pediatr Scand* 1982; **301** (Suppl): 107–19.
5. Phelan P, Hey E. Cystic fibrosis mortality in England and Wales and in Victoria, Australia. *Arch Dis Child* 1984; **59**: 71–83.
6. Walters S, Hodson ME, Britton J. Hospital care for adults with cystic fibrosis: An overview and comparison between special cystic fibrosis clinics and general clinics using a patient questionnaire. *Thorax* 1994; **49**: 300–6.
7. Frederiksen B, Laang S, Koch C, Holby N. Improved survival in the Danish centre-treated cystic fibrosis patients: Results of aggressive treatment. *Pediatr Pulmonol* 1996; **21**; 153–8.
8. Mahadeva R, Webb K, Westerbeek RC, et al. Clinical outcome in relation to care in centres specialising in cystic fibrosis: Cross-sectional study. *Br Med J* 1998; **316**: 1771–5.
9. Cystic Fibrosis Trust. Laboratory standards for processing microbiological samples from people with cystic fibrosis. Report of the UK Cystic Fibrosis Trust Microbiology Laboratory Standards Working Group. London, United Kingdom: Cystic Fibrosis Trust; September 2012.
10. Madge S, Khair K. Multi-disciplinary teams in the United Kingdom: Problems and solutions. *J Pediatr Nurs* 2000; **15**(2): 131–4.
11. Oxley H, Webb AK. How a clinical psychologist manages the problems of adults with cystic fibrosis. *J Royal Soc Med* 2005 98 (Suppl 45): 37–46.

12. Otley Groom V. Occupational therapy. In: Hodson ME, Geddes DM (Eds). *Cystic Fibrosis*. 2nd ed. London, United Kingdom: Arnold; 2000. pp. 419–24.

13. Hagedorn R. *Foundations for Practice in Occupational Therapy*. 3rd ed. London, United Kingdom: Churchill Livingstone; 2001.

14. Thorpe-Beeston JG, Madge S, Gyi K, Hodson M, Bilton D. The outcome of pregnancies in women with cystic fibrosis—Single centre experience 1998–2011. *BJOG* 2012; **119**.

15. McCallum PJ, Milunski JM, Cunningham DL. Fertility in men with cystic fibrosis. *Chest* 2000; 118: 1059–62.

16. Boylard DR. Sexuality and cystic fibrosis. *MCN AM J Matern Child Nurs* 2001; **26**: 39–41.

17. Bryon M, Madge S. Transition from paediatric to adult care: Psychological principles. *J R Soc Med* 2001; **94** (Suppl 40): 5–7.

18. Madge S, Bryon M. A model for transition of care in cystic fibrosis. *J Pediatric Nurs* 2002; **17**(4): 283–8.

19. Madge SL. National consensus standards for nursing children and young people with cystic fibrosis. *Pediatr Nurs* 2002; **14**(1): 32–5.

20. Barnes R. Why home healthcare is so important for patients with cystic fibrosis. *Br J Home Health Care* 2005; **1**(1): 14–5.

21. Thornton J, Elliott RA, Tully MP, Dodd M, Webb AK. Clinical and economic choices in the treatment of respiratory infections in cystic fibrosis: Comparing hospital and homecare. *J Cyst Fibros* 2005; **4**(4):239–47.

22. Kerem E, Conway S, Elborn S, Heijerman H. Standards of care for patients with cystic fibrosis: A European consensus. *J Cyst Fibros* 2005; **4**: 7–26.

23. Dodge J. Patient-centred cystic fibrosis services. *J Soc Med* 2005; **98** (Suppl 45): 2–6.

24. Littlewood J. Good care for people with cystic fibrosis. *Pediatr Resp Rev* 2000; **1**: 179–89.

25. Conway S, Balfour-Lynn IM, De Rijcke K, Drevinek P, Foweraker J et al. European Cystic Fibrosis Society standards of care: Framework for the Cystic Fibrosis Centre. *J Cyst Fibros* 2014; **13**: S3–S22.

42

Nursing

SUSAN MADGE AND KAMILLA DACK

NURSING CARE

INTRODUCTION

Advances in both medical management and provision of care over recent years have improved both quality of life and longevity. The multidisciplinary team (MDT) works together to ensure a holistic approach to the care of these patients with a complex disease. All specialist CF centers in the United Kingdom have at least one clinical nurse specialist (CNS) with expert knowledge of cystic fibrosis (CF). The role of the CNS is varied but in general offers care and support to patients attending hospital and those at home. In some centers, the CNS coordinates and facilitates community care in liaison with local or generic community nursing teams. However, other centers have a dedicated CNS who is able to offer direct care to patients in the community. The CNS, whether community or hospital based, can provide skilled support, advice, and care directly to the patient and family wherever it is needed. CNSs working in hospitals where there is no opportunity to work with a CF team are strongly advised to make contact with the nearest specialist CF center, both for their own support and to assure optimum care for their patients.[1]

This chapter will first discuss the role of the CNS—providing both a hospital and outreach service—and then describe the various key events throughout the life of a child and young adult where the role of the CNS is important in ensuring optimum clinical and psychosocial care. Further information on the role of the CNS (particularly the provision of an outreach service) can be found in Chapter 41 on specialist center care.

ROLE OF THE CNS

The UK Standards of Care of Children and Adults with Cystic Fibrosis in the United Kingdom[2] and the Standards of Care for Patients with Cystic Fibrosis: A European Consensus[3] state that the role of the CF CNS includes the following.

GENERAL INFORMATION

- The CNS must be registered with the UK Nurses and Midwives Council.
- The CNS must be a member of the UK CF Nursing Association.
- Those CNSs working with children must have undergone specific pediatric training.
- The CNS must have specialist knowledge and be experienced in the care of children or adults with CF.
- The CNS must maintain their Continued Professional Development through the attendance at courses and conferences.

ROLE

- The CNS must provide advocacy and psychosocial support, particularly at important times such as the notification of a screening result and diagnosis, first admission to hospital, first course of intravenous antibiotics, a secondary diagnosis (e.g., CF-related diabetes [CFRD]), transition, reproductive issues, pre- and postnatal care, transplant, and end of life issues.
- The CNS must provide home care support particularly for home intravenous antibiotic therapy.
- The CNS must provide education to others about CF including nurseries, schools, places of higher education, and work places.
- The CNS must act as a link between the patient and family, primary care and community services, and hospital.
- The CNS must act as a resource for training and education for other professionals involved in CF care.

- The CNS must contribute to research in all areas of CF, either through developing individual projects or participating in research carried out by the MDT.
- The CNS must take part in audit carried out on behalf of the CF service.

CNSs looking after children or adults with CF have a variety of additional responsibilities, not only to patients and their families but also to other staff involved in the care of those patients acting in a coordinating and liaising role between colleagues.[4] Specialist CF centers and patient groups have differing requirements; therefore, the CNS role varies not only between countries but also between centers within countries. It is inevitable, therefore, that the CNS role will develop to meet the needs of the local CF population.[3]

The CNS working in CF has a unique role in being involved with both patient and their family throughout a lifetime—from helping them to come to terms with the diagnosis to supporting them with end of life management. There are, however, certain key times in the patient's and family's life that more intensive support is required, for example; at diagnosis—whether as a newborn through screening, in later infancy, childhood, or as an adult, at first admission, transition from pediatric to adult care, planning a family, discussion about lung transplantation, and care at the end of life. The CNS should also be involved in providing support and information at times where there is often increased distress such as dealing with adolescence, adherence issues, fertility, and pregnancy, or following a secondary diagnosis (e.g., CFRD).

CF is a demanding disease to manage for the patient, the family, and the CF team. Patient health status, well-being, and satisfaction are the principal aims of the CNS and providing support and advocacy to the patient and family helps to achieve this. The CNS is actively involved in treatment decisions and monitoring care; however in addition to practical care (e.g., intravenous therapy), the CNS has a responsibility to ensure that every patient receives appropriate psychosocial care for their individual needs. The CNS coordinates care between patient and family, community services and hospital, both practically and through support and advice. Attention to these aspects of a nursing role should help to ensure patients receive lifelong support and good quality care.[5]

BOUNDARIES AND BURNOUT

The chronicity of the disease makes healthcare professionals working with children and adults with CF vulnerable to the pressure of a long-term professional relationship. This is most obvious when individuals, often mistakenly, start to blur professional boundaries and confuse the professional relationship with friendship. This long-term relationship can also lead to both an emotional and physical exhaustion as the extreme highs and lows take their toll.

Commonly there are two models of care adopted by professionals in the healthcare setting, the expert model where the carer assumes responsibility and the partnership model where professionals and patients negotiate care through mutual trust and collaboration. Management of CF demands a partnership model of care; however, working with a population of patients who have a lifelong, life-limiting disease demands a certain level of involvement. Supporting day-to-day management and managing acute crises requires a constant level of communication. It is inevitable and often helpful that a relationship of friendship and trust develops not only between the CNS and the patient/family but also among other members of the CF team.

There is a danger, however, that this relationship may change from a caring one to one that becomes more extreme and personal. Maintaining professional, caring boundaries for any member of the CF team can be difficult. In 2008, the UK Nursing and Midwifery Council stated that a nurse should maintain clear professional boundaries. In June 2012, they added further advice on the use of social networking, stating that nurses and midwives put their registration at risk if they are involved in any kind of content sharing online, including text, photographs, images, video and audio files. They added that nurses must not use social networks to build or pursue relationships with patients and service users, even if the patients are no longer under their care.[6]

The long-term and often emotional relationship that the MDT have with patients and families are at risk of becoming stressful and may lead to eventual burnout. Although childhood death is rare in CF, for those working in specialist adult CF centers dealing with the dying patient is inevitable. Due to the life-limiting nature of CF, the majority of deaths are in early adulthood (median age of death in the United Kingdom is 28 years[7]) and for the ward staff, junior doctors, and many members of the CF team this means working with patients within their peer group. Working closely with the adult CF population can, therefore, become emotionally draining and the CNS should ensure that support and supervision is available not only individually but also, if possible, for the MDT. Good support and regular communication within the team and supervision from colleagues outside the team will ensure that a caring relationship is maintained and that any member of the CF team is not put at risk.

DIAGNOSIS

Diagnosis through newborn screening is now common in many countries throughout the world. In the United Kingdom, the CNS plays an active role in talking to parents at diagnosis and then offering ongoing support and continuing education following the initial discussion. Where screening is not available most babies are diagnosed within the first year of life through identification of meconium ileus at birth (or suspected prenatally on ultrasound), failure to thrive, or repeated respiratory problems. Again, the CNS plays a similar role in offering ongoing support and education to the parents—this is discussed in more detail in Chapter 41.

Although professionals can be relatively positive in talking to parents about CF, it is inevitable that they will initially focus on the life-limiting nature of the disease. Receiving a diagnosis of CF is, therefore, devastating for parents, as it can be perceived as a death sentence for their newborn baby. Most parents will have never heard of CF and may not fully understand the implications of genetic inheritance; shock, panic, worry, blame, guilt, and confusion are often the most frequent reactions at this time.[8]

Not only will parents have been given devastating news, from diagnosis onwards, but also they will have to learn clinical skills that will become part of their daily lives. Performing airway clearance techniques or administering medication routinely to a well infant may feel unnatural and the parenting role may become confused with a more medicalized role at this early time. Individuals experience different reactions on an emotional and practical level at different times. The support, education, advice, and understanding that the CNS offers have therefore got to be individualized at a level and frequency to meet differing needs. Frequent contact between the CNS and the new parent is therefore essential, either in hospital, through home visiting, e-mail, or telephone.

The impact of this diagnosis on families—immediate and extended—cannot be underestimated. Reproductive issues for both the new parents and their siblings becomes an issue and the CNS play a key role in providing ongoing education and genetic counseling for both the parents and their families.

Although the majority of individuals with CF are diagnosed within the first year of life, there remains a minority who are diagnosed later. In the United Kingdom in 2012, there were 274 individuals diagnosed (range: 0–79 years), 24 as adults.[7] Diagnosis in adolescence and young adulthood is therefore not uncommon, and although 91% of the UK population are either homozygous or heterozygous for the Delta F508 mutation,[7] there are also a number of older adults with rarer mutations who are being referred from general respiratory or infertility clinics. Receiving a diagnosis of CF in adolescence, early or later adulthood can be devastating. For the adolescent or young adult, the introduction of the medicalized treatment regimens can be complicated. Much of the older CF literature describe a life expectancy of approximately 30 years and many late diagnosed young adults report feeling alarmed at this prognosis and, however well they feel, are terrified about dying at a young age. Young adults from various age groups find dealing with a much shortened life expectancy, coupled with a complex treatment regimen very hard to cope with. The CNS needs to spend a great deal of time supporting this particular group of individuals both practically, especially around issues of adherence, and psychosocially in managing life with this diagnosis.

PRESCHOOL

For many, after coming to terms with the diagnosis and learning how to carry out treatment regimens while adjusting back to family life, the early years can become almost normal. However, there are a few areas where CF management remains a nagging reminder of the disease.[9]

Armed with the knowledge that the recommended treatment regimens are planned to optimize their child's health, many parents follow a family routine that is centerd on CF care. For many parents, the child with CF may not be their first, not only are they having to organize life with a new baby and the demands of CF treatment, they are also looking after their other children. The CNS can be very helpful in supporting and guiding parents through the preschool period particularly with issues such as

- Administering medication
- Nutrition
- Pancreatic enzyme replacement therapy (judging the correct amount or refusal to take the enzymes) in conjunction with the dietitian
- Early treatment of chest infections and making decisions about when to ask for advice or start treatment
- Management of airway clearance and exercise in conjunction with the physiotherapist and clinical psychologist
- Starting nursery
- Dealing with siblings
- Planning further children

SCHOOL AGE

A child starting school for the first time can be a traumatic experience for any parent, control is suddenly lost and trust of other adults is demanded. As a parent of a child with CF this loss of control is even greater. Parents will have been exclusively carrying out CF treatment and monitoring their child's every cough and dietary requirement up until this point. Once at school another adult will have to be trusted to continue with this close monitoring. Issues such as following a CF eating plan at school, forgetting to take pancreatic enzymes, and involvement of the school nurse need to be addressed in advance.

Starting school is often not the only concern for parents at this time, there are mixed feelings about their child growing up and staying well. Starting school may also coincide with a change in treatment, for example, the introduction of nebulizer therapy, an admission to hospital for intravenous antibiotic therapy, or the commencement of enteral feeding. Coupled with additional treatments their child will be starting to assert his own independence and it is at this time that issues surrounding nonadherence can start to become more of a problem, especially with eating and physiotherapy.[10]

An established and trusting relationship with the CNS can be helpful for parents. Outreach to the home can be particularly useful as it gives parents time away from the clinical setting and allows them to discuss their anxieties in a safe environment. The CNS may also, with or without parents (but always with their permission), go to the school to talk about CF and how it relates to the child in particular, with teachers and school nurses.

Most school age children with CF are relatively well and take part in all the academic, sporting, and social activities provided by the school. Being an accepted part of a peer group is important, taking time off for outpatient visits or hospital admissions can interrupt this. Children have reported feelings of isolation and losing friends after repeated hospital admissions. Supporting treatment in the home such as intravenous therapy or enteral feeding often allows children to carry on at school. The provision of an outreach service can help as routine checks and early identification of problems can be carried out by the CNS in the patient's home, often after school has ended for the day. Some children, however, have to continue with their academic studies during admission to hospital. The hospital school teacher is invaluable at this time as a liaison between hospital and school and as a support for ongoing school work.

ADOLESCENCE

Adolescents with CF go through the same physical and emotional changes, experience the same rites of passage and have the same expectations as their healthy peers; this expectation is independent of the severity of lung disease.[11] To this end, the CNS should be able to have open and honest discussions about such issues as recreational drug use and the effects on CF, sexuality and safe sex, fertility, pregnancy, university, employment, body image, self esteem, and adherence to treatment regimens.[12,13] Relationships between adolescents and parents can become difficult at this time of life and it is often left to the CNS to encourage and support the promotion of self-care and responsibility, as well as answer some difficult questions.

Taking accountability for self-treatment involves young people with CF having access to accurate information about their disease and its treatment, and with this knowledge comes a greater understanding of their prognosis.[14] CNSs need to be sensitive and honest when giving information to young people with CF. Much of the information they (and their families) receive is from peers, the media, and the Internet; therefore, CNSs caring for this group of patients have a responsibility to ensure that the information they receive is correct and up to date. Preparing for complications such as hemoptysis, CFRD, the introduction of new drugs into the current treatment regime, and pregnancy are just a few of the possible topics where clear and accurate information are important. The CNS, therefore, plays a major role in the education of both the adolescent and their family of new treatments and complications that are part of adult life with CF.

Most children with CF will move from pediatric to adult care and it has been widely recognized that it is important to get the transition process right. Adolescents with CF not only have to deal with the usual changes of growing up but also have to deal with the challenges of assuming responsibility of care from their parents and transitioning of their care from a pediatric to an adult center.[15,16] Transition from pediatric to adult care happens at a time when the young person with CF is moving into adulthood in other areas of their life, such as further education or employment, forming relationships, and taking more responsibility for their own lifestyle. Transition, therefore, can be difficult for many reasons. CNSs involved with the transition process need to be aware of the many barriers that can prevent this process from being successful, such as the selection of a suitable age and time for transition, choosing an appropriate adult center, preparation of the parents as well as the adolescent, and poor communication between the pediatric and adult centers. The CF CNS often coordinates the process, ensuring clear lines of communication, involvement of the parents and adolescent in the decision-making process and an agreed process of transition between the pediatric and adult teams.[17–19]

Nowadays, children with CF are generally quite well and the majority of adolescents will never have needed an inpatient admission prior to transferring to adult services. However, it is often that the age of transition coincides with deterioration in health status and young people may find their first admission is to an unfamiliar ward where they do not know the staff. Many parents and young people consider the first admission for any kind of deterioration in health a life event, coupled with a change in hospital and CF team can often exacerbate their anxiety. For these individuals and their families, the first inpatient admission requires an increase in awareness and sensitivity from the ward staff and further support to both the patient and the family from the CNS liaising between the ward and the CF team.

Cross-infection is an important area of CF care, with most young people and their families aware of the problems and associated risks. All specialist CF centers have policies that have been written to meet the needs of their particular patient population.[20] Segregation is common practice in CF centers today and patients and their families will be used to safe cross-infection practices.[21] As young people become more independent, education about good hygiene and cross-infection practices are essential, with particular emphasis on hand washing, covering their mouths when coughing, and the risks of contact with others who have CF.

Death in the pediatric setting is rare due to the advances in CF care over the last decades and moving to an adult center not only brings these young people with CF into an environment where they will see others much sicker than themselves, it also signifies a step closer to death. CNSs need to be aware of the impact that a death can have on other patients in the ward at this time, and even though staff may not directly communicate a death to each patient, social networking, and texting between patients will. It is important to allow patients time to discuss their feelings and worries about their own mortality and be aware that these events can also impact on future hospital admissions.[11]

ADULTHOOD

CF is no longer a disease of childhood; today, more than half of the population of people with CF in the United Kingdom are adults and this number is increasing. Data from the UK CF Registry shows that of the 10,078 patients registered in 2012, 57.6% were 16 years or older (9.1% >40 years[7]). Similar figures have been reported in the most recent CF registries from Australia (49.3% >18 years) and the United States (49% >18 years).[22,23]

As with adolescents, adults with CF have the same anxieties and worries as their healthy peers. Studies from the United Kingdom, Canada, and Australia have all identified health, family, and financial matters as being concerns in the adult CF population.[24] As people with CF live longer, a greater number of them will live away from their parents, marry, become parents, own homes, work full time, and may also become carers themselves of their ageing parents. They will do all of these things while their disease progresses and their treatments become more complex and time consuming.[25,26] CNSs play a vital role in helping adults maintain a balance between treatment and lifestyle recognizing the need to help individuals adapt treatment regimens to suit them. This is most effectively done in collaboration with the MDT.

The CNS working with adult patients can have a varied role, which often includes:

- Educating employers and work colleagues.
- Liaison with government agencies and the work place to ensure maximum support (financial and practical) to enable patients to stay employed or retrain.
- Advocating on a patient's behalf with local social services.
- Educating and liaising with family doctors.
- Educating and liaising with local pharmacists.
- Negotiating easier access to classes at school or university.
- Advising patients on how to access services such as life insurance and mortgages, which may not have been such an issue in previous generations.
- Increasingly CNSs will work in collaboration with the family doctor, social services, and the CF team to support patients caring for their ageing parents.

As the adult CF population continues to increase, it is to be expected that more will become parents. CNSs working with adults with CF need to be aware of the reproduction options available to both males and females with CF to ensure that both men and women are able to make informed choices and are supported whatever their decision. These discussions should also involve the extended family if they plan to be involved with the care of future children in later years.

Although the majority of males with CF are infertile due to the absence of the vas deferens, many are able to father their own biological children using assisted conception techniques such as sperm aspiration and intracytoplasmic sperm injection (discussed in more detail in Chapter 28). Although the process is not influenced by health status, men with CF should be counseled before undergoing the process about life with a child, maintaining employment, managing treatment, deteriorating health, and eventual death leaving behind a single mother.

It has previously been thought that motherhood was a significant risk factor in the morbidity and mortality in women with CF. However, research has shown that with close monitoring, liaison with an obstetric team, and a reasonable lung function before conception, the outcome for both baby and mother can be good.[27-29] The CNS not only helps to coordinate this multidisciplinary approach to care but often carries out the care needed for a successful outcome.[30] Where possible, regular visits by the CNS in the community can provide invaluable support for the mother with CF both pre- and postnatally. These visits can be arranged to compliment regular appointments with the obstetric team allowing for close monitoring of the mother as well as improving communication between the two teams, thereby optimizing the care given.

Parents with CF who have children involve their children in CF in a variety of ways. Some try to keep the reality of the disease hidden away by carrying out treatments in separate rooms, not talking about CF and not taking the children to the hospital with them. Others involve their children from an early age through talking about the disease, carrying out treatment with the children around—often with the children helping—and taking them to hospital appointments with them. When providing care for adults with CF who have children, CNSs need to recognize the individual beliefs and attitudes of each patient and support them with a plan of care that will only involve their children if they wish it.[31]

ADVANCED DISEASE

It is widely recognized that complications such as pneumothorax, hemoptysis, and CFRD occur more commonly in older patients with CF.[32-34] Other complications in aging patients include osteoporosis, liver disease, cancers of the gastrointestinal tract, and arthropathy. These complications often develop at the same time as lung function starts to deteriorate, increasing the daily treatment requirements individuals have to maintain to continue with their level of health. CNSs providing an outreach service may have to manage one or more of these complications in the home. Complex medication regimens and organizing care to help maintain a lifestyle/treatment balance requires the CNS to plan care on an individual basis using their expert knowledge.

Respiratory disease is the main cause of morbidity and mortality in CF.[35] The use of oxygen therapy and noninvasive ventilation (NIV) are all commonly used in advanced disease to combat decreasing lung capacity. These treatments are not always readily accepted and part of the CNS role is to investigate the barriers to accepting these treatments and educate patients about the potential benefits of these treatments to promote independence.

When admissions become more frequent, longer in duration and the burden of treatment increases, patients or their families may wish to raise the issue of lung transplantation. The initial discussion can be a shock for both the patient and their families, and CNSs should allow plenty of opportunity to encourage discussion of these thoughts and feelings with various members of the team.[36] Early discussion with the team can raise many questions and concerns, for both patients and their families—individually or together—they may come to the CNS with queries or to seeking further information and support. The role of a CNS as advocate and educator for the patient is vital in this decision process.

Once the decision has been made, the CNS is heavily involved in the assessment process as well as supporting patients and families whether or not they have been accepted onto the list. Home visiting allows regular monitoring of patients without the ordeal of attending outpatient appointments with NIV, oxygen, or a wheelchair. Often when patients are waiting for a lung transplant, a trip to the hospital can leave them physically exhausted for the following 2 to 3 days. Regular assessment at home by the CNS allows for fewer hospital visits, regular physical and psychosocial assessment, and facilitates early admission, if required.

END OF LIFE

CF continues to be life-limiting; however, death in childhood, although uncommon, does occur. Conversely, although many young people with CF die before their thirtieth birthday, there are now a rising number of patients living with a very low lung function making short-term prognosis difficult.[37] Unlike other chronic diseases, the end stages of CF can be difficult to recognize, and during the terminal stages, symptom management can often be both active (continuing intravenous antibiotics) and palliative (commencing anxiolytics and analgesia). Although CF teams have traditionally provided a life time of care, palliative care specialists augment CF care by becoming usefully involved in symptom and end of life management.

Patients and their families have known about the prognosis of CF since diagnosis; however, even with some preparation and expectation, every death brings shock and great pain. Individuals with CF—children and adults—know when they are dying. They often need opportunities to discuss their fears and anxieties but may feel uncomfortable or protective talking about these issues with their family for fear of upsetting them or "letting them down." Advocacy allows the CNS to facilitate discussion between the patient and family, providing an opportunity for final words and goodbyes. Early discussion about an individual's wishes for the terminal stage of their disease is essential to aid appropriate care planning. Issues that may be raised include transplantation, wills, funeral arrangements, writing of letters or diaries to the family and where they would like to be when they die.[38] For some patients early discussion may be upsetting, but for others it can be a relief. The CNS needs to use judgment to assess each patient and family member individually when starting such conversations. When these discussions are well organized, patients' wishes can be documented and filed away until needed. CNSs also need be sensitive to the possibility that there may be more than one member of the family with the disease who may be affected by the end of life plans.[38]

Occasionally, there can be a lack of understanding between the patient and the CF team, again this is often due to a degree of protection. This can sometimes lead to misunderstanding and may prevent the patient and their family from making their wishes about any last requests known. The CNS can play an important role by ensuring the provision of accurate information for both the patient and the family enabling them to make choices, providing practical and emotional support for the patient and caregivers and liaising between the medical team and the patient.

Although the option of dying at home or in hospital is discussed with the patient (however old) and their family, the majority of both children and adults with CF are in hospital at the time of death. The ward has been described as a place of familiarity and security and children and adults have often said that they feel most comfortable spending their last days on the ward they have been admitted to frequently in the past.[39] Due to the complex nature of CF, it can often be difficult to determine when patients are in the final stages of their disease, with patients often receiving active treatment and medication until the last few hours of life. CNSs caring for patients at this stage are delivering a combination of preventative, therapeutic, and palliative care. These treatment regimens can be quite complex and the family may not be able to cope with such regimens in the home.

End of life management is a collaboration of care between the patient and their family, the CNS, the palliative care team, and the CF team. This collaboration provides optimum care for the patient and the family. It can also be helpful to access specialist advice providing the CNS with further ideas with which to better care for the patient.

In the United Kingdom, hospice facilities are not always available or appropriate for people with CF, with most based on an oncology model of care. However, unlike other patients with life-limiting diseases, people with CF may choose the security of hospital as a place to die. Many children and adults prefer the familiar surroundings of the ward with care being provided by staff who they may have known for many years. For the few who choose to die at home it is usually possible to liaise with local community palliative care/hospice teams. For this to be successful, the CNS plays a collaborative role, working closely with the palliative care team, the patient and family, and the CF team. Wherever the patient and their family choose for the end stages of life, the CNS offers emotional and practical support allowing the individual to die in comfort and with dignity.

BEREAVEMENT

Parents and carers of a child or adult with CF develop a close and trusting relationship with the CF team, often over many years. Although the CF team have a primary responsibility for the patient, there is no doubt that the sudden cessation of this relationship at death can cause additional feelings of loss to already bereaved families.[11] It is now widely accepted that ongoing bereavement care should be provided by the CF team—often the CNS.

People cope with grief in different ways, unfortunately in today's society we have little experience of death and therefore often do not know how to deal with our own or other people's sorrow. At a time when families most need support from each other, there can be difficulty in recognizing and accepting different reactions. Men and women respond differently, especially when their child has died (whatever age their child may have been). Mothers are more likely to experience a wide range of emotions including anxiety, anger, guilt, and despair. Fathers are more likely to focus their grief experiencing social isolation and hostility. As well as feeling different there may well be a mismatch in the highs and lows of coping and unfortunately this can lead to feelings of irritation and anger toward each other. The CNS plays a key role in these circumstances by providing individual emotional support and by helping parents to understand each other's grief reaction, thereby allowing them to support each other.

Although some families are willing to return to the hospital following a death, many find this very difficult. Visiting the family at home allows bereavement support to be offered in a safe and comfortable environment. Home visiting also allows other family members, siblings, or grandparents, for example, to receive some support. Unfortunately, although bereavement support is regarded as a role that CNSs or clinical psychologists take on, workload excludes this as a long-term commitment. Instead CNSs and clinical psychologists must be aware of alternatives and be ready to refer on to other agencies at an appropriate time.

THE FUTURE

The population of adults with CF is growing as deaths in childhood become rare and adults survive longer. The need for CNSs with expertise in CF will increase as the adult population demand increasing support and intervention allowing them to live full and active lives away from the hospital setting. Pharmacological and technological advances will continue to improve the management of CF care in the future however; with greater access to information people with CF are also exploring alternative options available to them. CNSs will have to become familiar not only with the current research and potential new therapies but also with the options of complementary and alternative therapies.

Unfortunately, CF will continue to remain a life-limiting disease for many years to come. An increasing life expectancy inevitably leads to an older and sicker group of adults. CNSs will find a rise in the numbers of patients they have to support through the end of their lives. Many of these adults will have partners, children, and grandchildren and bereavement care and support will become an important part of the CNS role.

CNSs in the future will find themselves providing a service that will help to enhance the treatment/work/life balance for many adults and will include increased support in the home, college, and workplace. This service, however, may not always be face to face; the CNS will have to become familiar with the developing e-technology of telemedicine, webcams, texting/messaging, and video phones (Skype, etc.). However, whether consulting by video link or face-to-face, the CNS will continue to offer both practical and emotional support to children and adults with CF, their parents, partners, and families.

REFERENCES

1. Madge S, Khair K. Multi-disciplinary teams in the United Kingdom: Problems and solutions. *J Pediatr Nurs* 2000; **15**(2): 131–4.
2. Cystic Fibrosis Trust. *Standards for the Clinical Care of Children and Adults with Cystic Fibrosis*. London, United Kingdom: Cystic Fibrosis Trust; 2011.
3. Kerem E, Conway S, Elborn S, Heijerman H. Standards of care for patients with cystic fibrosis: A European consensus. *J Cyst Fibros* 2005; **4**(1): 7–26.
4. Madge S, Dack K, Peres A. *Cystic fibrosis: The CNS specialist's role. Independent Nurse* 2011: 18–20.
5. Madge SL. National consensus standards for nursing children and young people with cystic fibrosis. *Paediatr Nurs* 2002; **14**(1): 32–5.
6. Nursing and Midwifery Council. *The NMC Code of Professional Conduct: Standards for Conduct, Performance and Ethics*. London, United Kingdom: Nursing and Midwifery Council; 2004.

7. Cystic Fibrosis Trust. *UK CF Registry.*London, United Kingdom: Cystic Fibrosis Trust; 2012.

8. Salm N, Yetter E, Tluczek A. Informing parents about positive newborn screen results: Parents' recommendations. *J Child Health Care* 2012; **16** (4): 367–81.

9. Geller DE, Madge SL. Technological and behavioural strategies to reduce treatment burden and improve adherence to inhaled antibiotics in cystic fibrosis. *Respir Med* 2011; **105** (Suppl 2): S24–31.

10. Madge S. Challenges for nurses. In: Bush A, Alton EWFW, Davies JC, Griesenbach U, Jaffe A (Eds). *Cystic Fibrosis in the 21st Century. Progress in Respiratory Research.* Vol. 34. Basel, Switzerland: Karger; 2006. pp. 286–92.

11. Madge S. Growing up and growing older with cystic fibrosis. *J R Soc Med* 2006; **99** (Suppl 46): 23–6.

12. Bolyard DR. Sexuality and cystic fibrosis. *Am J Matern Child Nurs* 2001; **26**(1): 39–41.

13. Roberts S, Green P. Sexual health of adolescents with cystic fibrosis. *J R Soc Med* 2005; **98** (Suppl 45): 7–16.

14. Arias Lorente RP, Bousono Garcia C, Diaz Martin JJ. Treatment compliance in children and adults with cystic fibrosis. *J Cyst Fibros* 2008; **7**: 359–67.

15. Nasr SZ. Cystic fibrosis in adolescents and young adults. *Adol Med* 2000; **11**(3): 589–603.

16. Madge S, Bryon M. A model for transition of care in cystic fibrosis. *J Pediatr Nurs* 2002; **17**(4): 283–8.

17. Flume PA, Taylor LA, Anderson DL, et al. Transition programs in cystic fibrosis centers: Perceptions of team members. *Pediatr Pulmonol* 2004; **37**(1): 4–7.

18. Bryon M, Madge S. Transition from paediatric to adult care: Psychological principles. *J R Soc Med* 2001; **94** (Suppl 40): 5–7.

19. Royal Brompton & Harefield guide to CF transition. www.rbht.nhs.uk/cf-transition/.

20. Henskens JE, VonNessen SK. Burkholderia cepacia in cystic fibrosis: Implications for nursing practice. *Pediatr Nurs* 2000; **26**(3): 325–8.

21. Conway S. Segregation is good for patients with cystic fibrosis. *J R Soc Med* 2008; **101** (Suppl 1): S31–5.

22. Cystic fibrosis in Australia 2012, 15th Annual Report from the Australian Cystic Fibrosis Data Registry.

23. Cystic Fibrosis Foundation. *Cystic Fibrosis Foundation Patient Registry, 2012 Annual Data Report.* Bethesda, MD: Cystic Fibrosis Foundation.

24. De Launiere L, Paquet F, Hébert Y. Socio-economic profile of the adult cystic fibrosis population of Quebec. *J Cyst Fibros* 2004;**3** (Suppl 1): 109.

25. Dobbin CJ, Bye PT. Adults with cystic fibrosis: Meeting the challenge. *Int Med J* 2003; **33**(12): 593–7.

26. Quon BS, Aitken ML. Cystic fibrosis: What to expect now in the early adult years. *Paediatr Respir Rev* 2012; **13**(4): 206–14.

27. Pernaut J, Audra P, Mossan C, Gaucherand P. Cystic fibrosis and pregnancy: Report of twin pregnancy and review of the literature. *Journal de Gynécologie Obstétrique et Biologie de la Reproduction* 2005; **34**(7): 716–20.

28. Boyd JM, Metha A, Murphy DJ. Fertility and pregnancy outcomes in men and women with cystic fibrosis in the United Kingdom. *Hum Reprod* 2004; **19**(10): 2238–43.

29. Thorpe-Beeston JG, Madge S, Gyi K, Hodson M, Bilton D. The outcome of pregnancies in women with cystic fibrosis—Single centre experience 1998–2011. *BJOG* 2013;**120**(3): 354–61.

30. Connors PM, Ulles MM. The physical, psychosocial and social implications of caring for the pregnant patient and newborn with cystic fibrosis. *J Perinat Neonatal Nurs* 2005; **19**(4): 301–15.

31. Edenborough FP, Borgo G, Knoop C, et al.; for the European Cystic Fibrosis Society. Guidelines for the management of pregnancy in women with cystic fibrosis. *J Cyst Fibros* 2008; **7** (Suppl 1): S2–32.

32. Flume PA, Yankaskas JR, Ebeling M, Husley T, Clark LL. Massive hemoptysis in cystic fibrosis. *Chest* 2005; **128**(2): 729–38.

33. Flume PA, Strange C, Ye X, Ebeling M, Husley T, Clark LL. Pneumothorax in cystic fibrosis. **Chest** 2005; **28**(2): 720–8.

34. Mackie AD, Thornton SJ, Edenborough FP. Cystic fibrosis related diabetes. *Diabet Med* 2003; **20**(6): 425–36.

35. Döring G, Flume P, Heijerman H, Elborn JS; for the Consensus Study Group. Treatment of lung infection in patients with cystic fibrosis: Current and future strategies. *J Cyst Fibros* 2012; **11**(6): 461–79.

36. Boehler A. Update on cystic fibrosis: Selected aspects related to lung transplantation. *Swiss Med Wkly* 2003; **133**(7–8): 111–7.

37. George PM, Banya W, Pareek N, et al. Improved survival at low lung function in cystic fibrosis: Cohort study from 1990 to 2007. *Br Med J* 2011; **342**: d1008.

38. Lowton K. 'A bed in the middle of no where': Parents' meanings of place of death for adults with cystic fibrosis. *Soc Sci Med* 2009; **69**(7): 1056–62.

39. Sands D, Repetto T, Dupont LJ, et al. End of life care for patients with cystic fibrosis *J Cyst Fibros* 2011; **10**(2): S37–44.

43

Physiotherapy

PENNY AGENT, NICOLA COLLINS, AND HELEN PARROTT

INTRODUCTION

As cystic fibrosis (CF) is a multisystem disease, physiotherapy for people with CF needs to deliver a comprehensive holistic treatment-management approach. Traditionally, the primary focus of physiotherapy has been airway clearance, and while this remains a core component of physiotherapy management, the role of the physiotherapist in CF has expanded to address the miscellany of issues presented by this multisystem disease. Specialist CF physiotherapists are expert autonomous practitioners who individually tailor the assessment and treatment of airway clearance, exercise (Chapter 36), postural and musculoskeletal issues, urinary incontinence, and inhalation therapy (Chapter 20) as a routine part of daily CF care. In addition, other important aspects may include support during pregnancy (Chapter 28), the management of respiratory failure with noninvasive ventilation (NIV) (Chapter 19), and terminal care (Chapter 46). Multiple aspects of physiotherapy are essential in the day-to-day management of CF and it is acknowledged that the holistic care required can be a huge burden for patients, and adherence to various treatments is challenging. Delivery of care must be flexible and adapted according to patient need, taking into account all relevant physical and psychosocial factors.

AIRWAY CLEARANCE

MUCOCILIARY AND AIRWAY CLEARANCE

Mucociliary clearance is a critical host defense mechanism of the upper and lower airways. Mucus transport depends on the integrity and function of the ciliated epithelium lining the airways, the properties of the mucus (quantity, viscosity, and rheology), and the shear forces generated by alterations in airflow from breathing. For airway clearance techniques to be effective, therefore, there must be an alteration in airflow and ventilation, allowing air to get behind or past the secretions[1] and the greater the shear force generated, the greater the movement of mucus.

Airflow can be affected by factors such as airway resistance, expiratory pressures, bronchial wall stability, and elastic recoil. Airway clearance techniques use various physiological concepts, such as asynchronous ventilation (faster filling times for healthier areas, slower for obstructed areas) where time constants and collateral ventilation allow for equal filling of alveoli (pendelluft), enhanced collateral channel ventilation (although absent in <1-year-olds), and the equal pressure point (EPP).[1] Inspiratory holds can be used to optimize filling time for obstructed areas promoting improved ventilation through collateral channels and interdependence. The EPP is the point at which the pressure within the airway is equal to the external pressure resulting in a zero pressure difference across the airway wall. Dynamic compression of the airways occurs downstream of the EPP toward the mouth, with the EPP being manipulated by the size of lung volume used for the forced expiratory maneuver. This principle defines the use of the forced expiration technique (FET) at varying lung volumes to cause a wave of compression to shear mucus through the airways (Figure 43.1).

In theory, airway clearance techniques reduce mucus plugging in CF and aid clearance of secretions containing inflammatory cell mediators and bacterial products in mucus, thereby reducing damage to airway epithelia and bronchial walls. In the short term, the aim is to reduce airway obstruction and resistance while improving airflow and ventilation. The long-term aims of practicing regular airway clearance are to delay disease progression and maintain optimal respiratory function, thereby maximizing quality of life.

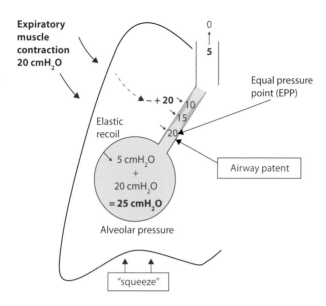

Figure 43.1 Equal pressure point (EPP): a static representation of a dynamic state, where the EPP moves dependent on the lung volume.

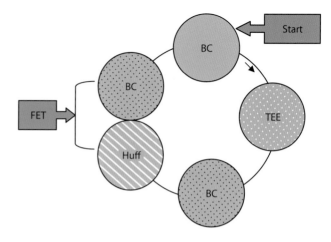

Figure 43.2 Components of the active cycle of breathing techniques (ACBT). BC, breathing control; TEE, thoracic expansion exercises; FET, forced expiration technique; huff, see text for explanation.

ACTIVE CYCLE OF BREATHING TECHNIQUES

The active cycle of breathing techniques (ACBT) consists of a flexible, repetitive cycle of breathing control, thoracic expansion exercises, and the FET (Figure 43.2). Each component of the cycle is clearly defined, but the length of each phase is flexible and should be adapted to individual patient need. ACBT is a useful airway clearance technique at all stages of the disease and can be introduced in young children as huffing/blowing games. As the ACBT is independent of a device and has no contra-indications for use, it is often recommended (along with autogenic drainage [AD]) as a first-line treatment technique, as long as the patient is able to follow instructions (Video 43.1).

Components of ACBT:

- Breathing control: tidal breathing using the lower chest, with minimal work of breathing (WOB). It is used between the more active parts of the cycle with its duration adapted according to patient need.
- Thoracic expansion exercises: active deep breathing exercises to full inspiration with a 3-second hold at end inspiration. Exhalation is passive and unforced.
- FET: one or two huffs (forced expirations) combined with breathing control.[2] Huffing to low lung volumes should be used first to assist in mobilizing and clearing peripherally situated secretions, followed by medium, and then high lung volumes when secretions have mobilized to the larger proximal upper airways.

ACBT has been shown to be effective and efficient in the mobilization and clearance of secretions[3,4] and short-term improvement in lung function.[5] It does not increase hypoxemia[6] and airflow obstruction[3,7] and is not further enhanced by the addition of devices, such as the Flutter,[7,8] positive expiratory pressure (PEP),[9] and high-frequency chest wall oscillation (HFCWO).[10] ACBT has been used in many short-term crossover trials in CF demonstrating equivalence in sputum cleared[8] and was demonstrated to have equivalent airway clearance effectiveness to AD, PEP, and oscillating PEP over a one-year study period.[11] A systematic review compared ACBT with other airway clearance therapies in CF, concluding that it was comparable to other therapies in outcomes such as patient preference, lung function, sputum weight, oxygen saturation, and number of pulmonary exacerbations.[12]

AUTOGENIC DRAINAGE

AD uses controlled breathing that aims to attain the highest expiratory airflows to move secretions from peripheral to central airways while avoiding coughing and significant airway closure/compression.[13–15]

Inhalation airflow velocity is slow, incorporating an end-inspiratory hold, to avoid inhomogeneous filling of the lungs and promote optimal filling of obstructed lung segments using collateral ventilatory channels. Exhalation airflow is linear and localized to generate shear forces within the airway to influence movement of secretions. The aim of AD is to achieve the optimal expiratory airflow, which is the highest expiratory flow velocity, without causing airway compression.[14] As AD requires breathing at different lung volumes, the expiratory airflow changes the position of the EPP and improves secretion clearance. AD can be performed in any position.

AD was traditionally taught as a 3-phase breathing regimen using low, medium, and high lung volumes to unstick, collect, and evacuate mucus[13] (see Figure 43.3, Video 43.2). However, more recently a more graduated "conveyor belt" approach is being described. The patient is also taught to localize their secretions using auditory, tactile, and proprioceptive stimuli to facilitate mucociliary clearance.[16]

Although four breaths are shown in Figure 43.3, more will usually be required for each phase for an actual treatment. Technique:

1. Clear the upper airway.
2. Take relevant inhaled medications to optimize airway clearance.
3. Assessment breath to localize secretions.
4. Slow inspiration through nose with open glottis, 2- to 4-second hold before exhalation.
5. Exhalation through nose or mouth with open glottis to the localized lung volume level.
6. Usually begins with functional, tidal, low lung volume breaths from expiratory reserve volume. This is repeated until secretions are audibly gathering in the airways.
7. At this point, the functional tidal volume is gradually raised toward mid to high lung volume as larger tidal volumes are taken.
8. Coughing should be restricted until the mucus has reached the large airways or the trachea. It can then be evacuated with a high lung volume huff or cough.

The AD technique can be optimized with an AD belt or therapist-applied manual pressure (overpressure) to the chest.

There is a paucity of evidence to support AD. AD was compared to ACBT combined with postural drainage in 18 adult CF patients. AD cleared mucus faster than the alternative technique. However, both methods improved ventilation, as measured by radio aerosol, and there was no significant difference in lung function between techniques.[17] A comparative 2-year crossover study compared AD to postural drainage and percussion, and no significant difference was demonstrated in pulmonary function between techniques although both groups improved. However, patients preferred AD.[18] In addition, when AD was compared to high-pressure positive expiratory pressure (Hi PEP) both techniques significantly improved lung function, AD to a greater extent, but AD also cleared less sputum.[19]

A randomized controlled trial of five different airway clearance techniques (ACBT, AD, PEP, and oscillating PEP) over 1 year found no significant difference between techniques in terms of pulmonary function (FEV$_1$)[11]; however, it may be questioned whether the groups in this trial were adequately powered to show differences. It is concluded that patient preference is one of the most important factors to consider when choosing an airway clearance technique, as patients are more likely to adhere to treatments they prefer.[11]

ASSISTED AUTOGENIC DRAINAGE

Assisted autogenic drainage (AAD) is used in infants or non-cooperative patients and moves their functional breathing level progressively toward their vital capacity by manual pressure (see Figure 43.4) or AD belt over the chest during inspiration. This stimulates the patient to exhale slightly more with each breath and guides the patient toward the desired lung volume to mobilize secretions. The abdominal wall is stabilized where necessary during the procedure and the cough is spontaneous.[21] Where appropriate, AAD can be combined with bouncing on a gym ball to relax the patient and enhance expiratory airflow velocity. Gastroesophageal reflux is not associated with this technique if the child is held in the upright sitting position.[21]

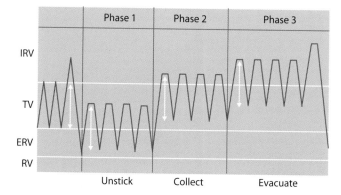

Figure 43.3 Physiological representation of the three phases of autogenic drainage. IRV, inspiratory reserve volume; TV, tidal volume; ERV, expiratory reserve volume; RV, residual volume. White arrows indicate size of respirations similar to normal tidal volume breaths.

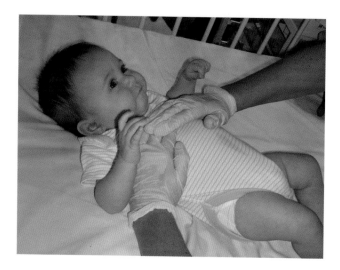

Figure 43.4 Assisted autogenic drainage in infants.

POSITIVE EXPIRATORY PRESSURE

PEP requires the patient to exhale against a mask (Figure 43.5a) or mouthpiece (Figure 43.5b) (with or without a nose clip) with resistance applied via a valved system. This resistance creates PEP in the airway, which temporarily increases functional residual capacity (FRC), encouraging collateral ventilation and alveolar interdependence to recruit closed airways. Airflow increases behind secretions obstructing the airway, increasing gas volume and pressure, thus facilitating mobilization of the secretions to the larger airways ready for FETs.[22]

PEP may also be helpful in supporting unstable airways by reducing dynamic compression during exhalation. This will again facilitate mobilization of secretions, which may have previously been "stuck" behind "floppy airways."[23]

A PEP of 10–20 cmH$_2$O during mid-expiration is thought to be optimal and can be measured by a manometer inserted into the expiratory limb.[24]

PEP is often carried out in sitting, but can be performed in any position, for 12–15 breaths followed by the FET (Video 43.3). PEP may also be combined with other airway clearance techniques, such as AD or postural drainage and percussion, or nebulizer therapy, such as hypertonic saline.[25] However, it must be recognized that although this may lower total aerosol deposition, it may be redistributed peripherally.[26]

PEP has been shown to be superior to postural drainage and percussion in terms of pulmonary function, in a 1-year study of 40 children with CF.[27]

Mortensten et al. (1991) found that both PEP and ACBT resulted in greater central and peripheral secretion clearance as measured by radio aerosol compared to controls.[28] However, comparing three different airway clearance techniques Lannefors and Wollner[29] found there was no difference in mucus cleared between postural drainage with thoracic expansion exercises, PEP and exercise (all techniques included FETs) as measured by radio aerosol although this study only had nine patients included and therefore may be significantly underpowered to detect changes.

In a comparative study of PEP and Flutter, PEP was found to be superior, as children using Flutter had a greater decline in lung function, and greater hospitalization and antibiotic use over 1 year. However, results for FEV$_1$ were not significant.[30]

A 1-year multicenter national study compared HFCWO to PEP.[31] PEP mask therapy was associated with significantly fewer pulmonary exacerbations and use of antibiotics than HFCWO; shorter treatment times were also reported for PEP.

A systematic review evaluated 25 studies that compared PEP to another form of airway clearance and found no significant difference in FEV$_1$ between techniques. However, in studies carried out for more than 1 month, patients tended to prefer PEP. It should be noted that the PEP studies included in this review were generally of poor quality and not adequately powered or did not include enough information to be included in a meta-analysis, and therefore results from these studies should be interpreted with caution.[32]

PEP was adapted for use with infants in the 1980s. It can be carried out in upright sitting in the caregiver's arms or seated on a gym ball with one hand holding the face mask (see Figure 43.6a). By listening and looking at the breathing

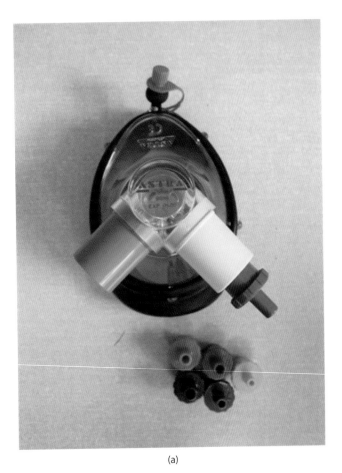

(a)

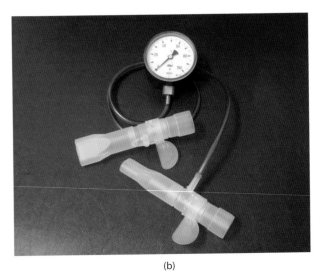

(b)

Figure 43.5 (a) Positive expiratory pressure (PEP) applied via a mask (Astra Tech, Stonehouse, United Kingdom). (b) PEP applied via a mouthpiece (Courtesy of PARI Medical Limited, West Byfleet, United Kingdom).

established in CF, and some authors may argue commencing therapy without obvious immediate benefit may worsen adherence.[61]

Whenever the physiotherapist decides to commence respiratory physiotherapy in the infant, there are a number of different treatment options available: modified postural drainage and percussion, infant PEP, AAD, and exercise. However, due to a paucity of trials, there is no evidence that one technique is superior to another.

Exercise should be encouraged from diagnosis and its importance throughout life highlighted. As the child becomes older, active participation in their physiotherapy is important to improve efficiency and effectiveness. Blowing games, huffing, and bubble PEP are useful and can lead to ACBT and airway clearance devices as appropriate.

POSTURAL DRAINAGE

Postural drainage uses gravity to drain individual lobes/segments of the lung.[63] Traditional head-down tilt postural drainage has gone out of vogue in recent years. This is not only due to evidence of gastroesophageal reflux being associated with the head-down tilt position,[64] but also due to patient-reported discomfort, changes in CF sputum viscosity, and the development of many other airway clearance techniques.[65] In fact, postural drainage in the head-down tilt position is generally only used on an individual patient basis with localized pathology. Modified postural drainage in the horizontal position has been shown to be equally effective,[65] and in infants, modified postural drainage was associated with fewer respiratory complications than the head down tilt position.[66] It is recommended that postural drainage should be combined with other airway clearance techniques such as PEP, ACBT, and AD.[52]

CONTINENCE

Urinary incontinence (the involuntary leakage of urine) is a problem that affects people with CF more than the healthy population.[67] It affects males (prevalence 5%–16%)[68] and to a greater extent females (30%–68%)[52,67] with CF. Onset of urinary incontinence has been reported in girls with CF as young as 9–11 years, and prevalence rates in females range from 30%–68%.[69]

Urinary incontinence is thought to be exacerbated by chronic cough, airway clearance demands, and physical exercise,[70] and is more common in worsening disease.[71] Urinary incontinence also has a significant impact on quality of life, and therefore it is vital that CF is identified and managed early by the CF physiotherapist, as treatment outcomes are favorable.[72] Most patients will be too embarrassed to bring it up on consultation unless the therapist asks directly.

Expert recommendations for the management of urinary incontinence include teaching patients "the knack" (contraction of the pelvic floor during activities such as sneezing, coughing, laughing), strength and endurance training

of the pelvic floor and lower abdominal muscles (3 sets of 10 pelvic floor exercises per day—pull pelvic floor upward toward diaphragm and hold for 3–5 seconds, then superimpose 3 quick contractions pulling each one higher up),[70] and optimal positioning during airway clearance to enhance pelvic floor function (feet flat on floor with 90 degree angle at hips and knees and neutral or extended lumbar spine).[73] In clinical practice, physiotherapists suggest avoid jumping on a trampoline after puberty and jog/step on it instead to avoid excessive downward pressure on the pelvic floor.

MUSCULOSKELETAL AND POSTURAL CONSIDERATIONS

Chronic and progressive respiratory disease leads to altered ventilatory mechanics and changes in chest wall structure. As a result, postural abnormalities and the associated pain have been identified in both adults and children[74] commonly including thoracic kyphosis and anterior glenohumeral joint positioning with tight pectoral musculature.[75]

Excessive coughing, gas trapping leading to hyperinflation, and breathlessness exert repetitive and abnormal forces on the musculoskeletal system over time. The development of secondary abnormalities is inevitable and often feature tight and sore trunk soft tissues and muscle, and pelvic floor insufficiency.[75] It has long been appreciated that the muscles in the trunk have a dual function of postural control and contribution to respiration,[76] so in time, optimal posture will be compromised to meet the demands of the hard working respiratory system. A vicious cycle of advancing disease, postural adaptations, and associated pain can occur. There are many factors that may contribute to musculoskeletal changes and pain, which must also be considered including poor nutrition, low bone mineral density, vitamin D and K deficiencies, long-term use of steroid therapy, infection and inflammation, and low physical activity levels.

There is an increasing body of evidence to support the role of musculoskeletal strategies for both the prevention and management of postural abnormalities and the associated musculoskeletal pain, and these should be considered from childhood. The authors of an observational study identifying postural changes in adults with CF reported that the angle of thoracic kyphosis was partly improved by simple postural education.[77] Reductions in the decline of FEV_1 and significant improvements in chest mobility, body strength, and subjective well-being were found in a 12-month interventional study where patients were given postural correction advice and exercises.[78] Improvement in pain and ease of breathing were achieved in a single-intervention study using manual techniques and massage in patients who presented with musculoskeletal concerns.[79]

There has been much work recently into the development of CF-specific musculoskeletal assessment tools to help identify the patients who would benefit from further advice and those who may require further input from and specialist musculoskeletal services.[52] Assessment and monitoring of musculoskeletal issues and the associated symptoms should be undertaken regularly by the CF specialist physiotherapist and can occur in the hospital, outpatient, or clinic setting.[52]

Basic postural and positioning advice should be individually tailored to each patient and take into consideration their activities within the home, school, and workplace. An awareness of appropriate postures during airway clearance techniques, inhalation therapy, and prolonged activities should be encouraged. Gentle early activity should be encouraged during recovery from an infective pulmonary exacerbation to ensure that poor posture secondary to increased coughing is not sustained. The annual review is an excellent opportunity to educate the patient and family on the importance of maintaining an active lifestyle and the positive impact that cardiovascular exercise and strengthening can have on bone mineral density and postural control.

TRANSITION AND INDEPENDENCE

Transition is detailed in Chapter 41 and is a process that should be undertaken over many years and openly discussed among the patient, family, and CF team, so that the family and adolescent are prepared for the move into adult CF care. Independence in carrying out treatments, including airway clearance, is an important part of transition. It is also a process that should be carried out slowly, in a planned and structured way, so that the child/adolescent is not suddenly given excessive responsibility which they are unequipped to manage, resulting in poor adherence to therapy.

ADHERENCE

Adherence to airway clearance is variable but is often reported as low.[80] Reasons for poor adherence include patients forgetting to do it, not feeling any immediate effect, time consuming, boring, and a burden.[81,82]

A questionnaire-based study of 63 adult CF patients actually reported a 60% high adherence rate to treatment and a 21% poor adherence rate. Lower education levels were strongly associated with poor adherence. PEP and Flutter were preferred techniques, whereas ACBT and AD showed moderate agreement and postural drainage and percussion showed low agreement.[83]

Education and understanding of the importance of airway clearance is paramount and patient preference in a chosen vital technique. Different techniques may suit different personalities at different times of their life. Treatment compromises that are adhered to may be more important than optimal techniques that are not performed.[33]

It is clear that caregivers are poor at predicting adherence among their patients as demonstrated in a study comparing adherence rates both predicted by clinicians and also from self-reports to electronic monitoring via a nebulizer-download facility (I-neb® nebulizer system).[84] Median adherence for self- and clinician reporting was 80% and 50%–60%, respectively; this is compared to actual adherence rates of 36% of prescribed treatment.

The therapist should work with the patient and family to understand how treatment can fit into their lifestyle, family dynamics, and cultural needs, so realistic regimens can be set. These should be adapted as appropriate throughout the patient's life.[84]

SPECIAL SITUATIONS

RESPIRATORY MUSCLE FATIGUE/COUGH

Respiratory muscles may fatigue in patients with severe disease and also be placed at mechanical disadvantage due to hyperinflated lungs and an altered thoracic cage. There is no evidence that respiratory muscle training improves a patient's functional capacity, although improvements in respiratory muscle strength are seen with this intervention.[85,86] As previously discussed, patients with respiratory muscle fatigue may benefit from positive pressure support during airway clearance to reduce their WOB.

An effective cough is vitally important to adequately clear the airway. It requires an inspiratory volume of 80%–90% of vital capacity, glottal closure for 0.2 seconds, and adequate contraction of intact expiratory muscles.[87] Any abnormalities in cough should be fully investigated by the CF team, and physiotherapy techniques may have to be optimized accordingly.

Patients with cough abnormality/weakness may also benefit from lung volume recruitment, breath stacking and a manually supported cough, or the use of mechanical insufflation–exsufflation devices, although none of these techniques have been studied in CF and are more commonly used in treating patients with neuromuscular disease.

Cough may also be abnormal due to malacic/unstable airways, premature airway closure, or vocal cord dysfunction; in these instances, PEP and Hi PEP may be useful for forced expirations and coughing, in combination with breathing control.[23] Stress incontinence may impact on patient's willingness to cough and should be assessed for. A tussis nervosa may also have to be considered in patients with abnormal cough, and multidisciplinary team working with speech and language therapy and psychology can be helpful. Cough suppression techniques may have to be taught in patients with irritable ineffective coughing, and directed effective coughing encouraged instead.

BREATHING PATTERN DISORDERS

Patients with CF, like those with and without respiratory disease, may, at some point in life, develop abnormal patterns of breathing. This may occur following an acute exacerbation or a life event such as a pregnancy, change in job role, or bereavement. Unfortunately, the associated symptoms of disordered breathing such as breathlessness, chest pains, tightness, and headache can be mistaken for the progression of CF lung disease. The assessment of breathing patterns and the impact on respiratory presentation is therefore an essential skill of the CF specialist physiotherapist and can play an important role in helping the wider medical team to identify the cause of symptoms.

Breathing pattern retraining programs have long been recognized as successful in realigning disordered patterns of breathing in other respiratory conditions such as asthma.[88–90] They focus on reducing the rate, depth, and volume of breathing through breathing awareness and relaxation. To date, there is no evidence to support the use of such approaches specifically in CF; however, in clinical practice, the knowledge of "normal" breathing patterns and mechanics can help to reduce anxiety, WOB, and maximize functional capacity. In addition, managing the symptoms of disordered breathing and normalizing abnormal patterns can avoid unnecessary increases in medical treatments.

PREGNANCY

CF teams are now more frequently required to support women with CF through one, if not multiple pregnancies, as part of routine CF center care. There are many maternal health-related factors that indicate the likely course and success of a pregnancy with preconception pulmonary function being one of the most important.[91,92] Females with an FEV_1 >60% predicted and above are at a lower risk of developing complications during pregnancy, delivery, and postpartum.[91,93] Knowledge of the physiological changes during pregnancy will assist the physiotherapist in planning any changes to airway clearance and exercise regimes (Table 43.1).

Women with CF may require many changes to their airway clearance during pregnancy to maximize treatment effect.[94] Positioning for airway clearance will require modifications potentially from an early stage in the pregnancy when nausea can impact on chest clearance and sitting, standing and head-up positions should be considered. Postural drainage in head-down tilted positions is not advised because the hormonal changes that occur can result in a reduction of the lower esophageal sphincter tone. This, combined with the growing weight of the baby and gravid uterus applying pressure on the stomach, can put the mother at increased risk of reflux at a time when there is a higher incidence of reflux symptoms.[95] Airway clearance techniques that allow upright positioning are well tolerated and combining or alternating between techniques, depending on symptoms, can also be useful.

Additional nebulized medications are commonly used during pregnancy when the use of systemic preparations is limited by concerns about possible teratogenicity. Proactive use of mucoactive agents such as RhDNase and hypertonic saline will help to optimize airway clearance when it is limited by physiological changes. Ensuring women are familiar with using a fast, and intelligent nebulizer system will be good preparation for the postpartum period where time is limited when caring for the newborn child.

Some women will require hospital admissions during their pregnancy to maintain health stability and nutritional status. This is an opportunity to review airway clearance and monitor the patient's WOB during pulmonary exacerbations and as the uterus continues to grow and impede lung excursion. Physiotherapists should have a low threshold for using positive pressure devices (such as IPPB and NIV) to reduce WOB, improve lung expansion as FRC reduces, and, therefore, enhance airway clearance effectiveness. If, on the rare occasion, the patient becomes more unwell toward or during the delivery period, NIV can also be used to support ventilation. Proactive assessment for ambulatory oxygen desaturation is recommended and supplementary oxygen can be used to avoid drops in fetal oxygen delivery.

Pregnant women should be advised to modify their exercise programs to avoid contact sports and reduce overheating and dehydration that can occur. Walking, swimming, and prenatal yoga are recommended forms of exercise that can be used to maintain fitness levels during pregnancy. The physiotherapist should also ensure that patients are given postural awareness advice, strengthening and stability work for the lumbosacral and pelvic floor regions and onward referrals to musculoskeletal and women's health services for further input if required.

Table 43.1 Physiological changes in pregnancy and the impact in CF

In Pregnancy	In a CF Pregnancy
Reflux	Reflux may lead to severe symptoms
Potential for gestational diabetes	CFRD may be present or gestational diabetes can lead to CFRD
Estrogen = increased mucous production	Mucous retention = increased infection risk
Progesterone = increased respiratory rate	Increased respiratory rate on the background of dyspnea
Reduced FRC by 10%–20%	Reduced FRC can lead to lung areas nearing closing volumes = atelectasis and hypoxia
Increased cardiac output, metabolic rate + oxygen consumption	High nutritional needs already exist, so pregnancy increases this further

The CF specialist physiotherapist is well placed to support the pregnant woman with CF in planning the support and care they will need postdelivery. Completing airway clearance and nebulized medication is essential to stabilize and improve pulmonary function once the baby has arrived; however, it can be the most challenging time as the CF mother will be torn between doing treatment and tending to her child. Providing advice on structuring family assistance, combining treatments (e.g., hypertonic saline and PEP), using nap times for airway clearance, planning who can clean equipment, etc. are useful topics to consider before the baby is due.

THE ASYMPTOMATIC ADULT WITH CF

There is little evidence to support the physiotherapist in deciding an appropriate management strategy for the asymptomatic adult with CF. Much of the evidence for airway clearance routines has been obtained by researching populations of CF adults with impaired lung function, chronically infected with *Pseudomonas aeruginosa*, and who have chronic sputum production.[11,96,97] It is reasonable to consider that patients with less characteristic presentations of CF, i.e., atypical disease, should require a different therapeutic approach to those patients with established lung pathology; however, the approach is likely to vary somewhat from center to center and from country to country.

Clearly, the first step in the clinical reasoning process is to have a robust approach to determining the presence of symptoms and/or disease in the adult population. There are different ways of determining this (see Chapter 10 for more details); however, concurrently, the CF specialist physiotherapist is well placed to inform decision making through the routine patient assessment. Observing spirometry technique, exercise testing, and assessing performance of the FET or airway clearance techniques can give valuable information about the presence of sputum, airway constriction, and breathlessness in the patient who claims to be asymptomatic. It is advised that when recommending routine airway clearance for the presence of suspected symptoms and/or lung disease, the physiotherapist should discuss the recommendations with the wider CF multi-disciplinary team (MDT) to ensure everyone follows a similar approach to care and attempt to evaluate the benefit to the patient over time. The truly asymptomatic patient is one subpopulation of CF adults that would benefit from an evidence base or consensus to support physiotherapy recommendations.

In the symptomatic patient with lung disease, there is some evidence to suggest that exercise strategies alone are inferior to airway clearance techniques in terms of sputum clearance.[98] In the asymptomatic patient, however, where there is no evidence of sputum retention, exercise advice and optimizing cardiovascular fitness should form the basis and focus of physiotherapy intervention. There is a wealth of evidence to support the impact of physical training programs on exercise capacity, strength, and lung function in people with CF.[44] Additional evidence in the asymptomatic population would further support the CF specialist physiotherapist in determining the best focus for our role with this patient group.

HEMOPTYSIS

Hemoptysis is the expectoration of blood from the lungs or bronchial tubes as a result of pulmonary or bronchial hemorrhage. Bleeding is sudden and usually arises from a bronchial artery, but reports also suggest aberrant origin of bleeding from nonbronchial collateral vessels or from anastomoses between the bronchial and nonbronchial circulation.[99]

From a physiotherapy perspective, the awareness of hemoptysis management is imperative, as the incidence of occasional mild hemoptysis is common in CF. There is a paucity of literature regarding the physiotherapy management, and guidance is drawn from clinical practice recommendations.[52,100] These recommendations advise alterations to practice according to the volume of blood expectorated (see Table 43.2).

Generally, airway clearance is beneficial in aiding the removal of purulent secretions contributing to pulmonary exacerbations[101] and also aiding the removal of blood products/clots, which heighten the inflammatory response and may cause atelectasis. Particularly in moderate or massive hemoptysis, modification of physiotherapy is prudent.[52] The benefits and risks of techniques must always be evaluated, and controlled breathing techniques such as ACBT or AD may be favored over positive pressure treatments, which may induce intrathoracic pressure changes and aggravate bleeding from friable vessels. A controlled FET to limit forceful coughing is advised to expectorate secretions. There is no evidence to suggest the cessation of inhaled therapies, and it is optimal to facilitate ease of clearance as much as possible, although if hypertonic saline induces uncontrolled coughing, then this should be used with caution during the acute episode. Although RhDNase has been suggested to present a risk, this remains unproven and evidence suggests a decreased incidence of hemoptysis in patients who use RhDNase.[101]

PNEUMOTHORAX

Spontaneous pneumothorax is defined as the presence of air within the pleural cavity, and in CF it usually occurs secondary to the underlying lung disease. Medical management is discussed in Chapter 14. There is no evidence advocating the physiotherapy adaptations required while managing patients with a pneumothorax, but clinical practice recommendations should be adhered to (see Table 43.3).

Table 43.2 Physiotherapy clinical practice recommendations for hemoptysis management

Blood streaking	Severe (≥250 mL/24 hours)
Reassurance and education	Urgent medical review
Continue with airway clearance	If actively bleeding, position into high side lying with bleeding side down
Care re cough force	Cease airway clearance and exercise until acute active bleeding resolved, then as per moderate hemoptysis
Avoid head-down tilt	
If recurrent: normal airway clearance and exercise	Optimize oxygen therapy and humidification
	May only cease airway clearance for ~2–3 hours post-acute active bleed as needed to clear blood clots and secretions (inflammatory)
Moderate (≤250 mL/24 hours)	**Post embolization**
Medical review	Ensure adequate analgesia and humidification
Maximize controlled airway clearance	Gentle mobilization
FET > coughing	Controlled breathing techniques – ACBT or AD
Cease manual techniques, head-down tilt	Gradually reintroduce normal airway clearance regime
Caution with all positive pressure (internal, external, oscillatory)	
Caution with hypertonic saline re-uncontrolled coughing	
Continue RhDNase	
Adequate humidification	
Mobility	

Sources: Adapted from Button B, Holland A. Physiotherapy for cystic fibrosis in Australia: A consensus statement. 2010, http://www.thoracic .org.au/imagesDB/wysiwyg/PhysiotherapyforCysticFibrosisinAustralia_1.pdf, page 49–50; ACPCF (Agent P, Morrison L, Prasad A). Standards of care and good clinical practice for the physiotherapy management of people with cystic fibrosis. Cystic Fibrosis Trust, 2011, http://www.cftrust.org.uk/aboutcf/publications/consensusdoc/Physio_standards_of_care.pdf, page 9.3–9.5.

Table 43.3 Physiotherapy clinical practice recommendations for pneumothorax management

Small	Large
Monitor shortness of breath	Extreme caution re-undrained pneumothorax—urgent medical intervention required
Cease positive pressure therapies	Intercostal drain in situ:
FET > Coughing (limit uncontrolled coughing)	Review positive pressure (IPPB, NIV, PEP)
Optimize humidification	Ensure optimal analgesia and humidification
Reduce exercise intensity	Drain incision site support during airway clearance and FET/Coughing
Avoid upper limb resistance exercises (due to intrathoracic pressure)	Avoid upper limb resistance exercises
Supplemental controlled oxygen at high flow rates	Encourage submaximal exercise
Post-op pleurodesis	**Post drain removal:**
Adequate analgesia	Avoid positive pressure and forced expiratory maneuvers to avoid recurrence or pleural fistula
Optimal humidification and inhalation therapy	
Early mobilization	
Use of controlled breathing techniques e.g. ACBT/AD	
FET > Coughing	

Sources: Adapted from Button B, Holland A. Physiotherapy for cystic fibrosis in Australia: A consensus statement. 2010, http://www.thoracic .org.au/imagesDB/wysiwyg/PhysiotherapyforCysticFibrosisinAustralia_1.pdf, page 52; ACPCF (Agent P, Morrison L, Prasad A). Standards of care and good clinical practice for the physiotherapy management of people with cystic fibrosis. Cystic Fibrosis Trust, 2011, http://www.cftrust.org.uk/aboutcf/publications/consensusdoc/Physio_standards_of_care.pdf, page 9.5–9.6.

EXTRAPULMONARY CONSIDERATIONS: CARDIAC, LIVER, AND RENAL

Patients with CF may experience a number of comorbidities, such as cardiac, liver, and renal disease associated with their CF. Physiotherapy interventions may need to be adapted accordingly and regular individual reassessment is essential.

Cor pulmonale is well recognized in patients with hypoxia and pulmonary hypertension, and oxygen therapy may give symptomatic relief. Physiotherapists should be cautious when exercising patients with secondary cardiac complications as it is often difficult to ascertain whether hypoxia has a respiratory or cardiac cause, and appropriate oxygen therapy should be provided, and additionally bi-level NIV may be required to support the cardiac/respiratory load.

In CF-associated liver disease, abdominal distension due to hepatosplenomegaly or ascites may restrict diaphragmatic excursion resulting in basal atelectasis. Airway clearance may need to be modified (avoid supine) and manual techniques (chest clapping and shaking) should be avoided in the presence of abnormal clotting.[52] If active variceal bleeding occurs, airway clearance may need to be temporarily discontinued or carried out with extreme caution. When exercising patients, careful monitoring of breathlessness and oxygen saturation is necessary, with consideration of anemia as a cause of dyspnea. In those patients with hepatopulmonary syndrome, right to left shunting occurs with hypoxemia.

Renal complications in CF may be due to renal colic, renal stones, and renal abnormalities in CF or due to secondary causes or associated conditions. Poor renal function can occur after repeated courses of antibiotics. Airway clearance and exercise regimes should be optimized with appropriate pain management (in cases of renal colic, renal stones), with consideration to secondary causes of dyspnea given.

CRITICAL CARE

There are no published studies to guide physiotherapy management of the intubated and ventilated patient with CF, but careful consideration should be given to optimizing airway clearance, humidification, and positioning for optimal ventilation and drainage of secretions. Rehabilitation should be commenced as soon as is practically possible with close liaison between the critical care and CF multidisciplinary team.[52]

TRANSPLANTATION

Lung transplant offers the chance of increased quality of life and survival to patients who have severe disease. Patients with CF may be waiting from a few weeks to years all the while requiring optimized medical management and to be in prime physical condition for surgery. It is crucial that their exercise and functional capacity, respiratory function, muscle strength, and postural alignment are optimized. "Pre-hab" (pretransplant rehabilitation) requires individualized physiotherapy programs coupled with appropriate short- and long-term goal setting, to match the patient's physical capabilities. These pre-hab programs need to be adapted to be appropriate for home use as well as during in-patient admissions for infective exacerbations. Regular exercise programs coupled with adjunctive NIV or oxygen therapy may be required to support patients' ventilatory demands and enable programs to be carried out.

Physiotherapy posttransplant can be varied and diverse and includes the management of the patient in the critical care unit, on the ward, and on-going as an out-patient.[52] Similar to pre-hab programs, posttransplant physiotherapy interventions focus on improving functional and exercise capacity (through cardiovascular and resistance work), range of joint movement, postural alignment, and inhalation therapy regimes. In the immediate postoperative period, adequate analgesia is vital to facilitate effective airway clearance and participation in rehabilitation. Patients experience vagal nerve denervation and have an impaired cough reflex post-transplant,[102] so appropriate assessment and airway clearance, if required, need to be taught. Caution must be applied when advising on exercise programs in patients who are on high-dose corticosteroid therapy (post episodes of rejection) due to the associated increased risk of tendonitis, tendon rupture, and osteoporotic changes.

TERMINAL CARE

The physiotherapist's relationship may change as lung disease advances and patients approach end of life. In the hospital setting, the physiotherapist may be required to continue airway clearance support often until hours prior to death.[103] This is in part to maintain patient comfort, but in many cases, it seeks to continue the routine of chest clearance that may have successfully existed for many years and is therefore a comfort to the patient and their families. Airway clearance may require adaptations to accommodate short, frequent sessions which will maximize symptomatic relief while minimizing fatigue and commonly require the addition of positive pressure devices to reduce work or breathing, i.e., IPPB or NIV.[103] In the majority of adult CF centers, the physiotherapists play a pivotal role in the instigation of NIV including "troubleshooting" settings to optimize ventilation and sleep and advising the patient on appropriate interfaces to maximize comfort. At this stage of a patients' life and with the appropriate knowledge, the physiotherapist can use NIV very effectively to manage symptoms of breathlessness and fatigue, often modifying settings to ensure functional mobilization and adequate airway clearance.

For some transplant-listed patients, coping with end-stage disease will coexist with the hope of receiving a lung transplant. In these cases, the experienced CF physiotherapist will be able to support the patient and family to find a balance between the burden of treatment required to remain clinically stable, including airway clearance and rehabilitation, and spending time with family and friends.

The familiar therapeutic relationship that exists between the patient and CF specialist physiotherapist at end of life can be useful when close communication with palliative care and hospice services are required. The physiotherapist may play a key role in assessing the success of symptom control strategies used by palliative care (see Chapter 36, terminal care) and in helping to access local hospice services if the patients are to be managed outside of the hospital setting.

HOME CARE PHYSIOTHERAPY

Standards of Care and Good Clinical Practice for the Physiotherapy Management of Cystic Fibrosis[52] recommend that the CF patient should have access to a physiotherapy home care service. Home care physiotherapy should be provided (if deemed appropriate) for people with CF at times of particular need such as change in therapy delivery or technique, during an exacerbation, in the event of palliative care at home, and during home intravenous antibiotics to support optimization of physiotherapy treatment.[52] This not only allows detailed assessment of physiotherapy regimes in the home setting but also provides support to the patient and wider family. It also gives the visiting physiotherapist an insight into how treatments fit into the patient's and family's life, and can address issues such as adherence. Focus on airway clearance and musculoskeletal and urinary incontinence can occur without the time pressure of the hospital appointment. In pediatrics, home care may also involve school visits where patients may be supported in carrying out their airway clearance at school. The individual may also wish to be supported in providing their teachers and peers with information about their diagnosis and the impact it has on their life. Education of the teachers is important so that opportunities for the patient to exercise can be encouraged and modified to suit the patient's individual circumstances.

CONCLUSION

Physiotherapy for CF requires a holistic approach with a focus on optimizing airway clearance, exercise capacity, musculoskeletal function, inhalation therapy regimes, and continence management. Physiotherapists adopt an autonomous assessment-based approach with high levels of clinical reasoning. Despite a general paucity of high-quality evidence in physiotherapy techniques for CF, there has been much progress in the design, quality and rigor, or studies in recent years. There is no "ideal" single best airway clearance technique, and frequent re-evaluation of the patient's individual needs enables the physiotherapist to adjust techniques in response to changing lung physiology and how the regime fits into the patient's daily routine. Physiotherapists recognize the burden of treatment that their holistic approach causes, so a fine balance is required in making regimes achievable.

Today's specialist CF physiotherapists should have a comprehensive toolbox of techniques and treatment approaches that create an individualized, evidence-based, creative multisystem approach to optimize health status and quality of life.

VIDEOS

- *Video 43.1 (http://goo.gl/E0ThMp)*: Video of ACBT.
- *Video 43.2 (http://goo.gl/LD0Vqc)*: Video of AD.
- *Video 43.3 (http://goo.gl/wNo1Rp)*: Video of PEP in practice—adult and infant.
- *Video 43.4 (http://goo.gl/ks42fO)*: Video of patient using Flutter.
- *Video 43.5 (http://goo.gl/fWvw0K)*: Video of patient using Acapella.

REFERENCES

1. Lapin CD. Airway physiology, autogenic drainage, and active cycle of breathing. *Respir Care* 2002; **47**: 778–85.
2. Thompson B, Thompson HT. Forced expiration exercises in asthma and their effect on FEV$_1$. *NZ J Physiother* 1968; **3**: 19–21.
3. Pryor JA, Webber BA, Hodson M et al. Evaluation of the forced expiration technique as an adjunct to postural drainage in the treatment of cystic fibrosis. *Br med J* 1979; **2**: 417–8.
4. Wilson GE, Baldwin AL, Walshaw MJ. A comparison of traditional chest physiotherapy with the active cycle of breathing in patients with chronic suppurative lung disease. *European Respir J* 1995; **8**(Suppl 19): 171S.
5. Webber BA, Hofmeyr JL, Morgan MDL, Hodson ME. Effects of postural drainage incorporating the forced expiration technique, on pulmonary function in cystic fibrosis. *Br J Dis Chest* 1986; **80**: 353–9.
6. Pryor JA, Webber BA, Hodson ME. Effect of chest physiotherapy on oxygen saturation in patients with cystic fibrosis. *Thorax* 1990; **45**: 77.
7. Pryor JA, Webber BA, Hodson ME, Warner JO. The Flutter VRP1 as an adjunct to chest physiotherapy in cystic fibrosis. *Respir Med* 1994; **88**: 677–81.

8. Hofmeyr JL, Webber BA, Hodson ME. Evaluation of positive expiratory pressure as an adjunct to chest physiotherapy in the treatment of cystic fibrosis. *Thorax* 1986;**41**: 951–4.

9. Pike SE, Machin AC, Dix KJ, Pryor JA, Hodson ME. Comparison of Flutter VRP1 and forced expirations with active cycle of breathing techniques in subjects with cystic fibrosis. *Netherlands J Med* 1999; **54**: S55–6.

10. Osman LP, Roughton M, Hodson ME, Pryor JA. Short-term comparative study of high frequency chest wall oscillation and European airway clearance techniques in patients with cystic fibrosis. *Thorax* 2010; **65**: 196–200.

11. Pryor JA, Tannenbaum E, Scott SF et al. Beyond postural drainage and percussion: Airway clearance in people with cystic fibrosis. *J Cyst Fibros* 2010; **9**: 187–92.

12. Robinson KA, Mckoy N, Saldanha I, OdelolaOA. Active cycle of breathing technique for cystic fibrosis. *Cochrane Database Syst Rev* 2010; Issue 11. Art. No.: CD007862. DOI: 10.1002/14651858.CD007862. pub2.

13. Chevaillier J. Autogenic drainage. In: Lawson D (ed.) *Cystic Fibrosis Horizons*. Chichester: John Wiley, 1984, p. 235.

14. Schöni MH. Autogenic drainage: A modern approach to chest physiotherapy in cystic fibrosis. *J R Soc Med* 1989; **82**(Suppl 16): 32–7.

15. Dab I, Alexander F. The mechanism of autogenic drainage studied with flow volume curves. *Monogr Paediatr* 1979; **10**: 50–3.

16. Chevaillier J. Autogenic drainage: The flow and breathing level modulation concept. In: International physiotherapy Group for Cystic Fibrosis (IPG/CF). *Physiotherapy for the Treatment of CF*. 4th ed. 2009. www.cfww.org.

17. Miller S, Hall D, Clayton C, Nelson R. Chest physiotherapy in cystic fibrosis: A comparative study of autogenic drainage and active cycle of breathing technique with postural drainage and percussion. *Thorax* 1995; **50**(2): 165–9.

18. Mcllwaine M, Wong L, Chilvers M, Davidson G. Long term comparative trial of two different physiotherapy techniques; postural drainage with percussion and autogenic drainage in the treatment of cystic fibrosis. *Pediatr Pulmonol* 2010; Wiley Online Library.

19. Pfleger A, Theissl B, Oberwaldner B, Zach MS. Self-administered chest physiotherapy in cystic fibrosis: A comparative study of high-pressure PEP and autogenic drainage. *Lung* 1992; **170**: 323–30.

20. Van Ginderdeuren F. Assisted Autogenic Drainage: Presented at Advanced airway clearance course at the European Cystic Fibrosis Conference, Dublin, June 2012.

21. Van Ginderdeuren F, Malfroot A, Verdonk J, Van Laethem S, Vandenplas Y. Influence of assisted autogenic drainage combined with bouncing on gastro oesophageal reflux in infants under the age of 5 months. *J Cyst Fibros* 2003; **2**(1): A251.

22. Groth G, Stafanger G, Dirksen H, Andersen J, Falk M, Kelstrup M. PEP (PEP mask) physiotherapy improves ventilation and reduces volume of trapped gas in cystic fibrosis. *Eur Physiopathol Resp Bull* 1985; **21**(4): 339–43.

23. Zach M, Oberwaldner B, Forche G, Polgar G. Bronchodilators increase airway instability in Cystic Fibrosis. *Am Rev Respir Dis* 1985; **131**: 537–43.

24. Falk M, Kelstrup M, Andersen Jet al. Improving the ketchup bottle method with positive expiratory pressure in cystic fibrosis. *Eur J Respir Dis* 1984; **65**(6): 423–32.

25. O'Connell O, O'Farrell C, Harrison M, Eustace J, Henry M, Plant B. Nebulized hypertonic saline via positive expiratory pressure vs jet nebuliser in patients with cystic fibrosis. *Respir Care* 2011; **56**(6): 771–5.

26. Laube B, Geller D, Lin T, Dalby R, Diener-West M, Zeitlin P. PEP changes aerosol distribution in patients with cystic fibrosis. *Respir Care* 2005; **50**(11): 1438–44.

27. Mcllwaine M, Wong L, Peacock D, Davidson A. Long term comparative trial of conventional postural drainage and percussion vs PEP physiotherapy in treatment of cystic fibrosis. *J Pediatric* 1997; **131**(4): 570–4.

28. Mortensen J, Falk M, Groth S, Jensen C. The effects of postural drainage and PEP physiotherapy on tracheobronchial clearance in cystic fibrosis. *Chest* 1991; **100**: 1350–7.

29. Lannefors L, Wollmer P. Mucus clearance with three chest physiotherapy regimes in cystic fibrosis: A comparison between postural drainage, positive expiratory pressure and physical exercise. *Eur Respir J* 1992; **6**: 748–53.

30. Mcllwaine M, Wong L, Peacock D, Davidson A. Long-term comparative trial of positive expiratory pressure vs oscillating positive expiratory pressure (flutter) physiotherapy in the treatment of cystic fibrosis. *J Pediatr* 2001; **138**(6): 845–50.

31. Mcllwaine M, Alarie N, Davidson G et al. Long-term multi-centre randomised controlled study of high frequency chest wall oscillation versus positive expiratory pressure mask in cystic fibrosis. *Thorax* 2013; **0**: 1–6.

32. Elkins M, Jones A, Van der Schans C. PEP physiotherapy for airway clearance in people with cystic fibrosis. *Cochrane Database Syst Rev* 2006; **2**: CD003147.

33. Lannefors L, Button B, McIlwaine M. Physiotherapy in infants and young children with cystic fibrosis: Current practice and future developments. *J R Soc Med* 2004; 97(suppl 44): 8–25.

34. Constantini D, Brivio A, Brusa D et al. PEP mask vs postural drainage in cystic fibrosis infants: A comparative trial. *Pediatr Pulmonol* 2001; suppl 22: A 400.

35. Oberwaldner B, Evans J, Zach M. Forced expirations against variable resistance: A new chest physiotherapy method in cystic fibrosis. *Pediatr Pulmonol* 1986; **6**: 358–67.

36. Thompson C, Harrison S, Ashley et al. Randomised cross over study of the flutter device and active cycle of breathing technique in non cystic fibrosis. *Thorax* 2002; **57**(5): 446–8.

37. Apps E, Kieselmann R, Reinhardt D et al. Sputum rheology changes in cystic fibrosis lung disease following two different types of physiotherapy: Flutter vs autogenic drainage. *Chest* 1998; **114**: 171–7.

38. Gumery L, Dodd M, Parker A, Prasad A, Pryor J. Clinical guidelines for the physiotherapy management of cystic fibrosis. CF Trust 2002.

39. Volsko T, Difiore J, Chatburn R. Performance of two oscillating PEP devices: Acapella vs. flutter. *Respir Care* 2003; **48**(2): 124–30.

40. Gondor M, Nixon P, Mutich R, Rebovich P, Orenstein D. Comparison of flutter device and chest physical therapy in the treatment of cystic fibrosis pulmonology exacerbations. *Pediatr Pulmonol* 1999; **28**(4): 255–60.

41. West K, Wallen M, Follett M. Acapella vs. PEP mask therapy: A randomised trial in children with cystic fibrosis during respiratory exacerbation. *Physiother Theory Pract* 2010; **26**(3): 143–9.

42. Morrison L, Agnew J. Oscillating devices for airway clearance in people with cystic fibrosis. *Cochrane Database Syst Rev* 2009; 21,1: CD006842.

43. Main E. Airway clearance research in CF: The 'perfect storm' of strong preference and effortful participation in long-term, non-blinded studies. *Thorax* 2013; **68**: 701–2.

44. Bradley J, Moran F, Elborn S. Evidence for physical therapies (airway clearance and physical training) in cystic fibrosis: An overview of five Cochrane Reviews. *Respir Med* 2006; **100**: 191–201.

45. Anderson J, Falk M. Physiotherapy in the paediatric age group. *Respir Care* 1991; **36**: 546–54.

46. Button B. Oscillating PEP. Presented at advanced airway clearance course at the European Cystic Fibrosis Conference, Dublin, June 2012.

47. Davies G, Banks A, Agent P et al. The use of high frequency chest wall oscillation during an acute infective pulmonary exacerbation of cystic fibrosis. Paper presented at North American Cystic fibrosis Conference, Orlando, 2012.

48. Newhouse PA, White F, Marks JH, Homnick DN. The intrapulmonary percussive ventilator and flutter device compared to standard chest physiotherapy in patients with cystic fibrosis. *Clin Pediatr* 1998; **37**: 427–32.

49. Natale JE, Pfeifle J, Homnick DN. Comparison of intrapulmonary percussive ventilation and chest physiotherapy. A pilot study in patients with cystic fibrosis. *Chest* 1994; **105**(6): 1789–93.

50. Homnick DN, White F, deCastro C. Comparison of the effects of an intrapulmonary percussive ventilator to standard aerosol and chest physiotherapy in patients with cystic fibrosis. *Pediatr Pulmonol* 1995; **20**: 50–5.

51. Varekojis SM, Douce FH, Flucke RL et al. A comparison of the therapeutic effectiveness of and preference for postural drainage and percussion, intrapulmonary percussive ventilation and high frequency chest wall oscillation in hospitalised cystic fibrosis patients. *Respir Care* 2003; **48**: 24–8.

52. Agent P, Morrison L, Prasad A on behalf of Association of Chartered Physiotherapists in Cystic Fibrosis (ACPCF). Standards of care and good clinical practice for the physiotherapy management of people with cystic fibrosis. Cystic Fibrosis Trust 2011 http://www.cftrust.org.uk/aboutcf/publications/consensusdoc/Physio_standards_of_care.pdf

53. Moran F, Bradley JM, Piper AJ. Non-invasive ventilation for cystic fibrosis. *Cochrane Database Syst Rev* 2009, Issue 1. Art. No.: CD002769. DOI: 10.1002/14651858.CD002769.pub3.

54. Holland AE, Denehy L, Ntoumenopoulos G. Non-invasive ventilation assistschest physiotherapy in adults with acute exacerbations of cystic fibrosis. *Thorax* 2003; **58**: 880–4.

55. Dwyer TJ. Randomised controlled two-centre trial of non-invasive ventilation-assisted chest physiotherapy during an exacerbation of cystic fibrosis. Paper presented at European Cystic Fibrosis Conference, Valencia, June 2010.

56. Placidi G, Cornacchia M, Polese G, Zanolla L, Assael B, Braggion C. Chest physiotherapy with positive airway pressure: A pilot study of short-term effects on sputum clearance in patients with cystic fibrosis and severe airway obstruction. *Respir Care* 2006; **51**(10): 1145–53.

57. van der Schans CP, van der Mark TW, de Vries G et al. Effect of positive expiratory pressure breathing in patients with cystic fibrosis. *Thorax* 1991; **46**: 252–6.

58. Morgan GE, Parrott H, Bilton D, Agent P. Positive pressure: A positive impact on airway clearance at home. *Pediatr Pulmonol* 2011; suppl 34: A385.

59. Hebestreit A, Kersting U, Basler B et al. Exercise inhibits epithelial sodium channels in patients with cystic fibrosis. *Am J Respir Crit Care Med* 2001; **164**(3): 443–6.

60. Dwyer TJ, Alsion JA, McKeough ZJ et al. Effects of exercise on respiratory flow and sputum properties in cystic fibrosis. *Chest* 2010; **138**: 1–8.

61. Prasad A, Dhouieb E. Clinical guidance for the physiotherapy management of screened infants with cystic fibrosis. *ACPCF Guidance Paper* 2008; number 4.

62. Prasad A, Main E, Dodds M. Finding consensus on the physiotherapy management of asymptomatic infants with cystic fibrosis. *Pediatr Pulmonol* 2008; **43**: 236–44.

63. Lorin MI, Denning CR. Evaluation of postural drainage by measurement of sputum volume and consistency. *Am J Phys Med* 1971; **50**: 215–9.

64. Button BM, Heine RG, Catto-Smith AG et al. Postural drainage in cystic fibrosis: Is there a link with gastro-oesophageal reflux? *J Paediatr Child Health* 1998; **34**: 330–4.

65. Cecins NM, Jenkins SC, Pengelley J, Ryan G. The active cycle of breathing techniques: To tip or not to tip? *Respir Med* 1999; **93**: 660–5.

66. Button BM, Heine RG, Catto-Smith AG et al. Chest physiotherapy in infants with cystic fibrosis: To tip or not? A five-year study. *Pediatr Pulmonol* 2003; **35**: 208–13.

67. Button B, Sherburn M, Chase J, McLachlan Z, Wilson J, Kotsimbos T. Incontinence (urinary and bowel) in women with cystic fibrosis compared to COPD and controls: Prevalence, severity and bother. *Pediatr Pulmonol* 2004; suppl 27: A359.

68. Gumery L, Hodgson G, Humphries N et al. The prevalence of urinary incontinence in the adult male population of a regional Cystic Fibrosis Centre. *J Cyst Fibros* 2002; **1**(suppl 1): 351A.

69. Prasad A, Balfour-Lynn I, Carr S, Madge S. A comparison of the prevalence of urinary incontinence in girls with cystic fibrosis, asthma and healthy controls. *Pediatr Pulmonol* 2006; **11**: 1065–8.

70. Button B, Sherburn M, Chase J, Stillman B, Wilson J. Effect of three months physiotherapeutic intervention on incontinent women with chronic cough related to cystic fibrosis and COPD. *Pediatr Pulmonol* 2005; suppl 28: A369.

71. Madge S, Agent P. Quality of life in women with cystic fibrosis and urinary incontinence. *J Cyst Fibros* 2008; 7: S100.

72. Miller J, Ashton-Miller J, deLancey J. A pelvic muscle precontraction can reduce cough related urine loss in selected women with mild stress urinary incontinence. *J Am Geriatric Soc* 1998; **46**: 870–4.

73. Sapsford R, Richardson C, Stanton W. Sitting posture affects pelvic floor muscle activity in parous women: An observational study. *Aust J Physio* 2006; **52**(3): 219–22.

74. Koch AK, Bromme S, Wollschlager B, Horneff G, Keyszer G. Musculoskeletal manifestations and rheumatic symptoms in patients with cystic fibrosis: No observations of CF-specific arthropathy. *J Rheumatol* 2008; **35**(9): 1882–91.

75. Massery M. Musculoskeletal and neuromuscular interventions: A physical approach to cystic fibrosis. *J Royal Society Med* 2005; **98**(suppl 45): 55–66.

76. Hodges PW, Gurfinkel VS, Brumagne S et al. Coexistence of stability and mobility in postural control: Evidence from postural compensation for respiration. *Exp Brain Res* 2002; **144**(3): 293–302.

77. Tattersall R, Walshaw MJ. Posture and cystic fibrosis. *J Royal Society Med* 2003; **96**(suppl 43): 18–22.

78. Demry A, Ben Ami S, Levi M et al. Chest strength and mobility training: A new approach to airways clearance. *J Cystic Fibr* 2006; **29**: 371.

79. Lee A, Holdsworth M, Holland A, Button B. The immediate effect of musculoskeletal physiotherapy techniques and massage on pain and ease of breathing in adults with cystic fibrosis. *J Cyst Fibros* 2009; **8**(1): 79–81.

80. Geiss S, Hobbs S, Hammersley-Maercklein G et al. Psychosocial factors related to perceived compliance with Cystic fibrosis treatment. *J Clin Psychology* 1992; **48**: 99–103.

81. Prasad A, Main E. Finding evidence to support airway clearance in cystic fibrosis. *Disabil Rehabil* 1998; **20**: 235–46.

82. Chappell F, Williams B. Rates and reasons for non-adherence to home physiotherapy in paediatrics. *Physiotherapy* 2002; **88**: 138–47.

83. Flores JS, Teixeira FA, Rovedder PM, Ziegler B, Dalcin Pde T. Adherence to airway clearance therapies by adult cystic fibrosis patients. *Respir Care* 2012; 58(2): 279–85.

84. Daniels T, Goodacre L, Sutton C, Pollard K, Conway S, Peckham D. Accurate assessment of adherence self reports electronic monitoring of nebulisers. *Chest* 2011; **140**(2): 425–32.

85. Houston BW, Mills N, Solis-Moya A. Inspiratory muscle training for cystic fibrosis. *Cochrane Database Syst Rev* 2008; **4**: CD006112.

86. Dekerlegand R, Hadjiliadis D, Myslinski M et al. The effect of inspiratory muscle training on respiratory muscle strength and functional capacity in adults with CF. *Pediatr Pulmonol* 2011; suppl 34: A393.

87. McCool FD. Global physiology and pathophysiology of cough: ACPP evidence-based clinical practice guidelines. *Chest* 2006; 129(suppl 1): 48S–53S.

88. Thomas M, McKinley RK, Mellor S et al. Breathing exercises for asthma: A randomised controlled trial. *Thorax* 2009; **64**(1): 55–61.

89. Holloway E, West R. Integrated breathing and relaxation training (the Papworth method) for adults with asthma in primary care: A randomised controlled trial. *Thorax* 2007; **2**(12): 1039–42.

90. Patel AS, Watkin G, Willig B et al. Improvement in health status following cough suppression physiotherapy for patients with chronic cough. *Chronic Resp Dis* 2011; **8**(4): 253–8.

91. Edenborough FP, Borgo G, Knoop C et al. Guidelines for the management of pregnancy in women with cystic fibrosis. *J Cystic Fibr* 2008; **7**: S2–S32.

92. Gilljam M, Antoniou M, Shin J, Dupuis A, Corey M, Tullis DE. Pregnancy in CF: Fetal and maternal outcome. *Chest* 2000; **118**: 85–91.

93. Edenborough FP. Women with CF and their potential for reproduction. *Thorax* 2000; **56**: 649–55.

94. Parrott H, Madge S, Thorpe-Beeston G, Agent P. Airway clearance requirements during pregnancy. *Pediatr Pulmonol* 2008; S31: 523.

95. Button BM, Roberts S, Kotsimbos T, Wilson J. Symptomatic and silent gastroesophageal reflux (GOR) in adults with cystic fibrosis: The usefulness of structured symptom questionnaire compared to 24 hr oesophageal pH monitoring to identify GOR. *J Cystic Fibr* 2003; **2**(1): 254A.

96. van der Schans CP, Prasad A, Main E. Chest physiotherapy compared to no chest physiotherapy for cystic fibrosis. *Cochrane Database Syst Rev* 2000, Issue 2. Art. No.: CD001401. DOI: 10.1002/14651858.CD001401.

97. Main E, Prasad A, van der Schans CP. Conventional chest physiotherapy compared to other airway clearance techniques for cystic fibrosis. *Cochrane Database Syst Rev* 2005, Issue 1. Art. No.: CD002011. DOI: 10.1002/14651858.CD002011.pub2.

98. Sahl W, Bilton B, Dodd M, Webb K. Effect of exercise and physiotherapy in aiding sputum expectoration in adults with cystic fibrosis. *Thorax* 1989; **44**: 1006–8.

99. Furnari ML, Salerno S, Rabiolo A, Caravello V, Pardo F. Case report: Bronchial to subclavian shunt in a CF patient. A potential pitfall for embolisation. *J Cyst Fibros* 2003; **2**: 217–9.

100. Button B, Holland A. Physiotherapy for cystic fibrosis in Australia: A consensus statement. 2010 http://www.thoracic.org.au/imagesDB/wysiwyg/PhysiotherapyforCysticFibrosisinAustralia_1.pdf.

101. Flume PA, Pulmonary complications of cystic fibrosis. *Respir Care* 2009; **54**(5): 618–27.

102. Duarte AG, Myers AC. Cough reflex in lung transplant recipients. *Lung* 2012; 190(1): 23–7.

103. Agent P, Tonkin V. A retrospective analysis of physiotherapy input during a standard admission compared to a terminal admission in adults with CF. *J Cyst Fibr* **6**(suppl 1): S63.

44

Nutritional aspects

SUE WOLFE AND SARAH COLLINS

INTRODUCTION

The dietetic management of cystic fibrosis (CF) is an integral part of the multidisciplinary approach to CF care. In the past poor growth and malnutrition were common features of CF[1] and although now not as common, still contribute significantly to increased morbidity.[2-9] Over the past 20 years, there have been many advances in both the respiratory and nutritional management of CF, which have had a significant impact on the nutritional status of patients. The introduction of national newborn screening (NBS) programs with the subsequent ability to start treatment early, in particular, has helped to improve the nutritional status of many patients.[10,11] Dietetic management aims to ensure that infants and children grow normally, achieving the 50th percentile for body mass index (BMI) by the age of 2 years and that adults have a normal BMI (females 22 kg/m^2 and males 23 kg/m^2).[4] It is also important that patients should have a normal body composition ensuring optimal muscle and bone strength and normal fat-soluble vitamin and essential fatty acid (EFA) status. Improving life expectancy has resulted in additional nutritional challenges, including managing CF-related diabetes (CFRD) and liver disease, renal complications, optimizing bone health and optimizing nutrition during pregnancy and pre- and post-transplantation.

To achieve an optimal nutritional status it is essential that all patients receive regular expert dietetic reviews, directed by CF center dietitians.[12] Advice should be age specific taking the patients' clinical condition, lifestyle, and culture into consideration.

NUTRITIONAL REQUIREMENTS

Energy requirements vary widely and depend on age, gender, nutritional status, lung function, and presence of pancreatic insufficiency (PI). Energy needs are generally quoted to be 110%–200% of those required by healthy individuals of the same age and gender.[4] Undernutrition results from an unfavorable energy balance between increased energy expenditure and losses and a reduced energy intake.

Increased energy expenditure

Infection, inflammation, certain drugs such as salbutamol,[13] deteriorating lung function,[14] and possibly a genetic component of CF[15] increase resting energy expenditure. An abnormal adaptive response to malnutrition also results in an increase in muscle protein catabolism and poor tolerance to acute infections.[16]

Increased energy losses

Despite adequate pancreatic enzyme replacement therapy (PERT), maldigestion resulting from bile salt deficiency, abnormal mucosal transport in the small intestine, and reduced pancreatic bicarbonate secretion may still contribute to increased energy losses due to malabsorption.[17] Inadequately treated impaired glucose tolerance or CFRD may also increase energy losses.

Reduced energy intakes

Many patients fail to meet recommended energy intakes with dietary fat providing approximately 35%–40% of the energy.[18-20] Anorexia is often present, especially during respiratory exacerbations and as disease severity increases resulting in dietary intakes that may be inadequate to support normal weight gain and growth. Other factors such as food dislikes, gastroesophageal reflux (GOR), increased sputum production, abdominal pain, vomiting, and psychosocial problems may also contribute.

It is important that children and adults with CF receive regular dietary reviews, and assessment throughout their life to ensure optimal nutritional status is maintained both when well and during periods of infection.

status for bone metabolism are also abnormal.[73] In view of these findings routine vitamin K supplementation is now recommended for all patients.[62,63,74,75]

ESSENTIAL FATTY ACIDS

Biochemical deficiency of EFAs, characterized by low levels of linoleic, α–linolenic acid, and omega-3 long-chain polyunsaturated fatty acids such as eicosapentaenoic acid and docosahexanoic acid, is common in CF.[76] Clinical symptoms of deficiency are rare; however, deficiency of EFAs may increase susceptibility to respiratory infections with staphylococcus and pseudomonas.[77] Deficiency may be partially caused by a defect in fatty acid metabolism related to the CF genotype.[78] The dose and type of EFAs required is unknown and therefore further work is needed before routine supplementation is recommended.[76]

WATER-SOLUBLE VITAMINS

In general, these vitamins are well absorbed in CF and supplementation is not necessary unless patients have inadequate dietary intakes.[21] Currently, the role of antioxidant vitamins is under investigation. Antioxidants may offset oxidative lung damage caused by persistent infection. Low levels of vitamin C[76] and impaired status of glutathione and carotenoids have been reported in CF.[33] Deficiency of these vitamins may disturb the protective antioxidant screen. The optimal dose and timing of antioxidant supplements is yet to be established.[79]

PROBIOTICS

Probiotics may have a role in the reduction of intestinal inflammation[80] and pulmonary exacerbation rate[81,82] in CF. Probiotics have been shown to be safe and effective in preventing *Clostridium difficile*–associated diarrhea in children and adults without CF receiving antibiotic treatment.[83] However, more research is needed to establish the ideal dosage and impact of using probiotics on health in the CF population.

PROVIDING NUTRITIONAL SUPPORT

Dietetic advice aims to achieve normal growth and nutritional status in all patients. Dietetic reviews and assessments should be performed regularly throughout life to ensure that an optimal nutritional status is maintained when well and during periods of infection. Advice should be tailored to the individual patients' needs, taking age, nutritional and pancreatic status, financial and family circumstance, religious and cultural dietary beliefs, and food preferences into account. Increasing the energy content of the normal diet, oral calorie supplementation, behavioral interventions, enteral tube feeding, and parenteral

nutrition (PN) have all been shown to improve weight gain in patients with CF.[84] Current European and UK nutritional management guidelines recommend a staged intervention approach to nutritional support partly based on weight, stature, and weight for stature.[21,33] The more recent North American guidelines have suggested that using BMI percentile positions in patients aged 2 to 20 years and BMI in adults is a more accurate predictor of nutritional risk.[4] Interestingly, a recent quality improvement approach to nutritional care has been developed, based on treating children with subtle nutritional deficits as well as those with obvious problems. This standardized approach, which ensured that all patients received the same high-quality care, resulted in significant improvements in nutritional outcomes.[85]

FEEDING INFANTS, TODDLERS, AND YOUNG CHILDREN

Age at diagnosis is a critical determinant of nutritional status. The most consistently observed benefits of NBS are nutritional.[86,87] National NBS for CF is now undertaken in the United Kingdom. Early diagnosis gives the opportunity to prevent nutritional problems, including failure to thrive, anemia, vitamin deficiencies, and hypoalbuminemia.[88]

Most infants with CF will thrive on either breast milk or a normal infant formula.[27,89,90] Demand breast-feeding should be encouraged as breast milk contains lipase and beneficial nutritional and growth factors. Exclusive breast-feeding has recently been shown to be associated with improved respiratory outcomes in the first 2[89] to 3[91] years of life. The North American, European, and UK nutritional management guidelines all recommend breast-feeding.[21,27,33]

For those who choose not to or cannot breast-feed, 150–200 mls (100–130 kcal)/kg/day of a standard infant formula will support normal growth in the majority of infants. If catch-up growth is required or malabsorption is difficult to control, energy requirements will be higher (see later). Approximately 15% of infants are born with MI. Although presentation with MI does not ultimately affect nutritional or respiratory status,[92,93] these infants are often nutritionally compromised in early infancy, especially if surgical resection is required.[94] Under these circumstances, a hydrolyzed protein, medium-chain triglyceride containing feed may be beneficial. A small percentage of infants may develop cows' milk protein intolerance, which should be treated with a hydrolyzed protein formula.[95]

Over 50% of the energy content of breast milk or infant formula is derived from fat and therefore infants (both breast-fed and formula fed) who present with obvious symptoms of malabsorption (pale, frequent, and oily stools) should commence PERT on diagnosis of CF (see Table 44.2). Delayed enzyme therapy at this stage will have a devastating effect on nutritional status. If the infant is breast-fed, care should be taken to ensure that the pancreatic enzyme preparations are not left on the nipple, which would result in soreness. The importance of regular growth assessment in the first few months of life when PERT is continuously adjusted and optimized cannot be overemphasized.

If weight gain is poor despite optimal PERT, in those infants who are breast-fed, increasing the frequency of breast-feeding or giving a complementary formula feed will help to increase the energy intake. In formula-fed infants, the use of a high-energy infant formula or carefully supervised feed concentration should be considered. Attention should be given to the protein:energy ratio of the feed and therefore the sole addition of fat and/or carbohydrate supplements should be avoided. The possibility of an additional diagnosis should also be considered.

Infants with CF may lose excessive sodium and chloride in their sweat[96] and failure to thrive may be related to, or exacerbated by, a poor sodium intake.[27,95,97] This may be a particular problem in hot climatic conditions if the infant is pyrexial or has excessive sodium losses through diarrhea or high stoma output.[95,98] The sodium content of breast milk and normal infant formula is relatively low (approximately 1.6 mmol/kg body weight for every 200 ml/kg fed). Deficiency, however, is difficult to determine, and urine sodium content (<10 mmol/L) gives an estimation of severe deficiency. Urine sodium : creatinine ratio (17–52) has been recommended as a more accurate assessment of sodium status in infants with CF.[99] The North American evidence-based guidelines for the management of infants with CF recommend routine sodium supplements for all infants with CF to a maximum of 4 mmol/kg/day.[27] The European and UK consensus guidelines on the nutritional management of CF do not recommend routine supplementation.[21,33] Both documents recommend that the need for sodium supplementation should be assessed on an individual basis taking climate and sodium losses into consideration. In most cases, supplementation with 1–2 mmol/kg should correct deficiency,[95] although more may be required in hot climatic conditions.[98]

Zinc deficiency may contribute to poor growth. In CF, deficiency can occur as a result of fat malabsorption. In one study zinc loss in the stool correlated with fecal fat losses[100] and in another study PERT improved zinc absorption.[101] North American guidelines for the management of infants with CF recommend that zinc supplementation is considered in infants with poor growth.[27]

GOR is relatively common in infants with CF[102] and can compromise growth and exacerbate respiratory symptoms. Treatments include thickening the feed, using a pre-thickened formula, using prokinetics, and reducing gastric acid[103] (see Chapter 22).

Weaning foods should be introduced at 4 to 6 months of age. Introducing meat at an early stage will help to improve the iron and zinc intake in breast-fed infants.[98] Full fat cows' milk should replace breast or formula feeds at 1 year of age. As the diet becomes more varied, the need for enzyme variation according to fat intake becomes greater (see above). Dietary counseling is essential throughout early childhood when long-term feeding habits are being established. It is important that mealtimes are positive experiences. Unfortunately food is often used as an effective tool to obtain parental attention and behavioral food refusal can develop.[104–106] Unless carefully handled, this behavior can persist for a number of years resulting in a poor dietary intake and growth. Attention to the behavioral aspects of feeding as well as providing nutrition education has been shown to be more effective in improving energy intakes and growth than nutrition education alone.[107–109] Most nutrition consensus documents now recommend that carers should be provided with written advice on encouraging positive eating behaviors.[4,21,27,33] This advice is summarized in Table 44.4.

ADOLESCENTS/ADULTS

Adolescence is a physically and emotionally demanding period associated with increased nutritional requirements due to rapid physical growth, pubertal changes, and increased physical activity. It is also a phase of developing independence, autonomy, and personal identity. There is a risk of disordered eating behavior in adolescents with

Table 44.4 Management of feeding behavioral problems

- Family meals should be encouraged, so meals become a social event. This will encourage good feeding behavior
- Food should be as attractive and fun as possible
- Distractions should be avoided, e.g., having the television on at mealtimes
- Food that the child is likely to eat should be offered before trying to increase the variety
- Small portions should be offered rather than over-facing the child and gentle encouragement should be given
- If a child is unwilling to try a new food, it should be offered 10–12 times before it can be concluded that the food is not liked
- Food refusal should be ignored. In the child's eyes any reaction given when the food is refused is attention and will encourage the bad behavior
- Praise should be given for "good" or "positive" mealtime behavior. Even small steps like taking a bite of a new food should be praised
- Mealtimes should be limited to 30 minutes. Allowing mealtimes to extend rarely results in more food being eaten. After 30 minutes food should be removed without comment and wait for the next routine meal/snack time
- A second meal should never be made if the first is refused
- A consistent approach should be observed by all involved with feeding the child

chronic illness[110] and therefore early identification and treatment of any eating disturbances in adolescents with CF is required.[111,112] Adolescence is also a time when treatment adherence may need addressing. Coping strategies have been shown to influence adherence to treatment, with positive/optimistic coping enhancing quality of life and facilitating treatment adherence.[113] Nutritional status needs close monitoring as the prevalence of malnutrition increases with age. Even in those with a normal BMI, a loss of fat-free mass occurs in those with severe lung disease.[114,115] Age-related complications of CF, e.g., CFRD and CF-related reduced BMD lead to increased dietary challenges to maintain optimal nutritional status throughout adulthood.

IMPROVING THE ENERGY CONTENT OF THE DIET

Patients should be encouraged to eat a high-fat diet with the liberal use of high-fat snacks and fried food if weight gain is poor. The CF dietitian should give advice on foods which will enhance weight gain such as the addition of butter, olive oil, cheese, and cream to foods. Encouraging small frequent meals and snacks will also help. A recent study has highlighted the overdependence on saturated fat intake.[116] This is potentially of concern, as increased life expectancy suggests that the diet should be as cardioprotective as possible. It may, therefore, be prudent to encourage the consumption of mono- and polyunsaturated fats. Serum EFA status may also be improved by the increased consumption of fat rich in linoleic (sunflower oil and docosahexaenoic acid) acid.[117]

THE USE OF ORAL NUTRITIONAL SUPPLEMENTS

If nutritional status remains poor despite encouraging a high-energy diet and ensuring optimal PERT, nutritional supplements may be beneficial for some patients.[4,118] A Cochrane review of three randomized clinical trials, including a total of 131 patients has suggested a lack of evidence of the value of these products for patients with CF.[119] The largest of these studies (102 patients) examined the efficacy of long-term supplement use in mildly malnourished children with good lung function.[120] In practice, prescribed on an individual basis, supplements are often used successfully to improve nutritional status.[121] There is a wide variety of prescribable supplements available in different presentations and flavors. These include bottled milk and juice-based drinks, milkshake powders, high-energy shots, and high-energy liquids and powders. It is important to ensure that the supplement is appropriate for the age of the patient that it is prescribed for. The quantity and timing of supplement intake is also important as they should provide additional nutrition to the diet and should not replace meals. Varying the type used helps to prevent taste fatigue, which is often reported with long-term supplement use.

ENTERAL TUBE FEEDING

Nasogastric (NG) or gastrostomy feeding is widely used in many CF Centers when oral dietary and supplement intake has failed to achieve an adequate nutritional status. Enteral tube feeding is reported to improve weight gain and nutritional status[117,122–128] and to stabilize or slow the rate of decline in lung function.[122,124,126,128,129] Early intervention is associated with improved outcomes[125,129,130] and therefore enteral tube feeding should be introduced as an early component of CF care.[27] Once started, tube feeding is often seen as a relief from stressful mealtime battles. However, more work is needed to examine the effect of this method of feeding on family function and quality of life. Despite its widespread use and reported nutritional and respiratory advantages, the Cochrane review concluded that the efficacy of enteral tube feeding has not been assessed by randomized control trials.[131] It is important to acknowledge, however, that performing such trials would be difficult due to ethical issues related to withholding an intervention when nutritional status necessitates it.

Patient preference and clinical status determine the route for enteral feeding. Some patients may prefer NG feeding; however, it is usually considered a less permanent method of nutritional support and used during respiratory exacerbations or prior to gastrostomy placement. The main disadvantages of NG feeding are that tubes may be unpleasant and difficult to pass, can be dislodged by coughing, GOR may be exacerbated, and it may have a negative effect on body image.[131] In view of these problems gastrostomy feeding through percutaneous gastrostomy tubes and low profile buttons is usually preferred for long-term nutritional support. Like NG feeding, gastrostomy feeding is also associated with complications such as nausea, vomiting, GOR, disturbed sleep, disturbed body image and leakage, granulation, and infection around the gastrostomy site. These complications are usually mild and transient.[131] If GOR is a problem, a Nissen's fundoplication may be indicated at the time of gastrostomy insertion.

Feeds are usually administered as continuous overnight infusions, as bolus feeds (gravity or pump assisted) during the day or a combination of both. The advantage of nocturnal feeds is that patients can be encouraged to continue to eat a high-energy diet throughout the day. A wide variety of enteral feeds are available and the feed chosen and the method and rate of administration should be appropriate to the patient's age, nutritional requirements, clinical condition, and lifestyle. The majority of patients tolerate a high-energy polymeric feed (1.5–2.4 Kcal/mL). If tolerance of these feeds is poor, an elemental or semi-elemental feed may be beneficial for some. All feeds, including elemental feeds, require PERT (see earlier) that should be determined on an individual basis. It is also important to monitor glucose intolerance at the time of introduction of enteral feeding and periodically thereafter. A small dose of insulin may be required to cover the feed.[21]

PARENTERAL NUTRITION

Parenteral nutrition (PN) is not routinely recommended as a method of nutritional support for patients with CF due to the risk of complications, difficulty of administration, and high cost.[23] Parenteral feeding may, however, be essential as short-term nutritional support following intestinal resection in infants presenting with MI,[96,23] following gastrointestinal surgery in older patients and in acute situations when enteral nutrition is not possible.[132] PN should only be used when enteral feeding is not tolerated and enteral feeding should be introduced as soon as possible to reduce the risk of cholestasis.

APPETITE STIMULANTS AND ANABOLIC HORMONES

Appetite stimulants have been used to try to improve the appetite in patients with CF. They should only be considered on an individual basis once all other reasons for inadequate growth or weight loss have been excluded.[133] Appetite stimulants should not be used in routine clinical practice.[134] Megestrol acetate has been found to improve weight and respiratory function.[135] Cyproheptadine hydrochloride has also been shown to improve the appetite in patients with CF.[136]

The anabolic agents insulin-like growth factor 1 and early insulin therapy[137] have also been studied in CF, but evidence of their value is poor. Growth hormone has been shown to improve weight gain and growth,[138,139] and creatine supplementation has resulted in improved muscle strength, patient well-being, and body weight.[140] However, most of the studies examining the use of adjunctive drugs have involved small patient groups and some have resulted in undesirable side effects.

NUTRITIONAL CHALLENGES

CYSTIC FIBROSIS-RELATED DIABETES (CFRD) (SEE CHAPTER 24)

CFRD is the most common comorbidity associated with CF. The aims of CFRD treatment are to maintain growth and optimize nutritional status, achieve good blood glucose control, and to avoid long-term complications.[141-144] Following diagnosis, patients should have a detailed dietary review and they should be advised on a diet appropriate to meet their nutritional requirements. If a high fat intake is required, then the emphasis should be placed on mono- and polyunsaturated fats. Intakes of protein and salt are not restricted. Some patients may be taught carbohydrate counting and how to adjust their insulin doses according to their carbohydrate intake. If they are not taught how to do this, patients should have regular meals containing complex carbohydrates and limit their simple carbohydrate intake to meal times. Patients receiving supplementary enteral feeds will need to have their insulin modified to optimize overnight glycemic

control. Insulin regimens should be tailored according to individual requirements taking into account their clinical and nutritional status, appetite, and level of physical activity.

BONE HEALTH

Reduced bone mineral density (BMD) is of particular concern in adolescent and adult patients,[145-148] but can occur in children.[149] Routine monitoring of bone health using dual energy xray absorptiometry (DXA) scans are recommended from the age of 8 to 10 years.[62,63,75] The many risk factors that contribute to the development of reduced BMD in patients with CF (see Chapter 26) should be addressed at routine clinic appointments. Nutrition-related factors include poor nutritional status[150] and delayed puberty, vitamin D, calcium and vitamin K[151] deficiencies. To a lesser extent, deficiencies of copper, phosphorous, magnesium, zinc, and protein and an excess of vitamin A may also have etiological roles.[75] Because of the multifactorial nature of reduced BMD in CF, it is impossible to establish a direct cause and effect for many of the risk factors.

The foundation for good bone health is established during infancy, childhood, and adolescence; therefore, there should be a focus on minimizing risk factors during these years. Particular attention should be given to achieving a normal nutritional status using the methods of nutritional support discussed above. There is currently some debate regarding the optimal plasma vitamin D levels for bone health, with consensus guidelines recommending a minimum plasma level of between 20 to 30 ng/mL (50 to 75 nnmol/L).[62,63,75] A high dietary intake of calcium is also recommended: 0–6 months 210 mg; 7–12 months 270 mg; 1–3 years 500 mg; 4–8 years 800 mg; 9–18 years 1300 mg; 19–50 years 100 mg; >50 years 1200 mg.[62] Dietary calcium is more effective than supplements, and this must be stressed to patients. The optimum vitamin K intake for bone health is still under debate. The European CF Bone Mineralisation guidelines recommend supplementation with vitamin K1: infants 0.5–2 mg; children >1 year, and adults 1–10 mg.[62]

PREGNANCY AND LACTATION

Nutritional status before and during pregnancy may be an important determinant of outcome.[152] Women with CF who plan their pregnancies and have preconceptional advice have significantly greater maternal weight gain and significantly heavier babies.[153,154] Advice regarding folic acid supplementation[155] and general food safety should be given. Dietary reviews should check nutritional adequacy with particular attention to ensure sufficient protein, calcium, and vitamin D intakes. It is important to maintain adequate vitamin D during pregnancy and breast-feeding, additional vitamin D supplementation may therefore be necessary.[156]

Nausea, vomiting, GOR, altered gastric motility, constipation, and diabetes may compromise nutritional status. There is an increased risk of developing diabetes during pregnancy in CF; therefore, an oral glucose tolerance test should be performed at the end of the first and second trimesters.[144] Careful and close monitoring of nutritional status and individual dietary advice is essential.[157] Nutritional intervention should be considered when weight gain is poor.

Care should be taken with vitamin A supplementation during pregnancy as high doses are teratogenic. Increased risks of birth defects have been associated with intakes greater than 10,000 IU (3,000 μg)/day.[158] Women with CF should take less than this and avoid excessive intakes of liver products because of their high vitamin A content.[21] Vitamin A levels should be checked at the start of each trimester.

Mothers with CF can successfully breast-feed[152] as their breast milk contains normal amounts of sodium and protein.[159] Maternal nutritional status should be carefully monitored during breast-feeding. Advice and nutritional support should be given to maintain an adequate dietary intake to meet the increased demands of breast-feeding.

TRANSPLANTATION

Poor nutritional status has been shown to compromise post-transplant survival[160–163] and is a risk factor for postoperative complications.[160,164,165] A detailed nutritional assessment should be conducted at the time of transplant assessment to optimize nutritional status. Nutritional support should be provided in the acute post-transplant period to maintain nutritional status. Patients also need to be taught about food hygiene and safety and dietary interactions with immunosuppressive drugs. Other complications which may require nutritional intervention post-transplant include hypertension, osteoporosis, hyperlipidemia,[166] diabetes, nephrotoxicity,[167] increased vitamin A and E levels,[168] and GOR. DIOS is also common in the early postoperative period and early medical intervention is essential.[169]

OVERWEIGHT AND OBESITY

Preventing nutritional failure is one of the primary concerns in the dietetic management of CF; however with improvements in survival and nutritional status, overweight and obesity exist.[170] The prevalence of overweight and obesity (BMI >25 kg/m^2) in adults homozygous for delta F508 has been reported at 10%.[171] Nutritional advice should be individualized to meet changes in nutritional requirements and dietary modifications may be required in children and adults to support long-term health and well-being. With improvements in treatments and survival, further research into the effects of overweight and obesity in CF is needed. Future management of children with CF should take into consideration the need to obtain an optimal body weight, which includes the prevention of malnutrition, overweight, and obesity.

RENAL DISEASE

Kidney disease is becoming increasingly common in CF.[172] CFTR is expressed in renal tubule cells;[172,173] however, renal disease is not considered a primary manifestation of CF. Renal disease tends to occur as a result of treatment with nephrotoxic drugs the commonest being aminoglycosides or immunosuppressive agents. Diabetes has also been implicated as a major cause of renal failure (see Chapter 27), patients with CF are also at increase risk of renal stones, especially calcium oxalate stones. Dietary modifications[174] are rarely required; however, close liaison with the renal team is important to avoid dietary restrictions, which would adversely impact on nutritional status.

LIVER DISEASE

Liver disease is a common complication associated with CF (see Chapter 23). Liver disease may exacerbate the risk of malnutrition due to increased requirements of protein and energy and increased fat malabsorption caused by cholestasis. Weight may not be a true reflection of nutritional status in patients with liver disease because of ascites or edema; other measures of nutritional status that are not affected by fluid retention such as mid-arm muscle circumference, triceps skinfold thickness, and handgrip strength may be more appropriate. Regular dietetic review and close liaison with the liver team is essential to maintain optimal nutritional status.

SUMMARY

Regular dietetic support is an integral part of CF care. The ultimate goal of nutritional management is that all patients should have a normal nutritional status. Patients should be seen by an experienced CF dietitian as soon as the diagnosis is made. Nutritional requirements should be assessed on an individual basis and be reviewed regularly so that nutritional interventions can be tailored to meet changes in clinical, physical, cultural, and psychosocial needs. The majority of patients with CF can achieve a good nutritional status from a high-energy and protein diet, although a normal diet may be adequate for some, especially those who are pancreatic sufficient. With increasing life expectancy, it is now important to consider healthy dietary principles such as the use of mono- and polyunsaturated dietary fat sources. The improvement in survival has also resulted in further dietetic challenges including the treatment of CFRD, pregnancy, renal disease, reduced BMD, and even obesity in some patients.

REFERENCES

1. Corey M, McLaughlin FS, Williams M, Levison H. A comparison of survival, growth and pulmonary function in patients with cystic fibrosis in Boston and Toronto. *J Clin Epidemiol* 1988; **41**: 583–91.
2. Vandenbranden SL, McMullen A, Schechter MS, et al; Investigators and Coordinators of the Epidemiologic Study of Cystic Fibrosis. Lung

function decline from adolescence to young adult-hood in cystic fibrosis. *Pediatr Pulmonol* 2012; **47**(2): 135–43.

3. Lai HJ, Shoff SM, Farrell PM. Recovery of birth weight z score within 2 years of diagnosis is posi-tively associated with pulmonary status at 6 years of age in children with cystic fibrosis. *Pediatrics* 2009; **123**(2): 714–22.

4. Stallings VA, Stark LJ, Robinson KA, et al. Clinical practice guidelines on growth and nutrition sub-committee; ad hoc working group. *J Am Diet Assoc* 2008; **108**: 832–9.

5. McPhail GL, Acton JD, Fenchel MC, et al. Improvements in lung function outcomes in children with cystic fibrosis are associated with better nutri-tion, fewer chronic pseudomonas aeruginosa infec-tions, and dornase alfa use. *J Pediatr* 2008; **153**(6): 752–7.

6. Pedreira CC, Robert RG, Dalton V, et al. Association of body composition and lung function in children with cystic fibrosis. *Pediatr Pulmonol* 2005; **39**(3): 276–80.

7. Stern M, Wiedemann B, Wenzlaff P; German Cystic Fibrosis Quality Assessment Group. From registry to quality management: The German Cystic Fibrosis Quality Assessment project 1995-2006. *Eur Respir J* 2008; **31**(1): 29–35.

8. Beker LT, Russek-Cohen E, Fink RJ. Stature as a prognostic factor in cystic fibrosis survival. *J Am Diet Assoc* 2001; **101**: 438–42.

9. Sharma R, Florea VG, Bolger AP, et al. Wasting as an independent predictor of mortality in patients with cystic fibrosis. *Thorax* 2001; **56**: 746–50.

10. Dijk FN, McKay K, Barzi F, et al. Improved survival in cystic fibrosis patients diagnosed by newborn screening compared to a historical cohort from the same centre. *Arch Dis Child* 2011; **96**(12): 1118–23.

11. Salvatore D, Buzzetti R, Baldo E, et al. An overview of international literature from cystic fibrosis reg-istries 2. Neonatal screening and nutrition/growth. *J Cyst Fibros* 2010; **9**(2): 75–83.

12. UK Cystic Fibrosis Trust Standards of Care Working Group. *Standards for the Clinical Care of Children and Adults with Cystic Fibrosis in the UK*. Bromley, England: Cystic Fibrosis Trust; 2011.

13. Vaisman N, Koren G, Goldstein D, et al. Pharmacokinetics of inhaled salbutamol in patients with cystic fibrosis verses healthy young adults. *J Pediatr* 1987; **111**: 914–7.

14. Dorlochter L, Roksund O, Helgheim V, et al. Resting energy expenditure and lung disease in cystic fibro-sis. *J Cyst Fibros* 2002; **1**: 131–6.

15. Bell SC, Bowerman AM, Nixon LE, et al. Metabolic and inflammatory responses to pulmonary exacerba-tions in adults with cystic fibrosis. *Eur J Clin Invest* 2000; **30**(6): 553–9.

16. Miller M, Ward L, Thomas BJ, et al. Altered body composition and muscle protein degradation in nutritionally growth-retarded children with cystic fibrosis. *Am J Clin Nutr* 1982; **36**: 492–9.

17. Littlewood JM, Wolfe SP, Conway SP. Diagnosis and treatment of intestinal malabsorption in cystic fibro-sis. *Pediatr Pulmonol* 2006; **41**(1): 35–49.

18. Woestenenk JW, Castelijns SJ, van der Ent CK, Houwen RH. Dietary intake in children and adoles-cents with cystic fibrosis. *Clin Nutr* 2013; **33**: 528–32.

19. White H, Morton AM, Peckham DG, et al. Dietary intakes in adults with cystic fibrosis—Do they achieve guidelines. *J Cyst Fibros* 2004; **3**: 1–7.

20. White H, Wolfe SP, Foy J, et al. Nutritional intakes and status in children with cystic fibrosis: Does age mat-ter? *J Pediatr Gastroenterol Nutr* 2007; **44**: 116–23.

21. UK Cystic Fibrosis Trust Nutrition Working Group. *Nutritional Management of Cystic Fibrosis*. Bromley, England: Cystic Fibrosis Trust; 2002.

22. Zhang Z, Lai HC. Comparison of the use of body mass index percentiles and percentage of ideal body weight to screen for malnutrition in children with cystic fibrosis. *Am J Clin Nutr* 2004; **80**: 982–91.

23. Lai HJ. Classification of nutritional status in cystic fibrosis. *Curr Opin Pulmon Med* 2006; **12**: 422–7.

24. Weidemann B, Paul KD, Stern M, et al. Evaluation of body mass index percentiles for assessment of malnutrition in children with cystic fibrosis. *Eur J Clin Nutr* 2007; **61**: 759–68.

25. Williams JE. Body composition in young children with cystic fibrosis. *World Rev Nutr Diet* 2013; **106**: 168–73.

26. King S, Wilson J, Kotsimbos T, et al. Body com-position assessment in adults with cystic fibrosis: Comparison of dual-energy X-ray absorptiometry with skinfolds and bioelectrical impedance analysis. *Nutrition* 2005; **21**: 1087–94.

27. Borowitz D, Robinson KA, Rosenfeld M, et al. Cystic Fibrosis Foundation evidence-based guidelines for management of infants with cystic fibrosis. *J Pediatr* 2009; **155** (Suppl 6): S73–93.

28. Walkowiak J, Nousia-Arvanitakis S, Agguridaki C, et al. Longitudinal follow-up of exocrine pancre-atic function in pancreatic sufficient cystic fibrosis patients using the fecal elasrase-1 test. *J Pediatr Gastroenterol Nutr* 2003; **36**: 474–8.

29. Borowitz D, Stevens C, Brettman LR, et al. Liprotamase long-term safety and support of nutri-tional status in pancreatic-insufficient cystic fibrosis. *J Pediatr Gastroenterol Nutr* 2012; **54**(2): 248–57.

30. Smyth RL, van Velzen D, Smyth AR, et al. Strictures of the ascending colon in cystic fibrosis and high strength pancreatic enzymes. *Lancet* 1994; **343**: 85–6.

31. Committee on Safety of Medicines. *Report of the Pancreatic Enzymes Working Party*. London: CSM; 1995.

32. Anthony H, Collins CE, Davidson G, et al. Pancreatic enzyme replacement therapy in cystic fibrosis: Australian guidelines. Pediatric Gastroenterological Society and the Dietitians Association of Australia. *J Paediatr Child Health* 1999; **35**(2): 125–9.

33. Sinaasappel M, Stern M, Littlewood J, et al. Nutrition in patients with cystic fibrosis: A European consensus. *J Cyst Fibros* 2002; **2**: 51–75.

34. Borowitz D, Gelfond D, Maguiness K, et al. Maximal daily dose of pancreatic enzyme replacement therapy in infants with cystic fibrosis: A reconsideration. *J Cyst Fibros* 2013; **12**: 784–5.

35. Wouthuyzen-Bakker M, Bodewes FA, Verkade HJ. Persistent fat malabsorption in cystic fibrosis: Lessons from patients and mice. *J Cyst Fibros* 2011; **10**(3): 150–8.

36. Taylor CJ, Hillel PG, Ghosal S, et al. Gastric emptying and intestinal transit of pancreatic enzyme supplements in cystic fibrosis. *Arch Dis Child* 1999; **80**: 149–52.

37. Domínguez-Muñoz JE, Iglesias-García J, Iglesias-Rey M, et al. Effect of the administration schedule on the therapeutic efficacy of oral pancreatic enzyme supplements in patients with exocrine pancreatic insufficiency: A randomized, three-way crossover study. *Aliment Pharmacol Ther* 2005; **21**(8): 993–1000.

38. Ng SM, Francini AJ. Drug therapies for reducing gastric acid in people with cystic fibrosis. *Cochrane Database Syst Rev* 2012; (4): CD003424.

39. Toouli J, Biankin AV, Oliver MR, et al. Management of pancreatic exocrine insufficiency: Australasian Pancreatic Club recommendations. *Med J Aust* 2010; **193**(8): 461–7.

40. Caras S, Boyd D, Zipfel L, et al. Evaluation of stool collections to measure efficacy of PERT in subjects with exocrine pancreatic insufficiency. *J Pediatr Gastroenterol Nutr* 2011; **53**(6): 634–40.

41. Bekers O, Postma C, Lombarts AJ. Determination of faecal fat by near infrared spectroscopy. *Eur J Clin Chem Clin Biol* 1995; **33**: 83–6.

42. Walters MP, Kelleher J, Gilbert J, Littlewood JM. Clinical monitoring of steatorrhoea in cystic fibrosis. *Arch Dis Child* 1990; **65**: 99–102.

43. Van der Neuker A, Pestel A, Tran TM, et al. Clinical use of acid steatocrit. *Acta Pediatr* 1997; **86**(5): 466–9.

44. Colombo C, Ellemunter H, Houwen R, et al. ECFS Guidelines for the diagnosis and management of distal intestinal obstruction syndrome in cystic fibrosis patients. *J Cyst Fibros* 2011;**10** (Suppl 2): S24–8.

45. van der Doef HP, Kokke FT, van der Ent CK, Houwen RH. Intestinal obstruction syndromes in cystic fibrosis: Meconium ileus, distal intestinal obstruction syndrome, and constipation. *Curr Gastroenterol Rep* 2011; **13**(3): 265–70.

46. Houwen RH, van der Doef HP, Sermet I, et al. ESPGHAN Cystic Fibrosis Working Group. Defining DIOS and constipation in cystic fibrosis with a multicentre study on the incidence, characteristics, and treatment of DIOS. *J Pediatr Gastroenterol Nutr* 2010; **50**(1): 38–42.

47. van der Doef HP, Kokke FT, Beek FJ, et al. Constipation in pediatric cystic fibrosis patients: An underestimated medical condition. *J Cyst Fibros* 2010; **9**(1): 59–63.

48. Kerrin D, Wolfe S, Brownlee K, Conway S. *Overnight Tube Feeds—Are Enzymes Necessary?* Abstract book. Stockholm, Sweden: International CF Congress; 2000. p. 118.

49. Armand M, Hamosh M, Philpott JR, et al. Gastric function in children with cystic fibrosis: Effect of diet on gastric lipase levels and fat digestion. *J Pediatr Res* 2004; **55**: 457–65.

50. Feranchak AP, Sontag MK, Wagener JS, et al. Perspective long term study of fat soluble vitamin status in children with cystic fibrosis identified by newborn screening. *J Pediatr* 1999; **135**: 601–10.

51. Yankaskas JR, Marshall BC, Sufian B, et al. Cystic Fibrosis Adult Care: Consensus Conference Report. *Chest* 2004; **125**: 1S–39S.

52. Greer RM, Buntain HM, Lewindon PJ, et al. Vitamin A levels in patients with CF are influenced by the inflammatory response. *J Cyst Fibros* 2004; **3**: 143–9.

53. Aird FK, Greene SA, Ogston SA, et al. Vitamin A and lung function in CF. *J Cyst Fibros* 2006: **5**: 129–31.

54. Hakim F, Kerem E, Rivlin J, et al. Vitamin A and E and pulmonary exacerbations in patients with cystic fibrosis. *J Pediatr Gastroenterol Nutr* 2007; **45**: 347–53.

55. Campbell DC, Tole DM, Doran RML, Conway SP. Vitamin A deficiency in cystic fibrosis resulting in severe xerophthalmia. *J Hum Nutr Diet* 1998; **11**: 529–32.

56. Tanumihardjo SA. Assessing vitamin A status: Past, present, and future. *Journal of Nutrition* 2004; **134**: 290S–3S.

57. Navarro J, Desquilbet N. Depressed vitamin A and retinol binding protein in cystic fibrosis correlations with zinc deficiency. *Am J Clin Nutr* 1981; **34**: 1439–40.

58. Penniston KT, Tanumihardjo SA. The acute and chronic toxic effects of vitamin A. *Am J Clin Nutr* 2006; **83** (2): 191–201.

59. Genaro Pde S, Martini LA. Vitamin A supplementation and risk of skeletal fracture. *Nutr Rev* 2004; **62**(2): 65–7.

60. Hall WB, Sparks AA, Aris RM. Vitamin D deficiency in cystic fibrosis. *Int J Endocrinol* 2010; 2010: 218691.

61. Wolfe SP, Conway SP, Brownlee KG. Seasonal variation in vitamin D levels in children with cystic fibrosis in the United Kingdom. *J Cyst Fibros*, 24th European CF Conference; 2001: 115.

62. Sermet-Gaudelus I, Bianchi ML, Garabedian M, et al. EuroCareCF: European cystic fibrosis bone mineralisation guidelines. *J Cyst Fibros* 2011; **10**: S16–23.

63. Cystic Fibrosis Trust Consensus Document. *Bone Mineralisation in Cystic Fibrosis*. Bromley, England: Cystic Fibrosis Trust; 2007.

64. Tangpricha A, Kelly A, Stephenson K, et al. An update on the screening, diagnosis, management and treatment of vitamin D deficiency in individuals with cystic fibrosis: Evidence based recommendations from the Cystic Fibrosis Foundation. *J Clin Endocrinol Metab* 2012; **97**(4): 1089–93.

65. Grey V, Atkinson S, Drury D, et al. Prevalence of low bone mass and deficiencies of vitamin D and K in pediatric patients with cystic fibrosis from 3 Canadian centres. *Pediatrics* 2008; **122**: 1014–20.

66. Wolfenden LL, Judd SE, Shah R, et al. Vitamin D and bone health in adults with cystic fibrosis. *Clin Endocrinol* 2008; **69**: 374–81.

67. Sexauer WP, Hadeh A, Ohman-Strickland PA, et al. Vitamin D deficiency is associated with pulmonary dysfunction in cystic fibrosis. *J Cyst Fibros* 2015; pii: S1569-1993(14)00303-8. [Epub ahead of print].

68. McCauley LA, Thomas W, Laguna TA, et al. Vitamin D deficiency is associated with pulmonary exacerbations in children with cystic fibrosis. *Ann Am Thorac Soc* 2014; **11**: 198–204.

69. Finklea JD, Grossmann RE, Tangpricha V. Vitamin D and chronic lung disease: A review of molecular mechanisms and clinical studies. *Adv Nutr* 2011; **2**: 244–53.

70. Borowitz D, Baker RD, Stallings V. Consensus report on nutrition for pediatric patients with cystic fibrosis. *J Pediatr Gastroenterol Nutr* 2002; **35**: 246–59.

71. Huang SH, Schall JL, Zemel BS, et al. Vitamin E status in children with cystic fibrosis and pancreatic insufficiency. *J Pediatr* 2006; **148**: 556–9.

72. Rashid M, Durie PR, Andrew M, et al. Prevalence of vitamin K deficiency in cystic fibrosis. *Am J Clin Nutr* 1999; **70**: 378–82.

73. Conway SP, Wolfe SP, Brownlee KG. Vitamin K status among children with cystic fibrosis and its relationship to bone mineral density and bone turnover. *Pediatrics* 2005; **115**(5): 1325–31.

74. Jagannath VA, Fedorowicz Z, Thaker V, et al. Vitamin K supplementation for cystic fibrosis (Review). *Cochrane Database Syst Rev* 2011; (1): CD008482.

75. Aris RM, Merkel PA, Bachrach LK, et al. Guide to bone health and disease in cystic fibrosis. *J Clin Endocrinol Metab* 2005; **90**(3): 1888–96.

76. Oliver C, Jahnke N. Omega-3 fatty acids for cystic fibrosis. *Cochrane Database Syst Rev* 2011; (80): CD002201.

77. Lloyd-Still JD, Bibus DM, Powers CA, et al. Essential fatty acid (EFA) and predisposition to lung disease in cystic fibrosis. *Acta Pediatr* 1996; **85**: 1426–32.

78. Freedman SD, Blanco PG, Zaman MN, et al. Association of cystic fibrosis with abnormalities in fatty acid metabolism. *N Engl J Med* 2004; **350**: 560–9.

79. Ciofu O, Lykkesfeldt J. Antioxidant supplementation for lung disease in cystic fibrosis. *Cochrane Database Syst Rev* 2014; (8): CD007020.

80. Bruzzese E, Raia V, Gaudiello G, et al. Intestinal inflammation is a frequent feature of cystic fibrosis and is reduced by probiotic administration. *Aliment Pharmacol Ther* 2004; **20**: 813–9.

81. Bruzzese E, Raia V, Spagnuolo MI, et al. Effect of Lactobacillus GG supplementation on pulmonary exacerbation in patients with cystic fibrosis: A pilot study. *Clinical Nutrition* 2007; **26**: 322–8.

82. Weiss B, Brujanover Y, Yahav Y, et al. Probiotic supplementation affects pulmonary exacerbation in patients with cystic fibrosis: A pilot study. *Pediatr Pulmonol* 2010; **45**: 536–40.

83. Goldenberg JZ, Ma SS, Saxton JD, et al. Probiotics for the prevention of Clostridium difficile-associated diarrhea in adults and children. *Cochrane Database Syst Rev* 2013; (5): CD006095.

84. Jelalian E, Stark LJ, Reynolds L, Seifer R. Nutrition intervention for weight gain in cystic fibrosis: A meta analysis. *J Pediatr* 1998; **132**: 486–92.

85. Leonard A, Davis E, Rosenstein BJ, et al. Description of a standardized nutrition classification plan and its relation to nutritional outcomes in children with cystic fibrosis. *J Pediatr Psychol* 2010; **35**(1): 6–13.

86. Simms EJ, Clark, McCormick J, et al. United Kingdom Cystic Fibrosis Database Steering Committee. Cystic fibrosis diagnosed after 2 months of age leads to worse outcomes and requires more therapy. *Pediatrics* 2007; **119**: 19–28.

87. Farrell PM, Lai HJ, Kosorok MR, et al. Evidence of improved outcomes with early diagnosis of cystic fibrosis through neonatal screening: Enough is enough! *J Pediatr* 2005; **147**: S30–6.

88. Shoff SM, Ahn HY, Davis L, Lai H; Wisconsin CF Neonatal Screening Group. Temporal associations among energy intake, plasma linoleic acid, and growth improvement in response to treatment initiation after diagnosis of cystic fibrosis. *Pediatrics* 2006; **117**(2): 391–400.

89. Jadin SA, Wu GS, Zhang Z, et al. Growth and pulmonary outcomes during the first 2 y of life of breastfed and formula-fed infants diagnosed with cystic fibrosis through the Wisconsin Routine Newborn Screening Program. *Am J Clin Nutr* 2011; **93**(5): 1038–47.

90. Ellis L, Kalnins D, Corey M, et al. Do infants with cystic fibrosis need a protein hydrolysate formula? A prospective, randomised comparative study. *J Pediatr* 1998; **132**: 270–6.

91. Colombo C, Costantini D, Zazzeron L, et al. Benefits of breastfeeding in cystic fibrosis: A single-centre follow-up survey. *Acta Pediatr* 2007; **96**(8): 1228–32.

92. Efrati O, Nir J, Fraser D, et al. Meconium ileus in patients with cystic fibrosis is not a risk factor for clinical deterioration and survival: The Israeli Multicenter Study. *J Pediatr Gastroenterol Nutr* 2010; **50**(2): 173–8.

93. Munck A, Gérardin M, Alberti C, et al. Clinical outcome of cystic fibrosis presenting with or without meconium ileus: A matched cohort study. *J Pediatr Surg* 2006; **41**(9): 1556–60.

94. Lai HC, Kosorok MR, Laxova A, et al. Nutritional status of patients with cystic fibrosis with meconium ileus: A comparison with patients without meconium ileus and diagnosed early through neonatal screening. *Pediatrics* 2000; **105**: 53–61.

95. Sermet-Gaudelus I, Mayell SJ, Southern KW. European Cystic Fibrosis Society (ECFS), Neonatal Screening Working Group. Guidelines on the early management of infants diagnosed with cystic fibrosis following newborn screening. *J Cyst Fibros* 2010; **9**(5): 323–9.

96. Arvanitakis SN, Lobeck CC. Metabolic alkalosis and salt depletion in cystic fibrosis. *J Pediatr* 1973; **82**(3): 535–6.

97. Ozçelik U, Göçmen A, Kiper N, et al. Sodium chloride deficiency in cystic fibrosis patients. *Eur J Pediatr* 1994; **153**(11): 829–31.

98. Kalnins D, Wilschanski M. Maintenance of nutritional status in patients with cystic fibrosis: New and emerging therapies. *Drug Des Dev Ther* 2012; **6**: 151–61.

99. Coates AJ, Crofton PM, Marshall T. Evaluation of salt supplementation in CF infants. *J Cyst Fibros* 2009; **8**(6): 382–5.

100. Krebs NF, Westcott JE, Arnold TD, et al. Abnormalities in zinc homeostasis in young infants with cystic fibrosis. *Pediatr Res* 2000; **48**(2): 256–61.

101. Easley D, Krebs N, Jefferson M, et al Effect of pancreatic enzymes on zinc absorption in cystic fibrosis. *J Pediatr Gastroenterol Nutr* 1998; **26**: 136–9.

102. Heine RG, Button BM, Olinsky A, et al. Gastro-oesophageal reflux in infants under 6 months with cystic fibrosis. *Arch Dis Child* 1998; **78**: 44–8.

103. Brodizicki J, Trawinska-Bartnicka M, Korzon M. Frequency, consequences and pharmacological treatment of gastroesophageal reflux in children with cystic fibrosis. *Med Sci Monitor* 2002; **8**: CR529–37.

104. Hammons AJ, Fiese B. Mealtime interactions in families of a child with cystic fibrosis: A meta-analysis. *J Cyst Fibros* 2010; **9**(6): 377–84.

105. Duff AJA, Wolfe SP, Dickson C, et al. Feeding behaviour problems in children with cystic fibrosis in the UK: Prevalence and comparison with healthy controls. *J Pediatr Gastroenterol Nutr* 2003; **36**: 443–7.

106. Stark LJ, Jelalian E, Powers SW, et al. Parent and child mealtime behavior in families of children with cystic fibrosis. *J Pediatr* 2000; **136**(2): 195–200.

107. Stark LJ, Opipari-Arrigan L, Quittner AL, et al. The effects of an intensive behaviour and nutrition intervention compared to standard of care on weight outcomes in CF. *Pediatr Pulmonol* 2011; **46**(1): 31–5.

108. Stark LJ, Quittner AL, Powers SW, et al. Randomized clinical trial of behavioural intervention and nutrition education to improve caloric intake and weight in children with cystic fibrosis. *Arch Pediatr Adol Med* 2009; **163**(10): 915–21.

109. Powers SW, Jones JS, Ferguson KS, et al. Randomized clinical trial of behavioral and nutritional treatment to improve energy intake and growth in toddlers and preschoolers with cystic fibrosis. *Pediatrics* 2005; **116**(6): 1442–50.

110. Neumark-Sztainer D, Story M, Falkner NH, et al. Disordered eating among adolescents with chronic illness and disability. *Arch Pediatr Adol Med* 1998; **152**: 871–8.

111. Abbott J, Conway, S, Etherington C, et al. Nutritional status, perceived body image and eating behaviour in young adults with cystic fibrosis. *Clin Nutr* 2007; **26**: 91–9.

112. Shearer JE, Bryon M. The nature and prevalence of eating disorders and eating disturbance in adolescents with cystic fibrosis. *J R Soc Med* 2004; **97** (Suppl 44): 36–42.

113. Abbott, J. Coping with cystic fibrosis. *J R Soc Med* 2003; **96**(Suppl 43): 42–50.

114. Bolton CE, Ionescu AA, Evans WD, et al. Altered tissue distribution in adults with cystic fibrosis. *Thorax* 2003; **58**: 885–9.

115. King SJ, Nyulasi IB, Strauss BJG, et al. Fat-free mass depletion in cystic fibrosis: Associated with lung disease severity but poorly detected by body mass index. *Nutrition* 2010; **26**: 753–9.

116. Smith C, Winn A, Seddon P, Ranganathan S. A fat lot of good: Balance and trends in fat intake in children with cystic fibrosis. *J Cyst Fibros* 2012; **11**(2): 154–7.

117. Maqbool A, Schall JI, Gallagher PR, et al. The relationship between type of dietary fat intake and serum fatty acid status in children with cystic fibrosis. *J Pediatr Gastroenterol Nutr* 2012; **55**(5): 605–11.

118. Woestenenk JW, Castelijns SJAM, van der Ent CK, Houwen RHJ. Nutritional intervention in patients with cystic fibrosis: A systematic review. *J Cyst Fibros* 2013; **12**: 102–5.

119. Smyth RL, Rayner O. Oral calorie supplements for cystic fibrosis. *Cochrane Database Syst Rev* 2014; (11): CD000406.

120. Poustie VJ, Russell JE, Watling RM, Ashby D, Smyth RL; CALICO Trial Collaborative Group. Oral protein energy supplements for children with cystic fibrosis: CALICO multicentre randomised controlled trial. *Br Med J* 2006; **332**(7542): 632–6.

121. Steinkamp G, Demmelmair H, Rühl-Bagheril, et al. Energy supplements rich in linoleic acid improve body weight and essential fatty acid status of cystic fibrosis patients. *J Pediatr Gastroenterol Nutr* 2000; **31**(4): 418–23.

122. White H, Morton AM, Conway SP, Peckham DG. Enteral tube feeding in adults with cystic fibrosis; patient choice and impact ov n long term outcomes. *J Cyst Fibros* 2013; 12: 616–22.

123. Bradley GM, Carson KA, Leonard AR, et al. Nutritional outcomes following gastrostomy in children with cystic fibrosis. *Pediatr Pulmonol* 2012; **47**(8): 743–8.

124. Best C, Brearley A, Gaillard P, et al. A pre-post retrospective study of patients with cystic fibrosis and gastrostomy tubes. *J Pediatr Gastroenterol Nutr* 2011; **53**(4): 453–8.

125. Truby H, Cowlishaw P, O'Neil C, Wainwright C. The long term efficacy of gastrostomy feeding in children with cystic fibrosis on anthropometric markers of nutritional status and pulmonary function. *Open Respir Med J* 2009; 3: 112–5.

126. Efrati O, Mei-Zahav M, Rivlin J, et al. Long term nutritional rehabilitation by gastrostomy in Israeli patients with cystic fibrosis: Clinical outcome in advanced pulmonary disease. *J Pediatr Gastroenterol Nutr* 2006; **42**(2): 222–8.

127. Van Biervliet S, De Waele K, Van Winckel M, Robberecht E. Percutaneous endoscopic gastrostomy in cystic fibrosis: Patient acceptance and effect of overnight tube feeding on nutritional status. *Acta Gastro-Enterlogica Belgica* 2004; **67**(3): 241–4.

128. Steinkamp G, von der Hardt H. Improvement of nutritional status and lung function after long-term nocturnal gastrostomy feedings in cystic fibrosis. *J Pediatr* 1994; **124**(2): 244–9.

129. Walker SA, Gozal D. Pulmonary function correlates in the prediction of long-term weight gain in cystic fibrosis patients with gastrostomy tube feedings. *J Pediatr Gastroenterol Nutr* 1998; 27: 53–6.

130. Oliver MR, Heine RG, Hang Ng, et al. Factors affecting clinical outcome in gastrostomy-fed children with cystic fibrosis. *Pediatr Pulmonol* 2004; 37: 324–9.

131. Conway SP, Morton A, Wolfe S. Enteral tube feeding for cystic fibrosis. *Cochrane Database Syst Rev* 2012; (12): CD001198.

132. Sciaky-Tamir Y, Armony S, Elyashar-Earon H, Wilschanski M. Prolonged TPN during pregnancy in a cystic fibrosis patient with chronic pancreatitis. *Eur J Obstet Gynaecol Reprod Biol* 2009; **143**: 62–3.

133. Nasr S, Drury D. Appetite stimulants use in cystic fibrosis. *Pediatr Pulmonol* 2008; **43**: 209–19.

134. Chinuck R, Dewar J, Baldwin DR, Hendron E. Appetite stimulants for people with cystic fibrosis. *Cochrane database System Rev* 2014; (7): CD008190.

135. Eubanks V, Koppersmith N, Wooldridge N, et al. Effects of megestrol acetate on weight gain, body composition, and pulmonary function in patients with cystic fibrosis. *J Pediatr* 2002; **140**: 439–44.

136. Homnick DN, Marks JH, Hare KL, Bonnema SK. Long-term trial of cyproheptadine as an appetite stimulant in cystic fibrosis. *Pediatr Pulmonol* 2005; **40**: 251–6.

137. Ripa P, Robertson I, Cowley D, et al. The relationship between insulin secretion, the insulin-like growth factor axis and growth in children with cystic fibrosis. *Clin Endocrinol* 2002; **56**: 383–9.

138. Hardin DS, Ellis KJ, Dyson M, et al. Growth hormone improves clinical status in prepubertal children with cystic fibrosis: Results of a randomized controlled trial. *J Pediatr* 2001; **139**: 636–42.

139. Hardin DS, Rice J, Ahn C, et al. Growth hormone treatment enhances nutrition and growth in children with cystic fibrosis receiving enteral nutrition. *J Pediatr* 2005; **146**: 324–8.

140. Braegger CP, Schlattner U, Wallimann T, et al. Effects of creatine supplementation in cystic fibrosis: Results of a pilot study. *J Cyst Fibros* 2003; **2**: 177–82.

141. Bridges N. Diabetes in cystic fibrosis. *Pediatr Respir Rev* 2013; **14** (Suppl): 16–8.

142. Kelly A, Moran A. Update on cystic fibrosis related diabetes. *Journal of Cystic Fibrosis* 2013; **12**: 318–31.

143. UK Cystic Fibrosis Trust Diabetes Working Group. *Management of Cystic Fibrosis Related Diabetes Mellitus*. Bromley, England: Cystic Fibrosis Trust; 2004.

144. Moran A, Brunzell C, Cohen R, et al. Clinical care guidelines for cystic fibrosis related diabetes. *Diabetes Care* 2010; **33**: 2697–708.

145. Javier RM, Jacquot J. Bone disease in cystic fibrosis: What's new? *Joint Bone Spine* 2011; **78**(5): 445–50.

146. Haworth CS. Impact of cystic fibrosis on bone health. *Curr Opin Pulmony Med* 2010; **16**(6): 616–22.

147. Buntain HM, Schluter PJ, Bell SC, et al. Controlled longitudinal study of bone mass accrual in children and adolescents with cystic fibrosis. *Thorax* 2006; **61**(2): 146–54.

148. Conway SP, Morton AM, Oldroyd B, et al. Osteoporosis and osteopenia in adults and adolescents with cystic fibrosis: Prevalence and associated factors. *Thorax* 2000; **55**: 798–804.

149. Lucidi V, Bizzarri C, Alghisi F, et al. Bone and body composition analyzed by dual-energy X-ray absorptiometry (DXA) in clinical and nutritional evaluation of young patients with Cystic Fibrosis: A cross-sectional study. *BMC Pediatr* 2009; **9**: 61.

150. Legroux-Gérot I, Leroy S, Prudhomme C, et al. Bone loss in adults with cystic fibrosis: Prevalence, associated factors, and usefulness of biological markers. *Joint Bone Spine* 2012; **79**(1): 73–7.

151. Fewtrell MS, Benden C, Williams JE, et al. Under carboxylated osteocalcin and bone mass in 8-12 year old children with cystic fibrosis. *J Cyst Fibros* 2008; **7**(4): 307–12.

152. Odegaad I, Stray-Pedersen B, Hallberg K, et al. Maternal and fetal morbidity in pregnancies of Norwegian and Swedish women with cystic fibrosis. *Acta Obstet Gynecol Scand* 2002; **81**: 698–705.

153. Kotloff RM, FitzSimmons SC, Fiel SB. Fertility and pregnancy in patients with cystic fibrosis. *Clin Chest Med* 1992; **13**: 623–35.

154. Morton A, Wolfe S, Conway SP. Dietetic intervention in pregnancy in women with CF—The importance of pre-conceptional counselling. *Isr J Med Sci* 1996; **32** (Suppl): S2.

155. Department of Health. Folic acid and the prevention of neural tube defects. Report from the Expert Advisory Group for Health Professionals. London: Department of Health; 1992.

156. National Institute for Health and Clinical Excellence. NICE Clinical Guideline 62—Antenatal care: Routine care for the healthy pregnant woman. London: NICE; 2008.

157. Edenborough FP, Borgo G, Knoop C, et al. Guidelines for the management of pregnancy in women with cystic fibrosis. *J Cyst Fibros* 2008: **7**; S2–32.

158. Rothman KJ, Moore LL, Singer MR, et al. Teratogenicity of high vitamin A intake. *N Engl J Med* 1995; **333**: 1369–73.

159. Gilljam M, Antoniou M, Shin J, et al. Pregnancy in cystic fibrosis. Fetal and maternal outcome. *Chest* 2000; **118**: 85–91.

160. Hollander FM, van Pierre DD, de Roos NM, et al. Effects of nutritional status and dietetic interventions on survival in cystic fibrosis patients before and after lung transplantation. *J Cyst Fibros* 2014; **13**: 212–8.

161. Hasse JM. Nutritional assessment and support of organ transplant recipients. *JPEN J Parenter Enteral Nutr* 2001; **25**: 120–31.

162. Madill, J., C. Gutierrez, J. Grossman, et al. Nutritional assessment of the lung transplant patient: Body mass index as a predictor of 90-day mortality following transplantation. *J Heart Lung Transplant* 2001; **20**(3): 288–96.

163. Lederer DJ, Wilt JS, D'Ovidio F, et al., Obesity and underweight are associated with an increased risk of death after lung transplantation. *Am J Respir Crit Care Med* 2009; **180**: 887–95.

164. Beck CE, Lin A, Robbins C, Dosanjh AK. Improvements in the nutritional and pulmonary profiles of cystic fibrosis patients undergoing bilateral sequential lung and heart-lung transplantation. *Nutr Clin Pract* 1997; **12**: 216–21.

165. Schwebel C, Pin I, Barnoud D, et al. Prevalence and consequences of nutritional depletion in lung transplant candidates. *Eur Respir J* 2000; **16**: 1050–5.

166. Nash EF, Stephenson A, Helm E, et al. Impact of lung transplantation on serum lipids in adults with cystic fibrosis. *J Heart Lung Transplant* 2011; **30**:188–93.

167. Maurer JR, Tewari S. Nonpulmonary medical complications in the intermediate and long-term survivor. *Clin Chest Med* 1997; **18**: 367–82.

168. Ho T, Samir G, Brotherwood M, et al. Increased serum vitamin A and E levels after lung transplantation. *Transplantation* 2011; **92**: 601–6.

169. Braun AT, Merlo CA. Cystic fibrosis lung transplantation. *Curr Opin Pulmon Med* 2011; **17**: 467–72.

170. Hanna RM, Weiner DJ. Overweight and obesity in patients with cystic fibrosis: A center-based analysis. *Pediatr Pulmomol* 2015; **50**(1): 35–41.

171. Kastner-Cole D, Palmer CN, Ogston SA, et al. Overweight and obesity in delta F508 homozygous cystic fibrosis. *J Pediatr* 2005; **147**: 402–4.

172. Nazareth D, Walshaw M. A review of renal disease in cystic fibrosis. *J Cyst Fibros* 2013; **12**: 309–17.

173. Morales MM, Falkenstein D, Lopes AG. The cystic fibrosis transmembrane regulator (CFTR) in the kidney. *An Acad Bras Ciênc* 2000; **72**: 399–406.

174. Terribile M, Capuano M, Cangiano G, et al. Factors increasing the risk for stone formation in adult patients with cystic fibrosis. *Nephrol Dial Transplant* 2006; **21**: 1870–5.

45

Psychology

ALISTAIR J.A. DUFF AND HELEN OXLEY

INTRODUCTION

The psychological effects of living with cystic fibrosis (CF) can be overwhelming for patients and their relatives. However, both can exhibit astounding emotional resilience to achieve good quality of life (QoL) in the face of adversity.

A new era of CF care has been forged from developments in diagnosis and management such that there is a remarkable improvement in the health of patients and increased survival.[1] With diagnosis commonly occurring in infancy via newborn screening, pediatric aspirations are that children and young people enter adulthood in excellent physical condition and with a good-enough QoL to engage fully in the opportunities of young adulthood. Twenty-first century cohorts of newborn patients are expected to live into their mid-50s,[2] with the further promise of treatments that are mutation-class specific and which address the underlying genetic defects, rendering CF a "plurality" of disease, each constituent with its own trajectory and outcomes. Consequently, for an increasing majority of children and teenagers with CF and their parents, descriptions of their psychosocial well-being published before the millennium are now somewhat redundant.

Contemporary cohorts of adults, some of whom have lived beyond their own expectations, now constitute the majority of the CF population in the United Kingdom. Many enjoy good QoL, many have jobs or are in further education, and some have families of their own. Median UK predicted survival is now almost 37 years.[3] However, median age of death in the United Kingdom is currently at 29 years[3] and predicted survival should not mask the fact that there remains considerable morbidity and early mortality in this group of patients. Although there remains hope that new pharmacological currently in clinical trials will lead to even better survival, anticipation will take time to be realized. Although increasing numbers of adults with CF have milder disease, for many, treatment remains complex, demanding, and time consuming, where optimal levels of adherence continue to compete with the activities of normal daily living.

Adults with CF have a range of additional challenges compared with their pediatric counterparts. There may be long periods of poor health and hospitalization, with a need to cope with declining function and the increased complications experienced by those growing older with CF. Juggling these issues, together with the demands of adult working/family lives (and sometimes concerns about who will provide the care needed in the future), can produce great challenges. This can result in significant emotional difficulties for many, which require specialist intervention. However, as with children and families, adults with CF also show great coping skills, and harnessing their resilience can help guide CF teams in maximizing patients' QoL as well as longevity.

Consequently, the psychological challenges of CF for patients and their families partly correspond to the era of care they were born into. The importance of psychological care within CF centers is undisputed and psychologically trained professionals are well-established members of the team. They have wide-ranging roles and responsibilities, which are extensively detailed in Standards of Care publications.[4,5] Furthermore, clinical trials and practice have benefited from utilizing the Cystic Fibrosis Quality of Life Scale[6] leading to an increase in the breadth of health outcome measures. Integrating patient reported outcomes has afforded expanded knowledge of the psychological, social, and emotional aspects of daily living with CF, not previously reflected in health indicators.

This chapter considers contemporary psychological aspects of CF in three sections. The first adopts a cohort model to consider infants, children, adolescents and adults, and their families. The second reviews one of the most clinically crucial psychological issues facing CF multidisciplinary teams (MDTs) today: adherence to treatment and other healthcare behaviors. The final section outlines key psychological treatments and management strategies, differentiating between those conducted generally by the team and specialized psychological therapies, delivered by the CF team psychologist.

time, forgetfulness, and running out of medication are often cited as the reasons for not adhering to treatment regimes. But once more, beliefs about the necessity of treatment are intermittent and often result in experimentation with cessation to test if a difference is seen.[54] When CF becomes more severe, despite good adherence, reduced QoL can lead to depression/low mood, which in turn affects motivation to take medicines and follow recommendations as directed. Demoralization, as opposed to depression, is seen in many people with physical illness, characterized by hopelessness and powerlessness[69] and leads to more entrenched patterns of poor adherence.

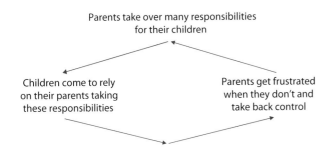

Figure 45.1 Parental conflict. Parents expect their children to take on those responsibilities but view their competencies negatively.[67]

Adherence to CF care, across all age groups is linked to four, well-established factors: (1) engagement and communication with the CF team, (2) knowledge, (3) assessment and measurement problems, and (4) regimen characteristics. These are detailed in Table 45.1.

DEMANDS OF HEALTH CARE

As morbidity increases so does the frequency of hospital attendances and admissions. Tackling this can be difficult particularly when an avoidant coping style (commonly seen in CF) has been utilized by the patient. Levels of activity and lifestyle become threatened and result in either the patient avoiding the care required to some degree or facing the "losses" and disruptions associated with exposure to the realities of CF experienced by others with more advanced disease. Advancing disease can also result in increasing need for surgical interventions (e.g., embolization and treatments for pneumothoraces) and use of intrusive medical devices (e.g., port-a-caths, gastrostomies, and noninvasive ventilation), leading to fear, anxiety, body image worries, and traumatic stress reactions. This can further disrupt optimal care and result in ambivalence about making decisions or giving consent. Teams need to understand these issues empathically and actively help manage the resulting emotions and behaviors.

Table 45.1 Multifaceted aspects of poor adherence

Factor	Elements	Responses
Engagement	Engagement with the team requires active attention to deliver optimal. Patient communication and relationships with the multidisciplinary team (MDT) will be influenced by beliefs about trust and autonomy or perceived interference with independent choices. Such conversations are investments in relationships with patients and parents. Patients are more likely to adhere if they feel supported by their MDT. Poor relationships with the MDT affect attendance and willingness to follow advice. As patients' confidence increases they switch from passive to active engagement in their health care. Actively engaged patients develop key knowledge and skills to manage health independently. Active engagement improves health outcomes and satisfaction.	Listen to and understand patient perspective about living with cystic fibrosis (CF). Respect patient choices, values, and decisions. Facilitate patients' consideration of the pros and cons of behavior change. Enhance the relationship with empathy and understanding. This helps patients discuss matters openly and honestly and helps them feel "connected" to team. *Do not:* • Argue for change • Openly confront resistance • Persuade, bribe, or cajole *Do:* • Invite patients' perspectives on their care • Accept that patients' treatment goals may vary from clinicians' • Reinforce any small changes or contemplation of change positively • Support patients' emerging confidence that they can adhere more

(Continued)

Table 45.1 (*Continued*) Multifaceted aspects of poor adherence

Factor	Elements	Responses
Knowledge	Gaps in patients/relatives knowledge and understanding are common. Knowledge is influenced by the quality of interactions with health professionals. Patients/relatives can be unwilling to express concerns and problems as part of an avoidant-coping style. Adolescents with CF engage in more risk-taking behaviors than healthy peers, whereas adults may not. Many adults do have incomplete understanding of infection risks. In older adults, treatment-specific knowledge is vital.	Give information about the illness and treatment using an information-exchange cycle.[71] Describe side effects and acknowledge problems associated with adhering to complex regimes. Underpin the long-term benefits of therapy rather than allude to any short-term gain. Pre-empt barriers to adherence by using goal setting and problem solving. Prepare for lapses in adherence by using implementation planning and monitoring.
Measuring	Unreliable measuring techniques account for inconsistency in adherence rates. No single measure of adherence will be accurate enough given the complexity of CF therapy and the required behaviors. Systematic review concludes that it is difficult to establish exactly what patients and parents are expected to do. Medical records often fail to contain reliable or consistent regimen information.	Provide a written treatment plan. Measure adherence using multimodal methods of assessment. Only use self-report measures in conjunction with at least one other measure. Electronic monitors have the greatest accuracy but are not yet a "gold standard" measure as they are expensive, prone to malfunction, and are not available for all CF treatments. In **large-scale studies**, pharmacy collection is the most feasible measure of adherence. In **clinical practice**, daily phone diaries should be used whenever possible as there is good correlation with electronic measures.
Regimen	Lower rates of adherence are most prevalent when: • Regimens are complex • There are adverse side effects • There are no perceived immediate benefits These factors alone are thought to account for huge variability in adherence rates to the different elements of CF care. The triumvirate of treatments which CF patients typically adhere to suboptimally are dietary recommendations, physiotherapy, and inhalation therapy.	Actively support efforts to routinized care. Adherence at weekend and during holidays can be less in adolescents and young adults. Where possible: • Consider "treatment holidays" • Negotiate what can be achieved initially and very gradually increase until optimal (or near-optimal) adherence is achieved • Introduce flexibility with dietary and physiotherapy regimens

SECTION 3: PSYCHOLOGICAL INTERVENTION AND MANAGEMENT

Psychological interventions are integral to optimizing CF health outcomes by improving adaptation, coping, and QoL; ameliorating emotional distress; inhibiting psychopathology; and optimizing engagement in healthcare behaviors. However, these responsibilities should not be undertaken by the psychosocial professional alone. The entire CF team must utilize some psychological skills to deliver effective care.

This section covers the four main aspects of delivering psychological care and support to patients/families: (1) psychological principles and skills underpinning care by the whole CF team, (2) screening and monitoring, (iii) interventions for adherence, and (iv) specialized psychological therapies.

PSYCHOSOCIAL CARE BY THE CF TEAM

The ethos of the team impacts on all aspects of patient care. Team members often have long and at times intense relationships with patients and families, seeing them frequently and sometimes in difficult circumstances. Teams need to deliver care that is both holistic and patient/family centered, paying attention to people with CF achieving a balanced QoL that has as much prominence as morbidity and longevity. Interdisciplinary working (i.e., working closely together with a shared philosophy, good communication, and willingness to address difficulties),[72] as opposed to multidisciplinary care (i.e., a team comprising different professionals), facilitates the integration of good psychological care.

Psychosocial support to patients and families needs to be provided by all members of the CF team in a "stepped" care way. At the primary level, basic skills can be utilized by everyone who has contact with patients,[73] based on a compassionate communication style, effective information giving, and recognizing and responding to distress. Specific training packages in this area have evaluated well.[74]

Relationships between healthcare professionals and patients/families need to be empathic, collaborative, and empowering. Good communication is a prerequisite for any CF team. Developing and nurturing communication skills, both verbal and nonverbal, is a tremendous investment in patients' well-being as they facilitate open discussion and information giving in a way that is individually meaningful to the patient, taking account of their needs for involvement, choice, and control in their care.[75,76] Practitioners in other illness groups regularly update these skills via a network of training, which have been shown to dramatic increase in clinician-expressed empathy.[77] These features were the hallmark of a US CF center, lauded for its health outcomes, where there was a huge emphasis on excellent collaborative communication and establishment of honest partnership with patients and families to identify and address problems creatively.[78] Teams need to continually review such efforts via quality improvement initiatives, which can focus on, for example, increasing outpatient efficiency and thereby the time available for consultations.[79] Skills for more specific situations should also be acquired by some team members; for example, breaking bad news (for which several techniques exist),[80] recognizing signs/symptoms of major psychological problems, and how to access emergency psychiatric services.

At the next level of psychological assessment and support, some staff use techniques such as relaxation training, problem solving, and "psychological first-aid" (e.g., in responding to expression of deliberate self-harm or suicidal ideation). Specialist psychological professionals should take a key role in developing and supporting the psychosocial skills of the CF team through training, strategic planning of team development, joint work, and case reflection/supervision, in addition to delivering higher level psychotherapeutic interventions to patients and families when required.

Working in a CF team generates great satisfaction for staff but can also result in huge emotional and physical demands. Striking the balance between patient care and self-care is, therefore, important and may need to be proactively addressed. In addition to sufficient training in specific psychological skills, opportunities for the team to meet to discuss difficult problems are essential, whether to do with patient care, patient/family/team dynamics or issues within the team. Such conversations may help after particularly stressful or upsetting events such as the death of a patient, in the context of team reviews.[81] "Clinical supervision" or reflective practice on casework that is routine for psychological therapists can be unfamiliar to other professionals, but its usefulness in managing challenging work is clear[82] and this can be incorporated into team-based "complex case meetings" held either regularly or as required. Whichever the forum, all CF teams need to find appropriate ways of supporting each other, managing stresses and functioning well as a group. The psychologically trained professionals in that team can play a significant role in ensuring this.

SCREENING AND MONITORING

Routine psychological surveillance is advocated in European Standards of Care.[5] In both pediatric and adult services, screening allows early identification of, and intervention for, emerging psychopathology to prevent the development of more severe problems, which then impact on health engagement and outcomes.

Psychological screening and assessment is increasingly becoming part of annual clinical review, which all UK CF patients should receive.[4,5] In the wake of TIDES data, an international guideline committee has recommended annual screening of depression and anxiety in adolescents and adults with CF (aged >12 years) and parent caregivers, using the PHQ-9 and GAD-7.[19] In the United Kingdom, the CF center service specification specifies that one of the essential roles of the team psychologist is to undertake annual assessment of every patient. Given the prevalence and risk factors associated with depression and anxiety, specific screening for these symptoms using internationally agreed measures is a logical step, and in the United Kingdom can form part of more comprehensive surveillance that is commensurate with a preventative/early-intervention ethos. The CF psychologist is ideally placed to evaluate the clinical significance of any elevated screening scores and make clinical decisions about initiating any strategies to address problems.

Other covered in psychological annual review can include other psychological problems present (or the risk factors for developing these), assessment of coping style, skills and resources, and assessment of healthcare behavior including a review of relationship with the CF team.

As well as during annual screening, patients/families with CF may benefit from routine assessment (and intervention as indicated) at certain points in the CF "illness trajectory." In pediatric services key times are postdiagnosis, going to secondary school, and transition to adult services. In adult services such points include: following diagnosis in adulthood, when there is a significant deterioration in health or emergence of new complications, at transplant referral, following traumatic medical events and when there is consideration of starting a family.

INTERVENTIONS FOR ADHERENCE

Specific psychological approaches for adherence difficulties stand much greater chance of success if they use combined or multimodal strategies, which are embedded in a strong team culture of openness and honesty. Actively listening to patients and engaging them in their health care helps achieve the "biting point" of having to act medically responsibly for care without "taking" responsibility for the patient.

Independent health care needs to be increased gradually from late childhood/early adolescence, and teams need to foster confidence in young patients by spending incrementally more time with them alone (away from their parents, but not exclusively so) during clinic visits. Here, the importance of optimal adherence is underlined by discussing precisely how this makes a difference to health and teaching young people how to express their views and concerns and formulate and ask questions during consultations. Teams also need to consider adherence in the context of what the patient wants to achieve in their lives (say, in the next 12 months). In this way, patients can start to explicitly link optimal adherence to better health and personal objectives.

Figure 45.2 presents an algorithm for considering what intervention might be appropriate and when.

Individual psychotherapeutic approaches to adherence depend on patients' readiness to change. Perceptual or emotional barriers are often present in those unwilling to openly recognize adherence problems or who lack motivation to change. The effectiveness of addressing these issues within the context of a motivational interviewing (MI) framework is gaining in both empirical and clinical strength.[70] There is emerging proof that CF-specific training in MI has lasting learning outcomes[83] and changes clinical practice.[84] For patients who are ready to make changes, a wide range of behavioral techniques (e.g. problem solving,[85] implementation intention planning, and reinforcement scheduling[71]) are gaining impressive ground. Several clinical trials are currently ongoing evaluating, for example, MI and problem solving, social networking, and web-based support.

Both perceptual/emotional and behavioral approaches to adherence are summarized in Table 45.2. Technical strategies (e.g., formulation and dosing options, and device technology and techniques) are also important when trying to improve adherence and need to be incorporated at every opportunity.[86]

Further work is now required to focus on accurately identifying who is and who is not adhering optimally. Self-reports and clinician reports of adherence do not achieve this when compared with electronic monitoring.[89] There also needs to be increased efforts to make interventions more practical for patients and their families. Use of technology, smartphone applications, online and text messaging, feedback loops, and web-based support streams are all under investigation. It has been suggested that using social media at the very least can help to transfer the locus of control to the patient and result in greater active engagement with health professionals.[90]

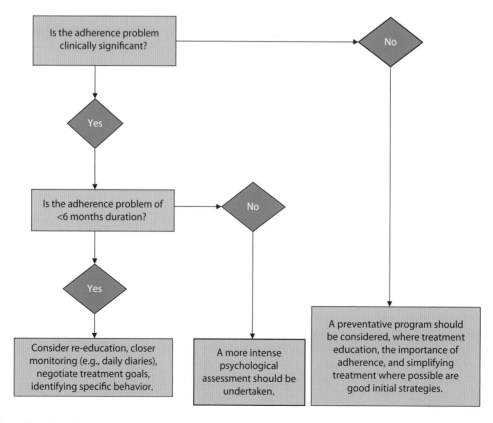

Figure 45.2 Algorithm for adherence interventions.

Table 45.2 Perceptual and behavioral strategies to improve adherence

	Approach	Aim	Activity
Perceptual	Motivational[71]	Utilize good relationships and agree on an agenda for discussion (expression of empathy). Develop discrepancy between thoughts and behaviors. Roll with resistance. Support self-efficacy when patient is ready to attempt change.	Use open-ended questions and reflective statements. Both patient and professional draw up a list of topics together, but the patient selects starting point. Explore health beliefs and perceptions. Use test results, weigh up pros and cons of increasing adherence. Avoid confrontation and return to empathic listening skill. Increase confidence and utilize behavioral strategies (see below).
	Personal construct[86]	Individuals interpret reality according to their own personal constructs of how the world works. Problems arise when these become redundant or do not alter to assimilate new information.	Acknowledges link between illness perceptions and self-identity and esteem. Aim to help patients change their constructs to a more viable option (e.g., by constructing an identity other than someone with CF).
	Cognitive[87]	Patients are encouraged to explore their thoughts and to link these to their emotional, behavioral, and physiological reactions.	Identify thinking "errors" and generate alternative, more balanced, thoughts.
Behavioral	Problem solving[85]	Assess negative impact of problems and generate alternative solutions.	Clarify and define the problem to be solved. Set realistic goal. Generate multiple possible solutions. List pros and cons for each solution. Select the best and most feasible solution (to be agreed by all stakeholders). Initiate and evaluate.
	Behavior modification[71,88]	Learn from observation and imitation, where desirable behaviors are reinforced. Reinforcement can be positive (a reward such as praise) or negative (avoiding something bad, such as illness). This is not to be confused with punishment, which can also be construed as positive (punishment such as being told off) or negative (losing a reward).	Set SMART goals (Specific, Measureable, Attainable, Relevant, and Time-bound). Identify: possible barriers, strategies to overcome them, and support. Implementation intention plans (defining the response if something goes wrong). Behavioral contracting. Incorporate into routines. Positive reinforcement of incremental success, varying the frequency of reinforcement schedule (from constant to intermittent) and the targets.

SPECIALIST PSYCHOLOGICAL THERAPIES

All CF teams must have specialized psychology provision to effectively deliver a range of well-established therapies and strategies considered central to achieving excellent health outcomes.[4,5,72]

Parental support following diagnosis

Postdiagnosis psychological support for parents can be provided in various ways, but is broadly achieved through a combination of didactic teaching sessions and group-based, peer interaction. For contemporary cohorts of parents of newborn infants with CF, the principal aims of psychological management at this point are to facilitate emotional processing of "loss," help parents balance the tasks of disease management with normal infant development by establishing good infant routines (including feeding patterns), and socialization. Parental confidence in engaging their child in social activity can be tempered by anxiety about exposure to environmental risks of infection and this needs to be openly discussed.[21] Acceptance and commitment therapy (ACT), and nondirective approaches are becoming viable and effective psychotherapeutic bases for this work.

Focused parent support groups can be particularly useful at this point, with ongoing, less-frequent opportunities for parents to meet being hosted by the team. Psychological surveillance needs to be established, either as part of annual review or on a case-by-case basis, for parents at risk of developing, among other things, insecure attachments, anxiety, depression or demoralization, post-traumatic stress symptoms (e.g., "flashbacks") role/parenting stress, and family functioning.

Behavioral problems

Anxiety alters the way in which parents raise their children, often resulting with unwanted behaviors being unwittingly reinforced. Behavior difficulties can impinge on CF treatment procedures (e.g., cough swabs, spirometry, swallowing tablets/medicines, using inhalation or resistance masks, and most commonly, venepuncture). The threats to effective care are enormous and as such, it is essential that CF psychologists attain competency in delivering the behavioral techniques known to be effective in ameliorating these problems.[88]

Perhaps the most common behavioral problem in childhood is feeding behavior. Combined behavioral and dietetic approaches are essential to both effect rescue from and prevent these difficulties. A randomized control trial of joint behavior therapy and nutritional education showed significant initial improvement in dietary intake but not in the longer term.[91] However, intensive behavioral and nutritional intervention remains effective, as is preventative parental work for preschool children with CF and need to be adapted to be incorporated into routine clinical practice.[92] Early referral for such interventions is thought to be crucial.[93]

Psychoeducation for patients and families

Given the reported gaps and misconceptions in CF-related knowledge of patients and relatives, teams need to continually implement education programs that inform, motivate, and support. There is a plethora of good CF information and registry data available (from the UK CF Trust, US CF Foundation, and other key medical websites). Evaluation of education programs is scant; however, a Cochrane review found some evidence to suggest that self-management education may improve knowledge in patients with CF but not in parents or caregivers. There was also some limited evidence to suggest that self-management education may result in positively changing a small number of behaviors in both patients and caregivers.[94] What is emerging as perhaps more important is the way in which information is given. The most clearly written and concise facts will not be heeded if there is no thoughtful engagement in the topic. Memory is the residue of thought and without thinking, no amount of repetition will increase learning or knowledge. The alternative is to engage in an information exchange, also known as the "elicit–provide–elicit cycle." Patients or carers are asked what they already know, then provided with some information with immediate follow-up questions about what they have retained and what their reactions are. This process actively absorbs people in processing information, significantly increasingly the likelihood it will be retained.[71]

A final essential strand of psychoeducational programs is preparing patients and relatives for developmental transitions (e.g., starting school and moving to high school, further education, or employment) and the transfer of or adaptations to treatment. Many centers now routinely use psychoeducational strategies prior to secondary school.

Individual psychological interventions (adolescents and adults)

For many emotional disorders, notably depression and anxiety, cognitive behavior therapy (CBT) is the treatment of choice for most.[95,96] The application of CBT in many chronic health conditions has been described elsewhere, together with details of this approach.[97] In essence, CBT approaches are collaborative, time limited, and structured ways of helping patients make changes to their thinking and behavior patterns to manage unwanted emotions. Complex psychological "formulations" (i.e., hypotheses about what is going wrong for a patient and why) are jointly built between psychologist and patient. Intervention then focuses on identifying unhelpful elements, and changes required. In CF, understanding the development and maintenance of emotional problems must include understanding of the role of CF itself, as this can be very significant, and the delivery of therapy may need to be modified significantly to be most effective.[98] Related "talking therapies" are emerging as useful for those with physical health problems including solution focused work[99] and several others (e.g., narrative approaches, mindfulness, compassion-focused therapy, and ACT—as outlined earlier) may have much to offer in CF psychological care. As in pediatric care, a systemic approach to problems may be needed (i.e., where appropriate, involving patients' partners, parents, and even children in therapeutic work).

Specifically tailored psychological treatment may be required for some of the adverse events experienced by people with CF. This requires both specialist knowledge of CF and how to utilize this in combination with any psychotherapeutic approaches used. For example, therapeutic work following major hemotypsis or pneumothorax may need to treat "post-traumatic" symptoms including maladaptive avoidance of activities, but simultaneously address the distinct reality of recurrence and effective management of this. Equally, at times of deteriorating health, psychological work may focus on improving coping strategies and problem solving while simultaneously addressing low mood and fear, in the face of the reality of CF.

At end-stage illness or transplant referral, significant psychological intervention is often required. Specifically adapted approaches might include using decision-making techniques (in conjunction with CF team), consideration of ability to emotionally cope with the transplant process, work on improving adherence or weight to a sufficient level, and managing the challenges of life on an active waiting list.[100] When lung transplantation is not an option, or does not occur as hoped, focus on anticipatory grief may be required, alongside psychological strategies for managing end-stage symptoms,[101] and work with family members.

Despite the rapid increase in CF services for adults and the work being done within these to deliver specialist psychological interventions of many kinds, little has been published on outcomes of such interventions with CF populations,[102] although generic proof of efficacy should be sufficient to determine benefits.

Finally, in addition to individual psychotherapeutic work, the team psychologist has an important liaison role where a more psychiatric approach is required. Coordinating care provided by the CF team and mental health services is important, as is guiding the CF team on identifying and managing psychosocial "risks" for patients and families (e.g., issues relating to child protection, self-harm, suicide, capacity to consent, and vulnerability).

CONCLUSIONS

With the dawning of a new era of CF care, patients with CF have significantly increased longevity. Yet, the challenge for medical teams is to ensure reciprocal enhancement in QoL. New ways of conceptualizing CF by genetic mutation class may determine different courses the disease may take and this requires a revision of how information is conveyed. New treatments present new psychosocial challenges for patients and their families as their burden of care changes. Continuing improved longevity in CF is dependent on a sequence in which the relationship between patient and health professional becomes the foundation to people with CF becoming active stakeholders in their care. It is only by achieving such an underpinning that new therapies will be adhered to optimally and as such, active listening and engagement skills are not the monopoly of psychosocial professionals and need to be adopted by the entire team.

Enough is known about which psychological interventions are effective to shape what may be helpful in the management of CF. Supporting parents after diagnosis and instilling hope for their child's future, screening for psychopathology, helping them manage behavior problems (both feeding and procedural) are key tasks in infancy and pre-school years. Optimizing the way in which children, young people and adults with CF, and their families obtain and retain information, as well as motivating and supporting their efforts to adhere to treatment is similarly vital.

Adolescents and adults also require specialist psychological intervention from time to time. Individual psychotherapy is effective in tackling psychopathology and CF psychologists have key roles in implementing and evaluating interventions, and targeting those thought to be most vulnerable. They are also able to guide and support the psychosocial care provided by other team members and help the team ensure that psychological care can be effectively and pragmatically incorporated into routine management.

There are many psychosocial aspects of CF that we are only beginning to understand. As with many aspects of CF care, increasing implementation of Quality Improvement/ Quality Management approaches has much potential to develop psychological care in CF in the future. The effects of family functioning on health outcomes are emerging, particularly with regards to adherence. Parent–child conflict has consistently emerged as a key factor in the establishment and maintenance of adherence difficulties. Health beliefs and illness perceptions are also important determinants of adherence, and coping strategies associated with more positive health outcomes and successful psychological adaptation must be explored further. MI is an effective intervention in other illness groups and offers a practical framework to health professionals working in CF without necessarily requiring further specific evaluation. When patients are motivated to change, MI contextualizes the emerging behavioral strategies, such as problem solving, solution-focused therapy, reinforcement scheduling, and implementation planning. What is now more important is how MI can practically be organized within teams.

Psychological aspects of CF care are of key importance in delivering effective and balanced services to patients and families, as a result of the substantial challenges CF poses and the complex nature of care. Adherence to treatment remains a particularly difficult issue in this field and the major contemporary psychological challenge. However in concluding, everyone working with CF patients and their families must salute the tremendous efforts they make to lead normal lives and maintain hope in the face of adversity.

REFERENCES

1. Simmonds NJ, Macneill SJ, Cullinan P, Hodson ME. Cystic fibrosis and survival to 40 years: A case-control study. *Eur Respir J* 2010; **36**: 1277–83.
2. Dodge JA, Lewis PA, Stanton M, Wilsher J. Cystic fibrosis mortality and survival in the UK: 1947-2003. *Eur Respir J* 2007; **29**: 522–6.
3. CF Trust. *Annual Data Report* 2013. July 2014. Available at https://www.cysticfibrosis.org.uk/media/316760/Scientific%20Registry%20Review%202012.pdf; accessed, February 20, 2015.
4. CF Trust. *Standards for the Clinical Care of Children and Adults with Cystic Fibrosis in the UK.* 2nd Edition. December 2011. Available at http://www.cftrust.org.uk/aboutcf/publications/consensusdoc/CF_Trust_Standards_of_Care_2011; accessed Febrary 20, 2015.
5. Smyth A, Bell S, Bojcin S, et al. European cystic fibrosis standards of care; best practice guidelines. *J Cyst Fibros* 2014; **13**: S23–S42.

6. Modi AC, Quittner AL. Validation of a disease-specific measure of health-related quality of life for children with cystic fibrosis. *J Ped Psychol* 2003; **28**: 535–46.

7. Moran J, Quirk K, Duff AJA, Brownlee KG. Newborn screening for CF in a regional paediatric centre: The psychosocial effects of false-positive IRT results on parents. *J Cyst Fibros* 2007; 6: 250–4.

8. Beucher J, Leray E, Deneuville E, et al. Psychological effects of false-positive results in cystic fibrosis newborn screening: A two-year follow-up. *J Pediatr* 2010; **156**: 771–6.

9. Castellani C, Southern KW, Brownlee K, Dankert-Roesle J, Duff AJA, Farrell M, et al. European best practice guidelines for cystic fibrosis neonatal screening. *J Cyst Fibros* 2009; **8**: 153–73.

10. Olshansky S. Chronic sorrow: A response to having a mentally defective child. *Soc Casework* 1962; **43**: 190–3.

11. Berge JM, Patterson JM. Cystic fibrosis and the family: A review and critique of the literature. *Fam Syst Health* 2004; **22**: 74–100.

12. Sheehan J, Massie J, Hay M, et al. The natural history and predictors of persistent problem behaviours in cystic fibrosis: A multicentre, prospective study. *Arch Dis Child* 2012; **97**: 625–31.

13. Modi AC, Quittner AL. Barriers to treatment adherence for children with cystic fibrosis and asthma: What gets in the way? *J Pediatr* 2006; **31**: 846–58.

14. Powers SW, Mitchell SR, Patton KC, et al. Mealtime behaviours in families of infants and toddlers with cystic fibrosis. *J Cyst Fibros* 2005; **4**: 175–82.

15. Stark LJ, Opipari LC, Jelalian E, et al. Child behaviour and parent management strategies at mealtimes in families with a school-age child with cystic fibrosis. *Health Psychol* 2005; **24**: 274–80.

16. Segal TY. Adolescence: What the cystic fibrosis team needs to know. *J R Soc Med* 2008; **101**: S15–27.

17. Szyndler JE, Towns SJ, van Asperen PP, McKay KO. Psychological and family functioning and quality of life in adolescents with cystic fibrosis. *J Cyst Fibros* 2005; **4**: 135–44.

18. Duff AJA, Abbott J, Cowperthwaite C, et al. Depression and anxiety in adolescents and adults with cystic fibrosis in the UK: A cross-sectional study. *J Cyst Fibros* 2014; **13**: 745–753.

19. Quittner AL, Goldbeck L, Abbott J, et al. Prevalence of depression and anxiety in patients with cystic fibrosis and parent caregivers: Results of The International Depression Epidemiological Study (TIDES) across nine countries. *Thorax* 2014; **69**: 1090–97.

20. Graetz BW, Shute RH, Sawyer MG. An Australian study of adolescents with cystic fibrosis: Perceived supportive and non supportive behaviours from families and friends and psychological adjustment. *J Adol Health* 2000; **26**: 64–9.

21. Ullrich G, Wiedau-Gors S, Steinkamp G, et al. Parental fears of Pseudomonas infection and measures to prevent its acquisition. *J Cyst Fibros* 2002; **1**: 122–30.

22. Sharpe D, Rossiter L. Siblings of children with a chronic illness: A meta-analysis. *J Ped Psychol* 2002; **27**: 699–710.

23. Foster CL, Eiser C, Oades P, et al. Treatment demands and differential treatment of patients with cystic fibrosis and their siblings: Patient, parents and sibling accounts. *Child Care Health Dev* 2001; **27**: 349–64.

24. Kuther T. Medical decision-making and minors: Issues of consent and assent. *Adolescence* 2003; **38**: 343–51.

25. Towns SJ, Bell SC. Transition of adolescents with cystic fibrosis from paediatric to adult care. *Clin Resp J* 2011; **5**; 64–75.

26. Hayes M, Yaster M, Haythornwaite JA, et al. Pain is a common problem affecting clinical outcomes in adults with cystic fibrosis. *Chest* 2011; **140**(6): 1598–1603.

27. Sharma I, Webb AK, Oxley H. Sleep problems in patients of an adult cystic fibrosis centre. *J Cyst Fibros* 2008; **7** (Suppl 2): S102.

28. Gee L, Abbott J, Conway SP, et al. Quality of life in cystic fibrosis: The impact of gender, general health perceptions and disease severity. *J Cyst Fibros* 2003; **2**: 206–13.

29. Gee L, Abbott J, Hart A, et al. Associations between clinical variables and quality of life in adults with cystic fibrosis. *J Cyst Fibros* 2005; **4**: 59–66.

30. Yohannes Y, Abebaw, Willgoss G, et al. Relationship between anxiety, depression and quality of life in adult patients in cystic fibrosis. *Respir Care* 2012; **57**: 550-6.

31. Riekert KA, Bartlett SJ, Boyle MP, et al. The association between depression, lung function and health-related quality of life among adults with cystic fibrosis. *Chest* 2007; **132**: 231–7.

32. Riekert KA Bartlett SJ, Boyle MP, Rand CS. The relationship between depression, disease severity and quality of life in adults with cystic fibrosis. *Am J Resp Crit Care Med* 2004; **169**: A392.

33. Cruz I, Marciel KK, Quittner AL, Schechter MS. Anxiety and depression in cystic fibrosis. *Semin Respir Crit Care Med* 2009; **30**: 569–78.

34. Goldbeck L, Besier T, Hinz A, et al (TIDES Study Group). Prevalence of anxious and depressive symptoms in German patients with cystic fibrosis. *Chest* 2010; **138**: 929–36.

35. Latchford GJ, Duff AJA. Assessing anxiety, depression and suicidal ideation in a single CF centre. *J Cyst Fibros* 2013; **12**: 794–796.

36. Duff AJA, Laurens H, Moore S, Povey L, Horton S. Deliberate self-harm and suicide in adults and parents of children with CF: A national survey of the experiences and training needs of the multi-disciplinary team. *J Cyst Fibros* 2005; **4** (Suppl 1): S112.

37. Goodwin RD, Pine DS. Respiratory disease and panic attacks among adults in the United States. *Chest* 2002; **2**: 645–50.

38. Tierney S. Body image and cystic fibrosis: A critical review. *Body Image* 2012; **9**: 1740–5.

39. Oxley H, Webb AK. How a clinical psychologist manages the problems of adults with cystic fibrosis. *J R Soc Med* 2005; **98** (Suppl 45): 37–46.

40. Iles N, Lowton K. What is the perceived nature of parental care and support for young people with cystic fibrosis as they enter adult health services. *Health Soc Care Commun* 2010; **18**: 21–9.

41. Delelis G, Christophe V, Leroy S, et al. The effects of cystic fibrosis in couples: Marital satisfaction, emotions and coping strategies. *Scand J Psychol* 2008; **49**: 583–9.

42. Didsbury J, Thackray E. *Cystic Fibrosis and Relationships*. Bromley, England: Cystic Fibrosis Trust; 2009.

43. Fair A, Griffiths K, Osman LM. Attitudes to fertility among adults with cystic fibrosis in Scotland. *Thorax* 2000; **55**: 672–7.

44. Havermans T, Abbott J, Colpaert K, De Boeck K. Communication of information about reproductive and sexual health in cystic fibrosis. Patients, parents and caregivers' experience. *J Cyst Fibros* 2011; **10**: 221–7.

45. Edenborough FP, Borgo G, Knoop C, et al. Guidelines for the management of pregnancy in women with cystic fibrosis. *J Cystic Fibros* 2008; **7** (Suppl 1): S2–32.

46. Widerman E. Knowledge, interests and educational needs of adults receiving a cystic fibrosis diagnosis after age 18. *J Cyst Fibros* 2003; **2**; 97–104.

47. Braithwaite M, Philip J, Tranberg H, et al. End of life care in CF: Patients, families and staff experiences and unmet needs. *J Cyst Fibros* 2011; **10**(4): 253–7.

48. Chapman E, Landy A, Lyon A, et al. End of life care for adult cystic fibrosis patients: Facilitating a good enough death. *J Cyst Fibros* 2005; **4**(4): 249–57.

49. Bourke SJ, Doe SJ, Gascoigne AD, Heslop K. An integrated model of provision of palliative care to patients with cystic fibrosis. *Pall Med* 2009; **23**: 512–7.

50. Sawicki GS, Dill EJ, Asher D, et al. Advance care planning in adults with cystic fibrosis *J Pall Med* 2008; **11**(8): 1135–41.

51. Robinson WM. A symptom based approach to palliative care in cystic fibrosis. *Prog Pall Care* 2011; **19**: 230–4.

52. Abbott J, Hart A, Morton A, et al. Health related quality of life in adults with cystic Fibrosis: The role of coping. *J Psychosom Res* 2008; **64**: 149–57.

53. Hofer M, Hirt A, Kurowski T, et al. Resilience, physical and psychical well-being and health related quality of life in adult CF patients. *J Cyst Fibros* 2012; **11** Suppl 138: 1569.

54. Jin J, Sklar GE, Sen Oh VM, Li SC. Factors affecting therapeutic compliance: A review from the patient's perspective. *Ther Clin Risk Manag* 2008; **4**: 269–86.

55. Bucks RS, Hawkins K, Skinner TC, et al. Adherence to Treatment in adolescents with cystic fibrosis: The role of illness perceptions and treatment beliefs. *J Ped Psychol* 2009; **34**: 893–902.

56. Horne R, Weinman JJ. Patients' beliefs about prescribed medicines and their role in adherence to treatment in chronic physical illness. *Psychosom Res* 1999; **47**: 555–67.

57. Horne R. Concordance, adherence and compliance in medicine taking. Report for the National Co-ordinating Centre for NHS Service Delivery and Organisation R & D (NCCSDO). December 2005. Available at http://www.medslearning.leeds .ac.uk/pages/documents/useful_docs/76-final -report%5B1%5D.pdf; accessed February 26, 2015.

58. DiMatteo MR, Giordani PJ, Lepper HS, et al. Patient adherence and medical treatment outcomes: A meta-analysis. *Med Care* 2002; **40**: 794–811.

59. Osterberg L, Blaschke T. Adherence to medication. *N Engl J Med* 2005; **353**(5): 487–97.

60. Arias Llorente RP, Bousoño García C, Díaz Martín JJ. Treatment compliance in children and adults with cystic fibrosis. *J Cyst Fibros* 2008; **7**: 359–67.

61. Briesacher BA, Quittner AL, Saiman L, Sacco P, Fouayzi H, Quittell LM. Adherence with tobramycin inhaled solution and health care utilization. *BMC Pulmonary Med* 2011; **11**: 5.

62. Eakin MN, Bilderback A, Boyle MP, et al. Longitudinal association between medication adherence and lung health in people with cystic fibrosis. *J Cyst Fibros* 2011; **10**: 258–64.

63. Quittner AL, Drotar D, Ievers-Landis CE, et al. Adherence to medical treatments in adolescents with cystic fibrosis: The development and evaluation of family-based interventions. In: Drotar D (Ed). *Promoting Adherence to Medical Treatment in Chronic Childhood Illness: Concepts, Methods and Interventions*. Mahwah, NJ: Lawrence Erlbaum Associates; 2000. pp. 383–407.

64. Riekert KA, Zhang J, Marynchenko M, et al. Pulmonary medication adherence among individuals with cystic fibrosis. *Ped Pulmonol* 2012; **S35**: 393.

65. HafetzJ, Miller VA. Child and parent perceptions of monitoring in chronic illness management: A qualitative study. *Child Care Health Dev* 2010; **36**: 655–62.

66. Dziuban EJ, Saab-Abazeed L, Chaudhry SR, Streetman DS, Nasr SZ. Identifying barriers to treatment adherence and related attitudinal patterns in adolescents with cystic fibrosis. *Ped Pulmonol* 2010; **45**: 450–8.

67. Butner J, Berg CA, Osborn P, Butler JM, Godri C, Fortenberry KT, et al. Parent-adolescent discrepancies in adolescents' competence and the balance of adolescent autonomy and adolescent and parent well-being in the context of type 1 diabetes. *Dev Psychol* 2009; **45**: 835–49.

68. Kettler LJ, Sawyer SM, Winefield HR, Greville HW. Determinants of adherence in adults with cystic fibrosis. *Thorax* 2002; **57**: 459–64.

69. Sansone RA, Sansone LA. Demoralization in patients with medical illness. *Psychiatry* 2010; **7**: 42–5.

70. European Cystic Fibrosis Society Consensus Statement. 2012. Clinimetric Properties of Adherence Measures. Available at http://www.ecfs.eu/projects/ahp-nursing-research/documents; accessed February 26, 2015.

71. Duff AJA, Latchford GJ. Motivational interviewing for adherence problems in cystic fibrosis. *Ped Pulmonol* 2010; **45**: 211–20.

72. Nobili RM, Duff AJA, Ullrich G, et al. Guiding principles on how to manage relevant psychological aspects within a CF team: Interdisciplinary approaches. *J Cyst Fibros* 2011; **10**: S45–52.

73. National Institute for Health and Clinical Excellence. *Supportive and Palliative Care for Adults with Cancer*. London: Department of Health, National Institute for Health and Clinical Excellence; 2004.

74. Connolly M, Perryman J, McKenna Y, et al. SAGE & THYME: A model for training health and social care professionals in patient-focussed support. *Pat Educ Counsel* 2010; **10**: 87–93.

75. Salmon P. *Psychology of Medicine and Surgery*. Chichester, UK: John Wiley & Sons; 2000.

76. Joint Report of Royal college of Physicians and Royal College of Psychiatrists. *Psychological Care of Medical Patients: A Practical Guide*. London, Royal college of Physicians and Royal College of Psychiatrists; 2003.

77. Fallowfield L, Jenkins V, Farewell V, et al. *Efficacy of a Cancer Research UK communication skills training model for oncologists: A randomised controlled trial*. Lancet 2002; **359**: 650–6.

78. Gawande A. The Bell Curve. What happens when patients find out how good their doctors really are? *The New Yorker*, December 2004. Available at http://www.newyorker.com/archive/2004/12/06/041206fa_fact; accessed February 26, 2015.

79. Locke Y, Harrison S, Baines R, et al. Transforming clinics to support adherence: An exercise in continuous quality improvement. *J Cyst Fibros* 2012; **11** (Suppl 1): S43.

80. Baile WF, Buckman R, Lenzi R, et al. SPIKES—A six step protocol for delivering bad news: Application to the patient with cancer. *Oncologist* 2000; **5**: 302–11.

81. Keene E, Hutton N, Hall B, Rushton C. Bereavement debriefing sessions: An intervention to support health care professionals in managing their grief after the death of a patient. J *Contin Nurs Educ* 2010; **36**(4): 185–9.

82. Allen R. Psychological care in physical health settings: The role of reflective practice with healthcare staff. *Clinical Psychology Forum* 2009; **199**; 24–8.

83. Duff AJA, Latchford GL. Motivational interviewing for adherence problems in cystic fibrosis: Evaluation of training healthcare professionals the learning outcomes of UK CF team training. *J Clin Med Res* 2013; **5**(6): 475–80.

84. Evans C, Barrett J, Osborne T, et al. Motivational interviewing and dietetics - a fresh approach to adherence issues. *J Cyst Fibros* 2012; **11** (Suppl 1): S123.

85. Nezu AM, Nezu CM, Perri MG. Problem solving to promote treatment adherence. In: O'Donohue WT, Levensky ER (Eds). *Promoting Treatment Adherence: A Practical Handbook for Health Care Providers*. New York: Sage Publications; 2006. pp. 135–48.

86. Geller DE, Madge S. Technological and behavioral strategies to reduce treatment burden and improve adherence to inhaled antibiotics in cystic fibrosis. *Respir Med* 2011; **105**: S24–31.

87. Heslop K. Cognitive behavioural therapy in cystic fibrosis. *J R Soc Med* 2006; **99** (Suppl 46): 27–9.

88. Bryon M. Behavior therapy and cognitive-behavior therapy. In: Bluebond-Langner M, Lask B, Angst DB (Eds). *Psychosocial Aspects of Cystic Fibrosis*. London: Arnold; 2001. pp. 318–28.

89. Daniels T, Goodacre L, Sutton C, et al. Accurate assessment of adherence: Self-report and clinician report vs electronic monitoring of nebulizers. *Chest* 2011; **140**: 425–32.

90. Hawn C. Take two aspirin and tweet me in the morning: How Twitter, Facebook, and other social media are reshaping health care. *Health Affair* 2009; **28**(2): 361–8.

91. Stark LJ, Quittner AL, Powers SW, et al. A randomized clinical trial of behavioural intervention and nutrition education to improve caloric intake and weight in children with cystic fibrosis. *Arch Pediatr Adolesc Med* 2009; **163**: 915–21.

92. Stark LJ, Opipari-Arrigan L, Quittner AL, et al. The effects of an intensive behavior and nutrition intervention compared to standard of care on weight outcomes in CF. *Pediatr Pulmonol* 2011; **461**: 31–5.

93. Opipari-Arrigan L, Powers SW, Quittner AL, Stark LJ. Mealtime problems predict outcome in clinical trial to improve nutrition in children with CF. *Pediatr Pulmonol* 2010; **45**: 78–82.

94. Savage E, Beirne PV, Ni Chroinin M, et al. Self management education for cystic fibrosis. *Cochrane Database Syst Rev* 2014; 9:CD007641. [Epub ahead of print] PMID: 25198249.

95. National Institute for Health and Clinical Excellence. Generalised anxiety disorder and panic disorder (with or without agoraphobia) in adults. Management in primary, secondary and community care. Clinical Guideline No. 113; 2011.

96. National Institute for Health and Clinical Excellence. Depression in adults with a chronic physical health problem—Treatment and management. Clinical Guideline No. 91; 2009.

97. Craig CA. *Cognitive Behaviour Therapy for Chronic Medical Problems*. Chichester, England: Wiley; 2001.

98. Moorey S. When bad things happen to rational people: Cognitive therapy in adverse life circumstances. In: Salkovskis (Ed). *Frontiers of Cognitive Therapy*. New York: Guilford Press; 1996. pp. 450–69.

99. Bray D, Groves K. A tailor made psychological approach to palliative care. *Euro J Pall Care* 2007; **14**(4): 141–3.

100. McDonald K. Living in limbo-patients with cystic fibrosis waiting for transplant. *Br J Nurs* 2006; **15**(10): 566–72.

101. Sage N, Sowden M, Chorlton E, Edeleanu A. *CBT for Chronic Illness and Palliative Care*. Chichester, England: Wiley, 2008.

102. Glasscoe CA, Quittner AL. Psychological interventions for people with cystic fibrosis and their families. *Cochrane Database Syst Rev* 2008; (16): CD003148.

FURTHER READING

Ernst MM, Johnson MC, Stark LJ. Developmental and psychosocial issues in cystic fibrosis. *Pediatr Clin North Am* 2011; **58**: 865–85.

46

Palliative and spiritual care

FINELLA CRAIG AND ANNA-MARIE STEVENS

INTRODUCTION

Palliative care is defined by the World Health Organization (WHO) as "an approach that improves the quality of life of patients and their families facing the problem associated with life-threatening illness, through the prevention and relief of suffering by means of early identification and impeccable assessment and treatment of pain and other problems, physical, psychosocial and spiritual. It is applicable early in the course of illness, in conjunction with other therapies that are intended to prolong life … and includes those investigations needed to better understand and manage distressing clinical complications."[1] There is emerging evidence for the beneficial role of a palliative care team in cystic fibrosis (CF), either working directly with the patient and family or indirectly through support and advice to professionals.[2,3] Based on this and in accordance with the WHO definition, the introduction of palliative care early in the illness trajectory of patients with CF should be promoted. Most studies, however, have focused on end of life care and advance care planning for adults[4-7] and there has been limited exploration of the early involvement of palliative care services.

This chapter will explore key issues in the delivery of palliative care to patients with CF, looking first at the adult population and then at the specific issues for children and young people (CYP).

PALLIATIVE CARE FOR ADULTS WITH CF

SYMPTOM PREVALENCE

Patients with CF experience a broad range of symptoms that are not necessarily determined by the severity of the pulmonary disease. Even those with mild disease commonly report chest pain, headaches, and abdominal pain.

Caregivers report that distressing symptoms are common during the last week of life, including dyspnea (100%), fatigue (96%), anorexia (85%), anxiety (74%), pain (67%), and cough (56%).[8] Patients with chronic disease report pain (84%) in an average of 2.1 locations, breathlessness (64%), and cough (83%) and 63% report that cough interferes with their sleep.[9] In addition to physical symptoms, psychosocial symptoms such as anxiety and depression are also prevalent.[7,10] CF is a chronic disease with a significant symptom burden.

SYMPTOM MANAGEMENT

The contribution that specialist palliative care services can make toward the control of patients' physical and psychological symptoms has been recognized,[11,12] but referral patterns are still poorly defined.[13] Management should combine the disease-specific knowledge of the CF team with the symptom management expertise of a palliative care team. The first consideration should always be to reverse the underlying cause of the symptom, where possible, alongside symptom management. Where the underlying cause is not reversible, or the burden in trying to do so outweighs potential benefits (such as remaining at home), symptom management will be the predominant intervention.

A holistic multidisciplinary approach is essential as social, psychological, and spiritual concerns impact on the symptom experience. Distraction and relaxation techniques, art and music therapies, and complementary therapies should be available. Some patients may also find homeopathy and alternative medicines beneficial.

Pain

Headache, abdominal pain, and chest pain due to infection and/or coughing are frequent. Good pain management will not only improve the patient's quality of life but also ensure that pain does not limit the ability to receive the necessary physiotherapy regime.

The control of pain is directed by the "Analgesic Ladder," which was presented by the WHO in 1996.[14] Although developed for the treatment of cancer pain, the principles apply to patients with acute and chronic pain from other causes:

Step 1: Simple analgesic, e.g., paracetamol, with an adjuvant if necessary. Adjuvant analgesics are defined as drugs with a primary indication other than pain that have analgesic properties in some painful conditions. Some adjuvant analgesics are useful in several painful conditions and are described as multipurpose adjuvant analgesics (antidepressants, corticosteroids), whereas others are specific for neuropathic pain (anticonvulsants, local anesthetics, or pain from bowel obstruction [octreotide], anticholinergics).

Step 2: Opioids for mild to moderate pain such as codeine, with an adjuvant if necessary.

Step 3: Opioids for severe pain such as morphine or oxycodone, with an adjuvant if necessary.

Pharmacological intervention should begin with simple analgesics on the first step of the ladder and proceeds upward as and when the pain reaches a higher level and the current analgesia is no longer effective. For patients with chronic persistent pain, analgesia should be administered regularly.

It is important to remember that the patient will experience different types of pain due to different etiological and physiological changes experienced in CF. Often the best practice is to combine the baseline analgesia with an appropriate adjuvant treatment to achieve maximum pain control. As there are so many variables in the selection of an appropriate adjuvant, discussion between the palliative care team and CF team is essential.

Breakthrough pain is a transitory increase in pain intensity to a level greater than the patients' well-controlled baseline or background level of pain. Breakthrough medication must be prescribed and can be given at times of pain exacerbation as well as in anticipation of an activity or procedure, such as physiotherapy, that is likely to be painful. Some patients will find fast-acting opiates, such as the sublingual preparations, particularly beneficial, although they tend to have a short duration of action. Any analgesia prescribed should be reviewed on a regular basis to ensure doses can be titrated in response to the needs of the patient.

It is important to remember that opioids can cause constipation and laxative therapy should be considered to ensure this symptom is avoided.

Adults with CF have an increased risk of bone fractures secondary to osteoporosis.[10] However, there is currently no clear evidence that the use of biphosphonates reduces the frequency of fractures or improves pain management.[15]

Cough

Cough is a complex and exhausting symptom that can be difficult to manage and has a significant impact on activities of daily living including eating and sleeping. Treatment includes alleviating infection and consideration of soothing cough elixirs such as simple linctus. If this is insufficient, adding an opioid such as codeine or morphine may be beneficial.[16]

Breathlessness

Treatment of the underlying cause of breathlessness, for example, a pneumothorax or respiratory exacerbation should always be considered. However, a proposed intervention may be influenced by, or influence, a patients preferred place of care. Complex intravenous antibiotic regimens, for example, may have little benefit at the end of life but may prevent a patient being discharged home. The burdens and likely benefits of any potential interventions should be discussed with the patient to support informed decision making.

Practical and supportive approaches, such as finding the optimum position and relaxation exercises may help, alongside symptom management. Patients with CF may benefit from noninvasive ventilation (NIV) as an adjunct to other airway clearance techniques. NIV used during sleep, in addition to oxygen, may improve gas exchange in moderate to severe disease, reducing nighttime breathlessness. The benefit of NIV during acute pulmonary exacerbations and in progressive disease remains unclear.[17] Other nonpharmacological interventions, such as cognitive behavioral therapy, may also be beneficial.[18]

The subjective sensation of breathlessness can be relieved using opioids, starting at very low doses (such as 30%–50% of the starting dose for pain), and titrated according to response. Patients may require regular or continuous dosing, with fast-acting preparations available to manage acute exacerbations.

Anxiety

If breathlessness is associated with anxiety, benzodiazepines such as lorazepam can help patients feel more relaxed and feel more in control.[19]

Unresolved confusion, fears, and anxieties can lead to increasing agitation as death approaches. Support to discuss and resolve these issues should precede the use of medications.

END OF LIFE CARE IN CYSTIC FIBROSIS

It is important to recognize that the role of palliative care is to support the CF team in caring for this group of patients. Decisions regarding ceiling of care and defining the ongoing treatment plan can at times be difficult to address due to the uncertainty of the disease and depending on the patient's response to treatments.

End of life care is an integral part of palliative care. The involvement of palliative care services early in the disease trajectory to support symptom management can be helpful in establishing relationships with patients and families while patients are still relatively well.

Most adults with CF have considered future care and are likely to have discussed this with their family.[8] However, less than one-third of patients have had any discussions about this with the clinical teams caring for them.[7] Although clinicians may feel apprehensive about initiating such discussions, patients and their families often welcome the opportunity to consider advance care planning and plan their preferred place of care and death. Palliative care services, working alongside the CF specialists, are ideally placed to support these discussions and facilitate patient preference. In considering DNaCPR it is important to make it clear to the healthcare team and, if appropriate, the patient and those close to the patient that a DNaCPR decision applies only to cardiopulmonary resuscitation. It does not imply that other treatments will be withdrawn or withheld. Other treatment and care will be provided if it is clinically appropriate and agreed to by a patient with capacity or if it is of overall benefit to a patient who lacks capacity.[20]

It is also important to recognize the holistic care needs of the patient with CF including spiritual support. In recent years there has been an attempt made to widen the definition of spirituality to not just focus on the religious side of support for the patient. For some patients, religion, prayer, and commitment to worship may be important, or for others searching for meaning or exploring transcendence can be meaningful.[21]

Institutions can deliver spiritual care in various ways through physical resources such as chapels, quiet rooms or prayer rooms and can also provide support from chaplains, faith healers, and volunteers. One of the key components of spiritual care relates to the expertise of the staff. Good communication between staff and patients while helping the patients to find meaning and "being there" for them all add to creating a spiritual environment.[21]

CHILDREN AND YOUNG PEOPLE WITH CF

Death in childhood from CF is rare and there is an expectation that most patients will survive into adulthood.[22] Despite this improving prognosis, however, CYP with CF will experience declining health, periods of acute deterioration necessitating increased medical interventions, hospitalization and school absence. The family will deliver increasing levels of health care at home and will face difficult decisions with regard to future treatments and potential outcomes.

Palliative care for children embraces a philosophy of life-long supportive care for CYP with life-threatening or life-limiting illness and their families, from diagnosis, throughout the disease trajectory and through bereavement.[23] The palliative care approach may be delivered by the CF team and by more universal teams such as the general pediatric team and community children's nurses. At times,

or throughout the illness trajectory, this may be supplemented by support from a specialist palliative care service.

The principles of palliative care are similar to those for adults, but the specific needs of CYP demands that they receive separate consideration. CYP are in continuous physical, emotional, and cognitive development, which will affect every aspect of their care from the dosage of medication to communication methods, education, and support. Some key areas that must be considered include:

- *Medication:* Many of the medications used in palliative care have been developed, formulated, and licensed for use in adults and may not be available in appropriate preparations for children. This presents additional challenges for symptom management.
- *Decision making and consent:* Parents legally represent their children in clinical, therapeutic, ethical, and social decisions. However, professionals must ensure that CYP are appropriately involved in discussions and decisions.
- *The family:* The social and emotional burden for the whole family is prolonged and complex. Parents (who are often the main carers), siblings, and grandparents will all require consideration and support.
- *Social needs:* CYP with CF, and their siblings, may have fewer opportunities for social interaction than their peers due to the demands of health care. It is essential that patients have access to peer groups and age appropriate play and leisure activities.
- *Education:* CYP, even with advanced disease, must have access to education in accordance with local statutory requirements. Schools may need additional support and training to care for the CYP at school, as well as to maintain social and educational links during periods of school absence.
- *Spiritual needs:* Many CYP will not have established their own belief systems and may need support as they explore this. This can become especially relevant as death approaches.

LIVING WITH CF

Families live with the conflict of maintaining hope and a semblance of day-to-day life despite persistent uncertainty—something that becomes more difficult in advanced disease and at times of acute disease exacerbation. Heavy nursing needs create a considerable burden of care. Hospital admissions cause practical difficulties, such as with making arrangements for care of other children as well as for the child in hospital. Long-term parental employment may be disrupted, placing additional financial pressure on the family. Parents can experience significant psychological stress, and depression, anxiety, sleep disturbance, and marital discord are not uncommon.[24] They may find it difficult to maintain discipline and boundaries and to balance their time and emotions between the child with CF and healthy siblings.

Supporting the family to maintain as normal a life as possible is essential. This includes maintaining social relationships, education, and activities outside the family. They should be offered assistance with care at home as well as access to respite, leisure, and social opportunities. School attendance should be facilitated, providing normality and structure, with social opportunities and peer group support, in addition to education.[25]

Siblings often feel excluded and isolated as parents may have little time for them, family life is disrupted and they have fewer opportunities for social activities.[25] They may develop feelings of low self-esteem, anxiety, and depression and may start to resent the sick child. Support should be provided individually, in the family unit and/or with other siblings in a similar situation. This type of support, especially access to sibling groups, may be available through a local children's hospice. Being routinely involved in the day-to-day care of the sibling with CF can also be helpful and can reduce feelings of exclusion.

COMMUNICATING WITH CYP

A natural reaction of parents is to protect their children by withholding what they perceive as frightening information and by excluding them from involvement in difficult decisions. However, even very young patients often understand more about their illness and its implications than their parents realize. Some may try to "protect" their parents by keeping their worries to themselves.[26]

Throughout their illness, CYP should be given opportunities to seek information, be included in discussions and decision making, and to express their feelings. Communication must be appropriate to their level of understanding about their illness and their concept of death, both of which will be influenced by their age, cognitive level, and previous experiences. It is important to remember that even some developmentally mature young people will choose to defer difficult discussions and decisions to their parents. Open discussion, allowing the young person to control the direction of conversation is essential. Using expressive media, such as play, art, and music can be hugely beneficial, particularly if the young person is reluctant or unable to express their fears verbally.

SERVICE PROVISION

CYP with CF must receive good care for their underlying condition, support to participate in a childhood that is as normal as possible, and support to achieve their developmental potential, as well as expert symptom management and palliative care support. Providing a joined-up three-tier service whereby CYP and their families can access universal services (e.g., education and child health), core pediatric and palliative care services (e.g., community nursing), and specialist CF and palliative care services is essential. Patients must have access to 24-hour care that is informed and appropriate to their current level of health need.[27]

CYP with CF predominantly access palliative care support via a combination of service models, all of which may be utilized throughout the illness trajectory:

Hospice care, where palliative care is delivered in an environment specifically suited to the needs of CYP and their families. Hospice care can often be used for short breaks as well as during times of crises and is not reserved only for end of life.

Community-based care delivered by community children's nurses, with support from local pediatricians. There may be additional palliative care support provided by hospital or hospice-based outreach teams, or dedicated community palliative care teams.

Outreach home care from specialist hospital-based services, when a specialist palliative care team and/or CF team provides care to the child at home, usually in conjunction with services based within the child's community.

Hospital inpatient care, where care is provided by CF teams or general pediatric teams with support from specialist palliative care or hospice outreach teams.

DEATH AND BEREAVEMENT

As their child's health deteriorates, parents should be encouraged to plan, with their CF and palliative care team, how crises should be managed and what medical interventions would be appropriate. This "advance care planning" should be regularly reviewed and adapted appropriately as the clinical situation changes. CYP should be given the opportunity to be involved in this decision-making process, taking into account their developmental level, understanding, and willingness (or not) to be included. When death is likely, parents and patients may value the opportunity of talking about what may happen leading up to and at the time of death and to consider place of care and death. Parents may need information about the practical details of what to do after their child has died, particularly if the death is likely to be at home. Some will want to consider and plan the funeral before death and some CYP will want to be involved in planning their own funeral, either with their parents or with support from professionals. Siblings may also benefit from being involved in these discussions.

Many CYP will not yet have established their own beliefs, values, and coping mechanisms. Thoughts of religious or spiritual beliefs may take on a new urgency for both parents and CYP as death approaches. They may look to a belief system to make sense of what is happening, or may reject a previously held belief system that has appeared to fail them. This can be particularly true for young adults, who have often reached a maturity whereby they will question previously accepted family beliefs in an attempt to explore and establish their own belief and value systems. Such rejection of a family belief system, as death approaches, can be especially difficult for parents.

Health professionals must support CYP to explore their own belief systems and this can often be facilitated by enabling them to talk openly with trusted adults or with religious representatives from a chosen faith group or a multifaith chaplain. Similar support should also be available for other family members. A common theme is the need to retain hope, but as death approaches the hope for cure may be redirected to hope for some sort of continuity after death, some sense of purpose, or that they will have left a meaningful mark on the world.

Grief following the death of a child has a depth and persistence that is often underestimated. Parents lose not only their child but also their hopes for the future. The whole family structure is altered and relationships are put under additional stress as each family member grieves individually. Grieving siblings often feel isolated and neglected as they cope with their own grief while living with grieving parents and siblings.

Parents value continuing support from professionals who have known their child and the opportunity to talk about their child and their grief. Some may benefit from referral to specialist bereavement support services or parent groups. Siblings may also need additional support, for example, through attending sibling bereavement groups or individually.

SYMPTOM MANAGEMENT[28]

In CYP, the symptoms experienced, principles of symptom management, and medications used are similar to adult practice. The main differences lie in symptom assessment, routes of drug administration, drug doses, and metabolism.

The ability of a young person to describe symptoms will vary in relation to their level of understanding, experience, and communication skills. Additional information must be sought from parents and carers and through a variety of techniques, such as play, art, or music therapy, or by using symptom assessment tools developed for young people.

Basic principles of drug administration

- Our recommendation is that a pediatric formulary is used for dosage information, such as (in the United Kingdom) the Association for Paediatric Palliative Medicine formulary[29] and British National Formulary for children.[30]
- The young person and family must be involved in developing an acceptable and achievable management plan. Drug choice will be influenced by the availability of suitable drug preparations in terms of dose, taste, availability of liquid formulation, tablet size, or liquid volume required. Complex regimens and large volumes of oral medication should be avoided.
- Long-acting preparations, including transdermal patches, are often most convenient and least intrusive.
- Buccal and sublingual routes can be a useful alternative to oral medications, but availability is limited to a few medications and they tend to be short acting.
- Parenteral drugs are usually given by continuous infusion in preference to bolus doses. Intramuscular drugs are painful and should be avoided.

Pain

The WHO analgesic ladder for children[31] is different to that for adults and recommends a two-step approach to pain management, omitting codeine which has been withdrawn from pediatric practice due to concerns regarding safety and efficacy. Paracetamol and ibuprofen are used in the first step for treating mild pain, and morphine or other strong opioids are used in the second step for management of moderate to severe pain. As in adult practice, adjuvants may be administered alongside analgesics when indicated. The administration of opioids to CYP often causes concern for parents and professionals. Parents may fear that they will precipitate their child's death or that introducing them too early will reduce later options for the management of pain and breathlessness. Clear explanation and support is essential to avoid the risk of medication being withheld or under-reporting of symptoms. The opioid side effects of nausea and vomiting, but not constipation, tend to be less frequent than in adults.

Respiratory symptoms

Drugs and other interventions, such as NIV, used in the management of cough and breathlessness are similar to those used in adult practice. There is some evidence to suggest a role for short courses of steroids in acute exacerbations of breathlessness.[32]

Anxiety and agitation

CYP may have unresolved confusion, fears, and anxieties that can lead to increasing agitation as death approaches. Professionals must provide opportunities for CYP to seek information, clarify misconceptions, and receive support. Medications should only be used as an adjunct to this.

Poor nutritional intake

Ensuring their child achieves a nutritional goal or target weight, often through supplemental feeding via gastrostomy, becomes part of the day-to-day life of the CF parent. At the end stage of the disease, however, large feed volumes may increase nausea, vomiting, and discomfort, so nutritional goals become harder to achieve. As death approaches, parents will need support to change the focus of feeding from weight gain to comfort and enjoyment. Parenteral nutrition should only be introduced if it is likely to be of long-term benefit and will not compromise the quality of the young persons' remaining life.

ADOLESCENT CARE

Specific challenges arise when adolescent development occurs alongside a life-threatening or life-limiting illness. The range and complexity of issues encountered in young adults with CF is immense. It includes issues relating to body image, risk-taking behaviors, independence, nonadherence to treatment, future treatments, and mortality.[33] Providing an appropriate environment for care, delivered by informed professionals, is essential. Transition to adult CF services, although relatively well developed, is not without challenges.[34] Transition to adult palliative care services, however, can be even more complex.[35] Many young people find that the adult hospice, with a focus on older patients, the acute management of complex symptoms, and care of the dying patient, is unable to provide the respite support and peer group interaction they experienced in the children's hospice. The development of appropriate services for young adults with palliative care needs remains a significant concern.

SUMMARY

Palliative care should not be withheld until death is imminent or disease-directed interventions have failed. It can, and should, begin in childhood and continue throughout the patient's life, alongside disease-directed treatments. A main focus of care, particularly in childhood, is support for day-to-day living and control of distressing symptoms. Early involvement of palliative care services, integrated with specialist CF services, will ensure that more patients and families can benefit from this support.

REFERENCES

1. World Health Organization. *National Cancer Control Programmes: Policies and Managerial Guidelines.* Geneva, Switzerland: World Health Organization; 2002.
2. Bourke SJ, Doe SJ, Gascoigne AD, Heslop K, Fields M, Reynolds D, Mannix K. An integrated model of provision of palliative care to patients with cystic fibrosis. *Palliat Med* 2009; **23**: 512–27.
3. Braithwaite M, Philip J, Tranberg H, et al. End of life care in CF: Patients, families and staff experiences and unmet need. *J Cyst Fibros* 2011; **10**: 253–57.
4. Chapman E, Landy A, Haworth C, Bilton D. End of Life Care for adult cystic fibrosis patients. Facilitating a good enough death. *J Cyst Fibros* 2005; **4**: 249–57.
5. Iles N, Lowton K. Young People with cystic fibrosis' concerns for their future. When and how should concerns be addressed, and by whom? *J Interprof Care* 2008; **22**: 436–8.
6. Mitchell I, Nakielna E, Tullis E, Adair C. Cystic Fibrosis: End stage care in Canada. *Chest* 2000; **118**: 80–4.
7. Sawicki G, Sellers D, Robinson W. Self-reported physical and psychological symptom burden in adults with cystic fibrosis. *J Pain Symptom Manag* 2008; **35**: 372–80.
8. Dellon E, Shores M, Nelson K, et al. Family caregiver perspectives on symptoms and treatments for patients dying from complications of cystic fibrosis. *J Pain Symptom Manag* 2010; **40**: 829–37.
9. Stenekes S, Hughes A, Gregoire MC, et al. Frequency and self management of pain, dyspnea and cough in cystic fibrosis. *J Pain Symptom Manag* 2009; **38**: 837–48.
10. Robinson W. A symptom based approach to palliative care in cystic fibrosis. *Prog Palliat Care* 2011; **19**: 230–5.
11. Edmonds PM, Stuttaford J, Penny J, et al. Do hospital palliative care teams improve symptom control? Use of a modified STAS as an evaluation tool. *Palliat Med* 1998; **12**: 345–51.
12. Stevens AM, Gwilliam B, A'Hearn R, et al. Experience with the use of the Palliative Care Outcome Scale. *Support Care Cancer* 2005; **13**: 1027–34.
13. Fadul N, Ahmed E, Palmer LJ, et al. Predictors of access to palliative care services among patients who died at a comprehensive cancer centre. *J Palliat Med* 2007; **10**: 1146–52.
14. World Health Organisation. *Cancer Pain Relief.* Geneva: World Health Organization; 1996.
15. Conwell LS, Chang AB. Bisphosphonates for osteoporosis in people with cystic fibrosis. *Cochrane Database Syst Rev* 2012; (Issue 4): CD002010.
16. Wee B, Browning J, Adams A, et al. Management of chronic cough in patients receiving palliative care: Review of evidence and recommendations by a task group of the Association for Palliative Medicine of Great Britain and Ireland. *Palliat Med* 2012; **26**: 780–7.
17. Moran F, Bradley JM, Piper AJ. Non-invasive ventilation for cystic fibrosis. *Cochrane Database Syst Rev* 2009; (1): CD002769.
18. Livermore N, Sharpe L, McKenzie D. Panic attacks and panic disorder in chronic obstructive pulmonary disease: A cognitive behavioral perspective. *Respir Med* 2010; **104**: 1246–53.
19. Clemens KE, Klaschik E. Dyspnoea associated with anxiety—Symptomatic therapy with opioids in combination with lorazepam and its effect on ventilation in palliative care patients. *Support Care Cancer* 2011; **19**: 2027–33.
20. General Medical Council. *End of Life Care: Treatment and Care After a DNACPR Decision.* London, United Kingdom: General Medical Council; 2010.
21. Urquhart DS, Lena PT, Francis J, et al. Deaths from cystic fibrosis: 10-Year analysis from two London specialist centres. *Arch Dis Child* 2013; **98**: 123–7.
22. Wright M. Good for the soul. In: Payne S, Seymour J, Ingleton C (Eds). *Palliative Care Nursing, Principles and Evidence for Practice.* New York: Open University Press; 2008.

23. Association for Children with Life-Threatening or Terminal Conditions and their Families (ACT) and the Royal College of Paediatrics and Child Heath (RCPCH). *A Guide to the Development of Children's Palliative Care Services*. United Kingdom: ACT; 2009.

24. Bluebond-Langner M. In the Shadow of Illness: Parents and Siblings of the Chronically Ill Child. Princeton, NJ: Princeton University Press; 1996.

25. Craig F, Boden C, Samuel J. Schooling of children with a life-limiting or life-threatening illness. *Eur J Pall Care* 2012; **19**: 131–5.

26. Bluebond-Langner M. *The Private Worlds of Dying Children*. Princeton, NJ: Princeton University Press; 1978.

27. Craft A, Killen S. Palliative care services for children and young people in England: An independent review for the secretary of state. England: Department of Health in England; 2007.

28. Jassal S. *Basic Symptom Control in Paediatric Palliative Care*. The Rainbows Children's hospice guidelines. Rainbows Hospice for Children and Young People; 2011. www.rainbows.co.uk; accessed March 13, 2015.

29. Jassal S (editor). *Association of Paediatric Palliative Medicine Formulary. Editor*. United Kingdom: ACT; 2012. www.act.org.uk; accessed March 13, 2015.

30. Paediatric Formulary Group. *BNF for Children (BNFc) 2012-2013*. London, United Kingdom: Pharmaceutical Press; 2012.

31. WHO. *WHO Guidelines on the Pharmacological Treatment of Persisting Pain in Children with Medical Illnesses*. Geneva, Switzerland: WHO; 2012.

32. Ghdifan S, Couderc L, Michelet I, Leguillon C, Masseline B, Marguet C. Bolus methylprednisolone efficacy for uncontrolled exacerbation of cystic fibrosis in children. *Pediatrics* 2010; **125**: e1259–64.

33. Withers AL. Management issues for adolescents with cystic fibrosis. *Pulmon Med* 2012; **2012**: 10 p.

34. Tuchman LK, Schwartz LA, Sawicki GS, Britto MT. Cystic fibrosis and transition to adult medical care. *Pediatrics* 2010; **125**: 566–73.

35. Craig F, Rajapakse CD, McNamara K, Williamson N. Investing in primary care as a bridge for transitional care. *Arch Dis Child* 2011; **96**(1): 1–2.

PART 7

Cystic fibrosis: The future

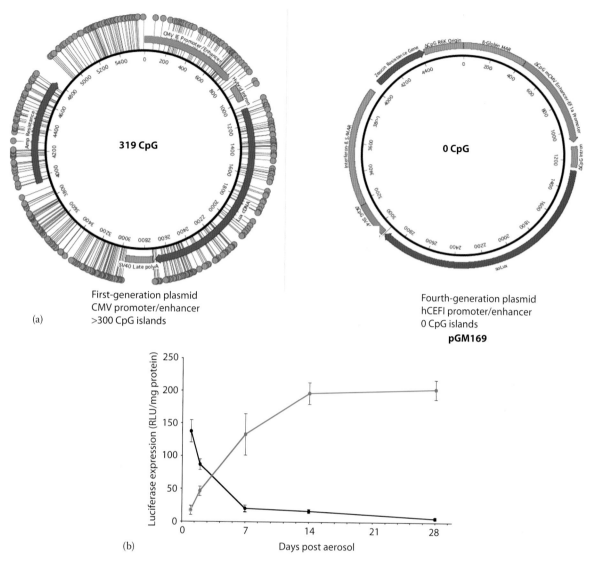

First-generation plasmid
CMV promoter/enhancer
>300 CpG islands

(a)

Fourth-generation plasmid
hCEFI promoter/enhancer
0 CpG islands
pGM169

(b)

Figure 47.3 Key modifications to the plasmid DNA. **(a)** Plasmid DNA carrying the CFTR complementary DNA (cDNA) was modified to prolong expression and reduce the risk of gene transfer agent-induced inflammation. The modification included the complete removal of proinflammatory cytosine phosphate guanine (CpG) dinucleotide motifs and the replacement of the viral cytomegalovirus promoter/enhancer (CMV) elements to a hybrid promoter consisting of a human CMV enhancer and the elongation factor 1α promoter (hCEFI). The final completely CpG-depleted plasmid carrying the CFTR cDNA under control of the hCEFI promoter is called pGM169. **(b)** Reporter gene expression in mouse lung after administration of plasmids regulated by the CMV promoter/enhancer (black) and the hCEFI promoter/enhancer (red).

view, appropriately pseudotyped lentiviral vectors are more likely to provide a step change in efficacy of gene therapy.

CELL THERAPY

The repopulation of airway epithelium following administration of gene-corrected stem/progenitor cells may be an alternative to classical gene therapy. Systemic and topical cell administration routes have been assessed and will be discussed below. In addition, recent progress in the field of lung and/or airway ex vivo bioengineering, which may in the future benefit CF patients, will be discussed.

INTRAVENOUS CELL THERAPY FOR THE TREATMENT OF CF DOES NOT HOLD MUCH PROMISE

The finding that, under certain circumstances, bone marrow (BM) or umbilical cord blood-derived stem cells (SCs) may have the capacity to transdifferentiate and repopulate various organs has triggered research into the development of SC-based therapies for a large number of diseases, including CF. It has been shown that these cells may have the capacity to induce expression of lung epithelial cell–specific markers when cultured appropriately (reviewed in Ref. [64]). In addition, Wong et al.[65] identified a population of cells positive for the Clara cell-specific marker Clara cell secretory protein (CCSP) in human and murine BM. The number of circulating CCSP positive BM cells increased after cell injury and these cells may be an interesting choice for cell therapy of lung disease. Wang et al.[66] have shown that mesenchymal stem cells (MSCs) of CF patients can, after ex vivo gene correction and coculture with primary CF airway epithelial cells in air–liquid interface cultures, generate CFTR-mediated chloride channel activity.

Several groups have attempted to assess if bone marrow stem cell (BMSC) can transdifferentiate into airway epithelium after intravenous administration, but results have been conflicting in part due to methodological artifacts.[64,67] Bruscia et al.[68] have reported that systemic administration of CFTR-positive BMSC into irradiated CF knockout mice may lead to very modest correction of the CF chloride transport defect in intestinal epithelium, but these studies have, to the best of our knowledge, not been reproduced in other laboratories. The same group also assessed if BMSC transplantation into newborn mice increased engraftment into various organs including lung, liver, and intestine but showed that detection of BM-derived epithelial cells remained a very rare event even in myeloablation newborn mice.[68] Along similar lines Loi et al.[69] showed that BM cells isolated from nonCF donor mice restored very low levels in CFTR expression in CF-knockout mice recipients. Combined data generated over the last few years illustrate that systemic administration of BMSC currently does not hold great promise for CF therapy.

TOPICAL CELL THERAPY HAS SUPERSEDED INTRAVENOUS APPROACHES

Interestingly, systemic administration of SC has been superseded by studies assessing topical administration of various types of SC, which maybe a more efficient route to deliver cell therapy to the airways. This was supported in studies by Wong et al.[65] and Rejman et al.[70] However, even after topical administration, the detection of transplanted cells in the recipient lung remained a rare event. Duchesneau et al.[71] extended these studies and showed that destruction of endogenous Clara cells with naphthalene 2 days prior to transplantation, in combination with busulfan-induced myoablation 1 day prior to transplantation, achieved maximal retention in the lung. However, the retention frequency of transplanted cells remained low and the differentiation status largely unresolved. In addition, it is unclear if and how these aggressive protocols can be translated into clinical applications. It has recently been reported that retention of BM-derived progenitor cells is increased in the presence of *Pseudomonas aeruginosa*-induced lung infection,[70] which may be particularly relevant for CF. However, despite more efficient retention after topical administration, the convincing detection and characterization of cells retained in the lung remains a problem. Although sensitive PCR-based methods can detect low levels of transplanted cells, these methods provide little information about engraftment and differentiation status of these cells. In contrast, microscopy-based methods even when coupled with sophisticated immunohistochemistry-based cell visualization and characterization suffer from low sensitivity and problems associated with reliable interpretation of images.

DIFFERENTIATION OF EMBRYONIC STEM CELLS INTO AIRWAY CELLS HAS BEEN SUCCESSFUL

In addition to adult SCs described above, embryonic SCs (ESCs) have been studied. Rippon et al.[72] published preliminary work following the fate of intravenously injected mouse ESCs and showed that a small number of transplanted, but not further characterized cells were detectable in the distal lung for a few days. Similarly, Leblond et al.[73] assessed intratracheal administration of murine ESCs and MSCs in uninjured and injured (2% polidocanol treated) murine lungs and showed some retention of not further characterized transplanted cells in injured but not uninjured murine lungs. Several studies have shown that, under certain circumstances, ESCs can be induced to express lung-specific proteins such as surfactant protein B and C as well as Clara cell protein 10.[74,75] Wang et al.[76] have shown that intratracheal administration of human ESC–derived alveolar type II cells improved survival and reduced inflammation and fibrosis in a bleomycin-induced murine lung injury model. Although it is currently unclear, if the protective effect is due to cell engraftment and differentiation or an undefined paracrine effects, this study is, to the best of our knowledge, the first to demonstrate amelioration of lung injury using ESCs.

Maybe more relevant in the context of CF is a recent study by Wong et al.[77] who showed that after careful optimization of culture conditions, human ESCs can generate conducting airway epithelium expressing functional CFTR. Combined with studies that have generated a human ESC line from a CF embryo[78] and induced pluripotent cells from dermal fibroblast of a CF subjects,[79] this technology may become powerful for disease modeling and drug screening. In the short term, these applications will certainly be more applicable than in vivo transplantation strategies.

EX VIVO BIOENGINEERING OF AIRWAYS HOLDS EARLY PROMISE

Ex vivo bioengineered lungs are a dream for the future. However, early steps toward lung tissue engineering have been taken. A variety of synthetic scaffold materials have been developed.[80] However, the use of decellularized lung scaffolds currently appears to be most promising to recapitulate and regenerate the complex lung structure. Protocols for the decellurization of rodent and nonhuman primate lungs have been developed,[81,82] and early

80. Song JJ, Ott HC. Bioartificial lung engineering. *Am J Transplant* 2012; **12**(2): 283–8.

81. Song JJ, Ott HC. Organ engineering based on decellularized matrix scaffolds. *Trends Mol Med* 2011; **17**(8): 424–32.

82. Bonvillain RW, Danchuk S, Sullivan DE, Betancourt AM, Semon JA, Eagle ME, et al. A nonhuman primate model of lung regeneration: Detergent-mediated decellularization and initial in vitro recellularization with mesenchymal stem cells. *Tissue Eng Part A* 2012; **18**(23–24): 2437–52.

83. Ott HC, Clippinger B, Conrad C, Schuetz C, Pomerantseva I, Ikonomou L, et al. Regeneration and orthotopic transplantation of a bioartificial lung. *Nat Med* 2010; **16**(8): 927–33.

84. Petersen TH, Calle EA, Zhao L, Lee EJ, Gui L, Raredon MB, et al. Tissue-engineered lungs for in vivo implantation. *Science* 2010; **329**(5991): 538–41.

85. Macchiarini P, Jungebluth P, Go T, Asnaghi MA, Rees LE, Cogan TA, et al. Clinical transplantation of a tissue-engineered airway. *Lancet* 2008; **372**(9655): 2023–30.

86. Jungebluth P, Alici E, Baiguera S, Le BK, Blomberg P, Bozoky B, et al. Tracheobronchial transplantation with a stem-cell-seeded bioartificial nanocomposite: A proof-of-concept study. *Lancet* 2011; **378**(9808): 1997–2004.

87. Moran A, Dunitz J, Nathan B, Saeed A, Holme B, Thomas W. Cystic fibrosis-related diabetes: Current trends in prevalence, incidence, and mortality. *Diabetes Care* 2009; **32**(9): 1626–31.

88. Kessler L, Bakopoulou S, Kessler R, Massard G, Santelmo N, Greget M, et al. Combined pancreatic islet-lung transplantation: A novel approach to the treatment of end-stage cystic fibrosis. *Am J Transplant* 2010; **10**(7): 1707–12.

48

Basic science: What will it deliver? Non-gene therapy treatments

JANE C. DAVIES AND FELIX RATJEN

INTRODUCTION

When the gene defect causative for cystic fibrosis (CF) was discovered in 1989, it was expected that this knowledge would result in new therapeutic approaches within 5 to 10 years. In reality, it has taken more than two decades until this fundamental knowledge could be translated in new therapies addressing the basic defect. Much has been learned about the function of cystic fibrosis transmembrane conductance regulator (CFTR) and the underlying pathophysiology of CF, but many aspects still need to be unraveled. This is highlighted by the recent resurgence of the debate surrounding airway surface liquid depletion as a primary defect in CF, and recent data from a CF pig model demonstrating that both sodium absorption and resultant airway surface liquid volume were in fact normal in newborn CFTR piglets.[1]

Regardless of the ongoing debates and the gaps in our knowledge, there has been considerable progress over the last decade or two. In particular, an understanding of the functional consequences of the various classes of *CFTR* mutation has resulted in the development of mutation-specific small molecules. Drugs with potential activity against at least class I to III mutations have moved into clinical trials or, in the case of the drug ivacaftor, into clinical care.[2] This is the start of a new era in CF; moving from symptomatic therapy of the downstream effects of CFTR dysfunction to treatments that address the basic defect directly. However, as we discuss below, it is unlikely that even the optimal therapeutic intervention would completely cure all manifestations of CF and therefore improving strategies to tackle the clinical hallmarks of CF lung disease, infection and inflammation, remains an important tasks for the future.

CFTR MODULATION

CFTR pharmacotherapy has certainly been the success story of recent years. Leading the field in terms of development phase is ivacaftor, a CFTR potentiator, initially developed for and studied in patients carrying at least one copy of the class III mutation, G551D. Results from clinical trials have been impressive: treatment not only improved measures of CFTR function such as nasal potential difference (nPD)[3] and sweat chloride but, much more importantly, had significant benefits on lung function, respiratory symptom scores, and pulmonary exacerbation rates.[2] Somewhat surprisingly and currently incompletely understood, there was also a significant gain in body weight. The effect size of lung function improvement exceeded that seen in any previous study evaluating a therapeutic intervention in CF and was certainly bigger than most people in the field had expected. These results have clearly demonstrated that CFTR-directed therapy can be highly effective and appear to have catalyzed a resurgence of enthusiasm among pharmaceutical companies developing small molecule therapies.

To date, however, the long-term efficacy of treatment on rates of lung function decline and on structural changes such as bronchiectasis remains unknown. The relatively small subgroup of patients for whom this drug is now licensed and the existing registries in the United States and Europe will allow these questions to be explored postmarketing. Compelling in vitro data suggest that this agent will have efficacy in other mutations where CFTR protein is present at the cell surface,[4] and trials are currently underway in nonG551D class III (gating) mutations, in the class IV mutation R117H, and in patients with some evidence of residual CFTR function. It is likely, therefore, that this drug will, in the future, have broader applicability.

Conversely, we already know that ivacaftor will offer no benefit for patients with the commonest CFTR mutation, deltaF508.[5] This mutation leads to a misfolded protein that also has multiple other problems including reduced function, decreased stability, and therefore a reduced residence time in the plasma membrane.[6] The folding defect alone has recently been shown to involve multiple steps and it is becoming clear that one drug alone is unlikely to address all of these abnormalities. Current studies with the CFTR corrector, lumacaftor (VX-809), support this view: the effect of this drug alone is limited and patients demonstrating very small reductions in sweat chloride and no improvement in nPD or lung function.[7] Even when combined with the potentiator, ivacaftor, the effect size on sweat chloride is significantly smaller than that observed in G551D patients receiving ivacaftor. Rather confusingly, recent data presented at conferences but at the time of writing, unpublished, seem to suggest that patients on the highest combined doses of these drugs had significant improvements in lung function despite this relatively minor sweat chloride response.[8] Interestingly, there was no correlation between forced expiratory volume in 1 second (FEV_1) and sweat chloride changes on an intrasubject basis in G551D either. This could reflect differential organ exposure, differing pharmacodynamic sensitivity to these drugs of perhaps even reflects that there is a much looser relationship between chloride transport and lung disease than is sometimes supposed, but clearly needs to be more fully understood. Many other corrector drugs are being developed and we should perhaps regard ourselves as being at the beginning of a long journey rather than having overoptimistic expectations that the rate of progress will be similar to the much easier task, potentiating CFTR already present at the cell surface.

Although the enthusiasm in the community is understandable, it is important to remember that not all drugs make it through to market and results of early phase studies should not be overinterpreted. This is highlighted by the recent example of ataluren, a drug developed to induce read through of class I (stop) mutations. This agent appeared to show considerable promise in early phase studies,[9,10] but a recent large, placebo controlled, phase 3 study failed to demonstrate a significant benefit on primary or secondary outcome measures (lung function, clinical symptoms, pulmonary exacerbations, and CFTR function measured by sweat chloride nPD).[11] Post hoc subgroup analysis appears to suggest an interaction with the commonly prescribed nebulized aminoglycoside antibiotic, tobramycin. Despite these disappointing results, the drug is being investigated further by PTC Therapeutics (South Plainfield, NJ) and may be of benefit in the future for well-defined patients. We highlight it as an illustration of the prudency in waiting for results of large control trials rather than raising expectations of treatment success based on small, early phase studies performed, particularly if results are inconsistent. Not every drug will be an ivacaftor and many drugs will fail to deliver their promise.

ION CHANNEL THERAPY

Although CFTR remains the ultimate target of CF therapy, another potential strategy is to address the imbalance of decreased chloride secretion and increased sodium absorption through either the epithelial sodium channel, ENaC, or alternative chloride channels. This is potentially attractive as all patients could benefit, regardless of their *CFTR* gene mutation. So far though, clinical development programs have been rather disappointing. A recent example is denufosol, an activator of calcium-activated chloride channels; in vitro, denufosol improved chloride secretion and inhibited sodium absorption.[12] Early clinical studies reported significant improvements in FEV_1 although of such a low magnitude to be of doubtful clinical significance[13,14] and a subsequent large confirmatory trial showed no clinical benefits.[15] There are a number of questions raised by this program including whether dose was in fact optimal but also whether overriding the ion transport defects of CFTR alone is sufficient or whether other CFTR functions are important in disease pathogenesis. Potentially, the timing of ion modulation therapy could be key: a study on the β-ENaC overexpressing mouse, which effectively recapitulates human CF lung disease demonstrated that amiloride a blocker of the ENaC ameliorated airway changes, but only if used preventatively. No benefit was seen once pathology had occured.[16] Although it does not appear likely that an effective ion channel therapy will become available in the near future, this treatment strategy should not be prematurely abandoned as it could still be a viable option and there is currently no guarantee that an effective CFTR pharmacotherapy will become available for the majority of CF patients.

AIRWAY HYDRATION

Osmotic agents such as hypertonic saline and mannitol have been introduced into clinical care and do have proven benefit both in terms of lung function and a reduction in exacerbations.[17,18] Although the assumption is that these agents improve airway surface hydration, this is difficult to prove and part of their effect may be to act as an irritant thereby improving cough clearance. Regardless of their mechanism of action, they are unlikely to act as disease-modifying agents and their effect size is relatively small. Improved efficacy could potentially be achieved by more targeted delivery to the small airways or extended exposure time such as overnight inhalation strategies. Although these options are currently being explored, it is not expected that even with optimized delivery, osmotic therapy will be efficacious enough to replace or offset the need to develop pharmacological modulators of ion channels including CFTR.

INFECTION AND INFLAMMATION

Until treatments targeting the basic defect are proved safe enough to be administered very early in life, these agents are likely to be only partially effective; even the most effective therapy cannot reverse irreversible structural damage such as established bronchiectasis, which we know can occur in early childhood. Improved treatment of infection and inflammation will, therefore, remain a priority. New antibiotics are unlikely to become available, but nonantibiotic approaches such as those disrupting biofilms, bacteriophage, antibody-based approaches, or enhancers of innate antimicrobial defense could become additional options. Aggressive treatment of infection is one of the main drivers of improved survival in CF, but in contrast, current strategies to treat airway inflammation are rudimentary and not in widespread use. In large part, the limited uptake of the nonsteroidal anti-inflammatory agent, ibuprofen, relates to concerns over side effects. Better ways to address the delicate balance of infection and inflammation therefore remain an important priority for the future. Recent experience has shown that being too aggressive in suppressing inflammation may have negative effects on infection as illustrated by a trial of an LTB4 receptor antagonist in which actively treated patients had a higher incidence of pulmonary exacerbations (ClinicalTrials.gov identifier: NCT00060801). There is a global and pan-disease concern that the development of conventional antibiotics is slowing down and that antimicrobial resistance mechanisms are outpacing us in this endeavor. What are the alternatives? In general, vaccine strategies targeted at *Pseudomonas aeruginosa* have been disappointing. A large trial is underway testing a novel form of passive immunity in the form of immunoglobulin Y generated in the yolks of hens' eggs (ClinicalTrials.gov identifier: NCT01455675). It is an attractive concept that a gargle, taken prophylactically, could protect against this infection, although results are awaited. Monoclonal antibodies are another approach, currently being explored. The widespread recognition, within the last decade, that *Pseudomonas* produce biofilms in the airway, which protect them from both host defense and exogenous antibiotics, has led to attempts to break this down, a mechanism which may, at least in part account for the efficacy of macrolide antibiotics. The interesting observation that nitric oxide (NO) breaks down biofilm via the cyclic diguanylate monophosphate pathway have led to attempts to use this gas, or perhaps more practically, NO donor molecules, synergistically with antibiotics.[19] Finally, bacteriophage, which bind specifically to bacterial cell walls and cause lysis, has undergone a resurgence in interest. Previously studied in poorly controlled and little reported trials in eastern Europe, they are now being tested for many infective diseases including of the gastrointestinal tract, skin, and outer ear. There are theoretical reasons why the development of bacterial resistance will be less likely than it is with conventional antibiotics, although this, and of course ability to deliver to the airway effectively and safely, need to be borne out in clinical trials. Perhaps a direction of travel will be the combination of conventional antibiotics with novel, nonantibiotic antimicrobials in synergistic formulations, which have both improved efficacy but also a lesser risk of evolving bacterial resistance. Similarly, finding the right balance between the two important drivers of CF lung disease, infection and inflammation, will remain a difficult challenge which may be best addressed with "double hit" agents that have effects on both mechanisms.

WHEN TO START NOVEL THERAPIES TARGETING THE BASIC DEFECT?

It is intuitively likely that these small molecule therapies will work best when introduced as early as possible, which in most cases would be immediately after diagnosis by newborn screening. Given that these therapies would be maintained for the entire lifespan of the patient, this poses significant challenges regarding the documentation of long-term safety. Current expertise in performing safety and efficacy studies in infants is limited. However, functional techniques such as infant lung function tests including those assessing ventilation inhomogeneity (lung clearance index assessed by multi-breath washout) are becoming available as are lower dose computed tomography imaging protocols. Particularly in young children in whom concerns over ionizing radiation rightly exist, nonradiation techniques such as hyperpolarized helium magnetic resonance imaging may hold future promise. Studies in this age group will almost certainly require a longer duration than current trials as the outcome measure will not be an improvement of clinical and functional status, but rather maintenance of health or a slowing of the natural history of the disease. Studies to aid a fuller understanding rates of progression are therefore essential; currently, the two groups focusing on this most closely appear to be generating somewhat discrepant results with regard to early structural changes.[20,21] Although regulators may accept pragmatic trials based on safety and biomarkers extrapolating from trials in older patients, we consider it is essential that efficacy trials are conducted in this age group; without them, not only do we deny the field an invaluable opportunity to observe the greatest magnitude of a potential disease modifying effect but we may also find clinicians (and very importantly, funders) unwilling to enable treatment for this age group.

WHAT WILL FUTURE THERAPY LOOK LIKE: POTENTIAL SCENARIOS

As pointed out above, correction of CFTR misfolding in deltaF508 patients is an extremely complex process. It is likely that one drug alone will be insufficient for optimal clinical effectiveness and that future successful treatments will be based on combinations of drugs targeting different steps and mechanisms of CFTR trafficking. Therefore, the future of patients with Phe508del mutation may lie in using multiple corrector drugs, possibly combined with a potentiator. The current evidence for ivacaftor suggests that an almost ideal potentiator is already available. On the other hand, drug development programs for correctors need to continue. In addition, basic science will be instrumental in helping us to better understand the crucial steps in CFTR processing and degradation so that drug targets can be based on mechanism rather than relatively crude measures such as high-throughput screening alone.

Current studies with available compounds already show that treatment response varies among patients and a complex treatment regimen of multiple correctors will likely not be equally efficacious in every patient. Understanding this variability will become increasingly important and could be achieved in a number of ways. Better definition of modifier genes involved in CFTR processing and ion transport could help to predict treatment responses and one could envision combining relevant testing on a gene chip that could be utilized to guide therapy. Alternatively, assays could allow for ex vivo testing of treatment response in tissues derived from patients. Studies are already under way to address this, but will likely either require airway derived tissue or patients' stems cells that are transformed into airway epithelial cells. Newer techniques allow these cells to be maintained in culture for extended time periods so different treatment combinations could be tested on cells of an individual patient before systemic or topical administration of the drug to the patient. This could move the field from personalized (genotype driven) to truly individualized therapy.

Although these in vitro tests could be helpful, it is unlikely that they will replace clinical response studies in patients. In view of multiple target therapy that will need to be tested, more sensitive outcome measures than those currently used in clinical trials are needed to perform these studies over shorter time periods with smaller sample sizes. Future trials may also require alternative study design such as $n = 1$ studies, which will be especially important for patients carrying rare mutations for whom larger trials will not be feasible.

Although it may be attractive to speculate that the future use of highly effective CFTR-modulating compounds could lead to a reduced (or removed) requirement for conventional treatments, it is crucial to bear in mind that current trial design tests these molecules as "add-on" treatments; we could find that the impressive efficacy observed in trials fails to translate fully into clinical benefits in the field if patients and clinical teams are too swift to withdraw standard treatment.

HOW WILL TREATING THE UNDERLYING DEFECT AFFECT OTHER ORGANS INVOLVED IN CF?

For the first time, systemic CFTR-modulating agents raise the potential for organs other than the lungs to be improved. It is intriguing to speculate on the reasons for improved weight in G551D patients on ivacaftor. It seems unlikely that in these patients, pancreatic exocrine insufficiency could have been impacted; in the majority of CF patients, significant pancreatic damage occurs prenatally and in the first of the two phase 3 trials to report this effect, patients were aged 12 years and above. It is possible that ion transport in the intestine, either chloride or perhaps more likely, bicarbonate, could have been improved. One could certainly speculate that these treatments would reduce the incidence or delay the onset of CF-related liver disease or diabetes, although this remains to be seen. As the vas deferens is to be the organ most sensitive to loss of CFTR function, as manifest by patients without CF but with congenital bilateral absence of the vas deferens, it is unlikely that any drugs initiated postnatally will impact on the infertility present in the majority of men with CF.

ALONGSIDE THE SEARCH FOR NEW DRUGS, HOW CAN WE FACILITATE PROGRESSION THROUGH CLINICAL TRIALS?

Over the last decade we have witnessed vast improvements in the way clinical trials are performed in CF, thanks in large part to the Trial Networks established in the United States, Europe, and Australasia. These networks design and propagate standardized procedures, which enhance data quality and increases recruitment numbers and rates. It is encouraging that the regulatory authorities are engaging with these groups to consider reforming trial design, in particular outcome measures for the relatively understudied groups such as infants and preschoolers, but there is still some way to go and outcome measures which are considered useful by investigators need to be validated before they will be accepted as alternatives to conventional lung function tests. Commercial sponsors are increasingly collaborating with investigators over optimal trial design and together, this triangulation of pharma, clinical, and academic medicine and regulatory bodies will, we hope, lead to the more rapid translation of successful ideas into clinical practice. CF is leading the field globally in the rational development of personalized medicine for a rare, life-limiting disease, but such research programs are expensive and have the potential to lead to drugs, which challenge budgets, particularly in countries with nationalized healthcare systems. As we enter this exciting new era in CF management, ongoing dialog with financial decision makers should smooth the way to a prescribing and funding environment within which the most effective therapies are readily available to those CF patients who could benefit.

REFERENCES

1. Chen JH, Stoltz DA, Karp PH, et al. Loss of anion transport without increased sodium absorption characterizes newborn porcine cystic fibrosis airway epithelia. *Cell* 2010; **143**: 911–23.
2. Ramsey BW, Davies J, McElvaney NG, et al. A CFTR potentiator in patients with cystic fibrosis and the G551D mutation. *N Engl J Med* 2011; **365**: 1663–72.
3. Accurso FJ, Rowe SM, Clancy JP, et al. Effect of VX-770 in persons with cystic fibrosis and the G551D-CFTR mutation. *N Engl J Med* 2010; **363**: 1991–2003.
4. Yu H, Burton B, Huang CJ, et al. Ivacaftor potentiation of multiple CFTR channels with gating mutations. *J Cyst Fibros* 2012; **11**: 237–45.
5. Flume PA, Liou TG, Borowitz DS, et al. Ivacaftor in subjects with cystic fibrosis who are homozygous for the F508del-CFTR mutation. *Chest* 2012; **142**: 718–24.
6. Lukacs GL, Verkman AS. CFTR: Folding, misfolding and correcting the DeltaF508 conformational defect. *Trends Mol Med* 2012; **18**: 81–91.
7. Clancy JP, Rowe SM, Accurso FJ, et al. Results of a phase IIa study of VX-809, an investigational CFTR corrector compound, in subjects with cystic fibrosis homozygous for the F508del-CFTR mutation. *Thorax* 2012; **67**: 12–8.
8. Boyle MP, Bell S, Konstan M, et al. The Investigational CFTR Corrector, VX-809 (Lumacaftor) co-administered with the oral potentiator Ivacaftor improved CFTR and lung function in F508DEL homozygous patients: Phase II study results. Poster session abstract presented at the 26th Annual North American Cystic Fibrosis Conference, Orlando, FL, October 2012.
9. Kerem E, Hirawat S, Armoni S, et al. Effectiveness of PTC124 treatment of cystic fibrosis caused by nonsense mutations: A prospective phase II trial. *Lancet* 2008; **372**: 719–27.
10. Sermet-Gaudelus I, Boeck KD, Casimir GJ, et al. Ataluren (PTC124) induces cystic fibrosis transmembrane conductance regulator protein expression and activity in children with nonsense mutation cystic fibrosis. *Am J Respir Crit Care Med* 2010; **182**: 1262–72.
11. Rowe SM, Tang L, Xue X, et al. The synthetic aminoglycoside nb124 suppresses CFTR premature termination codons more effectively than gentamicin and prior synthetic derivatives. Poster session abstract presented at the 26th Annual North American Cystic Fibrosis Conference, Orlando, FL, October 2012.
12. Yerxa BR, Sabater JR, Davis CW, et al. Pharmacology of INS37217 [P(1)-(uridine 5')- P(4)-(2'-deoxycytidine 5')tetraphosphate, tetrasodium salt], a next-generation P2Y(2) receptor agonist for the treatment of cystic fibrosis. *J Pharmacol Exp Ther* 2002; **302**: 871–80.
13. Deterding RR, Lavange LM, Engels JM, et al. Phase 2 randomized safety and efficacy trial of nebulized denufosol tetrasodium in cystic fibrosis. *Am J Respir Crit Care Med* 2007; **176**: 362–9.
14. Accurso FJ, Moss RB, Wilmott RW, et al. Denufosol tetrasodium in patients with cystic fibrosis and normal to mildly impaired lung function. *Am J Respir Crit Care Med* 2011; **183**: 627–34.
15. Ratjen F, Durham T, Navratil T, et al. Long term effects of denufosol tetrasodium in patients with cystic fibrosis. *J Cyst Fibros* 2012; **11**: 539–49.
16. Zhou Z, Treis D, Schubert SC, et al. Preventive but not late amiloride therapy reduces morbidity and mortality of lung disease in betaENaC-overexpressing mice. *Am J Respir Crit Care Med* 2008; **178**: 1245–56.
17. Elkins MR, Robinson M, Rose BR, et al. A controlled trial of long-term inhaled hypertonic saline in patients with cystic fibrosis. *N Engl J Med* 2006; **354**: 229–40.
18. Aitken ML, Bellon G, De Boeck K, et al. Long-term inhaled dry powder mannitol in cystic fibrosis: An international randomized study. *Am J Respir Crit Care Med* 2012; **185**: 645–52.
19. Yepuri NR, Barraud N, Mohammadi NS, Kardak BG, Kjelleberg S, Rice SA, Kelso MJ. Synthesis of cephalosporin-3'-diazeniumdiolates: Biofilm dispersing NO-donor prodrugs activated by β-lactamase. *Chem Commun (Camb)* 2013; **49**: 4791–3.
20. Mott LS, Park J, Murray CP, Gangell CL, de Klerk NH, Robinson PJ, Robertson CF, Ranganathan SC, Sly PD, Stick SM; AREST CF. Progression of early structural lung disease in young children with cystic fibrosis assessed using CT. *Thorax* 2012; **67**: 509–16.
21. Thia LP, Calder A, Stocks J, Bush A, Owens CM, Wallis C, Young C, Sullivan Y, Wade A, McEwan A, Brody AS; on behalf of the London Cystic Fibrosis Collaboration (LCFC). Is chest CT useful in newborn screened infants with cystic fibrosis at 1 year of age? *Thorax* 2014; **69**: 320–7.

49

The future: How will management change?

ANDREW BUSH AND DUNCAN GEDDES

INTRODUCTION

In this chapter, like latter-day Januses (the mythical two-headed god), we look back at what we wrote in the previous edition to see how well we predicted the future, and, undeterred by previous follies, look forward again to try to guesstimate how management will change.

DIAGNOSIS AND PREVENTION

In the previous edition, we predicted that cystic fibrosis (CF) prevalence would not fall, because widespread preconception screening for CF carrier status would never take off. It hasn't—but a fall in CF prevalence with screening has been consistently reported,[1–3] and there are a number of possible reasons. These include prenatal diagnosis and pregnancy termination in parents of affected children and also in their extended families; perhaps limitation of family size; and possibly, unrelated to screening, extended population mixing, and reduced consanguinity.

Since the last edition, universal newborn screening (NBS) has been introduced in the United Kingdom and is likely to extend across and beyond Europe. Of course, many areas of the world have been screening for decades! The main consequence has been for the most-part diagnosis at an early stage of disease; however, all may not be as well as might be thought. Furthermore, it must not be forgotten that missed diagnoses at screening are inevitable. Finally it should be noted that there are no fewer than 26 different screening strategies employed across Europe,[4] implying that there is a fair degree of uncertainty about the optimal method.

- Although determination and adoption of the optimal strategy for screening is highly desirable, we predict that this will not happen for many years to come.

How well is the newborn screened infant? Since the last edition it is now clear that NBS babies have abnormal lung function at 3 months of age.[5] What is not clear, and is obviously crucial, is what happens next? Clearly this is a key issue; if CF NBS infants go from strength to strength on conventional therapy, then any trials of novel therapy will have to enroll huge numbers to show any effect, unless we can prospectively delineate subgroups that are going to do less well. So we predict that before the next edition, the natural history of lung disease in optimally treated NBS infants will have been worked out, and we will be able to stratify at diagnosis a subgroup who will do well and thus would not be eligible for randomized controlled trials of treatment.

- However, we predict that determining the right end points for clinical trials in NBS infants will still be a work in progress.

Ignorance is bliss—but the age of innocence has gone. Nobody doubts the benefits of NBS, in terms of early institution of treatment to improve nutritional status and prevent lung disease, prevention of complications and thus treatment burden and fiscal cost, allowing future informed reproductive choices, and eliminating the long march to a diagnosis in the unscreened population. However, we have to acknowledge that we are creating disease. How should we describe the well infant, who has a raised immunoreactive trypsin, sweat chlorides less than 60, and two mutations in cystic fibrosis transmembrane conductance regulator (CFTR), one of which is not confirmed to be disease producing? One proposal was to use the term "genetic pre-CF," analogous to premalignant conditions, which in some cases may never actually progress to clinical disease.[6] The US CF Foundation have come up with the catchy phrase "Cystic fibrosis transmembrane regulator related metabolic syndrome" to describe this scenario.[7] Many clinicians would balk at this mouthful to describe a well infant, and particularly balk at trying to explain it to parents and reassure them that the child is well and may remain so for many years.

Sadly this is another prediction we got wrong—we thought that people would be less burdened with inappropriate diagnostic labels, and it is at least arguable that this new label moves in the opposite direction. Management guidelines have been published,[7] but if ever there was an area where individualized management is needed, it is this. Prolonged discussion time is needed to try to steer the family through this area, which is on the hinterland of disease.

- We predict that the CFTR-2 project (http://www.cftr2 .org/) will clarify the likelihood of many CFTR mutations actually causing disease, so that we will be able to reassure more parents about likely prognosis.
- We also predict that as molecular sequencing becomes more specific and combinations of mutations and single-nucleotide polymorphisms are found colocalized in many individuals that clinical prediction will become more, not less complex as the geneticists try to round up and explain the large number of genies currently lurking in the bottle.
- We speculate that ion current measurements will be increasingly used to try to diagnose (or otherwise) atypical cases of CF. This might include obtaining rectal mucosa for testing[9]; suction rectal biopsy is a routine investigation for suspected Hirschprung's disease and is a very simple procedure.

NEW TREATMENTS

Previously we discussed biomarkers, ethics and safety of research, reducing treatment burden, and novel therapies. Biomarkers have received a lot of attention in research, but in most areas we are long way away from what we need (further discussed below). Despite ever more demanding regulation, research continues to be high on the agenda, including the testing of medications in children, but no one has yet grasped the nettle of the issue of whether discarding a medication that is ineffective in adults may mean that something useful for children will have been lost. Treatment burden has been reduced to some extent with very fast nebulizers and dry powder devices, notably for antibiotics. Finally, anabolic therapies for nutritional failures and breeding pigs as a source of donor lungs still remains to be achieved, and indeed seem further away rather than nearer. Here, we discuss the past and future of conventional therapies (antibiotics, mucoactive drugs) and upstream therapies to correct the basic defect.

Antibiotics: out of left field. One prediction that is always correct is that the more dogmatically something is asserted by senior and venerated figures, the more likely it is to be wrong. Thus, we were taught that the lower airway is sterile in normal people, and CF bacteriology encompasses less than 10 microorganisms. Both assertions have been shown to be spectacularly wrong by molecular techniques, which detect many-fold more microorganisms than standard culture. The normal lower airway is teeming with bacteria,[8] and they are pivotal in the development of normal airway immune responses[9]; the CF airway also has a rich bacterial flora, including many obligate anaerobes.[10–15] It is clear that the multiplicity of bacteria, viruses, and fungi may interact in complex ways, either inhibiting or promoting the growth of particular pathogens. It would seem in general that bacterial diversity is a good thing, but otherwise we are struggling to understand the new microbiology of the airways. Clearly we should not abandon antibiotic strategies, which have stood us in great stead in the past,[16] but we need to be aware of the potential to cause whatever may be the airway equivalent of antibiotic-associated diarrhea; we know that we need lower airway bacteria for normal health.

- We predict that there will be a large number of longitudinal and intervention studies to try to understand the good and bad aspects of lower airway bacterial infection, but 10 years from now we will still be struggling to grasp the fundamental principles.

KISS—the way forward. Getting the basics right (KISS—Keep It Simple, Stupid) is obviously essential before starting novel, expensive, and potentially harmful therapies. The importance of this has been stressed in children with problematic severe asthma, of whom more than half do not need cytotoxics or monoclonal antibodies, but just to get the basics right.[17,18] Determining what the basics actually are will become increasingly difficult. The choice of nebulized antibiotics currently lies between colistin, tobramycin, and aztreonam lysine; coming on line are liposomal amikacin, ciprofloxacin, levofloxacin, and fosfomycin/tobramycin. In terms of mucolytics, we already have recombinant human deoxyribonuclease (rhDNase), hypertonic saline, and mannitol, with likely more to come. What is clear is that patients and professionals will have to make choices between these medications, because nebulizing everything is impractical in time and cost term. Furthermore, studies comparing different nebulized treatments will likely not be done because (1) there is an insufficient pool of patients; (2) they will not be seen as answering the great questions, such as how to correct the basic defect and will thus be of lower priority; (3) Pharma will not fund them, for fear of losing out; and (4) in any case, the results are utterly predictable, namely one antibiotic will not fit all and different individuals will respond better to different treatments (seen very clearly in trials of rhDNase, hypertonic saline, and mannitol). So this leads to our next prediction:

- A new focus in the next 10 years will be the development of robust protocols for N of one trials of conventional treatments, with the development of more sophisticated biomarkers than forced expiratory volume in 1 second (FEV_1) or asking the patient to fill in a questionnaire.
- On the negative side, we predict that medicalization of the healthy will increase as the numbers who are overtreated may approach or even overtake the numbers undertreated.

Back to basics: sorting out the upstream problem. In the last years, the emphasis has moved from firefighting the downstream complications of CFTR dysfunction to correcting the basic defect. The two approaches are gene therapy and the use of small molecules. Janus will not try to predict which approach will finally make CF a gastrointestinal disease of middle-aged people. Trials of gene therapy are ongoing, and it is likely that the current approach will be further refined and optimized before the final verdict can be delivered.

Small molecule therapy has come good in spectacular style, at least as far as the potentiator ivacaftor (Kalydeco, VX-770) is concerned.[19] The reductions in sweat chloride and increases in FEV_1 and body weight have been spectacular. Huge credit to the US CF Foundation, who funded a brutal high-throughput program that has screened around a quarter of a million compounds for biological activity in CF. However, as always, a great result throws up great questions. The best is the enemy of the good; ivacaftor has set a high bar of what we can achieve with small molecule therapy. For us, one of the bitterest lessons of the past years was the failure of denufosol.[20] As usual, it was subjected to the sort of excellent randomized controlled trials that are the hallmark of the CF community in the United States and Europe. With the retrospectoscope, that never-failing accurate diagnostic instrument, it is clear that in the totally understandable desire to offer hope to CF patients, we all blinded ourselves to the fact that changes reported in the initial trials, although statistically significant, were clinically small.[21,22] One lesson of ivacaftor is that we need big changes to make a difference, and at our peril do we fudge primary end points, torture the data with post hoc subgroup analyses, and blur the edges of statistical significance, because if we do not heed these lessons, history will repeat itself. We all want success for our patients, but we must, must, must be realistic. Great basic science and a great clinical result are not necessarily the same thing.

This is going to be particularly important as the use of ivacaftor spreads from *G551D* to the nine other gating mutations[23] and thence to nongating mutations. It is likely that effects will be seen, but we will need to be clear sighted, particularly in view of the cost (below), as to whether these effects are clinically worthwhile. So we hope we are right in predicting that

- There will be a new rigor in assessing novel therapies, and proof of concept (something has been achieved, there is a signal) and clinical reality (patients will get better with this treatment) will be kept separate

Ivacaftor was developed as a result of a brilliant but crude search strategy. The great prize is sorting out class 2 mutations such as *ΔF508*. Much more is known about the complexities of cotranslational and posttranslational folding of *ΔF508*, and the multiple check points between abnormal mRNA and producing a normal protein. So another prediction:

- The search for small molecule therapy for class 2 mutations will be refined, using a more designer molecule approach based on stoichiometric and other insights into the processing of CFTR.

Finally cost, the elephant in the room.[24] It must be acknowledged that pharmaceutical companies are not charitable foundations and deserve to make a profit. Second, governments will never take over and fund the sort of development programs that have led to ivacaftor. However, the cost implications of novel therapies are formidable; ivacaftor at the initially proposed cost of nearly $300,000 per patient per year would lead in the United Kingdom to 5% of the population raising the cost of CF care in the United Kingdom by 50%.[24] Cost-effective-speak does not help; if we had CF with one copy of *G551D* and the taxpayer was paying the money, it would be a great bargain for us! But by how much do you reduce the beneficial effects before the medication becomes of marginal benefit only? So our prediction:

- New molecules, combined with an aging CF population, will drive up the cost of CF and a grown-up, joined-up discussion about how we pay for this will be needed—but it will not happen!

Overall, small molecule therapy is a fantastic achievement in a very short time. Our final predictions in this section:

- The best of small molecule therapy is yet to come!
- Gene therapy will take longer to deliver, and new vectors look incredibly promising; Janus says that ultimately there will be a real head-to-head contest between gene therapy and small molecules, with real hard choices needing to be made.

NEW COMPLICATIONS

Our previous look to the future commented on the lack of drugs for CF liver disease, so no change there, then. We also commented on the need to focus prevention in early childhood, which to some extent will happen because of screening, although complication-specific strategies are lacking. Here we start with an old complication, which we predict will come increasingly into focus. CF is described as being punctuated by "exacerbations." The word "exacerbation" understates the importance of the problem, and "CF lung attacks" should be preferred.[25,26] In the case of CF, in one-third of so-called "exacerbations" spirometry never recovers[27,28] and they are also associated with an accelerated decline in lung function[29,30] and mortality.[31] We predict that this rather casual attitude will change, the word exacerbation will join colonization in the dustbin of history, and a CF lung attack will be seen as a needing a focused response to prevent further deterioration.

- CF lung attacks will lead to a focused response, reassessing the whole management package (by analogy with problematic severe asthma) and will cease to be seen as happenstance or a mere inconvenience.

Longevity has led to the unmasking of many CF complications, such as bone disease and insulin deficiency. Chronic renal impairment associated with insulin deficiency will likely become more important also. As a cohort of CF old age pensioners gathers numbers, will we need to be coping with CF vascular disease as a result of the high-fat diet or the obese CF patient. A fairly safe prediction is:

- CFTR dysfunction has a few more surprises to spring, and there will be at least one new organ system that will be discussed in a separate chapter in the next edition of the book.

Iatrogenic complications can be divided into acute and long-term complications, the latter an inexorable consequence of increased longevity. Acute complications, such as antibiotic allergy, are likely to remain a focus, but, giving a hostage to fortune, are only likely to gain new importance with new medications. However, it should be remembered, in the utterly justified euphoria about ivacaftor, that the studies have all been powered to show efficacy, but safety is still an imponderable. A 2% prevalence of a serious side effect such as malignancy could have been missed, and we have no medium-term toxicology studies either. Indeed, as we go to press, the possibility that ivacaftor may cause lens opacities has been raised so one prediction:

- There are no free lunches; the small molecule therapies have and will pay dividends, but there will be longer term side effects that we have yet to detect.

In terms of longevity, we need a new paradigm; safety issues in a disease characterized by death in the teenage years, as CF once was, and in a disease extending into old age, as now, are completely different. This we think we did get right last time around. Unsurprisingly, we have seen the selection of new organisms and increased antibiotic resistance in our old foes, and cumulative toxicity with nebulized aminoglycosides. We need to find a balance between not jeopardizing the gains of the past by pulling back on useful treatments and not creating new iatrogenic problems by overmedicating, particularly for prolonged periods of time. Janus predicts:

- We will discover new cumulative toxicities of medications and become aware of the need to be much more selective in our use of therapies; particularly given the likely increased vulnerability of the elderly to adverse effects of medications.

NEW PATTERNS OF CARE

As discussed previously, there is an increasing trend to use electronic media to monitor patients, which will continue, but these are still works in progress. Generally it is likely that conventional hospital care will be increasingly reserved for high dependency and intensive care cases, and everything else will be managed in the community. CF patients will disappear, to be replaced increasingly by normal people who want to lead normal unencumbered lives, but who happen to have CF. Increasingly, CF acute lung attacks will be managed in the community, with the provision of physiotherapy, dietetic advice, and the other adjuncts of management in the patient's home. Routine monitoring will increasingly be on Skype, with occasional home visits.

Another colossal elephant in the room is adherence,[31-33] which is notoriously poor in all chronic diseases, and in CF, as patients feel more and more like well people, it is likely to get worse. As discussed above, there is no point in prescribing expensive and potentially toxic medications if the basic treatments are not being accessed. There are a number of social media interventions being trialed to improve adherence, for example, text message alerts or tweets to try to remind patients that they need to take medication. A variety of incentives have been offered to reward adherence. The use of sticks as well as carrots might be explored—how about linking Facebook access to use of the nebulizer, for example? Facebook deprivation, although it might be classified a cruel and unusual punishment, would certainly cause young people to sit up and smarten up their approaches. However, "what one man can invent, another can discover" (Sherlock Holmes, *The Dancing Men*). So we predict:

- Electronic and social media will increasingly be used by healthcare professionals to aid compliance, and young CF patients will be increasingly good at circumventing these good intentions.
- More cheerfully, CF will be less and less a hospital disease.

MONITORING

The final section covers new technologies and better monitoring of old problems. We are able to do more and more tests; this does not mean that their performance is justified. In particular, we need to beware of the increasingly present VOMIT syndrome (**V**ictim **O**f **M**odern **I**maging **T**echnology).

The past attitude "we have nothing to offer you," well captured by Kevin Passey in Chapter 3, was rightly rejected and replaced by "everything that we can possibly do, must be done" and this resulted in a huge improvement in CF care and vastly improved prognosis. Now the extent of what can be done is so great that we need to review this approach. The Australasian bronchoscopy study,[34] an absolute model of its kind, demonstrated clearly that the aggressive use of fiberoptic bronchoscopy to monitor CF NBS infants yielded exactly no benefits. We need similar approaches for imaging technologies, in particular computed tomography (CT) scanning, which is done with ever-increasing frequency but without any evidence as yet of better outcomes. Although the radiation of an individual scan is reducing all the time, it is not zero, and there is an increased risk of cancer in CF. Our worrying prediction:

- If the frequency of performing CT scans continues to increase apace, we will have to deal with an epidemic of thyroid, esophageal, lung, and breast cancers in young CF patients.

Of course CT may be superseded by magnetic resonance imaging, especially as scan times become faster so babies can be scanned without anesthesia. However, the investigation will always be expensive and may throw up "abnormalities" of no consequence. Health commissioners will rightly want the cost of the tests justified in a setting of ever more expensive medications (above) and patients will question why they need to inconvenience themselves by spending a morning travelling for the tests and then undergoing them. The feasibility of a test is not necessarily the best indication for its performance. Janus says:

- There should be more studies of novel technologies along the lines of the Australasian bronchoscopy study—but they will not happen, because we will be dazzled by the headlights of new technologies!

Finally, monitoring of standard clinical decisions needs to move out of the nineteenth and twentieth centuries. It is ridiculous that we often make decisions about, for example, the length of a course of intravenous antibiotics by asking the patient how they feel! If we are to pull back on excessive treatments (above) while not losing the benefits of the past, we need to develop objective biomarkers of success, so we can pinpoint the patient who needs a long course and the one who perhaps only needs intravenous therapy for three days before switching to oral medications. Space precludes listing the many other decisions that are made in a ridiculously subjective manner. Adult asthma doctors have used sputum eosinophils to inform treatment decisions—so why cannot CF doctors do the same? So Janus's last prediction:

- We will develop objective biomarkers to inform clinical decision making in CF, but they will not be ready for discussion in the next edition!

SUMMARY AND CONCLUSIONS

The obvious first conclusion is that Janus would be well advised to take his two heads into retirement and be a prophet of the past not the future. A big theme is that we need critically to assess benefits and risks of new interventions and be rigorous in differentiating proof of concept from clinically relevant findings. We need to be ever more critical of new tests; what will we do with the results, will they influence management, and will they throw up irrelevant findings which, however, prompt yet more testing and attendant anxiety in the patient and expense to the Treasury? The main conclusion is that CF is changing rapidly in every aspect, and our students will be dealing with new problems in new ways that an increasingly outdated Janus can barely dream of now, even were he to summon supplementary heads to his aid. Never more have we so needed people with powers of acute observation and powerful intellects to undertake the clinical care of people with CF. Our final prediction, again along the lines of "tomorrow's rain will be wet," is that they will do it far better than us and far better than we can begin to imagine today.

REFERENCES

1. Cunningham S, Marshall T. Influence of five years of antenatal screening on the paediatric cystic fibrosis population in one region. *Arch Dis Child* 1998; **78**: 345–8.
2. Massie J, Curnow L, Gaffney L, Carlin J, Francis I. Declining prevalence of cystic fibrosis since the introduction of newborn screening. *Arch Dis Child* 2010; **95**: 531–3.
3. Scotet V, Duguépéroux I, Saliou P, Rault G, Roussey M, Audrézet MP, Férec C. Evidence for decline in the incidence of cystic fibrosis: A 35-year observational study in Brittany, France. *Orphanet J Rare Dis* 2012; **7**: 14.
4. Southern KW, Munck A, Pollitt R, Travert G, Zanolla L, Dankert-Roelse J, Castellani C; ECFS CF Neonatal Screening Working Group. A survey of newborn screening for cystic fibrosis in Europe. *J Cyst Fibros* 2007; **6**: 57–65.
5. Hoo A-F, Thia P, Nguyen TTD, Bush A, et al. Lung function is abnormal in 3 month old infants with cystic fibrosis diagnosed by newborn screening. *Thorax* 2012; **67**: 874–81.
6. Bush A, Wallis C. Time to think again: Cystic fibrosis is not an "all or none" disease. *Pediatr Pulmonol* 2000; **30**: 139–44.
7. Cystic Fibrosis Foundation, Borowitz D, Parad RB, Sharp JK, Sabadosa KA, Robinson KA, Rock MJ, Farrell PM, Sontag MK, Rosenfeld M, Davis SD, Marshall BC, Accurso FJ. Cystic Fibrosis Foundation practice guidelines for the management of infants with cystic fibrosis transmembrane conductance regulator-related metabolic syndrome during the first two years of life and beyond. *J Pediatr* 2009; **155** (6 Suppl): S106–16.
8. Hilty M, Burke C, Pedro H, Cardenas P, Bush A, Bossley C, Davies J, Ervine A, Poulter L, Pachter L, Moffatt MF, Cookson WO. Disordered microbial communities in asthmatic airways. *PLoS ONE* 2010; **5**: e857.

9. Herbst T, Sichelstiel A, Schär C, et al. Dysregulation of allergic airway inflammation in the absence of microbial colonization. *Am J Respir Crit Care Med* 2011; **184**: 198–205.

10. Rogers GB, Carroll MP, Serisier DJ, et al. Characterization of bacterial community diversity in cystic fibrosis lung infections by use of 16s ribosomal DNA terminal restriction fragment length polymorphism profiling. *J Clin Microbiol* 2004; **42** (Suppl 11): 5176–83.

11. Stressmann FA, Rogers GB, Klem ER, et al. Analysis of the bacterial communities present in lungs of patients with cystic fibrosis from American and British centers. *J Clin Microbiol* 2011; **49** (Suppl 1): 281–91.

12. Bittar F, Richet H, Dubus JC, et al. Molecular detection of multiple emerging pathogens in sputa from cystic fibrosis patients. PLoS ONE 2008; **3** (Suppl 8): e2908.

13. Sibley CD, Parkins MD, Rabin HR, et al. A polymicrobial perspective of pulmonary infections exposes an enigmatic pathogen in cystic fibrosis patients. *Proc Natl Acad Sci USA* 2008; **105**: 15070–5.

14. Tunney MM, Klem ER, Fodor AA, Gilpin DF, Moriarty TF, McGrath SJ, Muhlebach MS, Boucher RC, Cardwell C, Doering G, Elborn JS, Wolfgang MC. Use of culture and molecular analysis to determine the effect of antibiotic treatment on microbial community diversity and abundance during exacerbation in patients with cystic fibrosis. *Thorax* 2011; **66**: 579–84.

15. Stressmann FA, Rogers GB, van der Gast CJ, Marsh P, Vermeer LS, Carroll MP, Hoffman L, Daniels TW, Patel N, Forbes B, Bruce KD. Long-term cultivation-independent microbial diversity analysis demonstrates that bacterial communities infecting the adult cystic fibrosis lung show stability and resilience. *Thorax* 2012; **67**: 867–73.

16. LiPuma J. The new microbiology of cystic fibrosis: It takes a community. *Thorax* 2012; **67**: 851–2.

17. Bracken MB, Fleming L, Hall P, Van Stiphout N, Bossley CJ, Biggart E, Wilson NM, Bush A. The importance of nurse led home visits in the assessment of children with problematic asthma. *Arch Dis Child* 2009; **94**: 780–4.

18. Bush A, Saglani S. Management of severe asthma in children. *Lancet* 2010; **376**: 814–25.

19. Ramsey BW, Davies J, McElvaney NG, et al; VX08-770-102 Study Group. A CFTR potentiator in patients with cystic fibrosis and the G551D mutation. *N Engl J Med* 2011; **365**: 1663–72.

20. Ratjen F, Durham T, Navratil T, Schaberg A, Accurso FJ, Wainwright C, Barnes M, Moss RB; the TIGER-2 Study Investigator Group. Long term effects of denufosol tetrasodium in patients with cystic fibrosis. *J Cyst Fibros* 2012; **115**: 39–549.

21. Accurso FJ, Moss RB, Wilmott RW, Anbar RD, Schaberg AE, Durham TA, Ramsey BW; TIGER-1 Investigator Study Group. Denufosol tetrasodium in patients with cystic fibrosis and normal to mildly impaired lung function. *Am J Respir Crit Care Med* 2011; **183**: 627–34.

22. Deterding RR, Lavange LM, Engels JM, Mathews DW, Coquillette SJ, Brody AS, Millard SP, Ramsey BW; for the Cystic Fibrosis Therapeutics Development Network and the Inspire 08-103 Working Group. Phase 2 randomized safety and efficacy trial of nebulized denufosol tetrasodium in cystic fibrosis. *Am J Respir Crit Care Med* 2007; **176**: 362–9.

23. Yu H, Burton B, Huang CJ, Worley J, Cao D, Johnson JP Jr, Urrutia A, Joubran J, Seepersaud S, Sussky K, Hoffman BJ, Van Goor F. Ivacaftor potentiation of multiple CFTR channels with gating mutations. *J Cyst Fibros* 2012; **11**: 237–45.

24. Bush A, Simmonds NJ. Hot off the breath: 'I've a cost for'—the 64 million dollar question. *Thorax* 2012; **67**: 382–4.

25. FitzGerald JM. Targeting lung attacks. *Thorax* 2011; **66**: 365–6.

26. Bush A, Pavord I. Following Nero: Fiddle while Rome burns, or is there a better way? *Thorax* 2011; **66**: 367.

27. Sanders DB, Hoffman LR, Emerson J, Gibson RL, Rosenfeld M, Redding GJ, Goss CH. Return of FEV1 after pulmonary exacerbation in children with cystic fibrosis. *Pediatr Pulmonol* 2010; **45**: 127–34.

28. Sanders DB, Bittner RC, Rosenfeld M, Hoffman LR, Redding GJ, Goss CH. Failure to recover to baseline pulmonary function after cystic fibrosis pulmonary exacerbation. *Am J Respir Med* 2010; **182**: 627–32.

29. Sanders DB, Bittner RC, Rosenfeld M, Redding GJ, Goss CH. Pulmonary exacerbations are associated with subsequent FEV1 decline in both adults and children with cystic fibrosis. *Pediatr Pulmonol* 2011; **46**: 393–400.

30. Waters V, Stanojevic S, Atenafu EG, Lu A, Yau Y, Tullis E, Ratjen F. Effect of pulmonary exacerbations on long-term lung function decline in cystic fibrosis. *Eur Respir J* 2012; **40**: 61–6.

31. de Boer K, Vandemheen KL, Tullis E, et al. Exacerbation frequency and clinical outcomes in adult patients with cystic fibrosis. *Thorax* 2011; **66**: 680–5.

32. Latchford G, Duff A, Quinn J, Conway S, Conner M. Adherence to nebulised antibiotics in cystic fibrosis. *Patient Educ Counsel* 2009; **75**: 141–4.

33. McNamara PS, McCormack P, McDonald AJ, Heaf L, Southern KW. Open adherence monitoring using routine data download from an adaptive aerosol delivery nebuliser in children with cystic fibrosis. *J Cyst Fibros* 2009; **8**: 258–63.

34. Wainwright CE, Vidmar S, Armstrong DS, Byrnes CA, Carlin JB, Cheney J, Cooper PJ, Grimwood K, Moodie M, Robertson CF, Tiddens HA; ACFBAL Study Investigators. Effect of bronchoalveolar lavage-directed therapy on Pseudomonas aeruginosa infection and structural lung injury in children with cystic fibrosis: A randomized trial. *JAMA* 2011; **306**: 163–71.

Appendices

Appendix A

History of cystic fibrosis

JAMES M. LITTLEWOOD

INTRODUCTION

Cystic fibrosis (CF) is the most common life-shortening inherited disorder of Caucasian people. The incidence of around 1 in 2500 births is remarkably high as, until relatively recently, most affected children died in infancy or early childhood from pneumonia and malnutrition.

BEFORE THE 1930s

The first accurate description of the *swollen hardened gleaming white pancreas* likely to be due to CF was in an autopsy report on a supposedly "bewitched" 11-year-old girl in 1595 by Pieter Pauw, Professor of Botany and Anatomy at Leiden (1564–1617). From the middle of the seventeenth century there were many reports of infants who almost certainly had CF described in detail by Busch[1-3] even earlier than the well-known quotation of Rochholz that "The child will soon die whose brow tastes salty when kissed" in an almanac of children's songs and games from Switzerland.[4] Other versions of this prophecy include "If it tastes salty when someone is kissed on the brow then this person is hexed [bewitched]" in a dictionary of the Swiss–German language.[5] In 1838, Rokitansky[6] described the autopsy findings of ileal perforation and meconium peritonitis in a premature child likely to have had meconium ileus (although this is not of course completely synonymous with a diagnosis of CF). Landsteiner[7] gave a clear description of the pancreatic lesions in an infant with meconium ileus.

In 1888, Samuel Gee[8] described children with the appearances of severe intestinal malabsorption as having the "celiac affection" with an arrest of growth, a distended abdomen, and attacks of diarrhea with large, pale, foul-smelling stools. The cause was unknown but it became apparent that the syndrome was caused by a number of different conditions. The causative role of gluten in celiac disease, as we know it today, was not identified until 1950.[9] There were infants reported with the clinical syndrome described by Gee who at autopsy had definite histological changes in the pancreas and lungs.[10-14] The pancreatic histology of all these patients was typical of the changes that Dorothy Andersen[15] subsequently described using the term "cystic fibrosis."

THE 1930s

"CYSTIC FIBROSIS OF THE PANCREAS" RECOGNIZED AS A SPECIFIC ENTITY

Margaret Harper[16] of Sydney, who earlier had reported two children with congenital pancreatic steatorrhea, described a further eight children with clinical features compatible with CF. At autopsy, four had typical pancreatic changes.[17] Blackfan and Wolbach,[18] reviewing the histological changes in 11 children with vitamin A deficiency, noted 6 had extensive pancreatic lesions characterized by "dilatation of the acini and ducts, inspissated secretion, atrophy of the acini, lymphoid, and leukocyte infiltration to some degree and fibrosis"; they noted the lesions were "all identical and presumably representing a disease entity." In 1936, Fanconi et al.[19] described two children with "celiac syndrome" where "the changes in the lungs and pancreas, two vital organs, are so profound that their failure appears understandable." Blackfan and May[20] reported a further 35 infants with characteristic pancreatic histology and chronic lung infection, and other similar reports appeared in 1938.[21,22]

However, it was Dorothy Andersen[15] (Figure A.1), the pathologist at the Babies' and Children's Hospital at Columbia Presbyterian Medical Center in New York, whose 1938 publication resulted in CF being recognized as a specific entity. Andersen's meticulous study was initiated to review the clinical, laboratory, and autopsy findings of children with celiac disease to define the criteria for identifying those whose condition was caused by pancreatic disease.

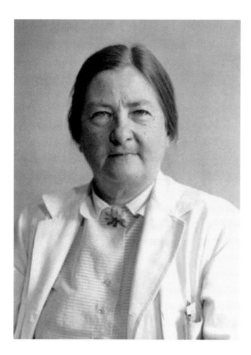

Figure A.1 Dorothy Andersen 1901–1963.

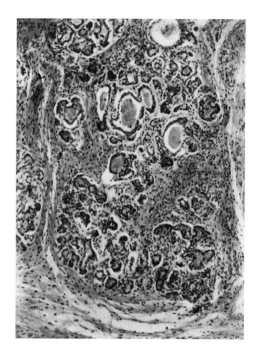

Figure A.3 Pancreas in an infant with cystic fibrosis at 6 days, showing dilatation of the acini and ducts, inspissated secretions, atrophy of the acini, leukocyte infiltration, and fibrosis. (From Andersen DH, *Am J Dis Child*, 56, 344–99, 1938. With permission.)

49 infants, and Andersen[23,24] suggested that vitamin A deficiency, resulting from the severe intestinal malabsorption, predisposed to the respiratory infections and bronchiectasis.

THE 1940s

A RECESSIVELY INHERITED MULTISYSTEM DISORDER

Despite Andersen's clear description of CF in 1938, "knowledge and recognition of the disease were almost nil for several years."[25] The few publications on CF came from North America; also Europe was heavily involved in the World War II. Charles May,[26] from the Babies' Hospital, New York, then a major in the US army, spoke on CF at a meeting of the Royal Society of Medicine in London and gave a succinct description of the 35 children with CF identified in Boston from 2800 pediatric autopsies over 15 years.

The familial incidence of CF was soon noted and a Mendelian recessive mode of inheritance recognized.[27,28] Sydney Farber, pathologist at the Children's Hospital, Boston, recognized that CF was a generalized disorder affecting organs other than the pancreas and introduced the term "mucoviscidosis." He concluded: "The inspissation of altered secretions in the pancreatic acini is only a part of a generalized disorder of secretory mechanisms involving many glandular structures but exerting its greatest effect on the pancreas."[29]

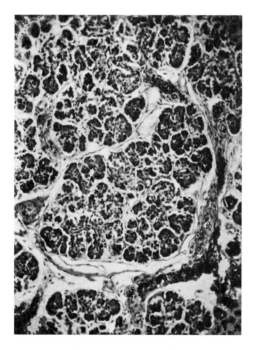

Figure A.2 Normal pancreas in an infant at 3 days.

She collected cases in which the presence of a definite pancreatic histological abnormality had been identified, and she described in great detail the clinical and autopsy findings of 49 such children—20 from her own hospital and others from colleagues and the literature. Andersen[15] described neonatal intestinal obstruction, later intestinal and respiratory complications and many other features, but particularly the striking characteristic pancreatic histology (Figures A.2 and A.3). The epithelial metaplasia characteristic of vitamin A deficiency was present in 14 of the

frequently in some CF centers and regimens for their use in CF were established. In some CF centers in the United States, the 50% survival increased to well beyond age 18 years and was attributed to improvements in antimicrobial therapy, routes of delivery, and increased therapeutic aggressiveness.[126] The increasing prevalence of *P. aeruginosa* respiratory infection and the use of gentamicin and tobramycin, and later carbenicillin and ticarcillin, all of which required systemic administration, resulted in the more general use of the intravenous rather than the intramuscular route.

CYSTIC FIBROSIS: "A NOT SO FATAL DISEASE"

Douglas Crozier[127] (who, in 1958, started the CF clinic at the Hospital for Sick Children, Toronto) reflected this improving outlook in his paper "Cystic fibrosis—a not so fatal disease." As early as 1972, his patients were advised to take a high-saturated-fat diet of whole milk, butter, eggs, and animal fats which did require them to take between 60 and 100 pancreatic enzyme capsules (Cotazym) each day, compared with the then conventional advice to have a low-fat diet to reduce unpleasant abdominal symptoms. Later, the better survival of these Toronto patients than others in Canada and in Boston was attributed to their superior nutritional state.[128]

THE DANISH APPROACH IS ASSOCIATED WITH AN IMPROVED PROGNOSIS

In some European clinics this lack of acceptance of the status-quo approach was also evident. For example, the Danish CF clinic in Copenhagen, where 80% of the country's 225 patients were treated, was established as a national CF center in 1968 by Erhard Flensborg.[129] In 1976, it was shown that the presence of chronic *P. aeruginosa* infection was closely associated with a poor prognosis.[130] Therefore, a policy of regular 3-monthly courses of intravenous antipseudomonal antibiotics for chronically infected patients was started and was associated with a fall in annual mortality from 10%–20% in 1976 to only 1%–2% in 1984–5.[131] Also, from 1981, cohort isolation of patients in the clinic was introduced—separating those with chronic *P. aeruginosa* from uninfected patients. Long-term inhaled colistin was introduced in 1987 for chronically infected patients,[132] and from 1989 inhaled colistin and oral ciprofloxacin was used to eradicate early *Pseudomonas* infection.[133] These treatment changes were eventually reflected by an impressive improvement in survival.[134]

LONGER SURVIVAL WITH WORSENING CHRONIC INFECTION COMPROMISED NUTRITION

As survival improved there was an increasing interest in the chronic nutritional problems that developed in the adolescents. A number of important studies in the late 1970s and early 1980s reported that the daily energy intake of people with CF, most of whom were on a restricted fat intake, was frequently even less than that recommended for healthy children of their age.[135] There was considerable interest in a nutritional supplement consisting of beef serum protein hydrolysate, a glucose polymer and medium-chain triglycerides (the "Allan diet") that was reported to improve weight gain,[136] a finding supported by subsequent trials.[137] However, the more effective new acid-resistant pancreatic enzymes were soon to become available, permitting most patients a normal fat intake—a more palatable way of increasing their energy intake. Toward the end of the 1970s, there was further evidence that a good nutritional state was shown to be associated with a better prognosis.[138] A new complication, recurrent acute pancreatitis, was reported in 10 adolescents and young adults, all of whom were pancreatic sufficient.[139]

Abnormalities of essential fatty acids had been noted by many authors from the 1960s[140] and subsequently[141] and were even suggested as the primary metabolic abnormality. Elliott[142] in New Zealand reported an unusually favorable clinical course in a child with CF treated with intravenous infusions of soya oil emulsion, which contains mainly linoleic acid, as well as in further treated children.[143]

IMMUNOREACTIVE TRYPSIN: A RELIABLE TEST FOR NEONATAL CF SCREENING

The measurement of IRT in the blood spots collected from newborns for metabolic screening was the first reliable test for neonatal CF screening.[81] The test was soon used in a number of neonatal CF screening programs and eventually in most combined with DNA testing.[144] However, it was apparent from the West Midlands and Wales UK study during the 1980s that early diagnosis following neonatal screening must also be followed by effective treatment, of the type available at a CF center, to show a long-term advantage for the screened infants.[145] Now that more effective treatment is available, early diagnosis is an established advantage in terms of growth[146] and even cognitive development.[147]

NATIONAL CF REGISTRIES: AN ESSENTIAL PROVISION TO MONITOR PROGRESS

Data collection was becoming increasingly important on both a national and local CF center basis. The CF Foundation's patient registry, developed by Warren Warwick from 1964 onwards,[148] had demonstrated a rise in median survival from 14 years in 1968 to 20 years in 1977. Also, Norman and colleagues published a series of papers between 1966 and 1975 recording the improving prognosis in the United Kingdom.[149] Between 1943 and 1964, 80% died by age 5 years and 90% by age 10 years, and 70% of infants with meconium ileus succumbed by age 3 months. Mary Corey had started data collection at the Toronto CF Clinic during the 1970s.[150] In 1995, the UK CF database (www.cystic-fibrosis.org.uk) replaced the original CF Survey started by the working party in 1982[151]; the UK CF database was replaced by CF Trust's CF Registry in 2007.

As a result of data from various registries, it became clear that, although there was a steady improvement in the condition and survival of many people with CF, there were significant differences in the treatment, condition, and even survival of patients attending different CF centers. In a study reflecting care through the 1970s, the median survival ages at three recognized US centers were 9.5, 18.1, and 22.8 years, respectively; it was considered that the differences reflected the different degree of supervision (number of clinic visits) and intensity of treatment (days of intravenous antibiotics) the patients received.[152] The philosophy of a comprehensive treatment program recommended by Matthews and his colleagues, by Shwachman, and subsequently by Crozier and others, had a major influence on CF care in the 1970s but unfortunately remained confined to a few CF centers and available to only a minority of people with CF.

INTERESTING BUT DISPARATE FINDINGS: A SEARCH FOR THE "CF FACTOR"

Scientists continued to search in vain for a lead to the basic defect. As one experienced CF center director observed: "Not professing to be a scientist or bench researcher, the unmet challenges that confront me every day as a clinician seem more distant and insolvable than they did thirty years ago."[153]

A unique protein band was described in CF serum electrophoresed through a pH gradient to its point of electric focus.[154] However, despite a great deal of research, neither isoelectric focusing nor using gels from isoelectric focusing to raise antibodies permitted accurate identification of the elusive "CF factor."[155] Lieberman et al.[156] described an elevated protein with lectin-like binding properties in the blood that was postulated to stimulate increased mucus production. A variety of other metabolic abnormalities were described. Extensive research into bronchial mucus and its glycoproteins led to no definite conclusions, which had a bearing on the etiology.[157] However, Yeates's work on mucociliary transport rates in humans did stimulate research into the epithelial transport of water and electrolytes.[158]

In summary, although during the 1970s some clinical progress was made in a few centers in controlling the secondary effects of the CF defect, generally progress was limited. Neither the location of the CF gene nor the underlying mechanisms of its serious pathophysiological effects were known.

THE 1980s

A DECADE OF EXCEPTIONAL CLINICAL AND SCIENTIFIC PROGRESS

At the start of the 1980s, the basic defect was unknown and the chromosome on which the CF gene was located had not been identified but by the end of the decade the CF gene and its main function had been identified.[159–161]

During the decade, prenatal diagnosis was pioneered by David Brock of Edinburgh,[162] which improved in accuracy when new linked probes were described in 1985[163] allowing families with an affected child to have reliable prenatal diagnosis in subsequent pregnancies.[164]

There were major advances in clinical care virtually all of which occurred at the increasing number of CF centers. CF center care was already well established in a few, but by no means all, cities in the United Kingdom but still available to only a minority of families. Survival was reported to be better in Victoria, Australia, where all patients had specialist CF center care than in England and Wales, where the majority attended the pediatric clinic at their local hospital.[165] These results prompted the formation of the British Paediatric Association's UK Working Party on Cystic Fibrosis in 1982, whose main recommendation was that all people with CF should have some contact with a specialist CF center, as only half the UK patients had such contact at the time.[166]

NEW TECHNIQUES OF PHYSIOTHERAPY

Various new devices and physiotherapy techniques were described during the decade,[167–169] and exercise received more attention. An increasing proportion of people with CF received treatment from physiotherapists experienced in CF. In the United States, the mechanical therapy vest proved increasingly popular with many patients but, even now, it is rarely used in the United Kingdom.[170]

MORE ANTIBIOTICS AND IMPROVED METHODS OF ADMINISTRATION

There was renewed interest in the use of nebulized antipseudomonal antibiotics after nebulized gentamicin and carbenicillin were shown to stabilize the condition of adults chronically infected with *P. aeruginosa*.[171] This proved to be a major advance despite some initial reservations regarding the development of bacterial resistance. Also there was a short report of successful eradication of early infection with *P. aeruginosa* using nebulized colomycin, thus delaying or preventing chronic *P. aeruginosa* infection.[172] The feasibility and success of early eradication of *P. aeruginosa* was later confirmed in an observational trial from Denmark using nebulized colomycin and oral ciprofloxacin (a treatment group was compared to a group who refused treatment, thus not formally randomized).[133] Early eradication gradually became established practice in Europe[173] and resulted in a significant reduction in the number of patients with chronic *Pseudomonas* infection in centers where early treatment was used.[174,175] Early eradication of *P. aeruginosa* eventually became accepted practice in North America following a controlled trial of inhaled tobramycin.[176]

During the decade there was earlier, more frequent and more effective use of intravenous antibiotics at all stages of infection.[177] Expert microbiological support, the use of two antibiotics, ensuring adequate blood levels, allowing for the altered pharmacokinetics in CF and also for the stage of the infection gradually became routine practice in most CF centers. Intensive courses of intravenous antibiotics became routine treatment for exacerbations of chest infection, and in Denmark regular 3-monthly 2-week courses of intravenous antibiotics were given to most patients who were chronically infected with *P. aeruginosa*.[178] New antipseudomonal antibiotics became available permitting a wider choice of treatment as bacterial resistance became more common (azlocillin from 1980, piperacillin from 1982, netilmicin from 1982, ceftazidime from 1983, aztreonam from 1986, and oral ciprofloxacin from 1986). With more frequent use of antibiotics, however, side effects were an increasing problem.[45,94,95]

There were improved techniques for establishing and maintaining intravenous access with heparin locks,[179] butterfly cannulas, percutaneous silastic catheters, long lines, and central venous catheters. Constant intravenous infusion pumps permitted maintenance of intravenous lines for many days at very slow flow rates (particularly useful in small children) and totally implantable venous access devices greatly reduced the stress and trauma of repeated venous access.[180,181] From 1984, EMLA local anesthetic cream was routinely applied before venepunctures—a major advance for all children requiring repeated venepunctures.[182] The increasing reliance on and more frequent use of intravenous antibiotics resulted in an increasing use of home intravenous antibiotics supervised by specialized CF staff—usually a CF Specialist Nurse.[183,184]

There were hopes that regular oral corticosteroids would reduce the damaging effects of inflammation,[185] but although children receiving alternate-day prednisone had better pulmonary function and reduced morbidity compared to controls, the frequent side effects precluded the more general use of oral steroids.

TREATMENT FOR CF-RELATED LIVER DISEASE

In 1989, Carla Colombo from Milan reported the beneficial effect of regular ursodeoxycholic acid treatment in improving liver function tests in CF-related liver disease.[186] Prior to this there had been no specific treatment for liver involvement. The suggestion by Kevin Gaskin that common bile duct stenosis was important in CF liver disease[187] was not supported by subsequent studies.[188] Liver transplantation has been used successfully in patients with CF and the results are surprisingly good. Lung function, far from deteriorating as a result of the long operation, improved in some patients.[189] Successful heart–lung–liver transplantations[190] and lung–liver transplantations have been performed.[191]

ACID-RESISTANT PANCREATIC ENZYMES: A MAJOR NUTRITIONAL ADVANCE

The nutritional state of many patients continued to improve due to the more widespread identification and correction of their inadequate energy intake.[192] The new acid-resistant enzymes were obviously more effective than the older

unprotected preparations.[193–195] Undoubtedly, these new enzymes were one of the major advances in treatment during the decade. They improved not only fat absorption and the nutritional state but also the symptoms and quality of life of many patients, most of whom could now tolerate a normal fat intake.[196]

MORE AGGRESSIVE NUTRITIONAL SUPPORT

Enteral feeding, first by the nasogastric route[197] and then by gastrostomy,[198,199] allowed rehabilitation of those with severe malnutrition, allowing reasonable nutritional state to be maintained even in many of the most severely affected patients (e.g., those awaiting transplantation). The first of a number of studies reported increased energy expenditure to be a major factor contributing to malnutrition.[200] Fat-soluble vitamin deficiencies were identified and corrected by appropriate doses of suitable supplements with varying success.[201–203] Oral gastrograffin was introduced as a treatment for meconium ileus equivalent—a treatment that is still widely used.[204]

ORGAN TRANSPLANTATIONS

A major advance, for those who had reached the end stages of their disease, was the successful introduction of heart–lung transplantation in 1985.[205,206] The possibility of successful treatment in the terminal stages of the condition had an obvious major influence not only on the prognosis but also on the treatment of severely affected individuals. The first results of heart–lung transplantations were quite remarkable and were related to surgical skills, to concentrated medical expertise in assessment and to aftercare, as well as to the availability of more effective immunosuppressive therapy to prevent organ rejection.[207] Later, double lung transplants became more popular.[208] Living-donor lung transplants have proved successful in some centers and will be chosen by some families, although now, fewer and fewer are being performed.[209]

INCREASING NEED FOR MORE CF CENTERS FOR ADULTS

As the population and age of people with CF increased, pediatric CF centers developed in most large cities in many countries. Toward the end of the 1980s, as a reflection of the improving survival, more CF centers for adults were required and gradually developed.[210] Arrangements for transition from pediatric to adult care received and continue to receive much attention.[211]

THE 1980s: SCIENCE

From epithelial transport abnormality to the identification of the gene

In 1981, Michael Knowles et al.[212] demonstrated an abnormal potential difference in the nasal mucosa of patients with

CF thus providing direct evidence of primary epithelial dysfunction. In 1983, Paul Quinton[213] showed that the chloride impermeability he had demonstrated in sweat glands was the basis for the raised sweat electrolytes in patients with CF. These were the most important advances to date in understanding the basic defect as a cell membrane transport problem and provided the first description of the basic cellular defect that has since been seen in all CF-affected cells. It was apparent that the problems with mucus were not due to abnormalities with its synthesis or composition, rather the fluid environment into which it was secreted.

Search for and identification of the CF gene

From the early 1980s, various groups attempted to identify the CF gene by using "reverse genetics," as the protein was unknown. Families with more than one affected child were studied. In 1985, using this technique, Eiberg in Copenhagen demonstrated a linkage to the enzyme paraoxinase, which exists in two forms but was present in the same form in 90% of CF siblings.[214] In the same year, Lap-Chi Tsui in Toronto, in a series of mouse hybrid experiments, demonstrated a marker on chromosome 7 linked to both paraoxinase and CF.[215] Other markers, known to be on chromosome 7, were closely linked to CF, the *Met* oncogenes, *Met H* and *Met D* from Ray White in Salt Lake City[216] and the DNA probe pJ3.11 from Bob Williamson's laboratory in London.[217] In 1989, the CF gene was eventually identified by teams headed by Lap-Chi Tsui, Francis Collins, and Jack Riordan and termed the "cystic fibrosis transmembrane conductance regulator." This was reported in three articles in a memorable issue of *Science*.[159–161]

Implications of identification of the gene

Since 1989, over 1800 different CF gene mutations have been described (www.CFTR2.org). There have been a number of practical benefits for the patients and their families. Carrier detection, accurate antenatal diagnosis, and incorporation of DNA testing into the many IRT neonatal screening programs have been major advances. Attempts to correlate phenotype and genotype have proved less successful than at first expected, but the major influence of environmental factors has been a confounding factor.[218] However, the definite correlation of so-called "mild" mutations with preservation of sufficient pancreatic function to achieve normal fat absorption (pancreatic sufficiency) and better clinical condition is now well established.[219] Also, certain mild mutations are associated with late-presenting disease often with normal pancreatic function and normal or near-normal sweat electrolytes.[220] An association of congenital bilateral absence of the vas deferens in infertile males has been associated with a high incidence of CF mutations, some with two mutations, the most common being *DF508/R117H*—somewhat blurring the edges of the traditional CF diagnosis.[221] A significant proportion of people with idiopathic pancreatitis, but who do not have CF, have been found to be carriers of a CF mutation.[222]

Now and the future

The improvements in clinical care at the CF centers, which characterized the 1980s, continue to the present. The realization that cross-infection with both *Burkholderia cepacia*[223,224] and *P. aeruginosa*[225,226] was a major problem had a profound influence on both hospital practice and the social lives of people with CF. Neonatal screening, early diagnosis and treatment before any chronic pulmonary damage, early eradication treatment of *Pseudomonas* to prevent or delay chronic infection, the introduction of effective new drugs such as recombinant human deoxyribonuclease,[227] antibiotic formulations designed specifically for inhalation,[228] and the widespread use of the macrolides[229] are likely to be reflected in a continuing improvement in health and survival of people with CF. However, the increasing number of adults with CF has resulted in more attention being given to problems of diabetes mellitus,[230] osteoporosis,[231] liver disease,[232] pregnancy,[233] and infertility.[234]

In 75 years CF has moved from a little known genetic condition, usually fatal in infancy and early childhood, to a complex multisystem disorder now affecting more adults than children. The abnormality of cell membrane transport has been recognized and finally the CF gene identified. The increasingly successful control of the secondary effects of the basic defect is due largely to advances in treatment developed at CF centers, which have resulted in clear treatment protocols[235,236] and efforts to ensure that these are available to all people with CF.[237] Treatment to correct or modify the basic defect by gene replacement or pharmacological means is showing considerable promise and likely to have a major influence on treatment regimens within a few years. In 2012, a multiple dose gene therapy trial started in the United Kingdom and the first specific treatment for a particular mutation (G551D) became available for patients.[238]

REFERENCES

1. Busch R. On the history of cystic mucoviscidosis. *Deutsche Gesundhs* 1978; **33**: 316.
2. Busch R. The history of cystic fibrosis. *Acta Univ Carol Med* 1990; **36**: 13–5.
3. Busch R. What do we know about the history of cystic fibrosis? *Quebec Adult CF Newslett* 2005; 28–30.
4. Rochholz EL. The child will soon die whose brow tastes salty when kissed. In: Weber JJ (Ed). *Almanac of Children's Songs and Games from Switzerland*. Leipzig, Germany; 1857.
5. Pfyffer JX. Zit bei 46: Zitierend aus dem Wörterbuch der Schweizerdeutschen. *Sprache* 1848; **7**: 899.
6. Rokitansky C von. *Sections-Protokoll und Gutachten*. Wien, Austria, 4, April 1838.
7. Landsteiner K. Darmverschluss durch eingedichtes Meconium Pankreatitis. *Zentralbl Allg Pathol* 1905; **16**: 903–7.
8. Gee S. On the coeliac affection. *St Bartholomew's Hosp Rep* 1888; **24**: 17–20.

9. Dicke WK, Weijers HA, van de Kamer JH. Coeliac disease: The presence in wheat of a factor having a deleterious effect in cases of coeliac disease. *Acta Paediatr Scand* 1953; **42**: 344–399.

10. Passini F. Pankreaserkrangkung als Ursache de Nichtgedeihens von Kindern. *Deutsch Med Wchnschr* 1919; **45**: 851–853.

11. Clarke CG, Hadfield G. Congenital pancreatic disease with infantilism. *Q J Med* 1924; **17**: 358–64.

12. Burghard E. Diseases of the pancreas in infancy. *Klin Wchnschr* 1925; **4**: 2305.

13. Gross F. Pancreatic atrophy in infancy and childhood. *Jahrb Kinderh* 1926; **112**: 251.

14. Hess JH, Saphire O. Celiac disease. Chronic intestinal indigestion: A report of three cases with autopsy findings. *J Pediatr* 1935; **6**: 1–13.

15. Andersen DH. Cystic fibrosis of the pancreas and its relation to celiac disease: A clinical and pathological study. *Am J Dis Child* 1938; **56**: 344–99.

16. Harper MH. Two cases of congenital pancreatic steatorrhoea with infantilism. *Med J Aust* 1930; **2**: 663.

17. Harper MH. Congenital steatorrhoea due to pancreatic defect. *Arch Dis Child* 1938; **13**: 45–56.

18. Blackfan KD, Wolbach SB. Vitamin A deficiency in infants: A clinical and pathological study. *J Pediatr* 1933; **3**: 679–706.

19. Fanconi G, Uehlinger E, Knauer C. Das coeliakie syndrom bei angeborener zystischer pancreasfibromatose und bronchiektasien. *Wien Med Wchnschr* 1936; **86**: 753–6.

20. Blackfan KD, May CD. Inspissation of secretion and dilatation of ducts and acini: Atrophy and fibrosis of the pancreas in infants. A clinical note. *Pediatrics* 1938; **13**: 624–37.

21. Thomas J, Schultz FW. Pancreatic steatorrhoea. *Am J Dis Child* 1938; **56**: 336–43.

22. Rauch S, Litvak AM, Steiner M. Congenital familial steatorrhoea with fibromatosis of the pancreas and bronchiectasis. *J Pediatr* 1939; **14**: 462–90.

23. Andersen DH. Cystic fibrosis of the pancreas, vitamin A deficiency and bronchiectasis. *J Pediatr* 1939; **15**: 763–71.

24. Andersen DH. The present diagnosis and treatment of cystic fibrosis. *Proc R Soc Med* 1949; 42: 25–31.

25. di Sant'Agnese PA. Experiences of a pioneer researcher: Discovery of the sweat electrolyte defect and the early medical history of cystic fibrosis. In: Doershuk CF (Ed) *Cystic Fibrosis in the Twentieth Century*. Cleveland, OH, AM Publishing; 2001. pp. 17–35.

26. May CD. Fibrosis of pancreas in infants and children. *Proc R Soc Med* 1943; **37**: 311–3.

27. Andersen DH, Hodges RC. Celiac syndrome. V: Genetics of cystic fibrosis of the pancreas with a consideration of etiology. *Am J Dis Child* 1946; **72**: 62–80.

28. Bodian ML (Ed) in collaboration with Norman AP, Carter CO. *Fibrocystic Disease of the Pancreas. A Congenital Disorder of Mucus Production (Mucosis)*. London: W Heinemann; 1952.

29. Farber S. Pancreatic insufficiency and the celiac syndrome. *N Engl J Med* 1943; **229**: 653–7.

30. di Sant'Agnese PEA, Andersen DH. Chemotherapy in infections of the respiratory tract associated with cystic fibrosis of the pancreas; observations with penicillin and drugs of the sulphonamide group, with special reference to penicillin aerosol. *Am J Dis Child* 1946; **72**: 17–61.

31. Harris R, Norman AP, Payne WW. The effect of pancreatin therapy on fat absorption and nitrogen retention in children with fibrocystic disease of the pancreas. *Arch Dis Child* 1955; **30**: 424–7.

32. Kennedy RLJ. Cystic fibrosis of the pancreas. *Nebr Med J* 1946; **31**: 493–6.

33. Shwachman H, Patterson PR, Laguna J. Studies in pancreatic fibrosis: Simple diagnostic gelatine film test for stool trypsin. *Pediatrics* 1949; **4**: 222–30.

34. Kessler WR, Andersen DH. Heat prostration in fibrocystic disease of the pancreas and other conditions. *Pediatrics* 1951; **8**: 648–56.

35. di Sant'Agnese PA, Darling MD, Perera G, Shea E. Abnormal electrolyte composition of sweat in cystic fibrosis of the pancreas: Clinical significance and relationship to the disease. *Pediatrics* 1953; **12**: 549–63.

36. Misch KA, Holden HM. Sweat test for diagnosis of fibrocystic disease of the pancreas: Report of a fatality. *Arch Dis Child* 1958; **33**: 179–80.

37. Gibson LE, Cooke RE. Test for concentration of electrolytes in sweat in cystic fibrosis of the pancreas utilizing pilocarpine by iontophoresis. *Pediatrics* 1959; **23**: 545–9.

38. Smalley CA, Addy DP, Anderson CM. Does that child really have cystic fibrosis? *Lancet* 1978; ii: 415–7.

39. Mearns MB. Cystic fibrosis: The first fifty years. In: Dodge JA, Brock DJH, Widdicombe JH (Eds). *Cystic Fibrosis—Current Topics*. Volume 1. Chichester, United Kingdom: John Wiley; 1993. pp. 217–50.

40. Reed JMW. Physiotherapy for chest diseases. In: Marshall G, Perry KMA (Eds). *Diseases of the Chest*, Volume 2. St Louis, MS: Butterworth; 1952. pp. 395–413.

41. Doyle B. Physical therapy in treatment of cystic fibrosis. *Phys Ther Rev* 1959; **39**: 24–7.

42. Docter JM. Unmet challenges in cystic fibrosis. In: Warwick WJ (Ed). *1000 Years of Cystic Fibrosis*. Minnesota: University of Minnesota; 1981. pp. 1–4.

43. Shwachman H, Kulczycki LL. Long-term study of 105 cystic fibrosis patients. *Am J Dis Child* 1958; **96**: 6–15.

44. Shwachman H. Therapy of cystic fibrosis. *Pediatrics* 1960; **25**: 155–63.

45. Shwachman H. Cystic fibrosis: Iatrogenic complications and related issues. In: Lloyd-Still JD (Ed). *Textbook of Cystic Fibrosis*. Boston, MA: John Wright; 1983. pp. 409–48.

46. Doggett RG, Harrison GM, Stillwell RN, et al. An atypical *Pseudomonas aeruginosa* associated with cystic fibrosis of the pancreas. *J Pediatr* 1966; **68**: 215–21.

47. West JR, Levin MS, di Sant'Agnese PA. Studies of pulmonary function in cystic fibrosis of the pancreas. *Pediatrics* 1954; **13**: 155–64.

48. Wessel HU. Lung function in cystic fibrosis. In: Lloyd-Still JD (Ed). *Textbook of Cystic Fibrosis*. Massachusetts: John Wright; 1983. pp. 199–216.

49. Gandevia B, Anderson CM. The effect of bronchodilator aerosol on ventilatory capacity in fibrocystic disease of the pancreas. *Arch Dis Child* 1959; **34**: 511–5.

50. Royce SW. Cor pulmonale in infancy and early childhood: Report on 34 patients, with special reference to the occurrence of pulmonary heart disease in cystic fibrosis of the pancreas. *Pediatrics* 1951; **8**: 255–74.

51. di Sant'Agnese PA. Bronchial obstruction with lobar atelectasis and emphysema in cystic fibrosis of pancreas. *Pediatrics* 1953; **2**: 178–90.

52. Keats TE. Generalized pulmonary emphysema as an isolated manifestation of early cystic fibrosis of the pancreas. *Radiology* 1955; **65**: 223–6.

53. Lurie MH. Cystic fibrosis of the pancreas and the nasal mucosa. *Ann Otol Rhinol Laryngol* 1959; **68**: 478–86.

54. Hiatt R, Wilson P. Celiac syndrome. VII: Therapy of meconium ileus, report of eight cases with review of the literature. *Surg Gynecol Obstet* 1948; **87**: 317–27.

55. Bishop HC, Koop CE. Management of meconium ileus, resection, Roux-en-Y anastomosis and ileostomy irrigation with pancreatic enzymes. *Ann Surg* 1957; **50**: 835–6.

56. Rasor R, Stevenson C. Cystic fibrosis of the pancreas, a case history. *Rocky Mt Med J* 1941; **38**: 218–0.

57. Jensen KG. Meconium ileus equivalent in a fifteen-year-old patient with mucoviscidosis. *Acta Pediatr* 1962; **51**: 344–8.

58. Gibbs GE, Gershbein LL. Incomplete pancreatic deficiency in cystic fibrosis of the pancreas. *Proc Soc Exp Biol Med* 1950; **37**: 320–5.

59. Di Sant'Agnese PA. Fibrocystic disease of the pancreas with normal or partial pancreatic function: Current views on pathogenesis and diagnosis. *Pediatrics* 1955; **15**: 683–97.

60. Kulczycki LL, Shwachman H. Studies in cystic fibrosis of the pancreas: Occurrence of rectal prolapse. *N Eng J Med* 1958; **259**: 409–12.

61. di Sant'Agnese PA, Andersen DH. Cystic fibrosis of the pancreas in young adults. *Ann Intern Med* 1959; **50**: 1321–30.

62. Lelong M, Joseph R, Le Tan Vinh, Bouvattier P. Cystic fibrosis of the pancreas and massive hepatic steatosis. *Arch Franc Ped* 1950; **7**: 234–40.

63. Webster R, Williams H. Hepatic cirrhosis associated with fibrocystic disease of the pancreas: Clinical and pathological reports of 5 patients. *Arch Dis Child* 1953; **28**: 343–50.

64. di Sant'Agnese PA. A distinctive type of biliary cirrhosis of the liver in patients with cystic fibrosis of the pancreas. *Pediatrics NY* 1956; **3**: 387–409.

65. di Sant'Agnese PA. Cirrhosis of the liver with portal hypertension in cystic fibrosis of the pancreas. *Bull NY Acad Med* 1955; **31**: 406–7.

66. Doershuk CF. The Matthews Comprehensive Treatment Programme: A ray of hope. In: Doershuk CF (Ed). *Cystic Fibrosis in the Twentieth Century*. Cleveland, OH: AM Publishing; 2001. pp. 63–78.

67. Matthews LW, Doershuk CF, Wise M, et al. A therapeutic regimen for patients with cystic fibrosis. *J Pediatr* 1964; **65**: 558–75.

68. Doershuk CF, Matthews LW, Tucker AS, et al. A 5-year clinical evaluation of a therapeutic program for patients with cystic fibrosis. *J Pediatr* 1964; **65**: 677–93.

69. Doershuk CF, Matthews LW, Tucker A, Spector S. Evaluation of a prophylactic and therapeutic program for patients with cystic fibrosis. *Pediatrics* 1965; **36**: 675–88.

70. di Sant'Agnese PA. *Year Book of Pediatrics, 1966/1967*. Gellis SS (Ed). Chicago, IL: Year Book Publishers; 1967. pp. 257–9.

71. Quinton PM. Physiological basis of cystic fibrosis: A historical perspective. *Physiol Rev* 1999; **79**: 3–22.

72. Andersen DH. Cystic fibrosis of the pancreas: A review. *J Chron Dis* 1958; **7**: 58–90.

73. Baggenstoss AH, Power MH, Grindlay JH. The relationship of fibrocystic disease of the pancreas to deficiency of secretin. *Pediatrics* 1948; **2**: 435.

74. Ayers WB, Stowens D, Ochsner A, Platou RV. Splanchnicectomy for cystic fibrosis of the pancreas: Analysis of results in 24 patients. *Pediatrics* 1951; **8**: 657–76.

75. Morrison C, Morrison R. National and international cystic fibrosis associations. In: Dodge JA, Brock DJH, Widdicombe JH (Eds). *Cystic Fibrosis—Current Topics*. Chichester, England: John Wiley; 1993. pp. 319–45.

76. Wiser WC, Beier FR. Albumin in the meconium of infants with cystic fibrosis: A preliminary report. *Pediatrics* 1964; **33**: 115–9.

77. Kopito L, Mahmoodian A, Townley IT, et al. Studies in cystic fibrosis: Analysis of nail clippings for sodium and potassium. *N Eng J Med* 1965; **272**: 504–9.

78. Lawson D, Westcombe P, Saggers B. Pilot trial of an infant screening programme for cystic fibrosis: Measurement of parotid salivary sodium at 4 months. *Arch Dis Child* 1969; **44**: 715–8.

79. Gurson CT, Sertel H, Gurkan M, Pala S. Newborn screening for cystic fibrosis with the chloride electrode and neutron activation analysis. *Helv Pediatr Acta* 1973; **28**: 165–74.

80. Shwachman H, Mahmoodian A. Reappraisal of the chloride plate test as screening test for cystic fibrosis. *Arch Dis Child* 1981; **56**: 137–9.

81. Crossley JR, Elliott RB, Smith PA. Dried blood spot screening for cystic fibrosis in the newborn. *Lancet* 1979; **i**: 472–4.

82. Hadorn B, Johansen PG, Anderson CM. Pancreozymin secretin tests of exocrine pancreatic function in cystic fibrosis and the significance of the result for the pathogenesis of the disease. *Can Med J* 1968; **98**: 377–84.

83. Barbero GJ, Siblinga MS, Marino JM, Seibel R. Stool trypsin and chymotrypsin: Value in the diagnosis of pancreatic insufficiency in cystic fibrosis. *Am J Dis Child* 1966; **112**: 536–40.

84. Anderson CM. Histologic changes in duodenal mucosa in coeliac disease: Reversibility during treatment with wheat gluten free diet. *Arch Dis Child* 1960; **35**: 419–27.

85. Valetta EA, Mastella G. Incidence of coeliac disease in a cystic fibrosis population. *Acta Pediatr Scand* 1989; **78**: 784–5.

86. Freye HB, Kurtz SM, Spock A, Capp MP. Light and electron microscopic examination of the small bowel of children with cystic fibrosis. *J Pediatr* 1964; **64**: 575–9.

87. Parkins RA, Eidelman S, Rubin CE, Dobbins WO. The diagnosis of cystic fibrosis by rectal suction biopsy. *Lancet* 1963; **38**: 851–6.

88. Lobeck CC, McSherry NR. Response of sweat electrolyte concentrations to 9 alpha-fluorohydrocortisone in patients with cystic fibrosis and their families. *J Pediatr* 1963; **62**: 393–8.

89. Doggett RG, Harrison GM, Wallis ES. Comparison of some properties of *Pseudomonas aeruginosa* isolated from infections in persons with and without cystic fibrosis. *J Bacteriol* 1964; **87**: 427–43.

90. Mearns MB. Simple tests of ventilatory capacity in children with cystic fibrosis. I: Clinical and radiological findings in 85 patients. II: Three-year follow-up on 50 patients. *Arch Dis Child* 1968; **43**: 528–39.

91. Phelan PD, Gracey M, Williams HE, Anderson CM. Ventilatory function in infants with cystic fibrosis: Physiological assessment of inhalation therapy. *Arch Dis Child* 1969; **44**: 393–400.

92. Mearns M, Young W, Batten J. Transient pulmonary infiltrations in cystic fibrosis due to allergic aspergillosis. *Thorax* 1965; **20**: 385–92.

93. Bernard E, Israel L, Debris MM, Tip M. Mucoviscidosis and idiopathic spontaneous pneumothorax. *J Fr Med Chir Thor* 1962; **16**: 105–9.

94. Zegarelli EV, Kutscher AH, Denning CR, et al. Coloration of teeth in patients with cystic fibrosis of the pancreas: II. *Oral Surg Oral Med Oral Pathol* 1962; **15**: 929–33.

95. Lietman PS, di Sant'Agnese PA, Wong V. Optic neuritis in cystic fibrosis of the pancreas: Role of chloramphenicol therapy. *J Am Med Assoc* 1964; **189**: 924–7.

96. Denton R. Clinical use of continuous nebulization in bronchopulmonary disease. *Dis Chest* 1955; **28**: 123–40.

97. Matthews LW, Doershuk CF, Spector S. Mist tent therapy of obstructive pulmonary lesion of cystic fibrosis. *Pediatrics* 1967; **39**: 176–85.

98. di Sant'Agnese PA. *Comment in Year Book of Pediatrics 1967/68.* Gellis SS (Ed). Chicago, IL: Year Book Publishers; 1968. p. 197.

99. Chang N, Levison H, Cunningham K, et al. An evaluation of nightly mist tent therapy for patients with cystic fibrosis. *Am Rev Resp Dis* 1973; **107**: 672–5.

100. Sproul A, Huang N. Growth patterns in children with cystic fibrosis. *J Pediatr* 1964; **65**: 664–76.

101. Kunstadter RH, Mendelsohn RS. Norethandrolone in children with and without cystic fibrosis of the pancreas. *Illinois Med J* 1961; **120**: 156–61.

102. Dooley RR, Moss AJ, Wright PM, Hassakis PC. Norethandrolone in cystic fibrosis of the pancreas. *J Pediatr* 1969; **74**: 95–102.

103. Gracey M, Burke V, Anderson CM. Treatment of abdominal pain in cystic fibrosis by oral administration of n-acetyl cysteine. *Arch Dis Child* 1969; **44**: 404–5.

104. Noblett HR. Treatment of uncomplicated meconium ileus by gastrografin enema: A preliminary report. *J Pediatr Surg* 1969; **4**: 190–7.

105. Hide DW, Burman D. An infant with both cystic fibrosis and coeliac disease. *Arch Dis Child* 1969; **44**: 533–5.

106. Rosan RC, Shwachman H, Kulczycki LI. Diabetes mellitus and cystic fibrosis of the pancreas: Laboratory and clinical observations. *Am J Dis Child* 1962; **104**: 625–34.

107. Milner AD. Blood glucose and serum insulin levels in children with cystic fibrosis. *Arch Dis Child* 1969; **44**: 351–5.

108. Johnson Sir R. *History of the Cystic Fibrosis Research Trust.* Twentieth Anniversary Meeting, Brighton, United Kingdom; 1984. pp. 3–6.

109. Batten J. Cystic fibrosis: A review. *Br J Dis Chest* 1965; **59**: 1–9.

110. Shwachman H, Kulczycki, Khaw Kon-Taik. Studies in cystic fibrosis: A report of sixty-five patients over 17 years of age. *Pediatrics* 1965; **36**: 689–99.

111. Denning CR, Sommers SC, Quigley HJ. Infertility in male patients with cystic fibrosis. *Pediatrics NY* 1968; **41**: 7–17.

112. Kaplan E, Shwachman H, Perlmutter AD, et al. Reproductive failure in males with cystic fibrosis. *N Eng J Med* 1968; **279**: 65–9.

113. Siegel B, Siegel S. Pregnancy and delivery in a patient with cystic fibrosis of the pancreas. *Obstet Gynecol* 1960; **16**: 438–40.

114. Chernick WS, Barbero GJ. Composition of tracheobronchial secretions in cystic fibrosis of the pancreas and bronchiectasis. *Pediatrics* 1959; **24**: 739–45.

115. Lev R, Spicer SS. An historical chemical comparison of human epithelial mucins in normal and in hypersecretory states including pancreatic cystic fibrosis. *Am J Pathol* 1965; **46**: 23–47.

116. Danes BS, Bearn AG. A genetic cell marker for cystic fibrosis. *Lancet* 1968; **18**: 1061–3.

117. Spock A. Abnormal serum factor in patients with cystic fibrosis of the pancreas. *Pediatr Res* 1967; **1**: 173–7.

118. Bowman BH, Lockhart LH, McCombs ML. Oyster ciliary inhibition by cystic fibrosis factor. *Science* 1969; **164**: 325–6.

119. Mangos JA, McSherry N. Sodium transport: Inhibitory factor in sweat of patients with cystic fibrosis. *Science* 1967; **158**: 135–6.

120. Wood RE. Pediatric flexible bronchoscopy: The inside story. In: Doershuk CF (Ed). *Cystic Fibrosis in the Twentieth Century*. Cleveland, OH: AM Publishing; 2001. pp. 112–9.

121. Mearns MB. Treatment and prevention of pulmonary complications of cystic fibrosis in infancy and early childhood. *Arch Dis Child* 1972; **47**: 5–11.

122. Mearns MB. Cystic fibrosis. *Br J Hosp Med* 1974; October: 497–506.

123. Lawson D. Panel discussion on microbiology and chemotherapy of the respiratory tract in cystic fibrosis. In: Lawson D (Ed). Proceedings of the fifth International CF Conference, Cambridge, 1969. Cambridge, London: Cystic Fibrosis Research Trust; 1969. p. 225.

124. Weaver LT, Green MG, Nicholson K, et al. Prognosis in cystic fibrosis treated with continuous flucloxacillin for the neonatal period. *Arch Dis Child* 1994; **70**: 84–9.

125. Stutman HR, Lieberman JM, Nussbaum E, Marks MI. Antibiotic prophylaxis in infants and young children with cystic fibrosis: A randomized controlled trial. *J Pediatr* 2002; **140**: 299–305.

126. Wood RE, Boat TF, Doershuk CF. Cystic fibrosis: State of the art. *Am Rev Resp Dis* 1976; **113**: 833–78.

127. Crozier DN. Cystic fibrosis: A not so fatal disease. *Pediatr Clin North Am* 1974; **21**: 935–48.

128. Corey M, McLaughlin FJ, Williams M, et al. A comparison of survival growth and pulmonary function in patients with cystic fibrosis in Boston and Toronto. *J Clin Epidemiol* 1988; **41**: 588–91.

129. Nielsen OH, Schiotz PO. Cystic fibrosis in Denmark in the period 1945–1981: Evaluation of centralized treatment. *Acta Pediatr* 1982; **71 (Suppl 301)**: 107–19.

130. Hoiby N. Antibodies against *Pseudomonas aeruginosa* in serum from normal persons and patients colonised with mucoid or non-mucoid *P. aeruginosa*: Results obtained by crossed immunoelectrophoresis. *Acta Pathol Microbiol Immunol Scand* 1977; **85**: 142–8.

131. Szaff M, Hoiby N, Flensborg EW. Frequent antibiotic therapy improves survival of cystic fibrosis patients with chronic *Pseudomonas aeruginosa* infection. *Acta Pediatr Scand* 1983; **72**: 651–7.

132. Jensen T, Pedersen SS, Garne S, Heilmann C, et al. Colistin inhalation therapy in cystic fibrosis patients with chronic *Pseudomonas aeruginosa* lung infection. *J Antimicrob Chemother* 1987; **19**: 831–8.

133. Valerius NH, Koch C, Hoiby N. Prevention of chronic *Pseudomonas aeruginosa* infection in cystic fibrosis by early treatment. *Lancet* 1991; **338**: 725–6.

134. Frederiksen B, Lanng S, Koch C, Hoiby N. Improved survival in the Danish Cystic Fibrosis Centre: Results of aggressive treatment. *Pediatr Pulmonol* 1996; **21**: 153–8.

135. Chase HP, Long MA, Lavin MH. Cystic fibrosis and malnutrition. *J Pediatr* 1979; **95**: 337–47.

136. Allan JD, Mason A, Moss AD. Nutritional supplementation in treatment of cystic fibrosis of the pancreas. *Am J Dis Child* 1973; **26**: 2–26.

137. Yassa JG, Prosser R, Dodge JA. Effects of an artificial diet on growth of patients with cystic fibrosis. *Arch Dis Child* 1978; **53**: 777–83.

138. Kraemer R, Rudeberg A, Hadorn B, et al. Relative underweight in cystic fibrosis and its prognostic value. *Acta Pediatr Scand* 1978; **67**: 33–7.

139. Shwachman H, Lebenthal K, Khaw P-T. Recurrent acute pancreatitis in patients with cystic fibrosis with normal pancreatic enzymes. *Pediatrics* 1975; **55**: 86–94.

140. Kuo PT, Huang NN. The effect of medium chain triglyceride upon fat absorption and plasma lipid and depot fat of children with cystic fibrosis of the pancreas. *J Clin Invest* 1962; **44**: 1924–33.

141. Strandvik B, Gronowitz E, Enlund F, et al. Essential fatty acid deficiency in relation to genotype in patients with cystic fibrosis. *J Pediatr* 2001; **139**: 650–5.

142. Elliott RB. A therapeutic trial of fatty acid supplementation in cystic fibrosis. *Pediatrics* 1976; **57**: 474–9.

143. Chase HP, Cotton EK, Elliot RB. Intravenous linoleic acid supplementation in children with cystic fibrosis. *Pediatrics* 1979; **64**: 207–13.

144. Southern KW, Littlewood JM. Newborn screening programmes for cystic fibrosis. *Pediatr Respir Rev* 2003; **4**: 299–305.

145. Chatfield S, Owen G, Ryley HC, et al. Neonatal screening for cystic fibrosis in Wales and the West Midlands: Clinical assessments after 5 years of screening. *Arch Dis Child* 1991; **66**: 29–33.

146. Farrell PM, Kosorok MR, Rock MJ, et al. Early diagnosis of cystic fibrosis through neonatal screening prevents severe malnutrition and improves long-term growth. *Pediatrics* 2001; **107**: 1–13.

147. Koscik RL, Farrell PM, Kosorok MR, et al. Cognitive function of children with cystic fibrosis: Deleterious effect of early malnutrition. *Pediatrics* 2004; **113**: 1549–58.

148. Warwick WJ, Pogue RE, Gerber HU, Nesbitt CJ. Survival patterns in cystic fibrosis. *J Chron Dis* 1975; **28**: 609–22.

149. Robinson MJ, Norman AP. Life tables for cystic fibrosis. *Arch Dis Child* 1975; **50**: 962–5.

the family is first approached by someone they are familiar with, and may trust, it is even more important that the first person to raise the diagnosis of CF made by newborn screening is well educated on current CF treatment and prognosis. The 2001 Victorian Government-initiated review of CF services in the state of Victoria (2001) highlighted that, in the state of Victoria (drainage population approximately 5 million persons, 65,000 livebirths per annum), one family doctor in 10 would see one person with CF in his or her lifetime. These figures raise the possibility that a person, perhaps experienced with the family but inexperienced in the latest up-to-date information on CF, will be the first person to discuss CF with the family. For this reason, preference is given for an experienced and well-trained genetic counselor to first approach the family by phone and suggest follow-up with the CF treatment team the following day. If geographical issues permit a home visit from a hospital-based CF clinical nurse consultant in association with a local doctor the family is already familiar with, this may be an alternative way to introduce the diagnosis.

Once the diagnosis of CF has been presented to the family, it is important to try to minimize the time before a face-to-face discussion occurs between members of the CF treatment team and the family. This will reduce the amount of disinformation that can be gained by families from out-of-date or misleading sources, such as medical information books in the local library or the Internet. One of the most powerful tools that patients and families can access for education and support about CF is the Internet, but the many excellent and helpful websites providing this service are indistinguishable to the inexperienced from dangerous and misleading sites.

DIAGNOSIS: INITIAL DIAGNOSIS INTERVIEW

Experience would suggest that parents do not retain much of the information provided during this initial interview, as it is understandably a very stressful time.[1] Recognition of this stress means that staff involved in this initial interview should be prepared to go over information several times and should also provide only relevant basics at the first meeting. The treating physician and clinic coordinator or nurse are ideally the two staff members who should be involved in this first interview. It is important that parental education levels, prior parenting experience and cultural issues be taken into account by the CF team when planning how to initially explain the diagnosis of CF. The same factors must also be taken into account when constructing the time frame for any educational period that may follow. An explanation of the basics of genetic inheritance is important to include at this early stage, stressing that no "blame" should be directed at one parent compared to another. In addition, it is important to outline that CF does not occur as a result of any risk-taking

behavior or other lifestyle issues. Smoking, alcohol intake, or recreational drug usage during or before pregnancy is not related to the birth of a child with CF, but have all been used at times by families to try to blame the occurrence of CF on partners or themselves. The basic pathophysiology of CF with general details regarding respiratory and gastrointestinal involvement should also be provided at this first meeting.

At the initial diagnosis interview families should be invited to attend an educational period over several days to meet all members of the CF treatment team. During this period, members of the treatment team provide education to the family on current and planned therapies, as well as assess the individual child for the presence of any clinical manifestation of CF—including cough, wheeze, steatorrhea, failure to thrive, and salt depletion. The outline of one such education week plan is set out in Table B.1.

Although this education period serves mainly to educate and empower family members, it allows medical staff to recognize early clinical manifestation of CF and to initiate appropriate therapy. Many pediatric hospitals have residential facilities for families (so-called "care-by-parent units"), which are ideal places for families to reside in during the education week. As the newly diagnosed infant is rarely acutely unwell and is often clinically asymptomatic, it is unnecessary for the child to be admitted to an acute bed of the hospital. However, using a residential facility attached to the hospital means that, between consultations with members of the CF team, the parents and related siblings can have quiet time to allow the new infant to feed and rest in quiet surroundings. We have found this to be a valuable resource by removing the family from distractions at home, such as work, enquiring friends, and so on, and it allows the family to concentrate on learning about CF in general and the therapies required. In a review of our education program, the residential basis for the education week was appreciated even by families who were in close geographical proximity to the hospital.[67] Of the 15 families interviewed as part of this review, 89% reported that not having to travel was a significant advantage.

The usual time between the first diagnostic interview and the commencement of the education week should be as short as possible for reasons outlined earlier. It is certain, however, that no matter how short this time period most families will attempt to access additional information regarding CF. In an attempt to provide up-to-date and accurate information on CF, a kit of educational material should be provided to the family at the first interview when the diagnosis is raised. In our clinic, families are given an education kit consisting of a set of booklets developed both within our own unit and from international CF support agencies. They discuss the basics of CF and its treatment, with particular emphasis on issues surrounding diagnosis and infancy. In addition, a DVD/video developed by our unit discusses the basics of CF. We have found this education pack to be invaluable in helping inform and educate other family members who did not attend the initial interview.

Table B.1 Outline of roles that various members of the cystic fibrosis (CF) care team play in the educational week for families of infants diagnosed by newborn screening, as used at the Royal Children's Hospital, Melbourne, Australia

Day 1	Physician	Answer questions from initial discussion. Query presence of any symptoms including diarrhea, abdominal discomfort, cough
	Counselor/nurse	Provide program for the week with appointment times and locations. Orient family to hospital
	Dietician	Assess nutritional status. Organize tests of pancreatic function (usually random stool or 3-day fecal fat analysis)
	Physiotherapist	Detailed respiratory assessment. Discuss role of physiotherapy and describe and demonstrate infant physiotherapy techniques. Teach the signs and symptoms of a respiratory exacerbation
Day 2	Counselor/nurse	Discuss grief, coping, and adjustment. Reinforce that the infant with CF is well, stress importance of normal parenting.
	Dietician	Discuss marital and family dynamics including sibling relationships. Arrange chest X-ray, blood tests, review results of screening tests for fat absorption and commence pancreatic enzyme therapy if indicated. Educate on principles of pancreatic enzyme replacement dosing and administration
	Physiotherapist	Demonstrate and teach modified drainage and percussion techniques. Discuss physiotherapy in the home setting including timing with feeds, involvement of siblings, and back care for carers
Day 3	Physician	Meet with family to answer questions. Discuss cross-infection issues. Offer meetings with grandparents and other family members. Contact local family doctor to discuss ongoing center-based care
	Counselor/nurse	Discuss community-based resources. Contact maternal and child health nurse and send out information package
	Dietician	Discuss vitamin and salt replacement. Assess efficiency of supplement enzyme therapy clinically and with random stool test
	Physiotherapist	Review parents' techniques and discuss importance of exercise in future development
Day 4	Physician	If required, meet with other family members including grandparents. Discuss genetic basis of disease and reassure that is not a lifestyle choice condition
	Counselor/nurse	Introduce CF community team—nurse and physiotherapist
	Dietician	Review end of 3-day fecal fat results, if performed, and commence therapy if required or, if enzyme therapy commenced, assess weight gain and feeding pattern for evidence of improved absorption. Discuss basis for high-energy high-fat diet
	Physiotherapist	Review and refine parents' techniques
	Genetic counselor	Revisit genetic basis of disease and arrange for blood testing of parents for genotype analysis. Discuss antenatal testing
	Community CF team	Introduce themselves to family and discuss role of community-based team. Set up first appointment for 1–2 weeks postdischarge
Day 5	Physician	Review outstanding issues. Discuss results of chest X-ray. Provide discharge medication. Reinforce concept of center-based care and encourage them to access team members at any time for information and advice
	Counselor/nurse	Contact local health providers including family doctor and primary pediatrician
	Other team members	Arrange clinic appointment for 2–3 weeks. Advise importance of cohorting in clinics and attention to attending on correct outpatient day as required or requested by parents

EDUCATION WEEK

There are two main aims to the education week. First, the family of the child needs to be educated about various aspects of the pathophysiology of CF, as well as the various therapies used. In addition, the medical team will need to spend time with the child and the family in assessing the specific CF phenotype that the child currently manifests. During the week, each member of the care team will introduce himself or herself and explain his/her role in CF treatments, and then spend time describing specifics of both pathophysiology and treatments in their relevant area of expertise. In addition, each member will assess the infant for the need for such therapies.

TEAM MEMBER ROLES

THE PHYSICIAN

In discussing the diagnosis of CF with parents and important balance between oversupply of information and missing important facts is essential. In the first interview during the education week any questions that have arisen since the initial diagnosis interview can be answered. These questions may stem from information that was unclear from the educational material provided or arise from questions raised by family members or other sources of information such as the Internet.

It is often necessary to set out early what is planned to be achieved in the education week. Parents will often, at this early stage, be keen to hear about research and discuss various "cures" that they may have heard about or hope exist. By setting out that the education week is simply to inform parents about CF and its various therapies, the parents can be directed to make the best use of the time during the week.

An open approach is vitally important at this early stage and willingness to answer any queries raised helps develop trust and faith in the treating team. It is important to try to keep the parents focused on issues relevant to their own child and the recent diagnosis of CF—the relevant therapies and plans for follow-up. Subjects such as research that may have been conducted on the Internet should be recognized but not allowed to become the focus of the discussions. Subsequent meetings with parents during the week allow additional time to raise specific points such as cross-infection issues, and cohorting, if such practices are employed at the particular clinic. The offer to speak to other family members in a group is often welcomed by grandparents or family members who are also of reproductive age. To ensure that there is a common level of understanding through all family members, such discussions with extended family members are generally best done with the immediate family, particularly mother and father, present. At the end of the interview on day 5, the opportunity for the parents to ask questions is again raised and there is discussion regarding the importance of regular contact and follow-up.

Although in many situations few or no respiratory symptoms or signs will be yet evident, respiratory assessment at this stage generally involves an assessment of lower airway pathogens and the commencement of antistaphylococcal therapy, which is generally continued for the first 12 months of life. Our unit's previous work on lower respiratory infections and inflammation in the newly diagnosed screened group showed that there was a much higher level of lower airway bacterial infection than expected. In a group of 45 newly diagnosed infants (32 by newborn screening) who had a bronchoalveolar lavage at a mean age of 2.6 months, 15 bacterial infections were diagnosed, 14 of which involved *Staphylococcus aureus*.[3]

THE CLINIC COORDINATOR OR CLINIC NURSE

Many centers have different roles for their clinical coordinator, who often have differing levels and types of training, ranging from trained nurse to social worker to academic psychologist. The role and extent of involvement in actual education about CF will depend on the specific training of the coordinator, but the major role will be one of support and advice for the family, as well as serving as the coordinator of the education week as a whole.

Counseling parents about the expected stresses and various emotions is an important role of the clinic coordinator. Although possibly not having formal psychological or counseling training, an experienced CF coordinator should be able to discuss issues with parents and refer to more formal services if this is considered necessary.

THE DIETITIAN

Although over 90% of adults and adolescents with CF have clinically apparent pancreatic insufficiency requiring supplemental pancreatic enzyme therapy, some infants diagnosed on newborn screening may have sufficient residual pancreatic exocrine function to have acceptable fat absorption at the time of diagnosis. Waters et al.,[4] in their review of the New South Wales screening program, found that of 78 patients diagnosed over a 7-year period, 49 (63%) were clinically pancreatic insufficient at diagnosis. Of the remaining 29 (37%), a further six (8%) developed pancreatic sufficiency over the following 4 years. Pancreatic insufficiency may already be clinically evident as diarrhea, abdominal cramping, irritability, and failure to gain weight; if a screening test such a random fecal fat microscopy analysis confirms the presence of abnormal levels of fat globules, pancreatic enzyme therapy can be started immediately. In such cases, by the end of the education week, similar repeat tests can confirm the correction of steatorrhea and improvement of clinical symptoms of malabsorption. The dietitian will also spend time discussing the basics of the high-energy diet and educating parents about enzyme therapy dosing and administration.

Breast-feeding mothers may worry that the need to introduce enzyme therapy means that breast-feeding has to be discontinued. The dietitian can encourage and support the mother through the first few feedings to try to ensure that breast-feeding is continued. In situations where breast-feeding cannot be continued, parents should be assured that adequate nutrition for the CF infant is achievable using commercially available formulas with pancreatic enzyme supplementation if required.

Deficiencies of fat-soluble vitamins A, D, E, and K have been demonstrated in pancreatic-insufficient individuals with CF, including infants diagnosed on newborn screening programs.[5] In a review of 127 infants diagnosed by the US CF newborn screening program in Colorado, deficiency of one or more fat-soluble vitamins was present in 44 of 96 patients (46%) at age 4–8 weeks. Vitamin A was deficient in 29% of cases, vitamin D in 23%, and vitamin E in 23%. During the education week, the dietitian should organize measurement of fat-soluble vitamins and commence therapy as necessary with an appropriate vitamin supplement.

THE PHYSIOTHERAPIST

Education, assessment, and initiation of airway clearance and aerosol therapy are the main role of the physiotherapist during the education week. Discussion with the parents of the importance of regular airway clearance and how this can be achieved and adjusted with advancing childhood age is provided. Commencement of any required aerosol therapy during the education week allows for several sessions to familiarize both the infant and parents with this treatment. Information about cross-infection issues and care, and cleaning of equipment can also be provided. The spectrum of future physiotherapy techniques—including the importance of regular exercise—is also raised at this early stage. Modified postural drainage techniques are introduced, and parents are encouraged to continue this for 20 minutes a day after discharge from the education week. This permits continued reinforcement of the technique to both the infant and parents. There is little evidence-based research available on the need for physiotherapy at this early stage.

THE GENETIC COUNSELOR

It is important for the genetic counselor to be available in the education week to answer queries about the inherited basis for CF. Family members of childbearing age may particularly wish to discuss the ramifications for, and options available for, themselves. In cases of compound heterozygotes diagnosed through follow-up sweat testing, the genetic counselor can organize genotyping of parents to attempt to identify the second gene mutation. Siblings of newly diagnosed infants are generally recalled for a sweat test following the diagnosis; the genetic counselor can explain why this is desirable, to ensure understanding of the inherited nature of CF.

THE COMMUNITY CF TEAM

Toward the end of the education week, introduction to the community-based CF team should be made. The team may include a nurse alone, or a nurse and physiotherapist will discuss with parents issues regarding CF treatment within the home and will organize a follow-up visit at home within 1–2 weeks at the end of the education week. It is important that the community team be introduced in the hospital setting, as this will reinforce to the family the concept of one CF treatment team across both hospital and community settings.

RESEARCH IN THE EDUCATION WEEK

Several centers initiate research projects in newly diagnosed patients from screening programs. It is important in this initial week to concentrate on educating and supporting the family rather than enrolling them in research programs. Many families will mistakenly believe that by enrolling in such research they may "cure" their child or at least be seen in a favorable light by the treatment team. Enrollment in research programs should not be raised until the family has a good understanding of CF and how it relates to their child. In addition, once a relationship has been established between the parents and the treatment team, a more informed and ethical acceptance, or decline, of involvement can be obtained. In our CF center, discussion about enrolment in early trials is always conducted by another CF Consultant and not the consultant who will take long-term supervision of the child's clinical care.

Although most centers obtain a standard anteroposterior chest X-ray of an infant during the educational week, some centers are increasingly utilizing high-resolution computed tomography (CT) scans in young infants as a way of examining, in detail, any structural problems that may already be present. This procedure will usually involve a general anesthetic to ensure proper films are available during expiration where early air trapping may be evident. Although some CT scans can be performed under sedation or even while the infant is asleep, these will not provide detailed information on air trapping and thus will be less helpful. Some centers will also perform infant lung function measurements on newly diagnosed babies; however, the information obtained from these studies, as well as from high-resolution CT scans, is yet to drive clinical therapy in any direction, and they are mostly seen as research tools. Some centers are keen to perform bronchoscopic alveolar lavage soon after the diagnosis of CF. Given that this procedure will require a general anesthetic, attempts to include it as part of the education week should be avoided if at all possible, to allow the parents to concentrate on learning about CF and how it clinically affects their child.

Enrollment in research projects should be raised at the earliest at the follow-up clinic appointment 2 weeks after the education week. Although it is inappropriate to attempt to enroll families in research at this early stage, many families will be reassured to learn that the unit they are now attached to has an active research program, and a general discussion of current research, without any offer or inducement to enroll in such projects will be informative to many families.

REFERENCES

1. Jedlicka-Kohler I, Gotz M, Eichler I. Parents' recollection of the initial communication of the diagnosis of cystic fibrosis. *Pediatrics* 1996; **97**: 204–9.
2. Sawyer S, Glazner J. What follows newborn screening? An evaluation of a residential education program for parents of infants with newly diagnosed cystic fibrosis. *Pediatrics* 2004; **114**: 411–6.
3. Armstrong D, Grimwood K, Carzino R, et al. Lower respiratory infection and inflammation in infants with newly diagnosed cystic fibrosis. *Br Med J* 1995; **310**: 1571–2.
4. Waters DL, Dorney SF, Gaskin KJ, et al. Pancreatic function in infants identified as having cystic fibrosis in a neonatal screening program. *N Engl J Med* 1990; **322**: 303–8.
5. Feranchak A, Sontag M, Wagener J, et al. Prospective, long-term study of fat-soluble vitamin status in children with cystic fibrosis identified by newborn screening. *J Pediatr* 1999; **135**: 601–10.

Index

Notes: Bold page numbers are used for figures, italic page numbers are used for tables.